NHS Staff Library at the L.G.I.

☎ **0113 39 26445**

This book must be returned by the date shown
below or a fine will be charged.

- 5 MAR 2008	
2 9 SEP 2008	
- 7 MAY 2010	
2 1 NOV 2011	
- 7 FEB 2017	
:- 4 JUL 2018	

Leeds Teaching Hospitals NHS Trust

Paediatric Surgery

Paediatric Surgery

Second Edition

Edited by

David M. Burge FRCS FRCPCH
Consultant Paediatric Surgeon

D. Mervyn Griffiths BM MCh FRCS
Consultant Paediatric Surgeon

Henrik A. Steinbrecher BSc MBBS MS FRCS FRCS(Paeds)
Consultant Paediatric Urologist

Robert A. Wheeler MS FRCS LLB
Consultant Paediatric and Neonatal Surgeon

Wessex Regional Centre for Paediatric Surgery,
Southampton University Hospital, Southampton, UK

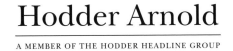

Hodder Arnold

A MEMBER OF THE HODDER HEADLINE GROUP

First published in Great Britain in 2005 by
Hodder Education, a member of the Hodder Headline Group,
338 Euston Road, London NW1 3BH

http://www.hoddereducation.co.uk

Distributed in the United States of America by
Oxford University Press Inc.,
198 Madison Avenue, New York, NY10016
Oxford is a registered trademark of Oxford University Press

Whilst the advice and information in this book are believed to be true and
accurate at the date of going to press, neither the authors nor the publisher
can accept any legal responsibility or liability for any errors or omissions
that may be made. In particular (but without limiting the generality of the
preceding disclaimer), every effort has been made to check drug dosages;
however it is still possible that errors have been missed. Furthermore,
dosage schedules are constantly being revised and new side-effects
recognized. For these reasons the reader is strongly urged to consult the
drug companies' printed instructions before administering any of the drugs
recommended in this book.

British Library Cataloguing in Publication Data
A catalogue record for this book is available from the British Library

Library of Congress Cataloging-in-Publication Data
A catalog record for this book is available from the Library of Congress

ISBN-10:   0 340 80910 8
ISBN-13:   978 0 340 80910 5

1 2 3 4 5 6 7 8 9 10

Commissioning Editor: Sarah Burrows
Project Manager: Colette Holden
Project Editor: Naomi Wilkinson
Production Controller: Joanna Walker
Cover Designer: Georgina Hewitt
Indexer: Indexing Specialists (UK) Ltd, Hove, UK

Typeset in 10/12 pts Minion by Charon Tec Pvt. Ltd, Chennai, India
www.charontec.com
Printed and bound in the UK by CPI Bath

What do you think about this book? Or any other Hodder Arnold title?
Please visit our website at www.hoddereducation.co.uk

Contents

Contributors

Amir Azmy MB BCh DS FRCS
Honorary Clinical Senior Lecturer
University of Glasgow
Glasgow, UK; and
Consultant Paediatric Urologist
Department of Paediatric Urology
Royal Hospital for Sick Children
Glasgow, UK

Srinivasan R Babu MS MCh FRCS
Specialist Registrar in Paediatric Surgery
Southampton University Hospital
Southampton, UK

Spencer W Beasley MS(Melb) FRACS
Clinical Professor of Paediatric Surgery
Christchurch School of Medicine
University of Otago
Christchurch, New Zealand

Mark Beattie FRCPCH MRCP
Consultant Paediatric Gastroenterologist
Paediatric Medical Unit
Southampton University Hospital
Southampton, UK

A Bianchi MOM(Malta) MD FRCS(Eng) FRCS(Ed)
Consultant Specialist Paediatric and Neonatal Surgeon
The Royal Manchester Children's Hospital
Manchester, UK

Thomas Boemers MD PhD
Head, Department of Paediatric Surgery and
 Paediatric Urology
Children's Hospital of Cologne
Cologne, Germany

Guy Bogaert MD PhD
Professor in Paediatric Urology
Department of Urology
University Hospitals
Leuven, Belgium

Victor Boston MD FRCSI FRCS(Ed) FRCS(Eng)
Consultant Paediatric Surgeon
Department of Paediatric Surgery
The Royal Belfast Hospital for Sick Children
Belfast, UK

David M Burge FRCS FRCPCH
Consultant Paediatric Surgeon
Wessex Regional Centre for Paediatric Surgery
Southampton University Hospital
Southampton, UK

SN Cenk Büyükünal MD
Consultant Paediatric Surgeon
Section of Paediatric Urology
Department of Paediatric Surgery
Cerrahpasa Medical Faculty
University of Istanbul
Istanbul, Turkey

Paul Chumas MD FRCS(SN)
Consultant Neurosurgeon
Leeds General Infirmary
Leeds, UK

Claire Clark MBChB MRCS(Ed)
Specialist Registrar in Paediatric Surgery
Royal Hospital for Sick Children
Edinburgh, UK

Tom Clarnette MD FRACS
Consultant Paediatric Surgeon
Department of Paediatric Surgery
Melbourne Children's Hospital
Melbourne, Australia

David Crabbe MD FRCS
Consultant Paediatric Surgeon
Department of Paediatric Surgery
Leeds General Infirmary
Leeds, UK

Sarah Creighton MD FRCOG
Consultant Gynaecologist
Elizabeth Garrett Anderson Hospital
University College Hospital
London, UK

Peter Cuckow MBBS FRCS(Paeds)
Consultant Paediatric Urologist
Department of Paediatric Urology
Great Ormond Street Hospital
London, UK

Eleri L Cusick ChM FRCS(Paed)
Consultant Paediatric Surgeon
Department of Paediatric Surgery
Bristol Royal Hospital for Children
Bristol, UK

Tolga E Dagli MD
Professor and Chief of Paediatric Surgery
Marmara University School of Medicine
Istanbul, Turkey

Mark Davenport ChM FRCS(Paeds) FRCPS(Glas) FRCS(Eng)
Reader in Paediatric Surgery
King's College Hospital
London, UK

Divyesh Desai MBS(Gen Surg) MCh(Urol)
Director of Urodynamics
Great Ormond Street Hospital
London, UK

HK Dhillon FRCS(Ed)
Associate Specialist in Perinatal Urology
Department of Urology
Great Ormond Street Hospital
London, UK

JAS Dickson FRCS(Eng) FRCS(Ed) FRCPCH
Retired Consultant Paediatric Surgeon
Sheffield, UK

Alan Dickson BSc MBChB FRCS(Ed)
Consultant Paediatric Urologist
Royal Manchester Children's Hospital
Manchester, UK

JC Djurhuus MD
Professor of Medicine
Institute of Experimental Clinical Research
University of Aarhus
Aarhus, Denmark

PG Duffy MB FRCS(I)
Consultant Paediatric Urologist
Department of Paediatric Urology
Great Ormond Street Hospital
London, UK

Evelyn H Dykes MB ChB FRCS(Paed)
Postgraduate Dean
North of Scotland Institute for Postgraduate Medical
  Education
Raigmore Hospital
Inverness, UK

Joanna Fairhurst MA(Cantab) MBBS MRCP FRCR
Consultant Paediatric Radiologist
Children's X-ray Department
Southampton General Hospital
Southampton, UK

Rodney Gilbert MMed FRCPCH
Consultant Paediatric Nephrologist
Department of Child Health
Southampton General Hospital
Southampton, UK

D Mervyn Griffiths BM MCh FRCS
Consultant Paediatric Surgeon
Wessex Regional Centre for Paediatric Surgery
Southampton University Hospital
Southampton, UK

Mark Griffiths MRCP FRCR
Consultant Paediatric Radiologist
Department of Paediatric Radiology
Southampton University Hospital
Southampton, UK

Constantinos Hajivassiliou BSc MBChB MD FRCS(Ed & Glas) FRCS(Paed)
Senior lecturer and Consultant Paediatric Surgeon
Department of Paediatric Surgery
Royal Hospital for Sick Children
Glasgow, UK

Ben Hartley MBBS BSc FRCS(ORL–HNS)
Consultant Paediatric Otolaryngologist
Great Ormond Street Hospital
London, UK

Catherine Hill BM MRCP FRCPCH
Senior Lecturer in Child Health
Community Clinical Sciences Division
Department of Child Health
Southampton University Hospital
Southampton, UK

David Howe DM FRCOG FRCS(Ed)
Consultant and Honorary Senior Lecturer in
 Feto-Maternal Medicine
Wessex Fetal Medicine Unit
Princess Anne Hospital
Southampton, UK

Alexander J Howie MD FRCPath
Department of Pathology
University College London
London, UK

Simon Huddart MA MBBS FRCS FRCS(Paed)
Consultant Neonatal and Paediatric Surgeon
Department of Paediatric Surgery
University Hospital of Wales
Cardiff, UK

Ieuan Hughes MA MD FRCP FRCP(C) FRCPCH FMedSci
Professor of Paediatrics
Addenbrookes Hospital
Cambridge, UK

John M Hutson BS MD(Monash) MD(Melb) FRACS FAAP(Hon)
Director of General Surgery
Royal Children's Hospital; and
Professor of Paediatric Surgery
University of Melbourne
Melbourne, Australia

J Michael S Johnstone MBChB FRCS(E)
Retired Paediatric Surgeon
Oakham, UK

TM Jørgensen MD
Professor in Paediatric Urology
Department of Urology
Aarhus University Hospital
Aarhus, Denmark

Edward Kiely FRCSI FRCS FRPCH
Consultant Paediatric Surgeon
Department of Paediatric Surgery
Great Ormond Street Hospital
London, UK

Lara Kitteringham MBChB FRCS(Paed)
Specialist Registrar in Paediatric Surgery
St George's Hospital
London, UK

Anthony Lander PhD FRCS(Paed) DCH
Consultant Paediatric Surgeon
Birmingham Children's Hospital
Birmingham, UK

Dorothy Lang FRCS(Glasg) FRCS(Lond)
Consultant Neurosurgeon
Department of Neurosurgery
Southampton University Hospital
Southampton, UK

Rachel Leaver BSc RN PGCE
Lecturer Practitioner
Middlesex Hospital
London, UK

Valerie Lewington BM MSc FRCP
Consultant Nuclear Medicine Physician
The Royal Marsden Hospital
Sutton, UK

Paul D Losty MD FRCSI FRCS(Eng) FRCS(Ed) FRCS(Paed)
Professor of Paediatric Surgery
Division of Child Health
The Royal Liverpool Children's Hospital (Alder Hey)
The University of Liverpool
Liverpool, UK

Gordon A MacKinlay MBBS LRCP FRCS(Ed) FRCS
Consultant Paediatric Surgeon
Royal Hospital for Sick Children
Edinburgh, UK

A Ewen MacKinnon MB BS FRCS(Eng & Glas) FRCPCH
Consultant Paediatric Surgeon
Department of Paediatric Surgery
The Children's Hospital
Sheffield, UK

Padraig Malone MB BSc MCh FRCSI FRCS
Consultant Paediatric Urologist
Department of Paediatric Surgery
Southampton University Hospital
Southampton, UK

Michael J Marsh MBBS MRCP MRCPCH
Director of Paediatric Intensive Care
Department of Paediatric Intensive Care
Southampton University Hospital
Southampton, UK

Hugh Martin MBBS FRACS FRCS(Eng)
Consultant Paediatric General and Burns Surgeon
Children's Hospital at Westmead
Westmead, Australia

SL McCarthy MBBS FRCS
Great Ormond Street Hospital
London, UK

Victoria McGrigor LRCP MRCS MBBS DCH FRCPCH
Consultant Community Paediatrician
Ashurst Education Centre
Ashurst Hospital
Southampton, UK

Vivien McNamara BMedSci BM BS FRCS(C/Th)
Specialist Registrar in Paediatric Surgery
Wessex Regional Centre for Paediatric Surgery
Southampton University Hospitals Trust
Southampton, UK

Isabella E Moore MA DM FRCPath
Consultant Paediatric Pathologist
Department of Cellular Pathology
Southampton University Hospitals Trust
Southampton, UK

Azad Najmaldin MB ChB MS FRCS(Ed) FRCS(Eng)
Consultant in Paediatric Surgery
Department of Paediatric Surgery
St James's University Hospital
Leeds, UK

Ole Henrik Nielsen MD
Consultant Paediatric Surgeon
Department of Paediatric Surgery
Juliane Marie Centre
Copenhagen University Hospital
Copenhagen, Denmark

Evelyn GP Ong BSc FRCS(Eng)
Specialist Registrar and Honorary Clinical Research
 Fellow
Institute of Child Health and Great Ormond
 Street Hospital
London, UK

Dakshesh H Parikh MBBS FRCS(Paed) MD
Consultant Paediatric Surgeon
Department of Paediatric Surgery
Birmingham Children's Hospital
Birmingham, UK

Simon Phelps MBBS FRCS(Paed Surg)
Specialist Registrar
Wessex Regional Centre for Paediatric Surgery
Southampton University Hospitals Trust
Southampton, UK

Agostino Pierro MD FRCS(Eng) FRCS(Ed) FAAP
Nuffield Professor of Paediatric Surgery
Institute of Child Health and Great Ormond
 Street Hospital
London, UK

Risto J Rintala MD PhD
Professor of Paediatric Surgery
Hospital for Children and Adolescents
University of Helsinki
Helsinki, Finland

S Rittig MD
Consultant Paediatric Nephrologist
Department of Paediatrics
Aarhus University Hospital
Aarhus, Denmark

Nicola P Smith MA MD MRCS(Eng)
Professor of Paediatric Surgery, Clinical
 Lecturer and Specialist Registrar
Division of Child Health
The Royal Liverpool Children's Hospital (Alder Hey)
The University of Liverpool
Liverpool, UK

Paul Spargo MBBS MRCP FRCA
Consultant Paediatric Anaesthetist
Anaesthetic Department
Southampton University Hospital
Southampton, UK

Richard Spicer MBBS MRCS LRCP(Eng) DCh FRCS(Eng) FRCPH
Consultant Paediatric Surgeon
Directorate of Children's Services
The Bristol Royal Hospital for Children
Bristol, UK

Henrik A Steinbrecher BSc MBBS MS FRCS FRCS(Paeds)
Consultant Paediatric Urologist
Wessex Regional Centre for Paediatric Surgery
Southampton University Hospital
Southampton, UK

Mark D Stringer MS FRCS FRCPCH
Consultant Paediatric Hepatobiliary/Transplant Surgeon
Children's Liver Unit
St James's University Hospital
Leeds, UK

Rajendra Surana MBBS MS FRCS(Paed)
Consultant Paediatric Surgeon
Welsh Centre for Paediatric Surgery
University Hospital of Wales
Cardiff, UK

Paul Sutherland MA BM BCh FRCA
Consultant Paediatric Anaesthetist
Anaesthetic Department
Southampton University Hospital
Southampton, UK

Paul KH Tam MBBS FRCS ChM
Professor and Chief
Division of Paediatric Surgery
The University of Hong Kong
Queen Mary Hospital
Hong Kong

Juan A Tovar MD PhD
Professor of Paediatric Surgery
Head, Department of Paediatric Surgery
Hospital Universitario 'La Paz'
Madrid, Spain

Atul Tyagi FRCS(SN)
Consultant Neurosurgeon
Leeds General Infirmary
Leeds, UK

W van't Hoff BSc MD FRCP FRCPCH
Great Ormond Street Hospital
London, UK

Suzie Venn MS FRCS(Urol)
Consultant Urologist
University College London
London, UK; and
St Richard's Hospital
Chichester, UK

Pieter Verleyen MD FEBU
Paediatric Urologist
AZ Groeninge Hospital
Kortrijk, Belgium

Jenny Walker MBChB ChM FRCS
Consultant Paediatric Surgeon
Department of Paediatric Surgery
Sheffield Children's Hospital
Sheffield, UK

Elizabeth B Whan
Locum Consultant Paediatric Surgeon
Southampton University Hospital
Southampton, UK

Robert A Wheeler MS FRCS LLB
Consultant Paediatric and Neonatal Surgeon,
Medical Lawyer
Wessex Regional Centre for Paediatric Surgery
Southampton University Hospital
Southampton, UK

Duncan Wilcox MD FRCS(Paeds)
Associate Professor in Paediatric Urology
The University of Texas
Southwestern Medical Center at Dallas
Dallas, TX, USA

Kenneth KY Wong MBChB PhD FRCS(Ed)
Assistant Professor
Division of Paediatric Surgery
The University of Hong Kong
Queen Mary Hospital
Hong Kong

CRJ Woodhouse MB FRBS FEBU
Professor of Adolescent Urology
The Institute of Urology
University College London
London, UK

Mark N Woodward MD FRCS(Paed)
Specialist Registrar
Department of Paediatric Surgery
Bristol Royal Hospital for Children
Bristol, UK

Preface

Textbooks of paediatric surgery tend to full into two main categories. There are those that are very detailed reference texts, often extending to more than one volume, which any specialist paediatric surgeon will wish to consult on a regular basis when dealing with uncommon conditions. Then there are small books designed for students, general practitioners and junior surgeons, usually covering common paediatric surgical conditions. There is a need for a textbook designed for trainees in paediatric surgery in order to provide them with the knowledge required to help them complete their training and to pass specialist examinations such as those in place in the UK, Europe and Australasia. This book is aimed at those trainees and with such examinations in mind.

In Part 1 of this book, we have included topics on basic science that underpin our clinical knowledge and how we implement it. In addition, the clinical chapters include sections of relevant basic science. We have also included topics such as communication skills and the child and the law, which are relevant to all doctors practising paediatrics.

Throughout the clinical sections, we have tried to identify the learning points for each chapter. Reading textbooks is not an easy task, and the text can be dry and lack direction. The learning points should focus the reader's mind on the important questions that they should ask themselves when they have finished reading the chapter. In addition, where relevant, we have included clinical scenarios, with the intention of focusing the reader's mind on how to implement their knowledge in a practical setting.

We have deliberately not included great detail about operative surgery. There are other texts that cover this issue well. We hope that the book will appeal to surgeons in training but also that it may be of interest to both specialist paediatric surgeons and surgeons who practise the general surgery of childhood.

The editors would like to acknowledge the understanding of their families during the gestation of the book and the help of the staff at Hodder Arnold.

Part 1

General principles of care

Congenital causes of disease

ANTHONY LANDER

Learning objectives

- To appreciate the relevance of developmental biology to our understanding of normal and abnormal anatomy.
- To revise the basic paradigm of cell biology and place it in the context of development.
- To understand something of the mechanisms underlying specification along the head–tail axis.
- To develop an insight into potential biological mechanisms behind structural anomalies.
- To be able to talk to parents about the aetiology of structural congenital anomalies.

INTRODUCTION

The application of molecular and cell biology to embryology and teratology has brought new insights into developmental biology, but the field is almost impenetrable for the busy surgeon. It is now necessary to understand not only comparative mammalian, in particular murine, development but also the development of *Xenopus*, chick, zebra fish and *Drosophila* in order to appreciate recent findings. This is because animals share homologous genes and developmental mechanisms. The mutation analysis work of Nusslein-Volhard on *Drosophila* in the 1980s gave us a head start in understanding mammalian development and was acknowledged with a Nobel Prize in 1995. The educated surgeon should understand something about master control genes, such as the well-conserved *Hox* genes.

The mapping of the entire human genome is now complete, and it is expected that the use of recombinant deoxyribonucleic acid (DNA) technology, antisense agents and transgenic techniques will lead to a better understanding of the genetic control of development and of the pathogenesis of many congenital anomalies. However, we must not lose sight of mechanisms not prescribed in the genes that influence development and play a role in teratology.

BASIC SCIENCE

Morphogenesis is the appearance of shape or form. It is of fundamental importance and must necessarily have been abnormal when structural congenital anomalies are seen. However, much happens before morphogenetic changes in tissues can take place. Cells have to be told what *type* of cell they are to be and *where* to go. Their *fate* has to be specified. Thus, key to *development* is the specification of cell fate.

Development is considered to be the gradual allocation of specific cells to more narrowly defined fates. Developmental biology asks: How are the cells chosen by position? What are the molecular and cellular events that constitute changes in cell fate?

Our understanding used to be limited to a description of the morphological changes that accompany embryogenesis. The driving forces of morphogenesis were a mystery. However, it is now apparent that mammals have made use of the regulatory cascades in gene expression that control morphogenesis in distant evolutionary ancestors, both for similar and quite different processes. It is also apparent that disruption of these mammalian regulatory genes can produce congenital anomalies. This disruption could be inherited as a gene defect, or it might be a consequence of interaction with an environmental agent.

MOLECULAR GENETICS AND DEVELOPMENT

The paradigm of molecular biology

> A gene is *transcribed* into *messenger ribonucleic acid* (mRNA), which is *translated* into a protein, which may be modified by *post-translational mechanisms*.

A cell type is somewhat defined by the genes it is expressing, because these dictate to a large extent the proteins produced. However, control of protein production is exercised at a number of levels in this system. The fundamental level of control exercised in development is at transcription.

Transcription factors offer the opportunity for control at the pretranscriptional level. These are proteins and thus gene products themselves; a good example is the *Hox* gene products. Control can be exerted after transcription into mRNA. Post-translational modifications can affect both function and transport of proteins. Thus, a cell may produce a specific mRNA but may not necessarily produce the protein.

An important group of transcription factors are genes containing the *homeobox*. The homeobox is 180 base pairs in length and codes for 60 amino acids whose conformational arrangement allows the protein to bind to DNA itself.

Imprinting

An allele is an allele is no longer tenable. For example, deletion of part of chromosome 15 (15q11–q13) gives rise to Prader–Willi syndrome when inherited paternally but to Angelman syndrome when inherited maternally. This is because the chromosomes themselves are modified in different ways when spermatozoa or ova are made. The maternal DNA is more highly methylated than paternally inherited DNA, and this difference may underlie the transmission of the different pathologies. Methylation affects cytosine bases, which precede guanosine bases and may affect some genes involved in intrauterine growth (*IGF2*, *IGF2r*, *WT1*). Some of these genes are activated and others are inactivated.

Murine pronuclei transfer experiments suggest that maternal chromosomes encourage embryonic development with reduced trophoblastic development, and paternal chromosomes encourage trophoblastic development. It is also worth noting that Huntington's chorea, spinocerebellar ataxia, myotonic dystrophy, neurofibromatosis I and II and Wilms tumour have different severities and ages of onset depending on the parent from whom the mutated gene is inherited. Genes with roles in these conditions may well be imprinted.

What types of gene product play roles in development?

There are a number of players in development, such as *growth factors*, *proto-oncogenes* and *transcription factors*, which also have jobs in the mature organism. Evolution has made use of similar sets of signalling systems and similar molecules in diverse places. Unfortunately, the names of these molecular species are based upon their historical discovery and can be uninformative and misleading. What is apparent is that some regulator genes in embryogenesis are also *tumour suppressor genes*. Recent advances have been as a result of mapping or cloning of the human homologues of specific regulatory genes or the discovery that their disruption is teratogenic.

Early on in fruit-fly development, maternally deposited mRNA may encode for diffusible growth factors or transcription factors that specify different subregions of the oocyte, zygote or embryo. These are called regulatory, selector or switch genes. Subsequently, zygotic genes are expressed. (In higher animals, there is less of a role for maternal effect genes, especially after cleavage.) One group of *Drosophila* zygotic genes, the *segmentation genes*, break up the embryo into similar segments. Similar mechanisms act in the segmentation of the *rhombomeres*, *pharyngeal arches* and *somites*.

GASTRULATION: PERHAPS THE MOST IMPORTANT PERIOD IN DEVELOPMENT

Gastrulation is the period in which the bilaminar germ disc develops the primitive streak and the node. Definitive endoderm and mesoderm then appear by movement of ectoderm through the primitive streak, so producing the trilaminar disc. In human, this happens during the third week, 15–22 days post-conception.

It is often perceived that a lot of the anomalies we deal with (e.g. oesophageal atresia, tracheo-oesophageal fistula, congenital diaphragmatic hernia, anorectal anomalies) have their origins during organogenesis. We imagine that primarily something has gone wrong with established blocks of tissues or tubes that we can visualize. The timing of putative teratological insults is then placed at these points during organogenesis. However, many of these anomalies may well have originated much earlier, during gastrulation, when cells are being told what to do and where to go. This is the time of *cell fate specification*. This is certainly so for a lot of defects, since they can be induced with brief exposure to teratogens during gastrulation in culture.

Gastrulation is a period and a set of processes. It covers the development of the conceptus from the *blastula*, which is the product of *cleavage* to the *neurula*, in which the scene is set for organogenesis. Gastrulation is characterized by the coordinated proliferation and movement of cells as individuals or in sheets, which fold, invaginate or delaminate as they are internalized from the surface of the conceptus. It is likely to be at this time that many cells receive information concerning their future fate or position. The body axes (head–tail, left–right) are set up, establishing the basic body plan.

At the end of gastrulation, these processes have generated *definitive endoderm*, surface and *neuroectoderm*, and the embryonic *mesoderm*. The thin column of mesoderm that appears most anterior to the node is the *notochord*. The notochord is an important dorsal mesodermal axial structure that is common to chordates. It influences vertebral and neural development. At the end of gastrulation, the floor plate of the neural tube is evident and the first somites are formed. Early primordia of heart and allantois indicate the beginning of organogenesis. These two structures are crucial to survival after gastrulation, as both size and metabolic demand soon exceed nutrient exchange by diffusion alone, and a heart and placentation are soon to become essential.

In amniotes, gastrulation starts with the *inner-cell mass*. The amniotic cavity develops on its dorsal surface and the inner-cell mass becomes a bilaminar germ disc of *epiblast* and *hypoblast*. The *primitive streak* (the organ of gastrulation) appears in the posterior (caudal end) of the epiblast. Only the epiblast contributes to embryonic tissue, giving rise to the ectoderm, amnion, definitive endoderm, and both embryonic and extra-embryonic mesoderm. The hypoblast is probably nearly all displaced into extra-embryonic endoderm by definitive endoderm, which passes through the streak. The hypoblast thus gives rise to extra-embryonic endoderm and yolk-sac endoderm. Other epiblast cells passing through the streak become mesoderm. At the end of gastrulation, the germ disc is trilaminar, with ectoderm, mesoderm and endoderm.

The specification of much of the mesoderm occurs during gastrulation, when cell movements allow many cells to pass through one 'organizing' region and so receive information concerning aspects of their future position and role.

The streak with its node are the organs of gastrulation. Cells that pass through the node extend along the (head–tail) anteroposterior (AP) axis to give the prochordal plate and notochord, anterior axial mesoderm, and both anterior and posterior midline endoderm. Cells passing through the lateral lips of the blastopore and the posterior streak form posterolateral mesoderm and endoderm, and extra-embryonic mesoderm in amniotes. Various genes may be switched on or off, and a function of the time spent in the region and exposure to various morphogens may be important in specifying cell fate.

The epiblast gives rise to all embryonic tissues, while the hypoblast is displaced by definitive endoderm to extra-embryonic yolk sac, with the exception of some posterior cells. The hypoblast cells are replaced by ectodermal cells passing mostly through the anterior end of the primitive streak to form definitive gut endoderm. Anterior hypoblast cells are displaced further anteriorly and into the visceral yolk-sac endoderm. Endodermal cells anterior to the node are displaced along the whole axis and into the anterior intestinal portal (foregut pocket); they are also found along the whole trunk and in the anterior and posterior yolk sac.

A *fate map* is defined at a specific time. It tells us the fate of cells from a region. In the mouse, maps have been based on clonal analysis using labels. Similar, but not topologically identical, fate maps have been constructed for other species.

Although species gastrulate in different ways, they end up with remarkably similar body plans. The need to gastrulate in different ways may relate to the size of the yolk and the need for amnion and extra-embryonic tissues. Often, later fetal stages look remarkably similar. During gastrulation, there are anatomical homologies: the mammalian and avian streak with the amphibian ventral and lateral blastopore lips, and the mammalian and avian node with the dorsal lip of the blastopore in the frog.

What are the mechanisms that drive gastrulation?

The organizer in *Xenopus* was described in the 1920s. It is the dorsal lip of the blastopore and lies for about 30 degrees either side of the midline; on ectopic transplantation, it is famous for being able to induce a second AP neural axis. Equally important is that the structures so induced have good dorsoventral specification. The organizer dorsalizes mesoderm and with the passage of time, as cells pass through, it is able to affect positioning along the head–tail (AP) axis.

Since the 1920s, some of the components and their evolutionary conservation have been described. For example, *Xenopus* genes expressed in the dorsal lip of the blastopore play a central role in executing Spemann's organizer phenomenon. Microinjection of mRNA from the gene into the ventral side of *Xenopus* embryos, where gene expression is normally absent, leads to the formation of an additional complete body axis, including head structures and abundant notochordal tissue. In addition, transplantation of the murine node has the same effect supporting the anatomical homology. Conjoined twins undoubtedly are formed at this stage of development.

Defects of gastrulation

Most defects of gastrulation are probably fatal. Body-plan anomalies and axial defects, whether genetic or teratogenic, have their origins in gastrulation. However, it may well be that many other anomalies arise from defects acting primarily at this time.

Overlapping *Hox* genes specify the anteroposterior axis

A universal positional information system was hypothesized in the 1970s, with the rules of interpretation varying between species, so leading to different pattern formation in different animals. This seems to be the case, at least for the head–tail axis, which is specified by the *Hox* code.

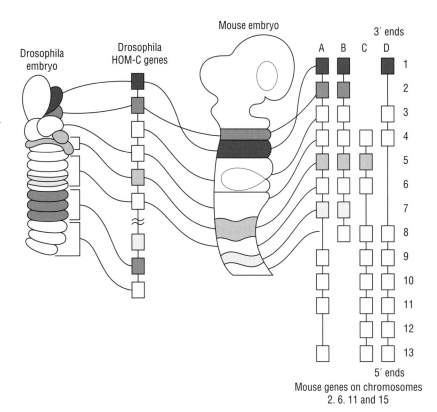

Figure 1.1 Drosophila *embryo and cranial limits of expression of the homeotic genes.*

Figure 1.1 illustrates the *Drosophila* embryo on the left and the cranial limits of expression of the homeotic genes. Organized in two clusters on *Drosophila* chromosome 3, these genes are known as the homeotic complex (*HOM-C*) genes. A common ancestor of this complex was duplicated twice, and mammals have four complexes of homeotic genes with similar sequence homology to the insect *HOM-C* genes.

Interestingly, the sequence of expression parallels the chromosomal location. In the fly, the thoracic and abdominal segments are specified; in mammals, rhombomeres and vertebrae are examples of specified segments. The expression pattern provides positional information that informs cells how far along the embryo they are. For example, in flies, the third thoracic segment expresses the *Ultrabithorax* (*Ubx*) gene. From this expression, the butterfly knows to develop wings, whereas *Drosophila* develops halteres. This is entirely consistent with Wolpert's universal positional information model.

Mouse *Hox* genes combinations and homeotic transformations

The mouse shown in Figure 1.2 illustrates the cranial expression boundaries of *Hox* genes in mice. The overlapping code specifies the development of individual somites or groups of somites. It is not clear whether the boundaries occur between the somites or between the recombined caudal and cranial halves of the prevertebral bodies. In mammals, the *Hox* genes are involved in the patterning of the vertebrae and are well characterized in craniofacial development. Some abnormal expressions of the *Hox* genes in mice cause cranialization of

caudal vertebral bodies, and other patterns of abnormal expression cause caudalization of cranial vertebral bodies. Their role in the regional specification of vertebrae makes it likely that they will be expressed abnormally in animal models of oesophageal atresia.

SOME SPECIFIC ANOMALIES

Duodenal and small-bowel atresias

The story of a solid phase in intestinal development, especially of the duodenum, continues in textbooks, but there is no evidence of a solid phase in the development of the gut. The aetiology of duodenal atresias and webs is unknown (Chapter 16), but the associations with multiple other anomalies suggest that it is an early problem. Jejunal and ileal atresias are seen without other malformations (except gastroschisis), and there is good evidence of a vascular aetiology. The association with gastroschisis is mechanical.

Hirschsprung's disease

The parasympathetic ganglia along most of the gut come from vagal neural crest cells (occipitocervical). Some hindgut ganglion cells are derived from the sacral neural crest. However, most sacral neural crest cells become glia and connective tissue. The concept of failure of craniocaudal neural crest cell migration in Hirschsprung's disease (HD, Chapter 17) has arisen from the chick in which the hindgut is populated by

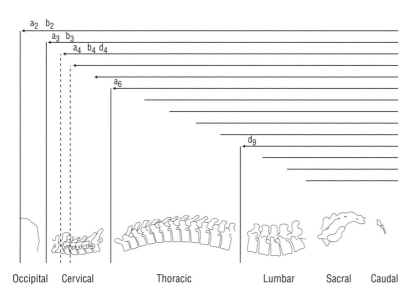

Figure 1.2 *The number of Hox genes expressed at any point along the head–tail axis tells vertebral-body cells what type of vertebral bodies they are to be. Only a_2b_2 are expressed in occipital bodies, but all are expressed in caudal bodies.*

neural crest cells three days after the foregut. In mammals, the process is almost simultaneous and occurs while the gut is very short, making a temporal migration problem in mammals less likely.

The neural crest cells have to be induced in the neural folds, detach, migrate, enter the gut wall, proliferate and differentiate. Problems could arise at any point of this pathway. The following conditions may provide clues:

Waardenburg disease types 1 and 2 may exhibit HD. In type 1, there is a mutation (*PAX3* chromosome 2q). The mouse mutant splotch (*Sp*) has hearing loss, pigmentation defects and Hirschsprung's disease and also has mutations in the *Pax3* gene.

The *RET* proto-oncogene is a tyrosine kinase receptor (chromosome 10q11.2). *Ret* mutants were reported in 50 per cent of a series of 35 familial cases of HD and in 16 of 45 (36 per cent) of cases of sporadic HD. Mice with a null mutation have HD and renal agenesis.

Interestingly, overactivity of the *RET* gene leads to multiple endocrine neoplasia type 2 (MEN2).

Endothelin-B receptor (EDNRB) maps to chromosome 13q22, and mutations have been reported in one of 17 cases of sporadic HD and in HD in association with Waardenburg disease. The mouse model here is the piebald lethal (*sl*) (also called spotting lethal).

The mouse mutant of *endothelin-3 ligand* (EDN3) is lethal spotted (*ls*). The human homologue is also abnormal in some cases of Waardenburg-associated HD. Interestingly, levels were found to be low throughout the colon in eight cases of HD.

Neural crest cells from *ls/ls* mice will invade wild-type colon in culture, but the reverse is not true. This suggests that the terminal colon is unreceptive to neural crest invasion in this mouse.

Renal development

The kidney proper develops from the metanephros, which appears at about five weeks. Its development illustrates reciprocal induction. The ureteric bud induces epithelial transformation in the mesenchyme of the metanephros to form nephric units. The reciprocal induction is that of the metanephros to induce branching of the ureteric bud. These inductive processes are driven by diffusible agents and do not need cell–cell contact. The agents now found to play roles in this reciprocal induction include *Hox*, *Pax* and zinc-finger gene products (e.g. *WT1*), growth factors and their receptors, and proto-oncogenes.

The craniocaudal overlapping *Hox* expression patterns may be pivotal in distinguishing the pre-, meso- and metanephros. *WT1* is required for ureteric bud sprouting, and the proto-oncogene tyrosine kinase receptor *c-ret* is needed for further growth and branching of the ureteric bud.

MULTICYSTIC DYSPLASTIC KIDNEY

Pathological cystic changes in multicystic dysplastic kidneys (MCDKs, Chapter 48) are associated with epithelial cells similar to those seen in the undifferentiated ureteric bud. There is a high expression of PAX2 (an oncogenic transcription factor) in these cells, and soluble paracrine factors may be driving the system, e.g. hepatocyte growth factor and insulin-like growth factor II. Interestingly, tissue around the cysts has a high rate of apoptosis (programmed cell death) with lack of *BCL2* and *PAX2*. Unfortunately, the current knowledge of these changes that accompany the pathology contributes little to our understanding of the problem.

URETERIC OBSTRUCTION

Bilateral obstruction causes oligohydramnios and lung hyperplasia. The role of antenatal surgical decompression of, for example, posterior urethral valves remains unproven due to a lack of controlled trials. Ureteric obstruction (Chapter 54) in the third trimester causes hydronephrosis, poor parenchymal growth and subcortical cysts, but earlier in gestation dysplasia is seen. But what is known of the molecular biology of obstruction-driven damage? Experimental murine ureteric obstruction causes enhanced apoptosis with abnormal expression of *BCL2*, *TGFβ1*, *angiotensin II* and *EGF*, each of which is implicated in normal metanephric development. Cause and effect are unclear, and the cascades of control are not established.

REFLUX

The loss of one murine *PAX2* allele results in a reduction of nephrons and a ureter predisposed to be a megaureter, possibly secondary to reflux (Chapter 52). The gene is also essential for retinal development in these mice. Since this pathology is evident when one allele is absent, the term *haplo-insufficiency* is used to describe a partial lack of functional protein. The dominant nature of the inheritance of reflux in some human pedigrees has led to a search for defects of this gene in affected families.

WT1 WILMS TUMOUR, DENYS–DRASH SYNDROME, WAGR

The normal gene product of the *WT1* locus is expressed in the metanephros, genital ridges and haematopoietic stem cells. Mutations in the gene are associated with Wilms tumour and genital anomalies in Denys–Drash syndrome (Chapter 42). Wilms tumour, aniridia, genital anomalies and retardation make up the WAGR association and may be related to disruption of closely linked genes. *WT1* is not the whole story, however, since lack of the normal imprinting that inactivates paternal *IGF2* gene can also lead to Wilms tumour in the picture of Beckwith–Wiedemann syndrome.

OTHER RENAL ANOMALIES

Some other renal anomalies are listed in Table 1.1.

Table 1.1 *Renal anomalies and genetic loci*

Syndrome	Genetic loci	Defined mutation
Bardet–Biedl	11q, 3p, 16q 15q	
Meckel	17q	
Di George	22q	
Autosomal recessive polycystic kidney disease	16p13.3	
Apert		*FGFR2*
Branchio-oto-renal		*Eyes absent* gene
Campomelic dysplasia		*SOX9* transcription factor in collecting ducts 17q24.3–q25.1
X linked Kallman		Signalling molecule
Denys–Drash		*WT1* transcription factor
		Missense mutation
Simpson–Golabi–Behmel		GPC3 (extracellular glycoprotein)

FGFR2, fibroblast growth factor receptor 2.

Morphogenesis of duplex renal development

A neat story explains the morphogenesis of 'absorption' of the mesonephric ducts and ureters into the bladder between weeks four and six, which accounts for the arrangement of duplex ureters. The first ureter to be 'absorbed' is the most caudal ureter, which drains the lower pole ureter (LPU). Its 'absorption' takes it most cranial into the bladder. The upper pole ureter (UPU) has its 'absorption' arrested before complete cranial migration and so ends its development in a caudal site, which will also be more medial than its partner. The ureter draining the UPU enters the bladder more caudally or opens outside the trigone (ectopic). The opening of the UPU is also more medial than the LPU. These observations are known together as the *Weigert–Meyer rule*. In addition, duplex kidneys demonstrate a relationship between the degree of renal dysplasia and the position of the ureteric orifice. This may relate to the ureteric branch meeting inadequately specified cranial metanephros. See Figure 1.3.

In boys, ectopic ureters can open into the prostatic urethra, the ejaculatory duct, the vas or the seminal vesicle. Ectopic

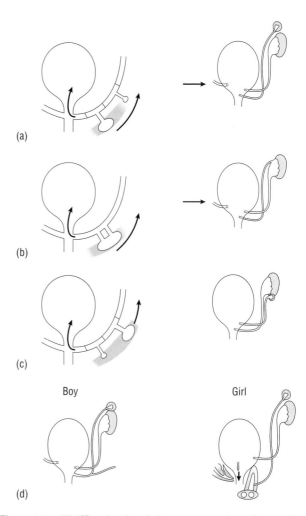

(a)

(b)

(c)

Boy   Girl

(d)

Figure 1.3 *Wolffian duct in relation to metanephros. See text for details.*

ureters in boys are always above the sphincter and do not cause wetting, but they can cause dysuria and infection. In girls, ectopic ureters can open into the vestibule, the vagina or, rarely, the uterus and so cause wetting.

Duplex renal development (Chapter 53, p. 465)

Figure 1.3 illustrates the Wolffian duct in relation to the metanephros. The Wolffian duct migrates into the bladder and the nephrogenic mass ascends. Figure 1.3a shows an LPU bud arising from the normal section and meeting good metanephric tissue; the UPU bud arises cranially and meets poor metanephros. After migration, the UPU opens caudally and the LPU opens normally into the bladder. Associated pathology includes a ureterocele with the UPU and reflux into the LPU.

Figure 1.3b shows two ureteric buds arising from normal Wolffian tissue and meeting good metanephros. Migration leads to crossing of the ureters. There may be reflux but the renal tissue may be normal.

Occasionally, as illustrated in Figure 1.3c, the UPU has arisen from normal tissue and the LPU has arisen from more caudal Wolffian tissue and met hypoplastic metanephric tissue. The lower pole then demonstrates dysplasia.

Figure 1.3d shows that if the UPU arises from the Wolffian region destined to be seminal vesicle, then the UPU is found to drain dysplastic renal tissue into the vesicle or a cyst in this region. In girls, the mullerian duct engulfs the Wolffian tissue before (left-hand side of the figure) and after (right-hand side of the figure) migration of the vaginal tissue into the vestibule. The ureter can then rupture and drain at any site in this region.

Sex determination

Analysis of the DNA of men with a 46,XX karyotype showed small amounts of Y chromosome had been translocated on to the X chromosome. This localized the sex-determining region (*SRY* gene) to the Y chromosome's short arm. The SRY protein drives the medullary sex cords to differentiate to Sertoli cells and secrete antimullerian hormone (AMH). Signalling from the SRY protein also causes mesenchyme in the genital ridges to differentiate into Leydig cells and secrete testosterone. The testosterone drives genital and brain changes.

Only 25 per cent of XY females have a disabled *SRY* gene. They can have a normal SRY gene but deletions at 9p or 10q or duplications of Xp. The story therefore is not as simple as it first appears. Furthermore, some XY individuals with the congenital skeletal dysplasia Campomelic dysplasia (see Table 1.1, *SOX9* mutations) are female. The SOX9 product is related to SRY and, when mutated, may block its action. Interestingly, the *WT1* gene discussed above may be upstream of *SRY*.

Limb anomalies

One of the confusions here is not the genes involved but the descriptive terminology:

Adactyly: no digits.
Ectrodactyly: absent digits.
Polydactyly: extra digits.
Syndactyly: fusion of digits.
Amelia, ectromelia: absent limb.
Meromelia: absent part of a limb.
Phocomelia: short, badly formed limb.
Hemimelia: short distal segment of a limb.
Acrodolichomelia: large hands or feet.

The axes of the limb are proximodistal, craniocaudal and dorsoventral. Left–right information is not needed to specify a limb. (A left–right agnosic cobbler could make pairs of shoes but could not satisfy the request to make only left shoes unless he or she had one to copy!)

PROXIMODISTAL AXIS

Overlapping *Hox* gene expression patterns illustrated in Figure 1.4 defines the upper-limb extremities. These gene expression patterns start distally with *Hox*-13 and progress more proximally as development advances, until *Hox*-9 appears and extends to the scapular region.

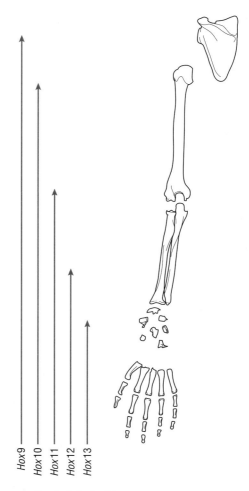

Hox9 Hox10 Hox11 Hox12 Hox13

Figure 1.4 *If cells find all of* Hox *9–13 expressed, then they become part of the hand. If only* Hox *9 and -10 are expressed, then the cells 'know' that they are in the region of the humerus.*

GENETIC THERAPY AND GERM-LINE THERAPY

Gene therapy is the insertion of new DNA into cells aiming to correct the instruction for making a protein. Consider conditions such as cystic fibrosis (CF) and severe combined immunodeficiency (SCID). Corrected copies of the *CF* gene, which codes for a transmembrane channel, can be inserted into pulmonary cells using a virus. SCID occurs when a particular enzyme is not produced. Some children have been treated with cells altered to carry the genetic instructions for making this enzyme, but it is too early to claim success. It will probably be too difficult to use genetic therapy for disorders that involve the actions of many genes. Also, for many health problems in which genes are involved, the genes are only partly responsible for what is wrong. In such cases, gene therapy may be only part of the solution.

The application of gene therapy in a treatment that could change the genes that a person passes on to their children is called germ-line therapy. Genes could be 'corrected' in the egg or sperm being using to conceive. The child that results would be spared certain genetic problems that might otherwise have occurred. It may even be possible to use germ-line therapy to remove a disorder from a family tree.

Table 1.2 *Timing of human embryonic development*

Day	Size of embryo (mm)	Development event
Week 1		
1		Fertilization
1.5–3		Cleavage 2–16 cells
4		Blastocyst enters uterus
5–6		Blastocyst hatches and implants
Week 2		
7–12		Implantation complete
13		Primitive streak develops, primary stem villi appear
Week 3		
16	0.4	Gastrulation: notochord forms
18	1–1.5	Neural plate and groove appear
20	1.5–2.5	First somites, neuromeres, primitive heart tube, early angiogenesis
Week 4		
22	2–3.5	4–12 somites, cranial neural folds fuse, cranial flexion, pulmonary primordia appear (asymmetric), 'heart pumps', first 2 pharyngeal arches and optic sulci form
24	2.5–4.5	13–20 somites, germ cells migrate, cranial neuropore closes, buccopharyngeal membrane ruptures
26	3–5	21–29 somites, caudal neuropore closes, pancreatic buds, urorectal septum forms, proximal limb buds, third to fourth pharyngeal arches form
28	4–6	30 somites, dorsoventral neural differentiation, cardiac septum primum, spleen, ureteric buds, lower limb buds, otic vesicle, lens placode, cranial motor nuclei
Week 5		
32	5–7	Spinal nerves, semilunar valves, greater and lesser curves of stomach, primary intestinal loop, metanephros, lens pit invaginates, cerebral hemispheres
33	7–9	Atrioventricular valves, cloacal folds, genital tubercle, hand plate, nasal pit invagination
Week 6		
37	8–11	Muscular ventricular septum, gut tube lumen occlude (?), major renal calyces, renal ascent, genital ridges appear, foot plate forms, retinal pigment, ears
41	11–14	Bronchopulmonary segments, cardiac septation completed, subcardinal veins, minor renal calyces, finger rays, dental laminae
Week 7		
44	13–17	Ossification, Sertoli cells, elbows, toe rays, intermaxillary process, eyelids, nipples
47	16–18	Septua primum and intermedium fuse, urogenital membrane ruptures
Week 8		
50	18–22	Intestinal loop completes anticlockwise rotation, in boys paramesonephric ducts regress
52	22–24	Pericardioperitoneal canals close
56	27–31	Chorionic cavity obliterated, superior vena cava established

WILL A PURELY GENETIC APPROACH EXPLAIN DEVELOPMENT?

It is a commonly held assumption that there is a mechanistic link between gene defects and their associated congenital anomalies and that this link is deducible by experiment and likely to be informative. The genes that are transcribed in early development are the focus of much research. They are undoubtedly important, but they are only part of the story. Unfortunately, there is great inertia behind the concept that a gene *x* is responsible for condition X. This leads to the assumption that finding gene *x* will necessarily be informative in understanding condition X. The genetic programme is played out in the physicochemical environment of the cell and the tissues of the conceptus. It must not be forgotten that non-genetic phenomena play very important roles in normal and abnormal development.

The assumption is questioned for four reasons: (i) The reductionist model in the physical sciences has failed, so why should it work in development? (ii) Certain phenomena crucial to early pattern formation cannot be specified by genetic information and so must be non-genetic, e.g. specifying left from right. (iii) Diverse anomalies often arise from indistinguishable insults. (iv) Indistinguishable anomalies often derive from diverse insults.

Timing of defects

We are often asked by parents 'Why did my child get this anomaly?', and many mothers are anxious that perhaps they should have done something different during the pregnancy to prevent the defect from arising. Although the timing of organ formation is as shown in Table 1.2, many anomalies seem to have their origins during gastrulation, or shortly thereafter, at a time when pattern formation and cell fate are established. We can say to these mothers that even though we do not know exactly how an anomaly occurred, it is likely to have had its origin well before they knew they were pregnant. Such reassurance may reduce the familiar misplaced sense of guilt that some mothers endure.

FURTHER READING

Larsen WJ. *Human Embryology*, 3rd edn. New York: Churchill Livingstone, 2001.

Lawrence PA. *The Making of a Fly: The Genetics of Animal Design*. Oxford: Blackwell, 1992.

Skandalakis JE, Gray SW. *Embryology for Surgeons*. Baltimore, MD: Williams & Wilkins, 1994.

Stephens FD, Smith ED, Hutson JM. *Congenital Anomalies of the Urinary and Genital Tracts*. Oxford: Isis Medical, 1996.

Wolpert L. *The Triumph of the Embryo*. Oxford: Oxford University Press, 1991.

Anatomy of the infant and child

JAS DICKSON

Learning objectives

- To appreciate the changes that occur with growth.
- To understand variations in the child, particularly in the neonate and infant, from adult positions and the relations of structures and organs.
- To learn practical sizes and relations of organs at different ages, e.g. body surface area, neonatal gut length, oesophageal length, bladder volume.

INTRODUCTION AND GROWTH

Why is there a place for a special chapter on paediatric anatomy? The anatomy of the child is essentially the same as that of an adult, but growth affects relative sizes and relations of structures change (Tanner 1978). Similar changes are seen in the embryo, but to a greater extent. The need is not simply to record the appropriate smaller sizes for tubes for use in children, such as endotracheal tubes, cystoscopes and endoscopes, but also to record the different positions and relations of structures.

The growth of a fetus into an adult has been well documented. Figure 2.1 shows the relative changes in body proportions during growth. The increase expressed by weight is greater than that in length, with the expansion of surface area lying in between (Table 2.1).

The fetus at birth can be described as a head, the size of which has been limited by the diameter of the birth canal, attached to an undeveloped body. The vascular system has to

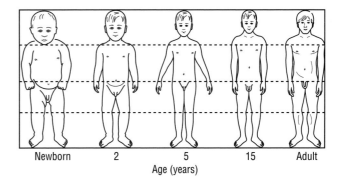

Newborn 2 5 15 Adult
Age (years)

Figure 2.1 *Relative changes in proportions during growth.*

develop to cope with the sudden increase in the partial pressure of oxygen of air-breathing life. The high oxygen levels are compensated for by free-radical scavengers and antioxidants. Immature capillaries are at risk from changes in blood pressure and circulation. These effects can be seen in the

Table 2.1 *Growth parameters*

Age	Weight (kg)	Length/height (cm)	Body surface area (m²)
Birth	3.5	50	0.21
1 year	10.0	76	0.44
5 years	19.0	110	0.75
10 years	30.5	138	1.08
Adult	70.0	175	1.85
Ratio of adult/ newborn	20:1	3.5:1	8.8:1

brain and retina, with periventricular haemorrhage in the brain and the retinopathy of prematurity (ROP; retrolental fibroplasia). During the last four weeks of intrauterine growth, the main deposition of fat in the subcutaneous tissues occurs. Glycogen storage in the liver increases and calcium and trace elements are deposited in the bones and liver.

After birth, there is least growth of the head and the greatest growth in the lower half of the body, following closure of the ductus arteriosus and the increase in post-ductal arterial blood flow. These changes mean that special charts are

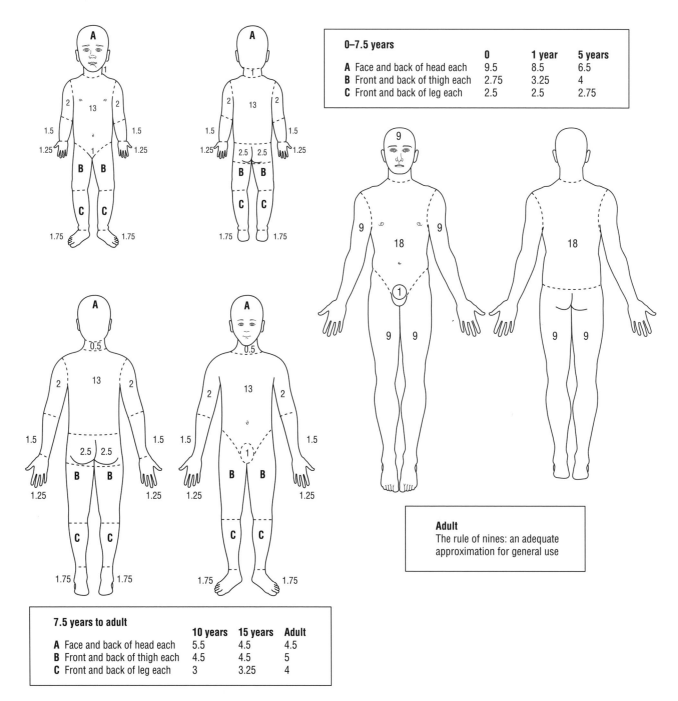

0–7.5 years			
	0	1 year	5 years
A Face and back of head each	9.5	8.5	6.5
B Front and back of thigh each	2.75	3.25	4
C Front and back of leg each	2.5	2.5	2.75

7.5 years to adult			
	10 years	15 years	Adult
A Face and back of head each	5.5	4.5	4.5
B Front and back of thigh each	4.5	4.5	5
C Front and back of leg each	3	3.25	4

Adult
The rule of nines: an adequate approximation for general use

Figure 2.2 *Changes in body surface area with age.*

required to assess the surface area affected in burned children (Figure 2.2). The simple 'rule of nines' is inadequate in children. The shape of the abdomen changes from being wider than it is long in the newborn to being longer than it is wide in the adult. Similarly, the ratio of the length from the xiphisternum to the umbilicus to that from the umbilicus to the symphysis pubis changes with growth of the lower half of the body (Figure 2.3). These changes have practical implications and explain partly the adult surgeon's preference for vertical midline incisions and the paediatric surgeon's preference for transverse supraumbilical incisions, particularly in the infant, for conventional abdominal surgery. Abdominal scars not only lengthen but also migrate. A gastrostomy placed in the epigastrium in the newborn ends up as a scar over the costal margin, and a transverse colostomy migrates round towards the loin (Figure 2.4).

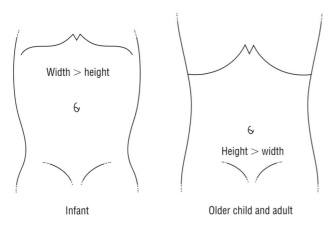

Figure 2.3 *Changes in proportion of anterior abdominal wall between infant and child.*

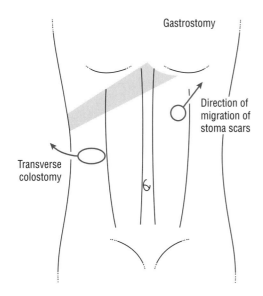

Figure 2.4 *Diagram demonstrating migration of scars due to growth of the patient.*

RADIOLOGICAL CHANGES

Skull

The comparison of drawings of the skull of an adult (Figure 2.5) and of a newborn (Figure 2.6) show similar changes, with much greater growth of the facial skeleton and mandible compared with the vault of the skull (Figure 2.7). The skull bones themselves show a major change from the thin single table of the infant to the much thicker calvarium with well-formed diploë between the two bony layers in the adult. This is

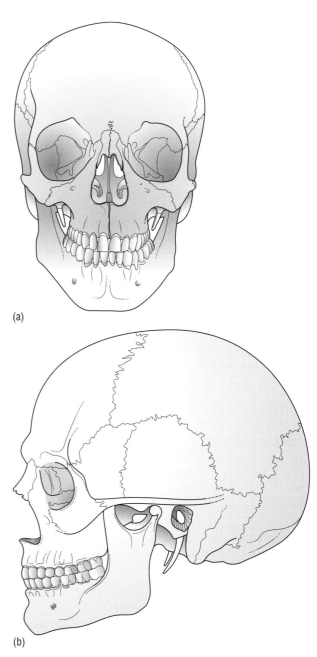

Figure 2.5 *Adult skull: note greater growth of facial bones compared with infant skull, covered in Figure 2.7. (a) Anterior view; (b) lateral view.*

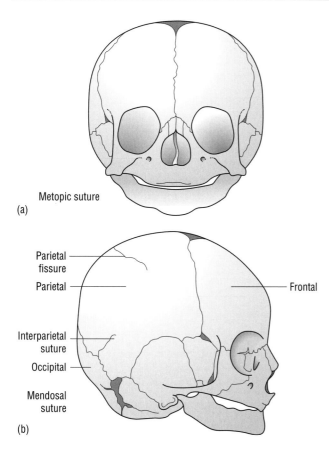

(a)

Metopic suture

Parietal fissure

Parietal

Frontal

Interparietal suture

Occipital

Mendosal suture

(b)

Figure 2.6 *Infant skull, showing congenital suture lines, which may be confused with fractures. (a) Anterior view; (b) lateral view.*

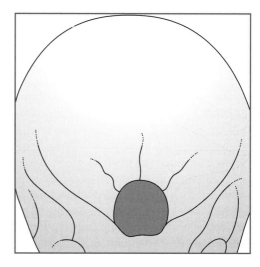

Figure 2.8 *Towne's view of skull, showing midline occipital suture and persistent membrane sutures laterally.*

important in the performing of a burr hole, as there is only one table to drill through in the infant. In Figure 2.6, in addition to the well-known suture lines, accessory suture lines are shown, which may cause confusion with skull fractures, i.e. the metopic suture in the middle of the frontal bone (Figure 2.6a) and a parietal fissure and the interparietal suture and, in the occipital bone, the mendosal suture (Figure 2.6b). On the Towne's view of the skull (occipital projection), the midline occipital suture entering the foramen magnum and persistent membranous fissures lateral to it are more difficult to differentiate from fractures and must be diagnosed with caution (Figure 2.8).

Neck

Among the problems seen on X-rays of the soft tissues of the neck in younger children is a false appearance of forward displacement of the oesophagus and trachea, suggesting a retropharyngeal abscess, which can occur in a crying, distressed child. The normal appearance is shown in Figure 2.9a; degrees of displacement, varying with inspiration and expiration, are shown in Figure 2.9b,c.

Chest radiographs

The major differences in the shape of the heart and the relative size of the heart and the chest of adults and infants are compared: in the infant, the heart lies more horizontally and occupies more of the chest (Figure 2.10) and the upper mediastinum is filled by the thymic shadow (Figure 2.11). The appearances of the thymus may be confusing; typical appearances are shown in Figure 2.11. In the older child, on deep inspiration, the heart may appear very narrow (Figure 2.12); this can also be produced, as in this case, by severe hypovolaemia.

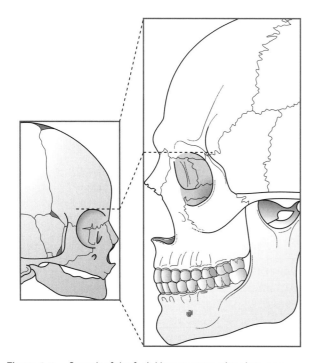

Figure 2.7 *Growth of the facial bones: comparison between neonatal and adult skulls.*

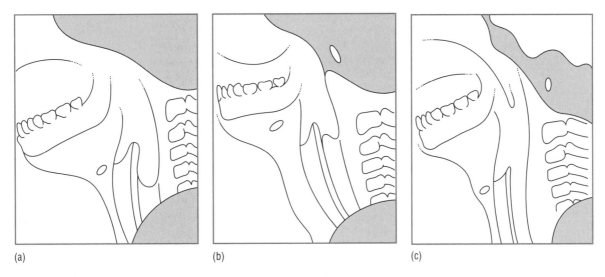

Figure 2.9   *Anterior displacement of oesophagus and trachea during inspiration and expiration: (a) at rest, (b) during inspiration and (c) during expiration.*

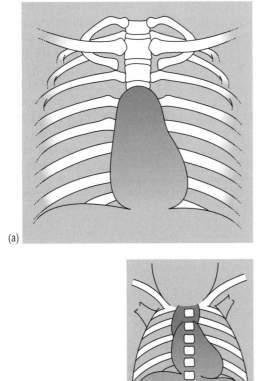

Figure 2.10   *Differences in chest X-ray of (a) a newborn compared with (b) an adult. Note the horizontal alignment of the heart in the newborn.*

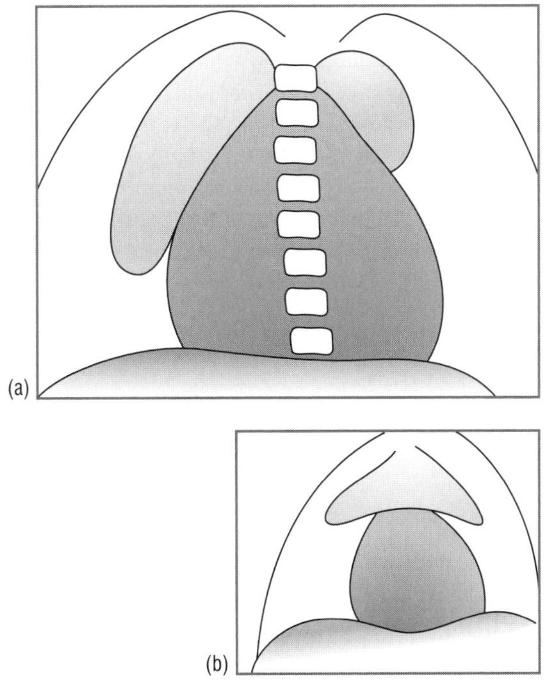

Figure 2.11   *The thymus has an obvious appearance in the infant and young child. (a) and (b) Typical thymus outlines on anteroposterior chest films.*

Abdomen

In the child, unlike in the adult, it is not possible to differentiate the large and small gut on its outline appearance, but the anatomical position of a loop may suggest its nature. In the

sigmoid colon in particular, it is often wise to confirm its identity by the use of contrast media.

RESPIRATORY SYSTEM

In the newborn, the ribs are aligned horizontally, tending to lie in a position of inspiration. Their descent to the more oblique position found in later life begins after the first year

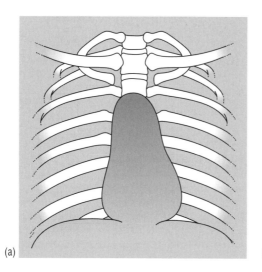
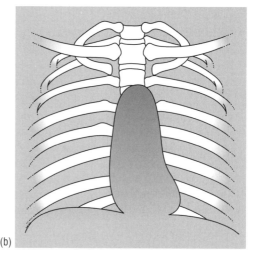

(a)   (b)

Figure 2.12   *Note the narrow heart in deep inspiration, which may be normal or a sign of hypovolaemia. (a) In the older child, on deep inspiration, the heart may appear very narrow. (b) Anteroposterior chest radiographs. Left expiratory view compared with right deep inspiration or severe hypovolaemia.*

of life. The adult configuration is achieved in later childhood. Thus, in the first year of life, it is not possible to increase the internal volume of the chest using the adult 'bucket-handle' movement of the ribs through the action of the intercostal muscles. Respiration depends predominantly on the function of the diaphragm. Abdominal distension interferes with diaphragmatic descent and causes respiratory distress.

Pleura

In early life, the pleura strips easily from the chest wall, permitting an extrapleural approach to mediastinal structures.

Upper air passages

For the first three months of life, the newborn baby is an obligatory nose-breather, owing to the tongue filling the oral cavity. This may be of value by ensuring warming and humidifying of the inspired air. The nasal passages contribute only 40–50 per cent of the airflow resistance, compared with around 63 per cent in the adult. This is important because of the effects on the airway of nasogastric and other tubes passed through one or both nostrils. Choanal atresia (Chapter 31, p. 264) or stenosis – congenital obstruction of the posterior nares – thus causes severe respiratory obstruction. If the atresia is unilateral, then it may be noticed when the one patent nostril is blocked by a nasogastric tube.

The infant epiglottis lies at an angle of 45 degrees to the posterior pharyngeal wall and during growth achieves the adult position closely approximated to the base of the tongue. It is soft, cartilaginous and often folded, and it may be rather short. The glottis lies with its aperture inclined more anteriorly than in the adult, opposite the lower border of the fourth

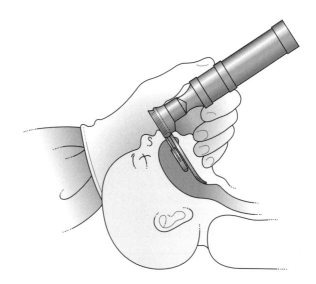

Figure 2.13   *Intubation of a neonate with a straight blade on the laryngoscope.*

cervical vertebra. During growth, it descends to lie in the adult position opposite the fifth and sixth vertebrae by the fourth year of life. Because of this high position, intubation is often performed most easily by using a straight laryngoscope blade. In the infant, the epiglottis should be picked up with the tip of the blade (Figure 2.13), whereas in older children, the tip is passed anterior to the epiglottis into the valleculae or glosso-epiglottic fossae.

The narrowest part of an adult's airway is the glottis, but in a child, the cricoid ring is narrower. The cricoid ring is a complete ring of cartilage, unlike the tracheal rings below it. By the age of 10–11 years, the adult configuration is achieved. The average cross-sectional area at the cricoid ring in the neonate is 28 mm^2, and 1 mm of oedema from infection or trauma will reduce this by 65 per cent.

Table 2.2 *Endotracheal tube sizes at certain ages*

Age (years)	Tube size (internal diameter, mm)
Preterm	2.5–3
Newborn	3.5
3–9 months	4.0
9 months–2 years	4.5
2	5.0
3	5.0
4	5.5
5	5.5
6	6.0
7	6.0
8	6.5
9	6.5
10	7.0
11	7.0
12	7.5
13	7.5

Trachea and main bronchi

The trachea at birth is 4 cm in length and 6 mm in diameter; in an adult, the average length is 12 cm and the average width 20 mm. The rate of growth is not linear, and spurts occur from the first few months of life to the third or fourth year and again around puberty. The trachea lies anterior to the vertebral column but to the right of the midline; the younger the child, the more it is to the right. Expected endotracheal tube sizes at certain ages are given in Table 2.2.

The right main bronchus is shorter than the left. At birth, the bifurcation of the trachea lies opposite the third to fourth thoracic vertebrae, but as growth proceeds it descends, until at six years of life it lies at the level of the fifth vertebra and at 12 years it lies at the level of the sixth thoracic vertebra.

Main bronchi

Because of the difference between the angles of the two main bronchi, it is more common for inhaled foreign bodies and other aspirated material to enter the right than the left main bronchus and from that the upper lobe bronchus at any stage of life. This is less true in younger children, in whom the angulation is less marked and mobility and flexibility are greater.

Lungs

Lung volume at birth is around 250 mL, whereas the adult volume is 6000 mL. The combined lung weight increases from 60 g at birth to around 750 g in adulthood. Bronchial segmental development is complete before birth. Postnatal development occurs in the acinar region. New alveoli form most rapidly in the first two years of life. They continue to form less rapidly during the first eight years of life and stop forming only with the cessation of growth of the chest.

GASTROINTESTINAL SYSTEM

Oesophagus

The oesophageal length can be measured from the lips at endoscopy, or from the nose, using a marked catheter. On measurement, it correlates as closely with age in months as with height and body surface area. The age formula, measuring from the lips, is

$$\text{Oesophageal length} = 21 + (0.136 \times \text{age in months})$$

which gives the length with an accuracy of 4 ± 4.1 cm. An alternative height formula used in pH measurement is

$$(0.207 \times \text{height in cm}) + 4.61$$

Using this measurement, a transnasal oesophageal probe should lie 2–4 cm from the oesophagogastric junction.

In the infant, the anti-reflux mechanism at the lower end of the oesophagus is less competent, probably because of relatively low pressure in the 'high-pressure' lower-oesophageal sphincter zone and the short length of the intra-abdominal oesophagus. These achieve more adult proportions from the second year of life.

Abdomen and contents

The changes in overall shape of the abdomen have already been alluded to (Figure 2.3). The liver and spleen are relatively large. The edge of the liver is normally palpable below the right costal margin in the infant and remains palpable across the epigastrium throughout childhood. A palpable spleen in a neonate may be normal.

Stomach

The relative capacity of the stomach is greater than in the adult. A 4-kg baby takes a feed of 120 mL (equivalent to 2 L in an adult). As a result, with crying and air-swallowing, the stomach can expand to take up the greater part of the abdomen. This distension becomes even greater in upper gastrointestinal obstructions, e.g. long-standing hypertrophic pyloric stenosis or duodenal atresia or stenosis. The pylorus normally lies to the right of the midline in the epigastrium but is very mobile. The transpyloric plane of the adult, said to pass through the pylorus, lies at the lower body of L1 on an X-ray and midway between the manubrial notch and the upper border of the symphysis pubis, but has no relevance to children. Analysis of the pyloric volume in patients with infantile hypertrophic pyloric stenosis and other vomiting children has shown that the size of the pylorus correlates well with the weight of the baby (Carver *et al.* 1987).

Small bowel

Gut function is well developed, even in preterm infants, with swallowing starting from 20 weeks' gestation, organized motor activity from 32 weeks' gestation and sucking from 35 weeks' gestation. Lymphoid tissue development follows the same pattern as elsewhere. The length of the small bowel from the duodenojejunal flexure to the ileocaecal valve is approximately 150 cm at 19–27 weeks' gestation, 200 cm at 27–35 weeks' gestation, and 300 cm ($\pm$40 cm) in a term newborn (Touloukian and Walker Smith 1983). These measurements were obtained at post-mortem after division of the mesentery, and actual lengths at laparotomy may be shorter. The adult length quoted is 1.5 m. Growth measured in experimental animals does not occur evenly or at the same rate as growth in height. The increase in length after gut resection is generally that expected from normal growth. The diameter does increase markedly and the mucosa hypertrophies.

Large bowel

The caecum may be relatively high at birth and continues to descend into the right iliac fossa during growth. In younger children, the appendix is more frequently retrocaecal. The shallow pelvis means that pelvic appendicitis is rare before the age of five years.

The caecum and ascending and transverse colon are supplied by the superior mesenteric artery through the ileocolic, right colic and middle colic arteries. The descending colon from the left third of the transverse colon is supplied from branches of the inferior mesenteric artery. Traditionally, the weakest part in the marginal artery of the colon has been assumed to be between the sigmoid vessels and the superior rectal artery critical point (Sudeck's point); however, the most tenuous link is actually at the junction of the superior and inferior mesenteric supply, between the ascending branch of the superior left colic and the middle colic vessels (Michels 1955).

The anal canal, which is 4 cm long in the adult, is 2–3 cm long in children and should be empty on digital examination. The anus of a newborn will take a 10–12 Hegar dilator, i.e. it is 10–12 mm in diameter, narrower than an average male adult little finger, but it will usually accept its gentle insertion without damage. A formula for anal size in the newborn is (el Haddad and Corkery 1985)

$$(\text{weight in kg} \times 1.3) + 7$$

GENITOURINARY SYSTEM

Bladder

The shallow pelvis of the newborn and young child means that the bladder is an abdominal organ, making suprapubic aspiration of urine a simple procedure, provided the bladder is palpable. The bladder capacity in millilitres can be estimated approximately from the formula

$$(25 \times \text{age in years}) + 25$$

Ovaries and uterus

At birth, the ovaries lie on the pelvic brim. Until the pelvic cavity enlarges, any increase in size from tumour or cyst formation will bring the ovaries into the abdomen as palpable or visible lumps. As the pelvic cavity enlarges, the fallopian tubes and uterus descend into it to take up the adult position by the menarche. The newborn uterus, under the influence of maternal hormones, is between 2.5 and 3.5 cm long. By six months, it has regressed to 80 per cent of its size at birth, regaining its neonatal size around five years. Growth to adult size occurs with puberty and just before menarche. Until then, there is no uterine flexion.

Male genitalia

The development of the penis and scrotum has been divided into five stages:

1 Infantile from birth to the onset of puberty. There is a slight increase in overall size but no change in appearance.
2 The start of scrotal enlargement.
3 Further increase in scrotal size. The penis increases in length.
4 Further increase in scrotal size and darkening of the scrotal skin. The penis enlarges and the glans develops.
5 Adult appearance.

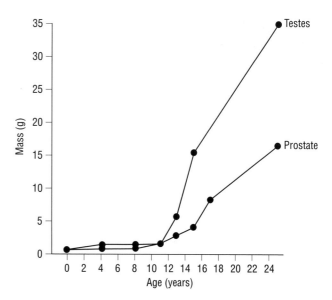

Figure 2.14 *Increase in mass of the testes and prostate gland during puberty.*

Testicular growth is minimal until the onset of puberty; then it progresses rapidly, this increase in size preceding the changes in the penis. The dramatic growth and increase in mass of the testes and prostate at puberty are shown in Figure 2.14.

CARDIOVASCULAR SYSTEM

For the first few years of life, the heart lies more horizontally than in the adult. With growth, the thorax lengthens and the heart elongates and descends to take up the adult position. The surface markings are as follows. The right margin lies to the right of the sternal edge from the second intercostal space to the junction of the sixth costal cartilage with the sternum. The left border runs obliquely from the second left intercostal space to the fourth intercostal space in the midclavicular or nipple line. The adult position is achieved in later childhood (Figure 2.10). The surface marking for placement of a ventriculoatrial shunt for hydrocephalus is the fourth right interspace. At birth, the foramen ovale is still valvular and is closed functionally by the increase in systemic pressure in the left atrium. In 75 per cent of children, this has fused by 12 weeks of age, but in up to 25 per cent, the 'foramen' remains probe-patent throughout life. The ductus arteriosus joins the left pulmonary artery to the arch of the aorta. It starts to close by muscular contraction after birth and should be obliterated to form the ligamentum arteriosum within a few weeks. Closure may be expedited by the prostaglandin antagonist indometacin and delayed by the prostaglandin epoprostenol.

Vascular access: venous

CENTRAL VENOUS ACCESS

Central venous access can be gained by direct puncture of the internal jugular, subclavian or femoral veins.

The internal jugular vein lies immediately deep to the sternomastoid muscle within the carotid sheath and is approached easily through the muscle (Figure 2.15). A point

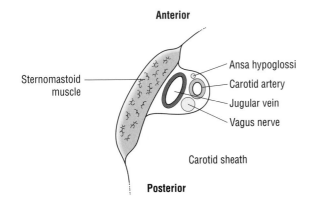

Figure 2.15 *Position of the internal jugular vein in the carotid sheath deep to the sternomastoid muscle.*

2–3 cm above the clavicle is chosen, over the medial third of the sternomastoid muscle, directing the needle towards the suprasternal notch. The subclavian vein at its junction with the internal jugular may be approached from above the clavicle. The needle is introduced in the angle between the clavicular head of the sternomastoid muscle and the clavicle and directed towards the sternal angle. From below, the needle is inserted 0.25–1 cm below the lower border of the clavicle, just lateral to its midpoint, and directed towards the upper border of the sternoclavicular joint. The lower border of the clavicle is felt and the needle is then directed just below that point, advancing slowly until the vein is entered. The femoral vein is identified lying just medial to the femoral artery, which is at the mid-inguinal point midway between the anterior superior iliac spine and the symphysis pubis, just caudal to the inguinal ligament.

PERIPHERAL VENOUS ACCESS

Peripheral veins are best identified by seeing and feeling them. The long saphenous vein at the ankle lies anterior to the medial malleolus of the tibia and can be palpated even when empty. In the cubital fossa, the laterally placed cephalic vein is easy to cannulate, but a central catheter inserted up it may be difficult to manipulate round the sharp bend near the clavicle, where it pierces the clavipectoral fascia to join the subclavian vein. Distally, the cephalic vein may be accessible as it passes from the venous arch on the back of the hand laterally around the lower part of the radius to enter the forearm. The medially placed basilic vein passes directly into the axillary vein. The external jugular vein crosses superficial to the sternomastoid muscle on its way from the neck to the subclavian vein. It is suitable for aspiration of blood and for injections but not for long-term use.

Vascular access: arterial

The radial artery at the wrist is favoured because of its free communication with the ulnar artery through the superficial and deep palmar arches and its superficial position on the radius. This communication can, and probably should, be checked before cannulating it, by occluding the artery by finger pressure to see whether this affects the colour of the fingers. The artery is palpable proximal to the wrist crease on the radius just lateral to the flexor carpi radialis tendon. When it is not palpable in very small babies, it can be seen by transillumination of the wrist.

The brachial artery in the mid-upper arm lies below the skin on the triceps and brachialis muscles midway between the medial borders of the biceps and the long head of the triceps muscles. It is accompanied by the median nerve. The femoral artery emerges into the thigh under the inguinal ligament at the mid-inguinal point and is separated from the pubic bone by the psoas muscle.

The dorsalis pedis artery, the continuation of the anterior tibial artery, is palpable on the dorsum of the foot over the first intermetatarsal space midway between the malleoli, just medial to the extensor hallucis longus tendon.

CENTRAL NERVOUS SYSTEM

Spinal cord

The spinal cord develops from the ectodermal neural plate. Failure of closure to form the neural tube explains the occurrence of spina bifida of the spinal cord and cranium bifidum and anencephaly. The floor of the normal fourth ventricle shows the appearance of a persisting unclosed neural tube. Neural tube closure should be complete by four weeks into gestation. The final development of the cord is not complete at birth and full myelination takes up to two years.

Up until birth, the vertebral column steadily outgrows the spinal cord, which recedes within the spinal canal. It has long been believed that this process continues throughout childhood. Advances in imaging, with ultrasound in the newborn and magnetic resonance imaging (MRI) at all ages, have made it easier to study the position of the conus (Wilson and Prince 1989). These studies showed that this is much more variable than was previously understood, and no evidence of differential growth after birth was found. The range for the vertebral level of the tip of the conus medullaris from birth to two years was from the T12 to the L2 disc space. A termination as low as L3 was found in normal subjects. The mean position lay over the body of L1 at all ages. A criticism of these findings is that they were not serial studies but were isolated in individual children. The deteriorating neural function associated with tethering of the cord by an abnormal filum terminale, lipoma of the cord or following repair of a myelomeningocoele suggests that the answer is not simple. In addition, the cord may recede dramatically when a tethered filum is divided.

Ventricular system

The lateral ventricles lie within the cerebral hemisphere, separated by the septum lucidum. They communicate through the foramina of Monro with the third ventricle, which lies in the midline between the thalami and communicates back through the narrowest part of the system, the cerebral aqueduct (of Sylvius), leading into the fourth ventricle, which is roofed by the cerebellum and has as its floor the hindbrain. The foramina of Magendie (central) and of Luschka (in the lateral recesses) in the fourth ventricle allow cerebrospinal fluid (CSF) into the subarachnoid space around the brain. The CSF is secreted by the choroid plexuses in the lateral, third and fourth ventricles and from the ependymal surface. It passes through the ventricular system and then over the surface of the brain, down the central canal of the spinal cord and over the surface of the cord. It is absorbed back into the bloodstream through the arachnoid granulations in the superior longitudinal (sagittal) sinus. Blockage at any point, including within the granulations or superior longitudinal sinus, causes hydrocephalus. In communicating hydrocephalus, there is free communication between the intraventricular systems and the subarachnoid space around the cord. CSF pressure can be obtained from lumbar puncture, and drainage is possible through a thecoperitoneal shunt. In non-communicating hydrocephalus, any attempt to lower the pressure around the cord may induce coning of the hindbrain into the foramen magnum and sudden death. Access to the ventricular system is relatively easy before the anterior fontanelle closes. A needle passed through a lateral angle of the anterior fontanelle vertically downwards towards the midline should hit the ventricle at 5 cm from the surface. Once the fontanelle has closed, a burr hole 1–2 cm from the midline is required. The choroid plexuses in the lateral ventricle lie posterior to the foramina of Monro, and an intraventricular catheter placed in the anterior horn of the lateral ventricle in front of this should not, in theory, become obstructed by the choroid plexus wrapping round it.

The cerebral veins cross the subarachnoid space from the relatively mobile cortex to drain into the rigid superior sagittal sinus. They run obliquely forwards, increasingly so posteriorly. This arrangement leaves them vulnerable to injury from rapid head movement, such as in a head injury or during severe shaking, leading to subdural bleeding and effusion.

Nerve biopsy

Two sites are suitable for obtaining a specimen of a peripheral nerve for neurological diagnosis. The sural nerve is found easily, as it lies posterior to the lateral malleolus midway between this and the tendo-achilles (calcaneus) and alongside the small saphenous vein. Complete division of the nerve causes anaesthesia only on the lateral side of the heel and foot. This can be reduced by splitting the nerve and sending only a half-thickness for biopsy. If motor fibres are required, then the most distal part of the deep peroneal (anterior tibial) nerve where it lies on the dorsum of the foot, lateral to the dorsalis pedis artery, can be taken. Anaesthesia is produced only in the web space between the first and second toes, and loss of power in the extensor digitorum brevis is not easily detectable.

REFERENCES

Carver RA, Okorie NM, Steiner GM, Dickson JAS. Infantile hypertrophic pyloric stenosis: diagnosis from the pyloric muscle index. *Clinical Radiology* 1987; **138**: 625–7.

El Haddad M, Corkery JJ. The anus in the newborn. *Pediatrics* 1985; **76**: 927–8.

Michels NA. *Blood Supply and Anatomy of the Upper Abdominal Organs.* London: Pitman, 1955.

Tanner JM. In: Falkner I, Tardrew F, Mourilyan J (eds). *Human Growth: A Comprehensive Treatise,* Vol. 2. New York: Plenum Press, 1978.

Touloukian RJ, Walker Smith GJ. Normal intestinal length in preterm infants. *Journal of Pediatric Surgery* 1983; **18**: 720–23.

Wilson DA, Prince JR. MR imaging determination of the location of the normal conus medullaris throughout childhood. *American Journal of Neuroradiology* 1989; **10**: 259–62.

FURTHER READING

Keats TE. *Atlas of Normal Roentgen Variants that may Simulate Disease,* 6th edn. St Louis, MO: Mosby, 1996.

Fetal medicine

DAVID HOWE

Learning objectives

- To understand the range of fetal medicine.
- To understand the diagnostic limitations of fetal medicine.
- To understand the interrelationships between specialists in fetal medicine, neonatal paediatrics and paediatric surgery in providing high-quality care.
- To be aware that the natural history of anomalies diagnosed prenatally may differ from that traditionally associated with postnatal diagnosis.

INTRODUCTION

Twenty years, ago the concept of a specialist in fetal medicine was virtually unknown. Obstetric care was focused on ensuring the wellbeing of the mother, since the fetus was inaccessible for diagnosis or treatment. Two areas of technical advance, real-time ultrasound and genetic diagnosis, have so altered our abilities that our whole concept of the fetus has changed and it is recognized as a patient, like any other, amenable to diagnosis and treatment.

Ensuring the best outcomes for fetuses with problems is possible only by close collaboration between a number of specialties, including fetal medicine, neonatal intensive care, paediatric surgery and paediatric cardiology. Specialists in each discipline need to understand their own abilities and limitations, and those of their colleagues, to ensure that parents are given accurate and consistent advice about the implications of any antenatal diagnosis for their child.

THE SCOPE OF FETAL MEDICINE

Fetal medicine falls into four main areas:

- Diagnosis and management of fetal malformations, with the greatest overlap with paediatric surgery.
- Diagnosis and management of other fetal conditions.
- Monitoring of fetal wellbeing.
- Prenatal screening and diagnosis of genetic conditions.

Diagnosis and management of fetal malformations

POSSIBILITIES AND LIMITATIONS OF ULTRASOUND

The great majority of antenatal diagnoses are now made during routine ultrasound screening of fetal anatomy, usually carried out at 19–20 weeks' gestation. A small number of anomalies, mainly neural tube and abdominal wall defects, will be forewarned by raised levels of maternal serum alpha-fetoprotein on 16-week serum screens. Until recently, there was no common agreement about what should and should not be checked during an anomaly scan, but in 2000 the Royal College of Obstetricians and Gynaecologists published guidelines to help standardize the procedure.

One of the recommendations was that parents should be given more explicit information about what might or might not be achieved by anomaly scanning. Many parents have an understandable expectation that anomaly screening will detect nearly all problems, whereas the reality is quite different. Overall, the antenatal detection rate of major fetal anomalies is around 75 per cent, but for some organ systems, the rate is much lower. Bricker *et al.* (2000) published a meta-analysis of the detection rate of fetal anomalies during routine screening (as opposed to detection rates in centres of expertise carrying out targeted scans), and some of these are shown in Table 3.1. The detection rate will be influenced by a number of factors, in particular how obvious an abnormality appears on a scan, but also including the mother's build (images are much less clear in obese women), the equipment used, the training and abilities of the ultrasonographers, and the time available to carry out the scans.

Some anomalies, such as neural tube and abdominal wall defects, are usually clear on scans, and the detection rates of these are above 90 per cent. Other problems may only be inferred by the absence of a normal structure in the fetus, e.g. absence of the fetal stomach suggesting an oesophageal atresia or absence of the bladder forewarning of a cloacal anomaly. Some abnormalities that might seem obvious to those not familiar with antenatal scanning are not diagnosable. This includes anomalies such as anorectal malformation: since the fetus does not empty its bowels during pregnancy, a low blockage does not produce obvious bowel distension. Finally, some abnormalities may not be apparent at 20 weeks and develop only later; duodenal atresia, which has a characteristic 'double-bubble' appearance on scan, may not become obvious until around 24 weeks' gestation and may be missed on a 19-week scan.

Recently, some other imaging methods have been used to help delineate fetal anomalies, but these have not yet entered routine practice. Magnetic resonance imaging (MRI) has been tried in some centres, particularly to assess neurological abnormalities, but often it does not add much information to that obtained with ultrasound. Three-dimensional ultrasound is now available and may be helpful in showing parents what an abnormality looks like, but it adds little to the ability to diagnose most problems.

MANAGEMENT OF ANOMALIES

When a fetal anomaly is discovered, the management follows the process shown in Figure 3.1.

ACHIEVING A DIAGNOSIS

The first imperative is to make as specific a diagnosis as possible to give the parents the most accurate information about the condition and its prognosis. Achieving a full diagnosis usually takes more than one visit, since in most cases there is a need for additional investigations. First, as much information as possible must be sought from scanning the fetus. If one abnormality is found, then often there will be others, which, if found, will greatly alter the prognosis. If additional anomalies are found, then they often worsen the chance of the baby surviving through neonatal surgery and increase the likelihood of the baby having an underlying genetic or chromosomal problem. For many abnormalities, it is appropriate to offer the parents karyotyping, since the risk of the baby having a chromosomal abnormality is at least as great as the risk if the maternal age is over 35 years, the conventional level of risk at which invasive testing is offered. Some anomalies,

Table 3.1 *Rates of detection of fetal anomalies on mid-pregnancy ultrasound*

System	Anomaly	Detection rate (%)
Central nervous system		76
	Anencephaly	97
	Spina bifida	67
Pulmonary		50
	Diaphragmatic hernia	45
Cardiac		17
	Ventricular septal defect	2
	Atrioventricular septal defect	42
	Single ventricle	56
Gastrointestinal		42
	Tracheo-oesophageal fistula	13
	Exomphalos	100
	Gastroschisis	100
Urinary tract		67
	Obstructive uropathy	67
	Renal dysplasia	63
Skeletal		24
	Limb-reduction defect	29
	Talipes	22
	Facial cleft	33

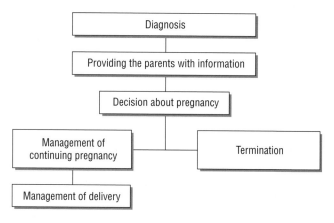

Figure 3.1 *Process of management of fetal abnormalities.*

such as cerebral ventriculomegaly, may be associated with other insults to the fetus, e.g. transplacental viral infections. Cytomegalovirus (CMV) and toxoplasmosis both cause fetal anomalies that may be apparent on scan.

DESCRIBING THE ABNORMALITY TO THE PARENTS

As the diagnostic process progresses, the parents must be kept up to date with information that is as accurate as possible. They need to have the scan abnormality described to them in terms that they can understand, and the implications for their child need to be discussed. When doing this, it is important to judge how ready they are to receive this information and to remember the need to describe normal anatomy, since many parents have a limited understanding of this. Immediately after a problem is recognized, many parents are in a state of shock and unable to take in complex information. It is often best in these circumstances to give them a limited amount of information and bring them back the next day, with a partner or friend present, to talk to them more fully, once they are ready to take in what is said.

PITFALLS FOR PAEDIATRIC SURGEONS COUNSELLING PARENTS ANTENATALLY

Paediatric surgeons may be invited to participate in the antenatal counselling of parents. This usually will be some time after the parents have first heard that there is a problem with their baby and when they are more receptive to the information given. The aspects they particularly wish to learn about from the paediatric surgeon may include the treatments available for their child's condition and the likely long-term outlook – in particular, mortality rates and whether their child will have residual problems or a disability.

There are several pitfalls for surgeons counselling in these circumstances. First, it is important that the information provided by the fetal medicine and surgical specialists is consistent, otherwise parents lose confidence in both. This requires regular communication, helped by agreed or shared written information for commonly encountered conditions. For uncommon conditions, it is often helpful to discuss what the parents will be told before counselling them. A second potential pitfall is the relative uncertainty of antenatal diagnosis. Ultrasound may reveal a fetal problem but fail to show associated conditions that will significantly alter prognosis. For instance, ultrasound may suggest the presence of oesophageal atresia but may not indicate an associated anorectal malformation in a baby with a VATER (vertebral, anorectal, tracheo-oesophageal, radial/renal) anomaly. Similarly, it will not be possible on ultrasound to determine the level of an oesophageal atresia or to differentiate it from a more serious laryngeal cleft. Thus, it is often necessary to discuss with parents a spectrum of possible diagnoses and prognosis. A third pitfall is to quote survival or complication rates from paediatric follow-up series when indicating the prognosis of a fetus with an antenatal diagnosis. Anomalies detected antenatally may be at the more severe end of the spectrum and may be associated with genetic or chromosomal problems, which will worsen the outlook. For instance, the survival rate of infants with congenital diaphragmatic hernia in paediatric series is around 70–80 per cent. For a fetus with an antenatally diagnosed diaphragmatic hernia, the survival rate through neonatal surgery is only 25 per cent overall and only 50 per cent if the baby has an isolated hernia with no associated chromosomal or structural anomaly. Many affected fetuses die *in utero* or soon after birth and before transfer to the surgical team, so those operated on have already been selected to have a better prognosis. Table 3.2 lists a number of conditions for which the advice given antenatally differs significantly from that provided postnatally.

Finally, there are an increasing number of medicolegal cases brought by parents of surviving children with disability, arguing that if they had been told all of the potential problems that their child would face, then they would not have continued the pregnancy. The arguments usually hinge on the information that they were given antenatally, and it is essential to keep clear contemporaneous notes of these discussions. Providing such information is hampered at present by the lack of high-quality follow-up studies of the long-term outcome of antenatally diagnosed conditions, and there is an urgent need for such studies.

TERMINATION OF PREGNANCY

Once the fetal abnormality has been discussed fully with the parents, they need to decide their plans for the pregnancy. In the UK, termination of pregnancy is permitted legally in a number of circumstances defined by the Abortion Act 1966, later modified by the Human Fertilisation and Embryology Act 1990. Termination may be performed at any stage in pregnancy where 'there is a substantial risk that if the child was born it would suffer from such physical or mental abnormalities as to be seriously handicapped'. After viability, usually taken to be 24 weeks' gestation, termination would only be offered in rare circumstances where the baby has a lethal or extremely disabling condition.

Up to 12 weeks' gestation, termination can be carried out as a simple operative procedure. Most anomalies will not be apparent by then, and after this stage the majority of units would terminate the pregnancy by giving the mother agents to induce miscarriage. Most units now give mifepristone, an antiprogesterone, 36 hours before admission to prepare the uterus and then induce contractions by giving prostaglandins in tablet or pessary form. In the great majority of women, this regime results in delivery within 24 hours of admission. Some women will need an evacuation of retained products of conception to empty the uterus of placental tissue that is not expelled spontaneously. After 21 weeks, it is usual practice to perform a feticide before induction by giving intracardiac potassium to prevent any possibility of the fetus being born alive.

Particular problems arise when a fetal anomaly is recognized in a twin or higher multiple pregnancy. If the pregnancy

Table 3.2 *Conditions for which prenatal advice differs from postnatal advice to parents*

Condition	Difference between antenatal and postnatal outcome
Facial cleft	When hare lip is evident on scan, it is often difficult to be certain whether the hard palate is also affected. Counselling will need to cover the surgery required in both circumstances.
Spina bifida	Ventriculomegaly seen in association with spina bifida may grow in proportion to the fetal head as pregnancy advances, or may increase rapidly, causing difficulty with delivery and worsening the outlook.
Diaphragmatic hernia	Overall survival of antenatally diagnosed cases is 25%, rising to 50% where isolated, i.e. normal chromosomes and no additional physical abnormalities apparent on scan. This compares with 70–80% survival in postnatal series.
Cystic hygroma	The abnormality referred to antenatally as cystic hygroma differs from the postnatal abnormality seen by surgeons. The antenatal abnormality is a fluid collection in the posterior neck, often septated. Sixty per cent of affected fetuses have chromosome abnormalities – usually Down or Turner syndrome. In the majority of cases, the hygroma resolves before birth in surviving fetuses. The abnormality seen postnatally by paediatric surgeons, usually confined to the anterior neck and unilateral, is rarely apparent before birth.
Congenital cystic adenomatoid malformation	This may enlarge during pregnancy, resulting in fetal hydrops or demise, although in the majority of cases the abnormality starts to resolve spontaneously and is smaller at delivery than in mid-pregnancy. Most are asymptomatic at delivery.
Sacrococcygeal teratoma	These may be solid or cystic. Solid tumours with a large blood supply may enlarge rapidly, resulting in high-output heart failure, causing fetal hydrops and intrauterine death.
Oesophageal atresia	This cannot be diagnosed with certainty but can be suspected from absence of the fetal stomach and the development of polyhydramnios. Most detected cases have atresia without fistula because the fetal stomach may be visible if there is an associated tracheo-oesophageal fistula.
Anorectal malformations	These are rarely apparent on scan, since the fetus does not routinely open its bowels during pregnancy, and a low obstruction will not cause evident bowel obstruction.
Exomphalos	The fetal bladder must be identified specifically, since ectopia vesicae may present as a lower abdominal wall defect.
Intra-abdominal cysts	Cysts arising from a number of structures in the abdomen appear identical on antenatal scan, so it is frequently impossible to be certain of the origin. Counselling should reflect this uncertainty.

is dichorionic, then a selective feticide can be performed to terminate the affected fetus, although there is about a ten per cent risk of causing miscarriage of both twins by doing so. If the twins are monochorionic, and thus sharing their circulation through a single placenta, then a cord-occluding method must be used to terminate the affected twin, since in these pregnancies the death of one twin can cause the death of, or harm to, the other.

MANAGEMENT OF CONTINUING PREGNANCY

Where the fetal abnormality is less severe and the parents opt to continue the pregnancy, then the main management issues are ensuring that the parents are informed and confident about the care their child will need, at the time of delivery and subsequently, to manage any antenatal complications that may arise, and to plan delivery to ensure that the child receives appropriate care.

During the anxious period after diagnosis of a problem, and before their child is born, most parents find it helpful to see the neonatal unit or the wards where their child will be cared for and to meet some of the staff concerned. Since this may be at a regional referral unit some distance from their home, this allows them to develop confidence in the team and to plan practical issues such as travel to and from the hospital.

Some anomalies may be associated with antenatal complications that require management. The most common problem is polyhydramnios, which can result from any condition that obstructs the gastrointestinal tract or inhibits swallowing in other ways, e.g. neuromuscular weakness. If the polyhydramnios is severe, then it may precipitate premature labour. In some cases, this can be ameliorated by giving the mother indometacin, which, in the fetus, reduces blood flow to the kidneys and lowers its urine output. Where this fails, the liquor can be removed by carrying out a large amniocentesis or amnioreduction. As with any invasive procedure, this may precipitate delivery, so the risk of intervention has to be balanced against the risk of labour if no action is taken.

MANAGEMENT OF DELIVERY

One of the most important aspects of care nearing the end of pregnancy is to plan the delivery to ensure that the child is born in appropriate circumstances. When a fetal anomaly is noted, many parents believe that the baby may benefit from delivery by caesarean section. In fact, this provides little benefit in the great majority of conditions, and the mode of delivery with few exceptions should be dictated by obstetric indications. There is little evidence that delivery by caesarean section is advantageous for gastroschisis, diaphragmatic hernia or spina bifida. If the baby has a large exomphalos containing liver and bowel, then the obstetricians may be anxious about this being damaged during vaginal delivery and opt for caesarean section; there may be similar worries with large sacrococcygeal tumours.

For children needing neonatal surgery, it may be helpful to deliver the baby in a unit with paediatric surgeons on site to avoid the need for early transfer. If the parents have some distance to travel, it may be practical to induce labour; this can help in planning neonatal cot availability. It is also important to ensure that the neonatal staff are aware that the delivery is due, and whether any special resuscitation or management is required at birth, so that this can be planned and the appropriate equipment gathered in advance.

Diagnosis and management of other fetal conditions

As well as management of anomalies, fetal medicine includes the diagnosis and management of other fetal conditions. The fetus is now a patient that may benefit from intrauterine treatment.

TRANSPLACENTAL DRUG THERAPY

The fetus may be treated by giving to the mother drugs that cross the placenta. The most widely used transplacental therapy is steroids given to mature fetal lungs and reduce the complications of prematurity. Drug therapy has also been used to treat fetal cardiac dysrhythmias. Both sustained bradycardias and supraventricular tachycardias may cause heart failure, visible in the fetus as hydrops, where fluid accumulates in tissues above and below the diaphragm. The fetus may develop heart block in a mother with lupus antibodies, which cross the placenta and destroy the Purkinje fibres. If the heart rate is very low, hydrops develops, which may improve with a combination of steroids and digoxin. Sustained fetal supraventricular tachycardias may also cause hydrops and may revert to sinus rhythm if treated with antidysrhythmics. Flecainide is usually the first choice in established hydrops. If transplacental therapy is unsuccessful, then the fetus may be treated by direct injection. Adenosine and amiodarone have both been used successfully to cardiovert the fetus.

DIRECT FETAL THERAPY

The most common form of direct fetal therapy is transfusion. This may be carried out to correct anaemia due to rhesus incompatibility or to treat parvovirus infection, which suppresses the fetal marrow. Alternatively, platelet transfusions may be required to correct thrombocytopenia caused by antiplatelet antibodies.

Fetuses with large pleural effusions may develop secondary hydrops and polyhydramnios. The effusions will also prevent development of the fetal lungs. Relieving the effusion by inserting a pleuro-amniotic shunt can preserve lung growth and relieve the hydrops. The shunt is a small double-pigtailed catheter, which is inserted through a wide-bore needle. These shunts also can be used to relieve bladder outflow obstruction.

Fetal therapy may be required in the management of monochorionic twin pregnancies that develop problems as a result of twin-to-twin transfusion. This causes circulatory overload in the recipient twin, resulting initially in polyuria causing polyhydramnios in that sac and eventually in fetal hydrops due to heart failure. If untreated, the polyhydramnios results in premature delivery; this can be prevented by serial amnioreductions, removing a litre or more of liquor on each occasion. In some cases, these also abate the process. Another treatment used in some centres is division of the connecting vessels between the placentas using fetoscopically directed laser.

The fetus may be damaged *in utero* by transplacental transmission of viruses and other microorganisms. *Toxoplasma gondii* and CMV are the most common agents that affect the fetus, and both may cause severe long-term problems, including brain damage, blindness and deafness. They may be diagnosed after the finding of fetal abnormalities such as cerebral ventriculomegaly, or they may be diagnosed by serological testing, possibly following a frank maternal illness. Amniocentesis and polymerase chain reaction (PCR) testing of the liquor for viral deoxyribonucleic acid (DNA) can help to determine whether the infection has crossed the placenta and thus increased the likelihood of fetal harm.

Monitoring fetal wellbeing

Another important role for fetal medicine is the monitoring of fetal wellbeing. This is achieved largely by biophysical methods. Ultrasound measurements will demonstrate that a fetus is not growing as expected, and scans can also be used to watch other indicators of fetal wellbeing, such as movements and breathing. Poor placental function is usually accompanied by high resistance to flow in the umbilical arteries, which can be demonstrated by Doppler assessment. As the placenta is a low-resistance system, there is normally forward flow in the cord throughout the cardiac cycle. With increasing resistance, forward flow stops in diastole; as the placenta deteriorates further, the end-diastolic flow becomes reversed. These changes are accompanied by redistribution of flow within the fetus to send blood preferentially to the heart and the head at the expense of other organs. The reduction in renal blood flow results in reduced liquor surrounding the baby and can also be demonstrated by Doppler examination of flow in the middle cerebral arteries and thoracic aorta.

Prenatal screening and diagnosis

This involves the antenatal detection of genetic and chromosomal disorders. Diagnosis is normally achieved using an invasive test such as amniocentesis or chorion villus sampling (CVS) to obtain fetal cells. Since these tests pose a small risk to the pregnancy, increasing emphasis has been placed in recent years on developing screening methods to identify women at greatest risk of having an affected child, to whom invasive testing is offered.

SCREENING FOR CHROMOSOME DISORDERS

The most common cause of congenital mental disability is Down syndrome, which affects about one in 650 births in unscreened populations. Many parents wish to have the condition identified antenatally to allow them to opt for termination of pregnancy. The risk of having a child with a trisomy increases with advancing maternal age, with an exponential rise above the age of 35 years, so this was the first indicator used. In the late 1980s, it was noted that women carrying affected fetuses had lower serum levels of alpha-fetoprotein, and this prompted a search for other similar serum markers. By taking blood at 16 weeks, a combination of serum markers is now used as a way to modify the age-related risk, to achieve higher specificity and sensitivity than age alone. This allows detection of Down syndrome in younger women and may allow some older women to avoid invasive testing and its attendant risks. Since then, it has also been noted that fetuses with trisomies tend to have greater oedema in the skin behind the occiput, or nuchal translucency, when scans are carried out between 10 and 14 weeks. Measurement of nuchal translucency is now offered in some units as another method of adjusting the maternal age-related risk of Down syndrome as a universal screening test. In women who accept these screening methods, the screening result is considered high-risk in about 75 per cent of those carrying an affected fetus, with a five per cent false-positive rate.

SCREENING FOR OTHER GENETIC CONDITIONS

Screening may be offered for some other genetic conditions to at-risk populations. Routine haemoglobinopathy screening is offered to non-Caucasian women, or to the entire population where the prevalence is high enough to justify this. Where both members of a couple are found to be carriers, they will be offered prenatal diagnosis.

For many other genetic conditions, prenatal diagnosis may be possible but is offered only where there is known family history. Cystic fibrosis is the most common single-gene disorder in the UK, but most families are unaware that they are at risk until the birth of an affected child. There have been pilot studies of population screening for the cystic fibrosis gene, but these have not become routine practice, not least because an alternative strategy of screening newborns might allow the disease to be treated more effectively, making termination a choice that parents would be less likely to make.

DIAGNOSTIC TESTS

Screening tests identify women as being at high risk of carrying an affected child, but definitive diagnosis or exclusion of the condition can be made only by obtaining cells from the pregnancy. The two most common tests are amniocentesis, in which liquor containing exfoliated cells is aspirated from the sac, and CVS, in which a sample is taken from the placenta. Both of these tests can be used to check the fetal karyotype and for DNA testing for single-gene disorders.

Amniocentesis is the easiest and safest procedure, but it cannot be done safely before 15 weeks' gestation because the amniotic membrane has not yet fused with the chorion. Using ultrasound guidance, a needle is inserted through the abdomen into the amniotic sac and 10–20 mL of liquor is aspirated. There is a procedure-related pregnancy loss rate of 0.5–1 per cent, as a result of miscarriage, membrane rupture or intrauterine infection.

CVS may be carried out in a similar fashion to amniocentesis, using a larger needle that is inserted into the placenta, or by inserting a transcervical catheter. The choice of method depends on operator preference and the position of the placenta within the uterus. A posterior placenta or a retroverted uterus may be more amenable to transcervical sampling. The test can be safely carried out from 10 weeks' gestation, but the pregnancy loss rate is around one to two per cent, higher than for amniocentesis.

SUMMARY

Recent advances in genetics and ultrasound have enabled us to consider the fetus as a patient amenable to investigation and treatment. Where fetal problems are identified, parents increasingly wish to discuss the treatment that their baby will require postnatally with paediatric surgeons, who can explain in detail what will be involved and what the outcome might be.

CLINICAL SCENARIOS

Case 1

During a routine mid-pregnancy scan, the fetus was noted to have its stomach within its chest, at the same level as the heart, which was deviated to the right. The mother was referred to the fetal medicine unit, where a diagnosis of left-sided diaphragmatic hernia was confirmed. The remainder of the baby was checked carefully to exclude other anomalies, and the mother was offered invasive testing to exclude chromosome anomalies. This confirmed a normal karyotype, and the mother was counselled that the likelihood of the baby surviving through delivery and neonatal surgery was about 50 per cent. To help her decide whether to continue the pregnancy, she met the paediatric surgical team to discuss in more detail what would be involved in caring for the child postnatally and what continuing morbidity it might face. The mother decided to continue the pregnancy and was scanned twice more to exclude the need to treat polyhydramnios and to check fetal growth and development. During the visits, she was able to see the neonatal intensive care unit and the post-natal surgical ward, enabling her to adapt more easily once the baby was born. Because she lived some distance from the tertiary unit, she was booked for delivery there. Induction of labour was arranged for 39+ weeks, in coordination with the surgical and neonatal units. She delivered the baby spontaneously, who was resuscitated by the attending neonatal team. Once the baby was stable, surgery was undertaken to close the diaphragm.

Case 2

A rhesus-negative mother with high anti-rhesus antibody titres following sensitization in a previous pregnancy was scanned regularly from 18 weeks' gestation. At 22 weeks, Doppler assessment of the middle cerebral artery showed increased peak systolic flow, suggesting that the baby was becoming anaemic. A fetal blood sample was performed from the cord vein where it enters the placenta, confirming that the baby was anaemic, with a haemoglobin of only 6 g/dL. The fetus was transfused with highly concentrated packed red cells, bringing the haemoglobin up to 14 g/dL. Further transfusions were carried out every fortnight until 32 weeks' gestation. The baby was delivered at 35 weeks. The baby had no detectable rhesus-positive blood at delivery and did not require exchange transfusions, but it did need top-up transfusions some weeks later due to persisting anti-rhesus antibodies.

REFERENCES

Bricker L, Garcia J, Henderson J, et al. Ultrasound screening in pregnancy: a systematic review of the clinical effectiveness, cost-effectiveness and women's views. Health Technology Assessment 2000; 4: 1–193.
Royal College of Obstetricians and Gynaecologists. Ultrasound Screening for Fetal Abnormalities. London: Royal College of Obstetricians and Gynaecologists, 2000.

FURTHER READING

Fisk N, Moise K, Jr. Fetal Therapy. Cambridge: Cambridge University Press, 1997.
James D, Steer P, Weiner C, Gonik B. High Risk Pregnancy, 2nd edn. London: WB Saunders, 1999.
Rodeck C, Whittle MJ. Fetal Medicine: Basic Science and Clinical Practice. London: Churchill Livingstone, 1999.
Wald N, Kennard A, Hackshaw A, McGuire A. Antenatal screening for Down's syndrome. Health Technology Assessment 1998; 2: 1–112.

Fetal surgery

CONSTANTINOS HAJIVASSILIOU

Learning objectives

- To understand the principles and techniques of prenatal intervention/fetal surgery.
- To understand the conditions that may be suitable for fetal surgery.
- To be able to discuss the principles on which the choice of patients is based.
- To understand the possible maternal and fetal complications of fetal surgery.
- To be able to offer preliminary counselling for families.

INTRODUCTION

Perhaps the first demonstration that a surgical procedure was possible on the fetus without inevitably precipitating abortion was that of *in utero* ligation of the mesenteric vessels in rabbits by Barnard and Louw approximately 50 years ago. The first published work reporting on the development of animal models of fetal surgery began to appear in the mid-1960s, with the first reports in humans appearing in the following decade. Although fetoscopy and intrauterine invasive procedures (e.g. amniocentesis, cord blood sampling) had been practised by obstetricians for some time, systematic reports on specific animal models and of early human attempts at fetal surgical procedures heralded the marked explosion of the field observed during the past 20 years, with a few centres performing fetal surgery first in the USA but then spreading to more units on both sides of the Atlantic.

In parallel to these developments, there has been a marked improvement in prenatal non-invasive imaging and diagnostic techniques, such as three-dimensional (3D) and, more recently, four-dimensional (4D) ultrasound, fetal echocardiography, including half-Fourier acquisition single-shot turbo spin echo (HASTE), and fast static and real-time magnetic resonance imaging (MRI). These techniques offer more accurate and reliable definition of fetal abnormalities in early pregnancy. This has resulted in further evolution of the criteria for consideration for fetal surgery, which initially was reserved for attempted correction of major anomalies with a devastating postnatal course, e.g. congenital diaphragmatic hernia (CDH), hydrops complicating sacrococcygeal teratoma (SCT) and cystic adenomatoid malformation (CCAM) of the lung.

As more and more conditions are considered suitable for prenatal intervention in this rapidly developing new field, non-lethal conditions are now being considered for fetal surgery, notably closure of spinal dysraphism.

In addition to the major cost implications that fetal surgery involves, it poses very major ethical dilemmas, mainly pertaining to the safety of the mother and the long-term prognosis of a surviving fetus.

RELEVANT BASIC SCIENCE

For the risks and benefits of a fetal surgical procedure to be assessed, it is essential that the natural history of the relevant disease process, especially the results of postnatal intervention, is known accurately and in detail.

Animal models

There can be valid physiological arguments for correcting certain malformations before birth. Animal experimentation and the development of such models in different species, most notably the pregnant ewe model both for open and fetoscopic surgical intervention, have been of great benefit in the development and application of fetal surgical techniques to humans. However, fetal surgery has proven difficult in primates and humans because the gravid uterus is exquisitely sensitive to induction of preterm labour and abortion caused by surgical manipulation. The feasibility of fetal intervention in humans has become a realistic objective following the development and rigorous refinement of both an anaesthetic and tocolytic regime in a primate model, to the point where operative mortality was almost equal to the expected spontaneous perinatal loss.

Fetal physiology: monitoring

The fetus is very sensitive to any physiological aberration, and its homeostasis should be preserved as far as possible during fetal surgery. To achieve this, accurate monitoring of fetal heart rate, temperature, oxygen saturation and electrocardiogram (ECG) and, ideally, access to the circulation are necessary. These have hitherto been difficult; however, both direct and indirect methods of monitoring, including implantable radiotelemetric devices, have been developed, and access to the circulation can be achieved through intraosseous needles. The latter have been shown to provide reliable sampling and pharmacological response to the administration of drugs, e.g. for resuscitation.

It is not known whether the fetus feels pain, but it will mount a significant stress response with hormonal and circulatory changes when painful stimuli are applied from 18–20 weeks. It is not known whether there are long-term neurodevelopmental sequelae. Pain relief for the fetus is provided by the maternal anaesthetic, unless the procedure is performed under sedation or local anaesthetic.

Resuscitation protocols, including chest compressions, drug choices and doses, have been developed following reports of fetal response to resuscitation attempts during fetal surgery.

Maternal considerations: complications

Anaesthesia during pregnancy, hysterotomy and subsequent delivery by caesarean section pose risks to the mother, who would otherwise usually be entirely healthy. Although early studies involving small numbers of patients suggest minimal risks and complications to the mother and her future reproductive potential, there is the possible risk of placenta accreta

in addition to reported cases of mortality and uterine rupture in subsequent pregnancies following hysterotomy for fetal surgery. Other complications include amniotic fluid leakage from the uterine surgical access ports, chorioamnionitis and chorionic membrane separation. Morbidity related to premature labour remains a serious problem, and the ability to control uterine contractions after hysterotomy, and the complications associated with current tocolytic drug regimes, remain the limiting factors in human fetal surgery.

Technical considerations

ANAESTHESIA AND EXPOSURE FOR OPEN FETAL SURGERY

Anaesthesia for fetal surgery involves two patients – the mother and the fetus. Maternal safety, avoidance of fetal asphyxia, adequate fetal anaesthesia and monitoring, and uterine relaxation are paramount. Anaesthetic considerations include the physiological changes of pregnancy, preterm labour, and the consequences of tocolytic drugs, maternal and fetal anaesthesia, and postoperative analgesia. Communication with the surgeon to determine the surgical approach and the need for uterine relaxation allows the anaesthetist to vary the anaesthetic technique, as required.

In summary, anaesthesia is induced with maximal uterine relaxation. A caesarean section is performed and the placenta and fetus are mapped ultrasonographically. The uterus and membranes are opened with a specially designed instrument, which applies haemostatic staples along the incision line, and the relevant part of the anaesthetized fetus is exposed and delivered. Amniotic fluid loss should be kept to a minimum, and all volume lost should be replaced as far as possible, with physiological solution if necessary, at the end of the procedure. Antibiotic solution is usually added to the liquor before closure of the uterine wall. Handling of tissues and operative time should be kept to a minimum.

THE EXIT PROCEDURE

The *ex utero* intrapartum treatment (EXIT) technique was developed to operate on the fetus just before delivery while still on placental support. The technique is necessary in cases where independent existence cannot be maintained after separation from the placenta. This would be necessary to secure the airway of a fetus with disease of the upper airways, e.g. congenital high airway obstruction syndrome (CHAOS) upper airway/cervical neoplasms, or to relieve the iatrogenic tracheal obstruction created by the application of a tracheal occluding device applied as part of the prenatal treatment for CDH (see below).

Once the fetal airway is secured and/or the tracheal occluding device has been removed, surfactant is administered. The fetus is ventilated and, once stable, the cord is divided, the placenta removed and the uterus closed, as described above.

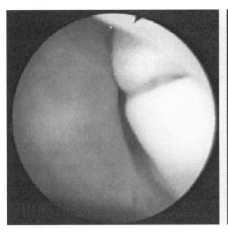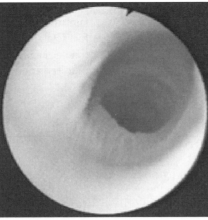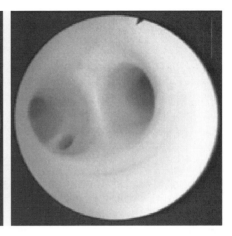

Figure 4.1 *Endoscopic view of fetal mouth, trachea (note anterior tracheal rings) and carina, with bronchial orifice in the fetal lung (130 days' gestation). See also Colour Plate 1.*

MINIMALLY INVASIVE FETOSCOPIC SURGICAL PROCEDURES

Fetoscopy is strengthening its position in fetal medicine and surgery. In addition to obstetrical fetoscopy and intervention, endoscopic fetal surgery techniques are being developed (Figure 4.1). The most common obstetrical fetoscopy procedures include surgical interventions on the placenta, umbilical cord and fetal membranes, coagulation of placental vessels and occlusion of the cord in the case of feto-fetal transfusion syndrome. Endoscopic fetal surgery techniques have been developed to minimize trauma to the uterus and fetus, thus reducing postoperative complications, notably premature labour and fetal loss. Fetal endoscopic surgery over the past decade has evolved towards shorter operating times, the use of smaller and fewer ports, minimizing the volume of amniotic fluid exchange and decreased blood loss. Most experience has been achieved in cases of twin-to-twin transfusion syndrome and CDH. However, complications still occur; they include premature rupture of membranes and premature labour, amniotic fluid leakage, chorioamniotic membrane separation, chorioamnionitis and fetal loss.

DISEASES AMENABLE TO FETAL SURGERY

All fetuses that may be candidates for prenatal intervention should be assessed thoroughly by diagnostic imaging as appropriate (ultrasound, ECHO, MRI). Karyotyping and other invasive diagnostic tests should be considered.

Bladder outlet/lower urinary tract obstruction

Obstructive uropathy (Chapter 55) leads to renal damage, oligohydramnios and lung hypoplasia, which may be fatal. Significant urethral obstruction accounts for approximately ten per cent of all patients who have a prenatal diagnosis of a urologic abnormality. In some of these patients, the process may be progressive; in others, lethal anomalies may coexist. Overall, approximately one per cent of fetuses diagnosed prenatally with urological problems will be suitable for prenatal intervention of the urinary tract (mainly some form of vesicoamniotic shunting).

Experimental models of obstructive uropathy suggest that relief of obstruction *in utero* prevents some of the dysplastic changes caused by obstruction. The development of prognostic criteria has aided in selection of appropriate fetuses for intervention. Favourable criteria include the composition of aspirated amniotic fluid (Na < 100 mEq/L, Cl < 90 mEq/L, osmolality < 210 mosmol) and amniotic fluid status, ultrasonographic appearance of the fetal kidneys and urine output on fetal bladder catheterization.

Following the first performance of the relief of bladder outflow obstruction in 1981, the selection criteria for prenatal intervention in cases of lower urinary obstruction have become much more stringent. This is because it has been shown that by the time the diagnosis was established or the procedure became technically possible, there was no improvement in the postnatal prognosis of the patient.

Thus, currently, in the absence of other lethal anomalies and if the diagnosis is made before lung maturity *in utero*, then a fetus with good prognostic criteria and normal renal appearance on scanning would be a candidate for a vesicoamniotic shunting procedure.

Cardiac surgery

Experience with, and results of, fetal cardiac surgical procedures are restricted to case reports and short series of patients. Despite marked improvements in fetal echocardiography, fetal cardiac surgery (both open and endoscopic) is still in its early stages of development.

Cleft lip and palate

There have been recent reports of successful cleft repair in animal models, utilizing the advantage of scarless healing of fetal tissues, resulting in macroscopically and microscopically normal architecture with potentially normal function. Cautious optimism is, therefore, being expressed, taking into consideration the risk–benefit analysis of fetal surgery for non-fatal conditions.

Congenital cystic adenomatoid malformation

Congenital cystic adenomatoid malformation (CCAM, Chapter 31) has a variable prognosis, depending on the size and histological type of the lesion. If it persists after birth, then it is excised in the early neonatal period. In severe cases complicated by hydrops, *in utero* death is almost inevitable.

Early reports of anecdotal success following fetal surgery despite high mortality have been strengthened by more recent data confirming the promise of successful outcome (60 per cent survival) of otherwise fatal space-occupying intrathoracic lesions treated by fetal surgery.

Congenital diaphragmatic hernia

The lung hypoplasia, which is probably both a primary and a secondary phenomenon of intrathoracic abdominal visceral herniation, and the associated pulmonary hypertension continue to evade attempts by postnatal intervention to reduce their frequently catastrophic consequences on neonatal survival. Bad prognostic criteria include polyhydramnios, associated anomalies, early diagnosis, high cephalothoracic ratio and a large volume of intrathoracic herniated viscera (including liver).

Like so many other 'firsts' in fetal surgery, successful open fetal surgery for correction of CDH (Chapter 30) took place at the University of California, San Francisco, USA. Closure of the diaphragmatic defect with a synthetic patch and also temporary cover of non-reducible abdominal viscera by a patch have been tried. These procedures are marred by the complications of open fetal surgery, in addition to the disastrous effects of manipulation of the liver out of the defect leading to occlusion of caval venous flow.

Although open fetal surgery for CDH showed relative promise, further developments are aimed at the early reversal of lung hypoplasia *in utero*. This entails occluding the trachea to block the egress of fluid secreted by the fetal lung. This in turn results in enlargement of the lungs and, to a variable degree, reduction of the herniated viscera back into the abdominal cavity. The fetus is delivered with the occluding device *in situ* and, while still on placental support, the device is removed and the airway re-established (EXIT procedure). Unfortunately, maintained tracheal occlusion results in severe reduction in the numbers of type II pneumocytes, with consequent depletion of surfactant and poor lung mechanics. This procedure is now possible using an intratracheal balloon placed percutaneously with the help of ultrasonography and fetal tracheobronchoscopy (Figure 4.2). These new modalities, including attempts to occlude the trachea for varying intervals and periodicity (Figure 4.3), are the subjects of randomized controlled trials.

Sacrococcygeal teratoma

Sacrococcygeal teratomas (Chapter 41) are generally managed by planned delivery and surgery in the early neonatal period. However, large tumours early in gestation may result in hydrops and fetal death, probably due to high-output cardiac failure in the fetus as a result of arteriovenous shunting through the tumour. Excision of the teratoma has been shown to be possible and presents another indication for fetal surgery, which may improve fetal survival. As these tumours can produce a pre-eclampsia-like syndrome, they pose a danger to both mother and fetus, which would make prenatal intervention during early pregnancy easier to justify. Percutaneous radiofrequency ablation is another treatment modality being investigated. Although promising, this still remains rather unrefined and is not easy to target.

Spinal dysraphism

Myelomeningocele (Chapter 40) is the most common congenital malformation of the central nervous system noted on prenatal ultrasound. The initial intent of *in utero* correction was to preserve distal neurological function by covering the exposed spinal cord. The ethical dilemmas of fetal surgery are disputed nowhere more fiercely than for the treatment of spina bifida and myelomeningocele. Spina bifida, although usually non-fatal, can have devastating functional and psychosocial consequences for the patient. Due to its significant postnatal sequelae, treatment *in utero* potentially could have a profound impact on the newborn: improved somatosensory evoked potentials with potential for preserved neurological function have been reported, although there has been little effect on sensorimotor function. The challenge is to define those patients that might benefit from such radical procedures before applying these techniques.

The criteria for consideration for *in utero* repair of myelomeningocoele at the University of California, San Francisco, included a normal karyotype; no other significant congenital anomalies or lumbar or lumbosacral defects; and gestational age/completion of repair by 24 weeks or less.

Prenatal repair was noted to result in an apparent reduction in hindbrain herniation and a possible decreased need for ventriculoperitoneal (VP) shunting. However, longer-term studies showed a steady increase in the need for a VP shunt, and after one year the prevalence of a shunt was similar between patients treated *in utero* and those treated in the neonatal period. Furthermore, no significant improvements in urodynamic parameters or anatomical anomalies of the urinary tract were observed after *in utero* repair of myelomeningocoele.

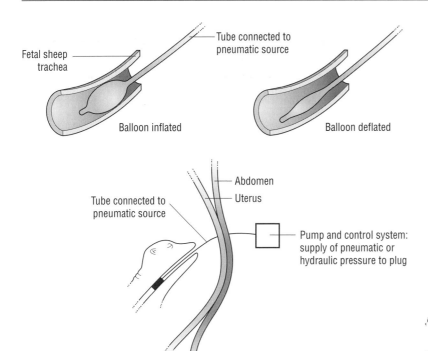

Figure 4.2 *Method of periodic tracheal occlusion in congenital diaphragmatic hernia (CDH).*

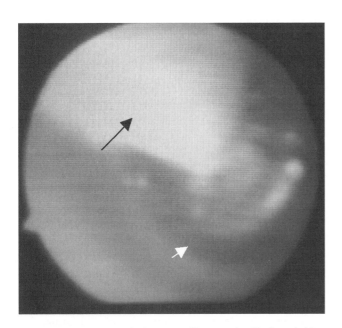

Figure 4.3 *Fetoscopic deployment of intratracheal balloon (white arrowhead) through flexible 3-mm fibre-optic endoscope. Hollow shaft of balloon catheter, black arrow.*

A randomized controlled trial is currently in progress in the USA, sponsored by the National Institutes of Health (NIH), to evaluate long-term outcome variables in patients with myelomeningocele treated *in utero* and to compare these with carefully selected matching controls treated by conventional methods. Fetal interventions will have to achieve significant measurable improvements in the control of hydrocephalus, mobility and continence over postnatal treatment to be justified.

Twin-to-twin transfusion

In this condition affecting monochorionic twins, one of the fetuses 'steals' blood flow from the other through abnormal placental vascular channels. In the vast majority of cases, eventually both twins die. Treatment options include fetoscopic laser ablation of the abnormal placental vessels and amnioreduction. The results of international randomized controlled trials are awaited.

Ventriculomegaly

The natural history of fetal ventriculomegaly is variable. Prognosis is poor if other anomalies coexist, is variable in progressive isolated ventriculomegaly, and is good in non-progressive isolated ventriculomegaly. Although intrauterine treatment of fetal cerebral ventriculomegaly has been largely abandoned, the above prognosis suggests that fetal surgery may have a role to play in carefully selected patients. However, there is no documented clear advantage of prenatal intervention compared with the currently available neonatal treatment options.

ETHICAL CONSIDERATIONS

Are the mother and fetus being used as experimental subjects? Is fetal surgery unnecessary, or is it simply the next logical step in the evolution of medical science?

Ethical issues in prenatal surgical intervention require special consideration because of the often conflicting interests of the mother and fetus, the mother being considered as an 'innocent bystander' exposed to a risk that does not clearly result in maternal benefit. Much time, effort and resources have been expended in the area of fetal surgery, and a lot of unwelcome media publicity has occurred in an area currently encompassing only a small number of patients. Physicians faced with the knowledge of the presence of a potentially treatable condition in a given fetus may feel the necessity of instituting treatment; however, the fact that treatment is possible cannot be taken as proof of its benefit. Over the past 20 years, an ethical framework for fetal surgery and fetal intervention has been developed, which continues to evolve as new procedures are developed, inevitably giving rise to new controversies.

The dilemmas and justifications are easier to resolve in cases where a catastrophic outcome is expected or where the fetal condition is known to be associated with maternal morbidity, e.g. pre-eclampsia syndrome with sacrococcygeal teratoma. Surgery for non-lethal fetal anomalies, e.g. repair of fetal myelomeningocele, represents the most difficult ethical challenge. Such procedures should be supported by the results of, and experience gained from, animal studies and require early evaluation by strict, carefully designed and controlled randomized clinical trials from which the benefit, if any, of the procedure to the fetal disease, and the effects on the mother, are evaluated to avoid premature dissemination of unproven therapies.

Before any risks, however small, are taken, all available information should be weighed carefully and discussed fully with the mother. Despite informed consent being obtainable, these procedures should be performed within an internationally agreed ethical framework.

Innovation in maternal-fetal surgery should be conducted and evaluated as research, and women must be considered research subjects in these trials. Centres of excellence should be established for conducting research and providing this highly specialized service, and efforts should be made to set at the earliest point proper controlled scientific studies. To this end, participation in the International Fetal Surgery Registry is encouraged. Such clinical studies should be conducted in concert with studies in appropriate animal models. The informed-consent process must ensure adequate comprehension and genuine willingness in those considering participation. Discriminatory and fearful attitudes towards individuals with disabilities should be addressed explicitly but objectively before making a decision to proceed with *in utero* intervention in an attempt to correct such disabilities. Furthermore, fetal surgery should not be performed for cosmetic indications unless, and until, there is reliable evidence that maternal-fetal surgery can be performed safely and long-term side effects on women and their offspring are minimal. Finally, funding of these studies and procedures should be considered in the context of the needs of society.

THE FUTURE

With the advent of minimally invasive access, monitoring and intervention techniques, there is little doubt that the future of fetal intervention relies on not open but fetoscopically performed procedures. Such minimally invasive techniques are associated with less stress for both the fetus and the mother and result in less likelihood of premature pregnancy loss. A clear demonstration of feasibility and safety of these procedures offering good prognosis would increase the choices available to treat affected fetuses. These are being combined with pharmacological means to improve lung maturation, e.g. administration of maternal steroids, to combat the effects of prematurity and lung immaturity.

The development of more effective and safer tocolytic regimes will undoubtedly reduce maternal morbidity and enhance the acceptance of these techniques. Fetoprotective drugs that could modify the fetus's metabolic response to stress are also being considered.

Finally, advances in stem-cell transplantation, gene therapy and tissue engineering may further augment the therapeutic armamentarium available to the physicians and surgeons looking after their yet unborn patients.

FURTHER READING

Fowler SF, Sydorak RM, Albanese CT, *et al*. Fetal endoscopic surgery: lessons learned and trends reviewed. *Journal of Pediatric Surgery* 2002; **37**: 1700–702.

Harrison MR, Albanese CT, Hawgood SB, *et al*. Fetoscopic temporary tracheal occlusion by means of detachable balloon for congenital diaphragmatic hernia. *American Journal of Obstetrics and Gynecology* 2001; **185**: 730–33.

Holmes N, Harrison MR, Baskin LS. Fetal surgery for posterior urethral valves: long-term postnatal outcomes. *Pediatrics* 2001; **108**: E7.

Myers LB, Cohen D, Galinkin J, Gaiser R, Kurth CD. Anaesthesia for fetal surgery. *Paediatric Anaesthesia* 2002; **12**: 569–78.

Sutton LN, Sun P, Adzick NS. Fetal neurosurgery. *Neurosurgery* 2001; **48**: 124–42.

The child in hospital

J MICHAEL S JOHNSTONE

Learning objectives

- To be aware of current recommendations regarding the provision of facilities for children in hospital.
- To be aware of the potential adverse effects of hospital admission on children and the ways in which these may be minimized.

INTRODUCTION

Conditions under which children are cared for in hospital the UK still vary. Although we strive for excellence for all children, first-class care remains elusive. The goal, of course, changes constantly as medicine advances, the patterns of illness alter and the expectations of the public are heightened. Nevertheless, in many parts of the country, children are now cared for in purpose-built and well-staffed departments. This has not always been so: during the twentieth century, much of the care of children fell below the acceptable level. Improvement was curiously slow until recent years. The improvement reflects a national determination to lift children's services, led by healthcarers but in response to the demands and expectations of today's parents.

The five areas listed below have been used as a framework for this chapter:

- historical aspects
- child-focused management
- facilities for children
- hospital admission
- special groups.

HISTORICAL ASPECTS

Recent improvement in the care of children in hospital was built on a solid foundation, notably the Platt Report (Platt Committee 1959), the formation of the National Association for the Welfare of Children in Hospital (NAWCH), the Court Report (Court Committee 1976), the United Nations (UN) Convention on the Rights of the Child, and the publication of *The Welfare of Children and Young People in Hospital* (Department of Health 1991) and *Children First* (Audit Commission 1993).

Platt Report

The Platt Report was remarkable and seminal to all that has followed. It was implicit that in the new National Health Service (NHS), patients received hospital care by right rather than patronage. Within this new structure, Platt focused attention on the emotional needs of the child. The hospital environment was to be open and friendly, and ward routine was to reflect the customary routine of the child. The pain of separation from the parent was recognized, and free visiting was recommended.

Details in the report referred to ward design, hospital staffing, and admission and discharge protocols.

National Association for the Welfare of Children in Hospital

Four mothers started NAWCH in 1963. They represented a wide group of parents who were concerned about the slow implementation of the Platt Report. Hospitals were lobbied and improvements demanded. In the mid-1980s, NAWCH broadened its focus to children in the community and changed its title to Action for Sick Children. Their Charter for Children, 1990, was endorsed by the Department of Health and the UK medical colleges and set standards for the care of children in hospital.

Court Report

The Court Report 1976 was a further outstanding contribution. This report examined the broader issues of childcare, embracing health services, social services and education. The report called for the integration of child health services, a child- and family-centred service with skilled help available and accessible, and a service that respects the child as a whole and as a continuously developing person. Although widely acclaimed, the report had surprisingly little impact and remains unfulfilled to this day.

Convention on the Rights of the Child

This convention enshrined the right of children to be cared for in a child-centred service. The convention had its origins in the words of Eglentyne Jebb, founder of Save the Children in 1925: 'I believe that we should claim certain rights for children and labour for their universal recognition.' The words were adopted in turn by the League of Nations in a Declaration of Rights of the Child (1926), the UN in 1959, and the UN convention in 1989. The principles of the convention are that it applies to all children without discrimination, that the best interests of the child are the prime consideration, and that the child's views must be taken into account. Articles of the convention are directed towards civil and political rights, the provision of nutrition, healthcare and education, and protection from exploitation at work and from physical, sexual and psychological abuse.

Welfare of Children and Young People in Hospital and *Children First*

The Welfare of Children and Young People in Hospital was published by the Department of Health (1991) to bring together the many and diverse documents on the care of children in circulation at that time. The document offered guidelines to NHS health authorities and trusts in their roles as providers and purchasers, respectively. *Children First* was, in effect, a consumer response by the Audit Commission to the Department of Health's guidelines. In *Children First*, a number of criticisms were listed, starting with the observation that previous recommendations such as the Platt Report had not been implemented. Further criticisms were the lack of attention to the special needs of children and their families, a shortfall in medical and nursing skills, and a lack of critical appraisal of treatment and hospital admission.

CHILD-FOCUSED MANAGEMENT

The NHS Plan 2000

Over the past ten years, there have been two major reforms in the NHS. The original structure was managed in a pyramidal system of management, matched by a cogwheel advisory structure based on consent. In 1994, under the reform Patients First, the internal market was introduced, with health authorities being the purchasers, and community and hospital trusts the providers, of healthcare. In 2000, the NHS Plan introduced a second far-reaching change. The purpose was to ensure high national standards and clear accountability, to devolve power to healthcare professionals and patients at the front line, and to break down outmoded professional barriers.

Central and local structures

Within the new structure, the Department of Health oversees development of healthcare through the National Strategic Framework. Two independent bodies – the Commission for Health Improvement and the National Institute for Clinical Excellence (NICE) – are responsible for inspection and setting standards, respectively. At an intermediate level, strategic health authorities, which have replaced area health authorities, provide strategic leadership and ensure delivery of health improvements.

At the local level, primary care trusts (PCTs) are the cornerstone of the NHS. They are responsible for improving health, for providing services to their community, and for forging partnerships with other PCTs and NHS trusts. It is a measure of their importance that they are funded directly from government. PCTs purchase hospital care through NHS hospital trusts. The primary role of the hospital trusts is to deliver service agreements, but they also have a role in teaching, research and development.

Implications for children

The NHS Plan has important implications for the care of children in hospital. Changes put forward were accelerated by a series of adverse reports on children's services, in particular the Kennedy (2001) Report. The post of National Clinical

Director for Children has been appointed. A Children's National Service Framework has been drawn up and is comparable to other priority areas in the NHS. There is to be a senior member of staff with responsibilities for children in each strategic health authority, PCT and NHS hospital trust. There is to be a greater integration of primary, community, acute hospital and specialist care across professional and agency boundaries, including social services.

Within an NHS hospital trust, children's services should form an independent directorate or, if too small, part of a joint directorate. Although answerable to the trust, the directorate has considerable independence, with its own budget and responsibilities for delivering care, staffing, performance, planning, training and governance. Guidelines on care are listed in *The Welfare of Children and Young People in Hospital* and enhanced by the Children's National Service Framework. There is an obligation to work within this framework.

A group of PCTs may purchase care from a single hospital. The commissioning may then need to be rationalized. One model is for a single PCT to take overall responsibility and to set up a children's board to bring together other interested parties. Likewise, children may be cared for in more than one hospital, and a single directorate in the main hospital may be given overall care. The provision of specialist services, which is particularly relevant to paediatric surgery, may depend on a critical population size. PCTs from different health authorities will then group together so as to match the population and agree on a single site for the service.

FACILITIES FOR CHILDREN

Children's hospital/unit

As noted above, the pattern and distribution of children's services in Britain remains uneven. A children's hospital may stand independently, or a children's unit may stand within a teaching or district general hospital. Less often, children are admitted to specialist hospitals. Where possible, children's facilities within a hospital should be brought together in a single and separate unit. If this is impractical in physical terms, then services should be managed as a single unit to ensure that a child ethos prevails.

Levels of service

The level of surgical service offered in a particular hospital remains the centre of vigorous debate. The very real convenience and advantages of a local service to a child and his or her family must be balanced against the ability to provide such a service safely. The pivot of the argument must be to provide the highest standard of care for the child. In widely different circumstances, the responsibility of the surgeon is to work within his or her level of competence, taking into account the strength of the unit. In *Looking Ahead* (Royal

College of Paediatrics and Child Health 2001), it is envisaged that in the future there will be a division of care between secondary and tertiary services rather than between a hospital and the community, the integration between hospital and community being such that separation becomes increasingly meaningless.

Secondary and tertiary surgical care

In practical terms, secondary-level care is based in a district hospital and provides for older children with straightforward problems. There needs to be a minimum population base of 200 000, a surgeon and anaesthetist trained and practised in the care of children, a children's ward with appropriately trained medical and nursing staff, and suitable imaging and pathology services.

Tertiary care is based on a regional centre or teaching hospital. Basic facilities as described above need to be supported by a range of specialist staff, a neonatal unit, an accident and emergency (A&E) department, a paediatric intensive care unit and a genetic unit. It is accepted widely that neonates and very young children, children with cancer, children with complex gastrointestinal and urological problems, and children needing intensive care should be admitted to such centres.

Hospital facilities

In hospital, a child may pass through a wide range of units, such as the A&E department, admission assessment, day care, inpatient wards, outpatient department, operating theatre and recovery area, intensive care, X-ray, radiotherapy, physiotherapy, play area and school. Ideally, each unit should have an area dedicated to the care of children and carry appropriately trained staff. In practice, the extent to which this is achieved depends on the size of the hospital, local policy, management focus, initiative, determination and sheer practicality.

OUTPATIENT DEPARTMENT

Paediatric outpatient departments should include a play area, a minor procedure room, privacy for breastfeeding, suitable furnishing, and ease of access for disabled people. The need for separation from adult patients seems obvious, but even today this is not always realized. There may be practical reasons for this, such as the need for specialist equipment or a consultant who sees children only occasionally.

ACCIDENT AND EMERGENCY DEPARTMENT

A quarter of patients attending A&E departments in the UK are children. They present with a range of problems, from minor febrile illness to major injury. Many children, particularly in inner cities, bypass normal primary care. In some hospitals, this practice is actively encouraged, and the departments are designed and staffed accordingly.

In major centres there will be departments dedicated to children, but in district hospitals this is not always feasible. In any department, however, it should be possible to reserve an area for children with prompt triage, a waiting and play space, and an examination room. Staff members in smaller departments often lack paediatric experience and expertise. As a result, there is a danger that children with serious medical problems, children at risk, and children with psychosocial problems may go unrecognized. There must be a well-rehearsed policy to deal with these difficult situations and ready access to supporting paediatric staff.

The report *Accident and Emergency Services for Children* (Royal College of Paediatrics and Child Health 1999) recommends that only hospitals with inpatient paediatric facilities should accept children, apart from those with minor injuries not requiring hospital admission. An exception is in geographically isolated trusts for which special arrangements must be made. The report also recommends that care is given within a child- and family-focused environment, separate from adults, with appropriately trained staff working in tandem with the children's unit, and there should be close liaison with the primary healthcare team.

In smaller hospitals, it is inevitable that there will be problems in offering emergency care. To counter these difficulties, the concept of a minor injury/illness service has been proposed for children with minor medical problems or injuries who need ready access to local services. Again, such a service must be child-sensitive in facilities and staffing. Minor problems envisaged are mild pyrexia, minor respiratory or gastrointestinal disorders, and superficial soft-tissue injuries.

DAY CARE

Day surgery for children is accepted practice, vigorously promoted and increasingly available. Surgical day care was introduced into clinical practice in Glasgow nearly 100 years ago, ironically in part to protect adults from 'nuisance'. The practice was promoted in the 1970s and finally came of age with the publication by Thorne (1991) of *Just for a Day*. Indications and protocols are well documented in numerous publications. The advantages of day care are seen as benefiting the child and family and cost-effectiveness. In fact, there is only marginal evidence to substantiate these claims. Other studies have found little difference in the psychological consequences of children treated on a day basis and those admitted overnight.

Quality day care demands high standards of medical and nursing skill and efficient organization. Inevitably, smaller units will care for both adults and children, but it should be possible to allocate children separate sessions and to make appropriate ward and staff adjustments. The structure of the unit should allow for children waiting for surgery to be separated from those recovering and to allow parents to remain with their children throughout. Anaesthesia and surgery should not be delegated to junior staff. Quick recovery is the key to good care and is best ensured by accurate surgery and effective pain control.

HOSPITAL ADMISSION

The child

It cannot be stressed too often that there are fundamental differences between the care of children and adults. Childhood is a period of growth and development, both physically and emotionally. During that period, the child is an integral and dependent member of a family structure. The differences must be respected. Just as physical illness can interrupt growth with long-term consequence, so too can emotional injury sustained either directly as a result of physical illness or indirectly as the consequence of management. The holistic approach to the child embraces the nature of the illness, the physical and emotional response of the child to illness, the place of the child within the family, and the consequence of the illness to both child and family.

Emotional stress

Hospital attendance is stressful for the child and the pattern of emotional disturbance is well described. Babies and toddlers aged between six months and three years are particularly vulnerable. Admission is complicated by the interplay of emotion between child and parent and anxious parents will transmit their fears. Children from disturbed homes may react more adversely. Emotional disturbance continues after the child returns home: there may be a pattern of eating problems, sleep disturbance, enuresis and regression of achievement levels. Surgical procedures are especially disturbing because of fears of death, concerns of pain and disfigurement, and loss of control of self. High levels of anger, aggression and withdrawal have been noted after hypospadias repair compared with appendicectomy.

There is good evidence that the stress of hospital admission can be reduced by skilled care. Constant explanation, support and reassurance are needed. The ward routine and environment should mirror, where possible, the pattern of life at home. A supportive relationship between parent and nurse will reduce both maternal anxiety and stress levels in children. Likewise, admission protocol, hospital design and ward ambience have all been shown to influence stress levels.

Is admission necessary?

Children should be admitted to hospital only if the care they require cannot be as well provided at home, in a day clinic or on a day basis in hospital (Platt Committee 1959). A close understanding and working relationship between the hospital and the community reduces the need for admission. While the term 'ambulatory paediatrician' may seem clichéd, it serves to focus attention on the principle of integration across boundaries of care.

Assessment unit

In acute paediatrics, many children are referred for admission with apparent serious illness. In some children, the problem may resolve in a matter of hours after a period of observation, prompt and simple investigation, and experienced medical attention. An A&E department may be too hectic for measured assessment, and the ward routine lacks flexibility. An assessment unit offers a middle road and has been used successfully in different centres. For example, in one hospital, midnight occupancy on the children's surgical ward fell by a quarter after such a unit was opened.

Admission protocol

The moment of admission is an anxious time for the child and parent. For children with elective problems, pre-admission visits to the ward can help to familiarize the family with details such as the hospital layout, the ward routine and the personal belongings that should be brought with the child. At the time of admission, a key nurse should meet the family in a play area or at the bedside. The child's home routine can be discussed in relation to the ward routine, and the child's particular likes and dislikes can be recognized. Familiar toys and photographs should be placed at the bedside. Ideally, the same nurse should provide continuity over the period of the child's stay.

By contrast, the emergency admission is less easy to manage. The child's resilience is reduced by apprehension, feeling unwell and, possibly, pain. The parents may be distressed and anxious. For the acutely ill child, prompt attention of both nurse and doctor will reassure the parent that a diagnosis is being sought and treatment started.

Ward policy

Best ward practice is structured carefully. A statement of policy, although apparently at first sight obvious, serves to reinforce the different elements of the structure. Such a policy can be illustrated and displayed for staff and parents. The policy might recognize the child as an individual with a right to express his or her own ideas and feelings. Furthermore, the child is part of a family with its own culture and individual needs, and it is recognized that hospital threatens this routine. In response to those needs, the ward offers pre-admission visiting, play specialists, qualified children's nurses, key nursing, a school, open visiting, a family routine and privacy.

Operation

A child, just like an adult patient, may approach surgery with equanimity or morbid fear; much depends on the individual and family background. The young child has no understanding of an operation and surgery is a sequence of events that are unfamiliar, alarming and possibly painful. By contrast, the older child may understand the nature of illness and the rationale of treatment, the extent of understanding depending on the child's age.

A child may have particular concerns about loss of consciousness, body image and loss of control. Fear of surgery can be aggravated by an earlier experience, unhelpful comments of friends, and watching television. Much can be done to allay these anxieties, and both the play specialist and the paediatric nurse have an important role. Regardless of whether the surgery is elective or emergency, time must be found to explain the procedure in simple and reassuring words to both the child and parent, to discuss how the child will feel after the operation, and to explain the care that will be needed postoperatively, e.g. dressings, splints, drips, catheters, drains and pain control.

Play and education

The role of play therapists in hospital is now recognized widely. Play is part of childhood and contributes to the intellectual, social and emotional growth of the child. Structured play not only creates a more normal situation for the child but also can be used for education and clinical assessment. Acting out an invasive procedure such as catheterization or blood transfusion on a model is a valuable way to prepare the child for such a procedure.

School, as with play, is also part of childhood. Hospital schooling not only gives continuity to learning but also provides stimulation and makes the hospital experience more normal. The Education Act 1944 empowers the local authority to provide appropriate education for all children of statutory age. Hospitals are obliged to provide school accommodation, although the local education authority meets the running costs. Many hospital schools have developed their roles to meet the particular education needs of children with disability and to provide an outreach service to a child's home. Under the Education Act 1981, children with special education needs may require statutory assessment. Among these are children with learning difficulties, children from disadvantaged social conditions, and children with medical conditions or treatment protocols that are likely to affect their learning. In the care of such children, there needs to be liaison with the education authority and social services.

SPECIAL GROUPS

Adolescents

Adolescents are a difficult group to define. Nevertheless, it is commonly accepted that the needs of adolescents are different from those of children and adults. Within adolescence, there may be a broad range of needs. For example, compare the needs of an immature 12-year-old boy with appendicitis with those of a 15-year-old girl with an ectopic pregnancy.

The age of this group should be interpreted flexibly but, in general, should include those in secondary education. There is general agreement that there is no need for exclusive specialization in adolescent medicine, but, where possible, adolescents should be brought together as inpatients, irrespective of specialty.

Although adolescents may be physically mature, their emotional needs are more akin to those of children. They should be nursed close to the children's unit or in a subunit of a children's ward. Schooling is important and they need their own recreation area. Although apparently confident, adolescents are often uncertain and insecure and in need of reassurance and the company of their own peer group. In particular, there may be concerns about body image and sexuality. Staff should be chosen with care, and it should be remembered that staff might be close in age to their patients, so they may identify with and feel threatened by their patients' problems.

People caring for adolescents must be mindful of difficult and sensitive areas. Emotional disturbance can present with anorexia. Complications of pregnancy and genitourinary infection may present with acute abdomen. The transfer of care of adolescents with chronic physical and mental disabilities to adult services needs to be integrated. Many will be seeking independence from home and carers, often within a supported framework. The transition can be eased through a young disabled unit.

Care and protection

People caring for children have a duty to recognize abuse and to make appropriate referral. The key is vigilance. There must be an explanation for trauma that is plausible and is recorded in the medical notes. Social services is the lead agency responsible for the protection of children at risk. However, all other agencies have responsibilities, including police, education, community health workers, healthcarers and voluntary services. The area child protection committee is a statutory body responsible to the local authority and should ensure openness and cooperation between the different agencies.

During the investigation of abuse, it is a fundamental premise that the child's interests are paramount. Moreover, there should be no delay, and the child's parents should be involved at all stages. The medical role relates to prevention, raising awareness, investigation of related medical problems, ongoing care, treatment and attendance at the child protection conference. Interagency cooperation is again emphasized. On the thorny question of confidentiality, the overriding principle is to protect the children, because their age and vulnerability mean that they cannot protect themselves.

At a practical level, each hospital must have a policy on how to handle suspected child abuse. Where there is serious concern, the problem must be referred to a senior paediatrician. Social services must be involved if there are suspicions of abuse. A register of children at risk should be available, either through the hospital A&E department or through social services.

Ethnic minorities

Care of children and family should take into account religious persuasion, racial origin and cultural and linguistic background (Children's Act 1989). A hospital is obliged to meet the needs of all the local population. In order to fulfil this obligation, the needs of minority groups have to be actively identified and met. To provide a sensitive service for minority groups, it has been argued that the cultural mix of the population should be reflected in the hospital staff.

Among minority groups, a number of difficulties are recognized. Within the service, there are particularly sensitive areas, such as communication, staff attitudes, and religious and cultural beliefs. Language is a problem, and the need for an interpreting service is self-evident. Stereotyping must be avoided. Religious beliefs and observances, particularly regarding the care of children after death, need to be appreciated and respected.

At a more practical level, there may be problems with diet, simple hygiene and identification. A range of food should be available for dietary needs and, where needed, brought to the hospital by the family. For most children, hygiene means the traditional soap-and-water scrub, but for others, the time and order of washing follows religious custom. Naming systems may be confusing, e.g. a child may have added names to indicate gender, generation and status. Finally, of course, disease patterns vary: an acute abdomen may be caused by sickle cell disease and an abdominal mass by tuberculosis.

Refugees and asylum-seekers

Refugee children comprise a vulnerable group. Curiously and confusingly, a refugee child or minor, as defined by the Home Office, is a person under the age of 18 years. Such children are entitled to NHS care. The guidelines highlight a number of important issues. Neonatal screening and primary immunization may be incomplete. Refugee children may suffer from emotional distress and malnutrition. Age may be uncertain, and therefore development charts need to be interpreted with caution. Depending on the country of origin, there may be risk of human immunodeficiency virus (HIV)/acquired immune deficiency syndrome (AIDS), and tropical and infectious diseases, including tuberculosis, hepatitis B and C, malaria and schistosomiasis. Interpreters should be available for language problems. The child and family are entitled to confidentiality.

REFERENCES

Audit Commission. *Children First: A Study of Hospital Services*. London: HMSO, 1993.
Court Committee on Child Health Services. *Fit for the Future*. London: HMSO, 1976.

Department of Health. *Welfare of Children and Young People in Hospital.* London: HMSO, 1991.

Kennedy I. *Learning from Bristol.* London: The Stationery Office, 2001.

Platt Committee, Ministry of Health. *The Welfare of Children in Hospital.* London: HMSO, 1959.

Royal College of Paediatrics and Child Health. *Accident and Emergency Services for Children.* London: RCPCH, 1999.

Royal College of Paediatrics and Child Health. *Looking Ahead: Paediatric and Child Health – the Next Ten Years.* London: RCPCH, 2001.

Thorne R. *Just for the Day: Caring for Children in the Health Services.* London: NAWCH, 1991.

Imaging

MARK GRIFFITHS

Learning objectives

- To understand the imaging techniques available and the differences between them.
- To understand the appropriate use of imaging.
- To understand the appropriate imaging modalities for specific clinical situations and why a specific imaging modality is chosen.

INTRODUCTION

The ability to image disease processes and their complications plays a central role in the management of surgical patients. The confirmation of clinical suspicion or proposition of alternative diagnoses enables appropriate surgical planning, including the avoidance of inappropriate intervention. The choice of imaging technique, however, needs to be tailored to answer the clinical question posed and should be the least traumatic to the patient undergoing investigation.

Each imaging technique has its strengths and weaknesses. The technique used will determine the information available from the examination and hence what conclusions can be drawn. Thus, it is important to understand the techniques involved in image production and the potential for misinterpretation of positive and negative findings.

Different imaging techniques also require differing levels of patient cooperation and preparation. A clinical decision to employ a less specific technique may be appropriate in light of a patient's ability to cooperate with an examination or the requirement for sedation or anaesthesia.

Imaging of renal abnormalities is discussed in Chapter 49.

IMAGING TECHNIQUES

Plain films

Plain radiography is often the first imaging undertaken to aid in the diagnosis of a sick child. A chest radiograph may reveal consolidation in a lower lobe as a cause of abdominal pain or the presence of pleural effusion complicating pneumonia. In the abdomen, free gas or intestinal obstruction may be demonstrated, as may diagnostic features, such as intramural and portal gas in necrotizing enterocolitis (Figure 6.1). Plain films, however, are two-dimensional representations of three-dimensional structures, with only limited soft-tissue discrimination, and their limitations should be recognized. A normal abdominal radiograph would not exclude intussusception or malrotation but could exclude obstruction or toxic dilation in the presence of active ulcerative colitis (Figure 6.2).

Plain films are the initial imaging of choice in trauma, with a standard series of chest, pelvic and cervical spine images being acquired in the presence of major trauma.

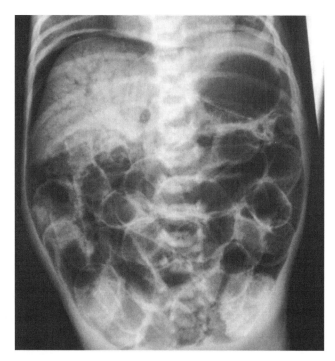

Figure 6.1   *Abdominal radiograph of premature neonate, demonstrating free intraperitoneal air beneath the hemi-diaphragms. The free air and intraluminal air outline both sides of the bowel wall (Rigler's sign), and gas is seen within the portal veins within the liver. There is gas within the bowel wall, indicating necrotizing enterocolitis, which has been complicated by perforation.*

Contrast screening

Fluoroscopy – continuous screening with image display on a display monitor – enables real-time visualization of movement of contrast materials within the body. Contrast materials used include air, carbon dioxide, barium and compounds containing iodine or gadolinium molecules. These materials absorb the X-ray beam differentially compared with the surrounding soft tissues, enabling their visualization. The choice of contrast material depends on the organ under examination, since their properties of absorption, viscosity and conspicuity by fluoroscopy vary.

CONTRAST AGENTS

Barium
Barium is a non-absorbed material that provides high contrast and hence is used extensively in examination of the gastrointestinal tract. Depending on its dilution, barium has a high viscosity and thus can be used to coat mucosal surfaces. Due to its density dilution within the small bowel, it has only a minor effect on visualization. Barium is not absorbed; therefore, its presence within the peritoneum following perforation may lead to granuloma and adhesion formation. In the lungs, it is cleared only by cilia or macrophage action. Its

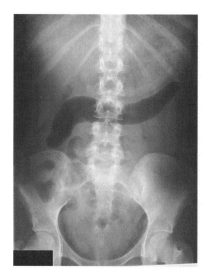

Figure 6.2   *Plain abdominal radiography, showing gas-filled transverse colon. There is no stool within the colon, and there is bowel-wall thickening, with loss of the normal haustration. The appearance is in keeping with active colitis.*

high viscosity may lead to failure to visualize small sinuses or fistulae, unless the solution is diluted, but this makes it less visible on the image.

Iodine-containing solutions (water-soluble contrast agents)
These may be used within any organ. They are less viscous than barium but are less visible on screening and may dilute more quickly. They are absorbed and hence may be used in sinuses and do not pose a problem within the peritoneum. They will affect lung function on direct contact by altering the surface tension, but they are cleared rapidly. They may be used intravascularly and hence are used for vascular enhancement, both in angiography and computed tomography (CT). They are excreted predominantly by the kidney and hence can be used to demonstrate the renal pelvicalyceal system. The risks involved in intravascular use of these compounds are mainly from anaphylactic reactions and, rarely, impairment of renal function.

Air and carbon dioxide
These may be used as negative contrast agents, most commonly for visualization of bowel. Air is an ideal agent for reduction of intussusception due to its low viscosity. It has fewer complications than barium if inadvertent bowel perforation and peritoneal contamination occur.

Gadolinium
This may be used as an X-ray contrast material, but its high cost means that its use is limited to magnetic resonance imaging (MRI) and X-ray examinations in which the patient has a known allergy to iodine-based contrast agents.

UPPER-GASTROINTESTINAL STUDIES

These may be performed with barium or water-soluble contrast agents. Real-time fluoroscopy of the oropharynx may be recorded to demonstrate aspiration and oropharyngeal movement. The patient is required to swallow the contrast material to examine the oropharynx and oesophagus, although nasogastric tube introduction may be used to examine the stomach and duodenum if necessary. Views of the oesophagus are obtained in orthogonal projections to enable examination of intrinsic and compressive lesions. Continuous fluoroscopy can be used to assess peristalsis and bolus propagation. Barium may be mixed with solid food material to further assess motility. Fluoroscopic examination with barium within the oesophagus can be used to assess tracheal calibre and tracheomalacia during respiration.

Examination of the upper gastrointestinal tract may be performed in single contrast, in which only a positive contrast agent is placed in the intestine, or double contrast, in which a positive agent and a negative agent such as carbon dioxide are used. Studies on neonates and young children are normally performed as single-contrast studies and hence mucosal detail is not delineated. Single-contrast studies provide detail of anatomy, intrinsic and extrinsic compressive lesions, and lesions protruding into the lumen of the organ. Definition of the position of the duodenojejunal (DJ) flexure requires visualization of the first bolus of contrast through the duodenum with the patient lying flat, as rotation of the patient may project the DJ flexure away from its true position. Rotation of the patient should be assessed by the position of the anterior ribs or heart compared with the spine.

SMALL-BOWEL STUDIES

The small bowel may be examined with barium, often with the addition of a propulsive agent such as metoclopramide or a small quantity of gastrograffin. These agents decrease small-bowel transit time and thus help to prevent dilution of the contrast agent and flocculation by the small-bowel secretions.

LARGE-BOWEL STUDIES

The large bowel may be examined with water-soluble or barium solutions introduced rectally. Gastrograffin may be used to delineate meconium and treat meconium ileus, its osmotic potential and soap-like effect producing expulsion of the viscid meconium.

Ultrasound

Ultrasound examination is a dynamic investigation that uses high-frequency vibration and the effect of tissue impedance on reflection of these waves to produce cross-sectional imaging of soft tissues. The examination is generally tolerated well by patients, requiring only the application of warmed acoustic coupling gel and gentle pressure with the transducer. For examination of the renal tract and pelvis, the patient must have a full bladder; for examination of the gallbladder, the patient must be fasted. Any organ that can be accessed without bone or gas between it and the transducer can be imaged; for example, in the neonate the brain may be imaged through the open fontanelle.

Doppler examination may be used to assess blood flow and may quantify flow, such as within cardiac shunts. Colour-flow imaging can be used to view flow patterns over a large area and for mapping areas for more detailed Doppler examination.

Computed tomography

CT provides cross-sectional imaging of the body by using finely collimated X-ray beams and the effect of the body's absorbance of the X-ray beam while it is rotated about the body. Modern CT scanners may produce 64 or more axial images during a rotation of the X-ray tube around the patient, this often being performed within one second. During the acquisition of the data, the patient must be still, and thus cooperation or sedation is required. Each axial slice may be collimated down to a width of less than 1 mm. Once acquired, the data may be manipulated to vary the appearance of the image to demonstrate different organ densities, providing detailed information for tissues such as lung and bone. Processing of the data may also be used to reformat the images into different planes of orientation for viewing, and volume data manipulation may be used to produce angiographic and surface-rendered images. CT imaging does, however, have a high radiation burden for the patient; for example, an abdominal CT examination is equivalent to approximately 500 chest radiographs. Its use, therefore, must be limited to situations in which the information cannot be acquired by other means.

Enhancement of the vessels by the use of an intravenous contrast agent is often required, with timing of the scan in relation to the injection being critical. Vessel enhancement can help to distinguish vessels from lymph nodes and highlight abnormalities of perfusion within the liver, spleen and kidneys. Aberrant vessels may be demonstrated and, in the setting of trauma, extravasation of contrast may demonstrate active bleeding.

Nuclear medicine imaging

Radiolabelled contrast agents and their movement within the body can be imaged using a gamma camera, although spatial resolution is not as high as with other imaging modalities. Nuclear medicine studies are particularly helpful in assessing the function of organs, such as renal (^{99m}technetium-labelled dimercaptosuccinic acid; DMSA) and hepatic (hydroxy-iminodiacetic acid; HIDA) excretion imaging. They can also be used to target specific organs and tissues. Because technetium is taken up by gastric mucosa, it can be used to diagnose bleeding from a Meckel's diverticulum, some of which contain ectopic gastric mucosa. Positron-emission tomography (PET) is a technique that links accurate localization of tracer with high metabolic rate and is used to help identify active regions of tumour growth.

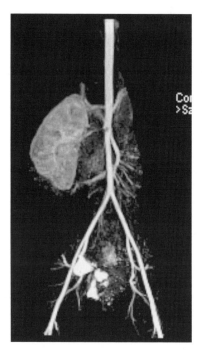

Figure 6.3 *Magnetic resonance imaging angiogram of the abdominal aorta taken following timed injection of gadolinium, after a left nephrectomy for a Wilms tumour, showing irregularity of the aorta at the site of previous intervention but normal distal aorta and iliac vessels. The superior mesenteric artery and remaining renal artery can be visualized.*

Magnetic resonance imaging

MRI produces images using rapidly changing magnetic gradients to induce resonant changes in magnetic dipoles of protons. These changes depend on the local environment of the proton and hence the changes can be used to interrogate proton density. This enables high soft-tissue contrast to be obtained, and, with alteration of acquisition parameters, signals from specific tissues may be suppressed or highlighted. Scan plane orientation may be altered without patient movement. Contrast given intravenously can be used to produce angiographic images and to assess perfusion of tissues (Figure 6.3). MRI has an advantage over CT in that no ionizing radiation is used to produce the images, but acquisition times may be long – up to several minutes for one selection of images – and movement at any stage will distort the whole sequence of images. Sedation or anaesthesia therefore may be required for younger patients. The small diameter of the bore of the magnet within which the patient must be positioned may induce claustrophobia, although wider-bore magnets and semi-open systems are being developed.

IMAGING DIFFERENT REGIONS OF THE BODY

The different methods of imaging have specific roles in different parts of the body. These are summarized in Table 6.1.

Cranial imaging

The open anterior fontanelle in the neonate makes ultrasound imaging of the brain possible, allowing assessment of

Table 6.1 *Main uses of the different cross-sectional imaging methods in different body regions*

Body region	Ultrasound	CT	MRI
Head	(Neonate only) Haemorrhage Ventricular dilation	Haemorrhage Trauma	Migrational anomalies Space-occupying lesions
Chest	Heart structure and function Pleural collections Diaphragm function	Chest wall Mediastinal masses Lung parenchyma Trauma	Heart Great vessels Blood flow
Abdomen	Fluid-filled structures (kidney, gallbladder, cysts) Pyloric stenosis Appendicitis Inflammatory bowel disease Trauma (FAST) Varices	Solid organs Trauma Malignancy assessment Vascular anatomy	Solid organs Intraspinal tumour extension
Musculoskeletal	Soft tissues Joints Lesion vascularity	Trauma	High-resolution soft-tissue imaging Ligaments Intervertebral discs

CT, computed tomography; FAST, focused abdominal sonography for trauma; MRI, magnetic resonance imaging.

ventricular size and intraventricular or parenchyma haemorrhage. Serial measurements to assess progression of hydrocephalus are possible without radiation burden to the child. Assessment of abnormal developmental anatomy (e.g. posterior fossa in Dandy–Walker syndrome, absence of the corpus callosum) is also possible. Ultrasound, however, is less useful in the assessment of extra-axial spaces, where CT is better, or the assessment of white-matter migrational abnormalities, where MRI is more accurate. Once the fontanelle has closed, cranial ultrasound imaging cannot be performed, due to the high reflectivity of the skull bones. In this case, CT is used in the assessment for acute haemorrhage or trauma, and MRI is used for the investigation of space-occupying lesions and migrational abnormalities. MRI may also be used to determine flow within vessels and the ventricular system.

Chest imaging

The mainstay of investigation of chest disease is the chest radiograph, which allows assessment of the lung parenchyma, lung vascularity, mediastinal contour and soft tissues of the chest wall. Free air (pneumothorax) is seen easily, as may be the cause of the air leak (Figure 6.4), and inhaled radio-opaque foreign bodies can be identified accurately (Figure 6.5). Ultrasound imaging is limited to assessment of the heart and soft tissues of the chest wall and investigation of pleural masses and collections, since the ultrasound beam is reflected by air/tissue interfaces within the lung. In the assessment of pleural collections, ultrasound may indicate the location of fluid (e.g. anterior or posterior) and also can measure pleural thickening and demonstrate the presence of loculation, both of which may influence management. Ultrasound-assisted drainage catheter placement also may be performed. Assessing diaphragmatic movement in eventration or phrenic nerve palsy is a valuable role of ultrasound. Masses abutting the diaphragm, such as pulmonary sequestrations, are usually imaged easily by ultrasound, and Doppler can detect feeding vessels.

MRI can provide anatomical imaging of the heart and great vessels and functional imaging of blood flow though stenoses, ducts and cardiac defects without the need for contrast administration.

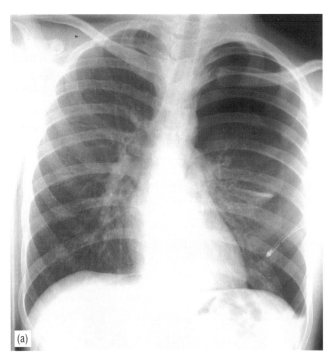

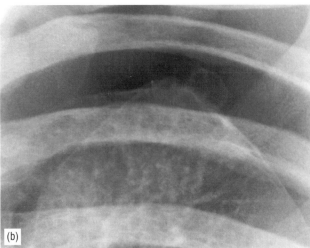

Figure 6.4   *(a) Chest radiograph, demonstrating a left pneumothorax with an intercostal pleural drain in situ. (b) Coned view of the apex of the lung within the left pneumothorax. An apical bulla can be seen as a predisposing factor for developing a pneumothorax.*

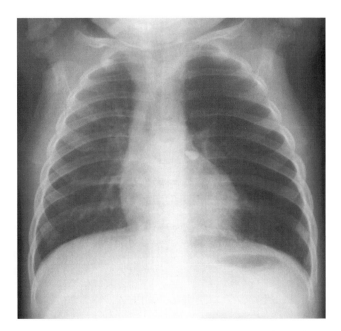

Figure 6.5   *Chest radiograph, showing hyperinflation of the left lung, with a radiodenisty projected over the left main bronchus. This was found to be an inhaled tooth at bronchoscopy, causing hyperinflation due to a ball-valve-like effect in the bronchus.*

CT can be used to image the chest wall, mediastinum and lung parenchyma. The use of intravenous contrast will highlight normal and aberrant vessels and define lymph nodes. Computer reconstruction of the data enables surface-rendered images of the inside of the trachea and airways, enabling virtual bronchoscopy (Figure 6.6). However, without inspiratory and expiratory imaging, dynamic collapse of the airways cannot be visualized. Dynamic visualization of tracheomalacia or bronchomalacia may be performed with fluoroscopy; although the trachea may be visualized adequately adjacent to contrast introduced into the oesophagus, the main bronchi and more distal airways require water-soluble contrast to be introduced directly into the bronchial tree (bronchography).

Barium contrast studies can be used to assess oropharyngeal movement in patients with difficulty feeding or possible aspiration. Video of continuous fluoroscopy of the oropharynx can be reviewed at slow frame rates for a full assessment of the complex movement in real time. Contrast introduced into the oesophagus may demonstrate an H-type tracheo-oesophageal fistula, but to evaluate this fully, a prone head-down examination with screening from the side while introducing contrast via a tube within the oesophagus is required (tube oesophagogram) (Figure 6.7). Extrinsic compression of the oesophagus by an aberrant vessel or intrinsic abnormality such as a web, stricture or achalasia can be demonstrated by contrast, although suboptimal oesophageal distension may prevent their detection.

Abdominal imaging

Imaging of abdominal pathology demonstrates the need for tailored investigation. Examination of the lumen and mucosa of a viscus requires the presence of either a natural contrast agent, such as air within bowel loops on an abdominal radiograph or bile within a gallbladder on ultrasound, or

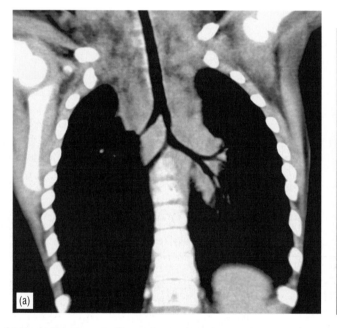
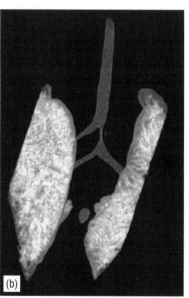

Figure 6.6 *(a) Coronally reformatted image from a chest computed tomography examination. The image delineates the presence of a bridging bronchus crossing to supply the right lower lobe from the left main-stem bronchus. (b) Surface-rendered image of the airways, with the remainder of the chest structures removed digitally, demonstrates the relationship of the main airways with the lungs.*

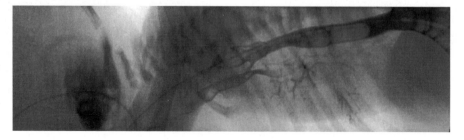

Figure 6.7 *Lateral view of the chest, with the patient prone, taken during instillation of water-soluble contrast into the oesophagus by a nasogastric tube. Contrast is seen to pass into and outline the trachea by way of an H-type tracheo-oesophageal fistula.*

an appropriate contrast agent introduced into the lumen, such as barium during an enema examination. Ultrasound can be used to examine the intra-abdominal organs, provided that air between the organ under investigation and the probe can be excluded. CT can examine both the solid organs and the lumens of bowel loops, but this incurs a large radiation burden. MRI can be used to examine the solid organs without radiation, and techniques are being developed for angiography and urography. However, patient cooperation is required in MRI because of the long scanning times.

Neonatal bowel obstruction

The imaging technique used depends on whether the obstruction is in the upper or lower gastrointestinal tract. A plain film is used to determine this by assessing the number of filled bowel loops. Upper-intestinal obstruction can be delineated by the introduction of air into the stomach via a nasogastric tube. Barium may be unhelpful in complete upper-intestinal obstruction and may lead to aspiration of barium into the lungs. However, barium is the contrast of choice to diagnose malrotation by delineating the position of the DJ flexure, which defines the position of the root of the small-bowel mesentery. To exclude malrotation, the DJ flexure must confidently be seen to be to the left of the vertebral body's left pedicle at the level of the gastric antrum, with the patient positioned flat (Figure 6.8).

Ultrasound may demonstrate malposition of the superior mesenteric artery relative to the vein and suggest the diagnosis of malrotation, but a normal relationship on ultrasound does not exclude malrotation.

In low gastrointestinal obstruction, a barium enema should be performed to assess colonic size and the level of obstruction. If meconium ileus is found, then diluted gastrograffin can be introduced, but to aid decompression the gastrograffin must surround the meconium and thus must be seen within the dilated loops of bowel. Gastrograffin has both lubricant and osmotic effects, and precautions must be taken to prevent the baby becoming dehydrated.

Pyloric stenosis

Pyloric stenosis (Chapter 22) can be confirmed confidently by ultrasound examination by visualization of a lengthened pylorus (>14 mm) with wall thickening (>4 mm) (Figure 6.9). Dynamic imaging will also show that the pylorus

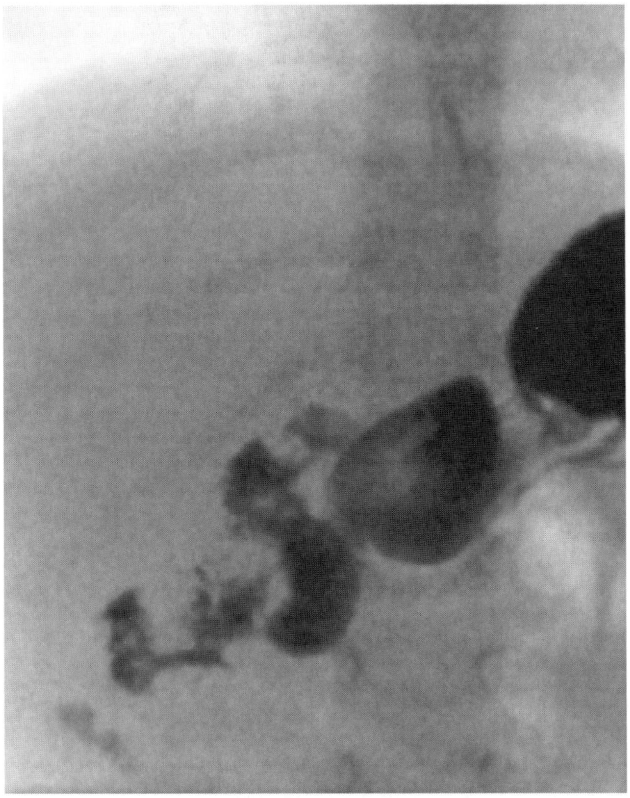

Figure 6.8 *Barium has been introduced into the stomach via the gastric tube and is seen to delineate the duodenojejunal flexure to the right of the spine, with the proximal small bowel also right-sided. The appearance confirms malrotation.*

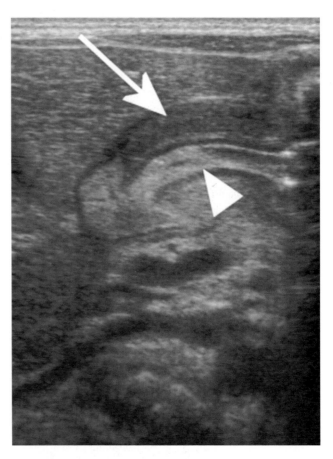

Figure 6.9 *Longitudinal ultrasound image of an enlarged pylorus, showing the hypoechoic enlarged muscle layer (arrow) beneath the echogenic mucosal layer (arrow head).*

remains closed despite the presence of fluid within the antrum of the stomach.

Acute abdominal conditions

APPENDICITIS

An abnormal appendix is detected by ultrasound in at least 70 per cent of patients with appendicitis (Chapter 27). The inflamed appendix is seen as a blind-ending tubular structure that is non-compressible and measures 6 mm or more in transverse diameter. There may also be secondary signs of inflammation, with oedema of the surrounding omentum. Visualization of a normal appendix is more difficult. CT performed with rectal contrast can identify a higher percentage of abnormalities in suspected appendicitis, but the significant radiation dose must be considered. Complications of appendicitis, such as an abscess and appendix mass, may be visualized readily by ultrasound, and examination of the pelvic organs through the distended bladder can identify the ovaries and uterus and pathology originating from these.

INFLAMMATORY BOWEL DISEASE

Bowel thickening may be seen in the presence of inflammatory bowel disease (Chapter 25), and ultrasound may be used to localize the region of inflammation to large or small bowel and may identify no contiguous inflamed segments in keeping with skip lesions.

INTUSSUSCEPTION

An intussusception (Chapter 23) is seen as a mass comprising a set of concentric rings, with alternating high and low echogenicity of the muscle and mucosal layers of the bowel wall, which is sometimes described as having the appearance of a doughnut (Figure 6.10). Ultrasound may be used to monitor reduction of intussusception, although more commonly fluoroscopic screening of air or barium under pressure is used. Success rates for the reduction of intussusception with air enema are in excess of 70 per cent. Ultrasound can also visualize the presence of a lead point as the cause of an intussusception. Ultrasound frequently is used to exclude intussusception in doubtful cases.

ABDOMINAL TRAUMA

Ultrasound examination of the abdomen has become an increasingly common investigation to detect intraperitoneal fluid and has superseded diagnostic peritoneal lavage (Chapter 29). Focused abdominal sonography for trauma (FAST) examinations aim to detect free fluid, which is an indication of intra-abdominal bleeding. The examination is not performed to define solid-organ injury. FAST scanning is used in conjunction with continued observation of the patient and may be repeated; if free fluid is found, then either formal ultrasound examination or CT should be performed. Ultrasound may miss some solid-organ injuries, and CT of the abdomen with intravenous contrast enhancement is more accurate.

Hepatobiliary disorders

Ultrasound can identify:

- liver enlargement and alteration of the normal parenchyma echo texture, as seen in inflammatory and infiltrative disorders;
- focal liver abnormalities, e.g. abscess, tumour;
- biliary tract calculi;
- gallbladder wall thickening, as occurs with cholecystitis and veno-occlusive disorders;
- abnormalities of the biliary tree, e.g. choledochal cysts, biliary atresia;
- the direction of flow within the portal and hepatic veins: reversal of flow may be seen with advanced liver disease, and collateral flow in gastro-oesophageal varices can be identified;
- splenic size, which may be monitored without radiation effects.

MRI can also be used to visualize the biliary tree and the hepatic vascular anatomy.

Abdominal masses

Ultrasound is the investigation of choice for the initial imaging of abdominal masses. It can identify readily whether a mass is solid or cystic and, with Doppler, can define blood flow though the mass. The appearance of the wall of a cystic mass may be diagnostic. The presence of defined layers within a cyst that have the appearance of muscle and mucosal layers of bowel indicate a duplication cyst (Figure 6.11), whereas complete colour-flow filling of the mass would be in keeping with an aneurysm or vascular malformation. The location of the mass can be assessed readily, and the organ of origin usually can be identified by ultrasound, although if the mass is large such assessment is more difficult.

A cystic lesion within the pelvis may be related to:

- the bladder or ureters (urachal cyst, ureterocele);
- the ovaries (benign or malignant disease);
- the bowel and mesentery (duplication cyst, mesenteric lymphatic cyst);
- the neural canal (anterior meningocele);
- the uterus and internal genitalia (haematocolpos).

Dynamic ultrasound scanning can be used to visualize movement of a mass relative to an organ or vessel, and this movement can be used to exclude involvement by the mass.

CT is the best imaging method to stage abdominal malignancies (Figure 6.12). It can also be used to assess lung parenchyma for metastases. CT may be used to examine areas that cannot be visualized by ultrasound due to technical problems. Vessels supplying or being displaced by a tumour may

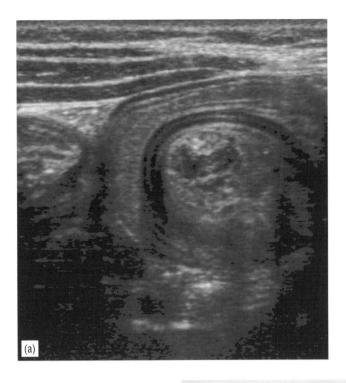

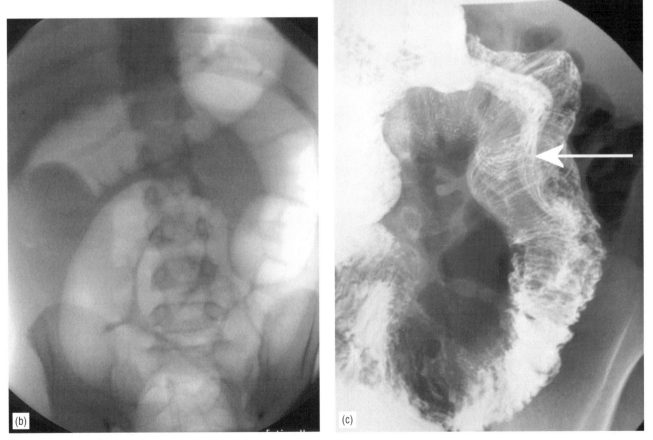

Figure 6.10 *(a) Ultrasound image of an intussusception, demonstrating the multiple concentric rings of bowel wall, in keeping with an intussusception. (b) Demonstrates the colon to be distended with air introduced rectally, with the intussusception demonstrated as a filling defect at the hepatic flexure. (c) Demonstrates barium within a loop of small bowel, which has intussuscepted into the distal small bowel. This shows the coiled spring appearance, with the lumen of the intussuscepted bowel being indicated by the arrow.*

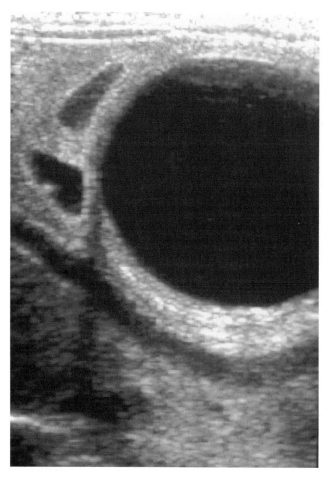

Figure 6.11 *Ultrasound demonstrates a cystic lesion within the upper abdomen adjacent to a normal fluid-filled bowel loop. This cystic lesion has a defined wall thickness, consisting of several layers. This layered wall appearance is in keeping with a duplication cyst.*

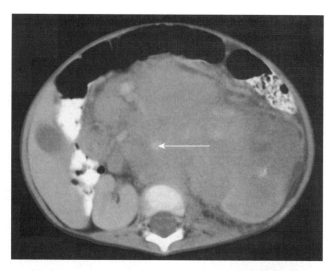

Figure 6.12 *Axial computed tomography image through the abdomen, demonstrating a large retroperitoneal mass. The mass encases the aorta (arrow) and is seen to be displaced from the vertebral body. The high density of the aorta is due to the presence of intravenously injected contrast. The mass was proven to be a neuroblastoma. High-density material within the bowel loops is orally ingested dilute water-soluble contrast.*

be highlighted by the administration of intravenous contrast. Such contrast is particularly useful in defining lesions within the liver and kidneys, due to the differences in perfusion of masses compared with normal tissues.

Staging of abdominal tumours requires determination of whether a mass is locally invasive, whether local or distant nodes are enlarged, and whether metastases are present. CT will identify fairly small lesions (e.g. contralateral lesions in a patient with Wilms tumour). CT can formally identify the segments of the liver involved by a hepatoblastoma and thus identify tumours that could be resected. CT may readily demonstrate vessel encasement by a neuroblastoma and extension within the spinal canal, which may be impossible to visualize with ultrasound. MRI is the best investigation in order to demonstrate neural compression by an invading tumour, such as neuroblastoma.

Musculoskeletal imaging

Plain X-rays are the initial investigation of choice in bone pathology. Fractures may be identified readily, and their

healing can be monitored on follow-up radiographs by observing periosteal reaction and callus formation. Fluoroscopy can be used to image fracture manipulation and to show the joint surface and mobility during an arthrogram. Ultrasound may be used to examine the soft tissues and in the investigation of joints, where it can show the integrity of ligaments and tendons and the presence of joint effusions. Synovial thickening may be demonstrated in inflammatory disorders.

Ultrasound examination of soft-tissue swellings can define easily whether a lump is cystic or solid. It may also be possible to define the origin of the lump by its location and attachment to adjacent structures, such as the neurovascular bundle. In suspected haemangioma, Doppler may be used to assess vascularity of the lump.

MRI of musculoskeletal abnormalities provides high soft-tissue definition and may provide multiplanar imaging, enabling accurate assessment of ligaments and tendons, as well as information about bone marrow and muscles. MRI images can be adjusted to highlight oedema and thus may be useful in spinal trauma and infection to assess ligamentous or disc abnormalities, which may not be visualized on X-ray imaging, and can assess neural compression by visualizing directly the spinal cord and nerve roots (Figure 6.13).

Intervention

Ultrasound, CT and fluoroscopy may all be used to visualize structures for biopsy and needle access and to guide instrumentation. Ultrasound may be used to visualize a needle

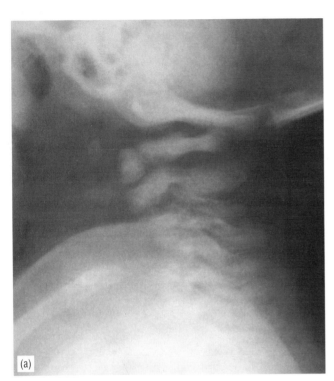

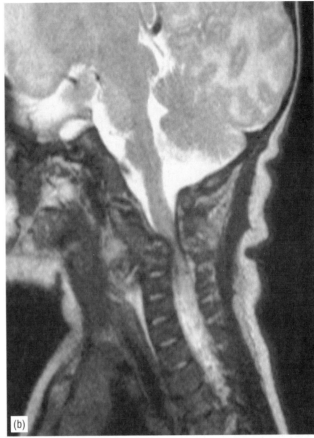

Figure 6.13 *(a) Lateral view of the cervical spine of a neonate, showing acute kyphosis with loss of disc space at the C5 level. (b) Magnetic resonance image, demonstrating loss of disc signal of C5–6 and increased signal within the vertebral bodies adjacent, with a prevertebral soft-tissue mass. This is in keeping with an infective discitis. There is compression of the spinal cord at this level.*

path and to guide vascular access, by visualizing vessels and their compressibility in real time. Echogenic needle tips have been developed to aid visualization with ultrasound. The introduction of CT fluoroscopy has enabled real-time visualization of needle movement with CT, enabling drainage or biopsy of structures that are difficult to visualize with ultrasound, such as those hidden by gas or bone, e.g. in the chest and retroperitoneum.

FURTHER READING

Ebel K-D, Blickman H, Willich E, Richter E. *Differential Diagnosis in Pediatric Radiology*. Stuttgart: Thieme; 1999.

Kuhn JP, Slovis T, Haller J. *Caffey's Pediatric Diagnostic Imaging*, 10th edn. St Louis, MO: Mosby; 2003.

Swischuk LE. *Imaging of the Newborn, Infant, and Young Child*, 5th edn. Philadelphia, PA: Lippincott Williams & Wilkins; 2004.

7

Transport of sick infants and children

MICHAEL J MARSH

Learning objectives

- To understand the intricacies of critical-care transport.
- To understand the organizational aspects of critical-care transport.
- To be able to communicate effectively with a regional transport service.
- To be able to provide clear advice to a transport service regarding specific surgical requirements.

INTRODUCTION

The concept of regionalized critical care has developed over the past 30 years with the adoption of the principle that the transfer of a patient to a unit able to deliver a higher level of care should improve the morbidity and mortality through the receipt of expert critical care and specialist expertise, including surgery. A documented improvement in morbidity and mortality in critically ill neonates, infants and children along with evidence of the safety of the transport process when performed by specialized teams has further promoted regionalization of specialist services. The goal of the critical-care transport team is to provide high-quality intensive care throughout the transfer process, effectively providing an intensive-care bed on the move. Most children become critically ill near to their homes and undergo resuscitation and stabilization at the local hospital. If the individual's needs exceed the local expertise, then an inter-hospital transport by an expert team is required to maximize a good outcome.

There are three groups of patients needing critical-care transport that directly concern the paediatric surgeon:

- Children who have been the victims of trauma resulting in either severe traumatic brain injury or poly-trauma.
- Term and preterm neonates with either major congenital anomalies or complications of the neonatal period, such as necrotizing enterocolitis.
- Infants and older children who have either a severe form or a complication of a condition such as appendicitis or volvulus.

ORGANIZATION

General principles of transport

Most people think that it is safer to perform an intra-hospital transfer, e.g. from a paediatric intensive care unit

Table 7.1　*Relative merits of local versus regional transport when considering an infant or child requiring urgent surgical intervention*

Local team transport	Regional team transport
Saves time	Journey time doubled
Lacks appropriate staff	Dedicated staff
Lacks equipment	Appropriate equipment
May lack expertise and training	Expert, well-trained

(PICU)/neonatal intensive care unit (NICU) to a radiology department or theatre, than to perform an inter-hospital transfer from hospital A to hospital B. Hence, the former are frequently done without due attention to vital issues, in particular the personnel and equipment involved along with sufficient attention to details, including communication. This can result in poor practice, where staff prepare inadequately, have insufficient handover and leave vital equipment behind and therefore put the patient at risk. The absence of a vehicle in the intra-hospital transfer is the only significant difference. Hence, the same principles and standards should be applied to both intra- and inter-hospital forms of transport. Meticulous preparation and training by a team of experts is the key to success.

Regional considerations

The makeup of a regional transport team has many influences, including local geographic factors such as the distances needed to travel, the size of the area covered and the presence of any difficult-to-access sites, such as islands or remote mountainous sites. Sufficient consideration needs to be given to all these factors when planning individual critical-care transport. The need to use air transport can have profound effects on the constitution of a team, the logistics of the process and the costs involved.

There are occasions when consideration also needs to be given to the potential benefits of utilizing a local transport team rather than the specialist regional team. There are situations when the overriding need of the child, following initial resuscitation and stabilization, is the early access to surgical expertise, e.g. an expanding acute extradural haematoma. In this situation, the senior medical staff involved must weigh the risks and benefits of the two options (Table 7.1).

A transport system should also encourage and support the early transport back to the local hospital of neonates, infants and children. This is especially true for neonates, where the benefits gained from the family's support can be enormous. In addition, it enables the efficient use of the tertiary services that frequently have limited resources to cope with the demands.

TEAM CONSTITUTION

A large number of people, performing both administrative and clinical roles, need to be involved in a successful transport service, although the number performing the transport itself can be as small as three.

Medical director

The medical director has overall responsibility for the service and, along with a deputy, should be available for consultation on a 24-hours-a-day basis. Such people are trained in paediatric critical care or neonatology and transport medicine. Their most important roles are as follows:

- audit of clinical cases, critical incidents and service performance;
- running the outreach programme to referring hospitals;
- managing a quality-improvement programme;
- approval of all equipment and medication;
- development of policies and protocols;
- selection and training of team members.

Transport coordinator

The transport coordinator is usually a qualified and very experienced critical-care nurse and is responsible for the daily activities of the team and the organization and maintenance of the equipment. Along with the medical director, the transport coordinator collects audit data and helps to develop and manage the service. This may be a full-time dedicated role or, more commonly in the UK, the nurse in charge of either the PICU or NICU. In a large service, the transport coordinator improves the performance and the ease of access to the service for the referring hospitals.

Duty consultant

The duty consultant must be available 24 hours a day and is usually trained in paediatric critical care or neonatology. He or she is expert in the care of critically ill neonates, infants and children and has overall control of the individual patient transport. The duty consultant decides ultimately on the membership of the team and the mode of transport for each case. If they are not physically involved in the transport, then they must maintain supervisory contact of the team during the transport.

Transport doctor

The doctor may be either a consultant or a senior trainee with the relevant skills and experience required to care for a critically ill patient (Box 7.1).

Transport nurse

The transport nurse is a PICU- or NICU-trained nurse, usually with considerable experience in clinical care. For most transports in the UK, the nurse works in collaboration with a doctor; however, there is an increasing number of nurse-led transports, particularly in neonatal medicine. In this case, the nurse must have the qualities and skills listed in Box 7.1.

Transport paramedic/technician/driver/pilot

Depending on local resources and the individual case, any or all of the above may be involved. It is important to stress that both the driver and the pilot should make decisions regarding transport based on their training and knowledge and the weather conditions, and must not be influenced by the patient's clinical condition. Drivers should be discouraged from exceeding speed limits and going through red lights, as these practices put all team members and the patient at increased risk. In addition, the time saved, which is only likely to be a few minutes, by such practices is not likely to benefit the patient. When time is critical to outcome, it is an easy referral process, a rapid response for the team leaving, and an efficient handover at the referring hospital that gain time.

It has been recommended that, ideally, the transport team should include a critical-care technician who is responsible for setting up and maintaining all equipment used, including ventilators, monitors, infusion pumps and incubators. Few teams in the UK have such personnel and, hence, the doctor and nurse may have to fulfil this role.

The team constitution should be decided by the duty consultant based on the condition of the patient and the mode of transport to be used. Ideally, every team should have a doctor, a nurse, a critical-care technician and a dedicated driver. There may be additional doctors and nurses present for training purposes or because the clinical condition of the patient dictates the extra personnel.

There is controversy as to whether the presence of a doctor makes a difference to outcome. In neonatal transfer, there is no evidence that the presence of a doctor improves outcome and, hence, a significant number are performed by neonatal nurse practitioners; however, some services insist on a doctor being present in more complicated neonatal cases. If the transport is nurse-led, then the nurse must have extra expertise, including stabilization, management of critical illness, monitoring, endotracheal intubation, intraosseous and central access, and insertion of a chest drain. In paediatric intensive care, there is no evidence to support the safety of excluding

a doctor. Therefore, with rare exceptions, paediatric critical-care transport teams invariably include a doctor, although this may change in the future.

EQUIPMENT

Although equipment is vitally important to a successful and effective transport service, it is beyond the scope of this book to provide exhaustive lists; these can be found in the texts suggested in the list of further reading. However, it is useful to understand the principles involved in selecting the equipment and the categories into which they can be classified (Box 7.2).

In essence, everything necessary to continue the stabilization and management of a critically ill neonate, infant or child is required. There must also be sufficient stores to be able to deliver care for at least twice the anticipated duration of the transfer. The equipment is packed in a number of lightweight and easily accessible bags, with associated comprehensive equipment checklists. As with trolleys, equipment should be movable by usually two, and a maximum of three, people.

Equipment categories

- *Airway*: everything necessary to non-invasively and invasively maintain airway, including tracheostomy.
- *Vascular access*: everything necessary to obtain, secure and maintain peripheral, central and intraosseous access.
- *Other supplies*: including dressings, fixation devices, chest drains, urinary catheters and special equipment necessary for individual case, e.g. clear plastic wrap for gastroschisis.
- *Monitor*: with both invasive and non-invasive abilities, e.g. Propaq (Drager Medical, Lubeck, Germany).
- *Ventilator*: this can be compressed-gas-driven (mostly suitable for older children), e.g. Oxylog 1000 (Drager

Medical), or electrically driven, e.g. Oxylog 2000 (Drager Medical).

- *Defibrillator*: but used extremely rarely.
- *Immobilization device*: spinal board, vacuum mattress.
- *Transportation device*: trolley, incubator, pod.
- *Reference guides*: paediatric formulary, Broselow tape.

VEHICLES

In the UK, the vast majority of inter-hospital critical-care transports can be done by road using a land ambulance. As a

---

Box 7.3 Factors to be considered when selecting mode of transport

Severity of patient's illness
Post-resuscitation stability
Urgency for which specialist care is required
Transit times between the hospitals involved
Availability of vehicles
Personnel's abilities
Weather and traffic conditions
Geography
Safety
Cost

---

general principle, if the region covered by a transport service is urban, then road transport is all that is likely to be necessary. If the region is rural and involves journeys in excess of 100 miles (150 km), then it is also necessary to have access to both fixed-wing and rotary aircraft. The duty consultant is responsible for reviewing these three options and for making the final decision as to what is most appropriate. In order to do this, a number of variables must be considered (Box 7.3), remembering that the safety of the team and the patient are paramount.

Although air transport can be invaluable, it is very costly, and in a resource-limited service due consideration must also be given to this fact. The relative merits of all forms of transport are summarized in Table 7.2.

COMMUNICATION

The transport of a critically ill neonate, infant or child is complex and involves a large number of hospital professionals in at least two different institutions. If a road ambulance and either form of air transport are utilized for the transfer, then the numbers of people involved increases considerably. Good communication is vital to ensure rapid, safe and efficient transport of the critically ill patient to the receiving hospital. When the patient requires the expertise of a paediatric surgeon, the surgeon plays a pivotal role in this complex clinical communication. There are many aspects of the transfer

---

Table 7.2 *Advantages and disadvantages of different transport vehicles*

	Road ambulance	Rotary-wing aircraft	Fixed-wing aircraft
Advantages	One-transfer door-to-door service	Rapid, takes 30–50% of road-transport time at 120–180 mph, and should be considered for journeys <150 miles	Rapid transport over distances >150 miles
	Ease of training	Easy access to difficult and remote locations	May carry more personnel
	Readily available	Smoother flight	
	Large cabin space with good access to patient		
	Affordable – to own, lease, maintain Adequate space	Decreases odds of a crash	Fly above or around bad weather
	Family members can also travel		
Disadvantages	Motion sickness	May require multiple patient transfers	Negative effects of high altitude if not pressurized
	Some limitations to access and what can be performed whilst moving	In event of crash, less survivable	Loading patient difficult
	Traffic delays	Costly: £2000/hour	Require airport
	Transport times longer	Unobstructed landing site required	Always require multiple journeys
	Vibration and noise 70–75 dB	Increased noise and vibration 90–110 dB	Substantially higher costs
		No pressurization, so altitude effect above 2500 m	
		Fuel capacity limits range to 150 miles	
		Weight restriction limits personnel	

that the surgeon needs to be aware of but not necessarily involved in directly, but there are other aspects in which the surgeon is a key player (Table 7.3). It should always be remembered that communication is an active two-way process and both parties are responsible for the quality and content of the information transferred.

RECORD-KEEPING, DOCUMENTATION AND AUDIT

All parties involved in critical-care transport should keep accurate notes of the referral, advice given and management throughout the transport. This enables accurate and meaningful audits to be performed and, hence, facilitates ongoing quality improvement of the service. Currently, few surgeons keep written records of the initial referral and the advice given at this stage. Individuals should be encouraged either to produce their own documentation of this process or to enter this information on to the transport team's notes.

SPECIAL PRINCIPLES

Although it is beyond the scope of this book to deal with details of transport in depth, there are a number of situations that are worth highlighting, as additional knowledge, care or equipment may be necessary.

Neonates

PHYSIOLOGICAL ISSUES

In any newborn, term or preterm, considerable efforts may be necessary to maintain the central body temperature. Ideally, a thermo-neutral environment should be provided, although in physiological extremes, this can be extremely difficult, e.g. an extremely low-birth-weight infant who needs air transport in the middle of winter. In order to achieve this, a vast array of techniques and equipment may be utilized:

- incubator or pod
- radiant heater
- plastic wraps
- insulating blankets
- heat shields
- chemically activated heat packs/mattress
- Central and peripheral continuous temperature monitors
- control of environmental temperature, e.g. ambulance cabin.

An understanding of the normal physiological changes that are associated with the adaptation to breathing at birth, and how these may go wrong, is important. The development of persistent pulmonary hypertension of the newborn (PPHN) is well documented when the newborn becomes critically ill. In conditions with associated pulmonary hypoplasia (e.g. congenital diaphragmatic hernia, renal dysplasia), an element of pulmonary hypertension is almost inevitable and has a

Table 7.3 *Communication and responsibilities for the paediatric surgeon involved in organizing critical-care transport*

Communication	Key information transfer
Referring doctor to paediatric surgeon	Diagnosis or clinical problem, time of onset of condition, physiological state, recommended immediate actions
Paediatric surgeon to duty transport consultant	All of the above, plus name of referring doctor, institute and contact numbers. Details of recommended immediate actions and further actions or surgical concerns relevant to transfer and likely definitive surgical interventions
Duty consultant to transport team	All of the above, plus anticipated critical-care interventions, plan of management for the transfer, team constitution, and mode of transport. Agree communication plan for the transfer
Transport team to referring team	Medical and nursing members of the transport team should make direct contact with the referring team in order to obtain up-to-date data on physiological condition, treatments and problems. Additional advice and contact numbers should be given, along with details of planned transfer and family members
Transport team to receiving PICU/NICU	If the receiving institute is not the transport team's base unit, then a summary of all the above should be given before the transfer. An update should be given to the receiving PICU/NICU immediately before leaving the referring hospital and before arriving at the receiving unit
Transport team to paediatric surgeon	At any time in the process, the surgeon should be consulted for any clarification of management or additional advice. At handover, a summary of the patient's conditions, management and interventions should be given to the surgeon before their assessment

NICU, neonatal intensive care unit; PICU, paediatric intensive care unit.

significant effect on mortality. In these cases, the transport team's work is complicated further as the team needs to have the ability to deliver and monitor inhaled nitric oxide during transport.

The management of fluids and electrolytes is challenging, especially in very low-birth-weight infants, and this can be complicated further by the presence of a congenital abdominal-wall defect and the need to transfer the infant immediately after birth.

SOCIAL ISSUES AND OUTCOME

Due consideration should always be given to the family of a neonate who is critically ill and requires transfer to a specialist centre. It is important to remember that although the family often wishes to travel with the child, it is the responsibility of the duty consultant and transport team to decide whether they are able to transfer them along with the patient.

Whatever the surgical condition of the neonate, it is important to remember the overriding effect that gestation has on outcome. Therefore, when deciding on treatment options, including the use of a specialist transport service, gestation must be taken into account, especially at the extremes of potential viability.

Aviation physiology

If air transport is to be used, then the transport team must be trained in aviation physiology. It is also important for the surgeon to be aware of the basic laws of physics and understand the potential effects of aviation on a patient. Equipment can also be affected during aviation, although this is the concern of the transport team rather than the surgeon.

Boyle's law states that at a constant temperature, the volume of a gas varies inversely with pressure:

$$P_1V_1 = P_2V_2$$

where P_1 and V_1 represent the initial pressure and volume, respectively, and P_2 and V_2 the resultant pressure and volume, respectively. Hence, with an increase in altitude (i.e. the barometric pressure falls), the volume of a gas will increase. Although the effects are not usually severe during flight, a patient with intestinal obstruction or free air in any anatomical space may be severely compromised. The surgeon must consider the likelihood of these surgical problems and discuss them adequately with the transport team if air transport is to be used.

OUTCOME

Specialist teams perform the majority of critical-care transports safely and effectively. A clear understanding of the individual roles and responsibilities along with rapid and efficient communication help to ensure that patients receive the most appropriate care during transport before delivery of definitive surgical care. Involvement of surgeons in critical incident reporting and audit of the transport services will help to maintain standards and deliver quality-improvement programmes.

CLINICAL SCENARIOS

Case 1

A term infant weighing 2.2 kg is born with an undiagnosed gastroschisis but no other congenital anomalies are evident. On referral to the surgical team, advice is given to wrap the intestines in cling film whilst attending to stabilization. The paediatric transport team is informed and makes arrangement to transfer the child breathing spontaneously in an incubator. On discussion with the referring NICU, the infant is tachycardic (175 beats/min) but normotensive. The infant is thought to be hypovolaemic, and advice is given to administer a fluid bolus. On arrival of the transport team, the infant remains tachycardic (160 beats/min) and has a central temperature of 35.5 °C. Two additional fluid boluses are given, and the infant is placed in a transport incubator with additional insulation blankets. Transfer is uneventful and definitive surgery is performed four hours after arrival in the surgical institute.

Case 2

A four-year-old child is a back-seat passenger in a road-traffic accident involving a head-on collision. The Glasgow Coma Scale (GCS) was 11 at the scene. A lap-belt only was noted. The child was immobilized and transferred to the local hospital. In the emergency department, the GCS was 8, so the child was intubated and ventilated immediately after a rapid-sequence induction. The cardiovascular system is stable. A subsequent computed tomography (CT) scan of the head revealed diffuse axonal injury with a small frontal lobe haematoma but no mass effect. The cervical spine X-ray was normal, the chest was normal (including a CT scan), and the abdomen was soft and non-distended, but there was a fracture of the left femur. The transport team was mobilized whilst stabilization was continued. Transfer was complicated by cardiovascular instability requiring 20 mL/kg of colloid. On assessment in the PICU, the abdomen was mildly distended. A double-contrast CT scan of the abdomen reveals a retroperitoneal rupture of the duodenum, and thoracoabdominal spine X-rays reveals a Chance fracture at L2/3. A laparotomy was performed, revealing, in addition to the duodenal rupture, a compression injury to the jejunum; a 15-cm resection and primary anastomosis was performed before fixation of L2/3.

FURTHER READING

Jaimovich DG. *Handbook of Pediatric and Neonatal Transport Medicine.* Philadelphia, PA: Lippincott Williams & Wilkins 2002.

Macnab AJ. Optimal escort for interhospital transport of pediatric emergencies. *Journal of Trauma* 1991; **31**: 205–9.

Martin T. *Handbook of Patient Transportation.* London: Cambridge University Press, 2001.

Pollack MM, Alexander SR, Clark N, *et al.* Improved outcomes from tertiary center paediatric intensive care: a statewide comparison of tertiary and nontertiary care facilities. *Critical Care Medicine* 1991; **19**: 150–59.

Warren J, Fromm RE, Orr RA, *et al.* Guidelines for the inter- and intrahospital transport of critically ill patients. *Critical Care Medicine* 2004; **32**: 256–62.

8

Paediatric anaesthesia

PAUL SPARGO AND PAUL SUTHERLAND

Learning objectives

- To understand the principles of preoperative assessment and preoperative preparation of children.
- To understand the principles of anaesthesia for neonates, infants and children.

INTRODUCTION

Paediatric anaesthesia has evolved as a separate subspecialty of anaesthesia over the past 50 years. The Association of Paediatric Anaesthetists of Great Britain and Ireland was founded in 1973. Although there is a trend towards greater specialization, anaesthetists working in general hospitals must retain the core knowledge and skills to provide immediate care to children. Improvements in training and monitoring have led to a greatly improved level of safety.

It is not the purpose of this chapter to provide an in-depth account of the anaesthetic management of neonates, infants and children. Emphasis is given to the basic principles of anaesthesia for these groups, their preoperative assessment and preoperative preparation. These topics are of greatest relevance to the practising surgeon.

APPLIED BASIC SCIENCES

Airway anatomy

There are important differences in the anatomy of the respiratory system of the infant compared with the older child (Table 8.1). The U-shaped epiglottis projects posteriorly at an angle of 45 degrees above the glottis. It must be elevated to see the vocal cords, and hence a straight-bladed laryngoscope is recommended during tracheal intubation. In older children and adults, a curved blade is preferred. In younger children, the cricoid cartilage, a circular ring of cartilage, is the narrowest part of the airway. In view of this, uncuffed tracheal tubes usually are used in children under ten years of age, and a small gas leak around the tube is desirable. In this way, mucosal compression with subsequent oedema is prevented. A small decrease in tracheal diameter leads to a dramatic increase in resistance to flow.

Respiratory physiology

The ribs of infants extend horizontally and the diaphragm is less domed than in adults, with a much more limited excursion. Changes in minute ventilation can be effected only by changes in respiratory rate, as the tidal volume is fixed. The volume of gas in the lungs at the end of a normal expiration, the functional residual capacity (FRC), is an important reservoir for oxygen. The opposing forces of the cartilaginous chest wall and the elastic recoil of the lungs determine the FRC. A high respiratory rate and the narrow larynx help to maintain

Table 8.1 *Differences between infant and adult airways*

Infant airway compared with adult airway	Importance
Relatively large occiput	Intubation achieved most easily with patient lying on a flat surface with no pillow; shoulder roll sometimes helps
Short neck Small jaw	
Relatively large tongue	Easily obstructs pharynx, making intubation more difficult
Glottis situated at level of C3–4 and rather anterior	Larynx may be better viewed with a straight-bladed laryngoscope and gentle external laryngeal pressure
Large, floppy epiglottis	Laryngoscope blade passed beyond epiglottis; vocal cords visualized by anterior and upward movement, lifting epiglottis out of the way
Narrowest part of the larynx at the level of the cricoid cartilage	Uncuffed tracheal tubes used
Short trachea	Inadvertent endobronchial intubation possible

Table 8.2 *Changes of normal physiological variables with age*

Age	Heart rate (beats/min)	Blood pressure (mmHg)	Blood volume (mL/kg)
Neonate	140	70/40	90
1 year	120	80/50	80
5 years	100	100/60	70

Box 8.1 Preoperative assessment: important features in the preoperative history

Age
Birth history
Previous anaesthetic history
Family history of anaesthetic problems
Concurrent medical problems:
　Respiratory, e.g. upper respiratory tract infection, asthma, apnoea
　Cardiac
　Neurological, e.g. epilepsy, cerebral palsy, anatomical abnormalities
　Gastrointestinal (gastro-oesophageal reflux is of importance)
　Renal
Drug history
Allergies

FRC by limiting gas escape during expiration and encouraging gas trapping. A reduction in FRC can result in airway closure and intrapulmonary shunting. General anaesthesia itself reduces FRC. Bradypnoea, or brief periods of apnoea, may result in hypoxaemia by allowing gas escape and shunting to occur. Basal oxygen consumption is proportionately higher in children than in adults, with the result that hypoxaemia occurs more quickly when the oxygen supply to the lungs is interrupted.

Cardiovascular physiology

The change from fetal to neonatal circulation is precipitated by a rapid fall in pulmonary vascular resistance. However, the pulmonary vascular pressures of the neonate are labile and may, in some circumstances, remain elevated. Hypoxia, hypercarbia and acidosis also cause pulmonary vasoconstriction and will encourage right-to-left shunting through a patent foramen ovale (PFO) or a patent ductus arteriosus (PDA). The cardiac output of the neonate is dependent principally upon heart rate, as contractility has little capacity for change. Normal values for heart rate, blood pressure and blood volumes at different ages are given in Table 8.2. The neonatal parasympathetic nervous system is fully functional at birth, although the development of the sympathetic nervous system is not complete until four to six months of age. The stimulation of reflexes involving receptors in the upper airway, e.g. during laryngoscopy, tends to elicit bradycardia. Up to 50 per cent of five-year-old children may still have probe-patent

PFO and, therefore, are at risk of systemic air embolus if air is injected into the systemic venous circulation.

Pharmacology

There are important differences in the pharmacokinetics and pharmacodynamics of drugs in infants, children and adults. Infants have a reduced plasma protein binding and a larger total body water and extracellular fluid volume. Neonates have an immature blood–brain barrier, different receptor affinities and underdeveloped metabolic and excretory systems. As a consequence, the potency of some anaesthetic drugs changes with age. Neonates and infants are more susceptible to the effects of sedative drugs, opioids and non-depolarizing muscle relaxants. The relatively high alveolar ventilation of neonates and infants increases the rate of uptake and excretion of inhalational anaesthetic agents. Neonates and infants may be more sensitive to the cardiovascular depressant effects of volatile agents.

PREOPERATIVE ASSESSMENT

Careful preoperative assessment is the basis of good anaesthesia and takes the form of a detailed medical and surgical history, physical examination and investigations (Boxes 8.1

> **Box 8.2 Preoperative assessment: important features of the clinical examination**
>
> Assessment of airway and dentition
> Respiratory system
> Cardiovascular system
> Basic neurological assessment in some patients

Table 8.3 *American Society of Anesthesiologists (ASA) classification of physical status*

Classification	Physical status
I	Normally healthy patient
II	Patient with mild systemic disease
III	Patient with severe systemic disease that is not incapacitating
IV	Patient with incapacitating systemic disease that is a constant threat to life
V	Moribund patient who is not expected to survive 24 hours with or without an operation

Emergency cases are designated by the addition of 'E' to the classification number.

and 8.2). It is useful to assess the general medical fitness of the patient. The American Society of Anesthesiologists (ASA) classification of physical status grades patients according to severity of systemic disease (Table 8.3). A history of problems during previous anaesthetics is of particular importance. These may range from postoperative nausea and vomiting or sore throat, to airway difficulties, to rare inheritable conditions such as malignant hyperpyrexia or suxamethonium apnoea, and so anaesthetic problems in other members of the family may be of importance. A history of drug allergy must be sought; precise details are important because clinical symptoms or signs may be ascribed to a drug in the absence of good evidence of true drug sensitivity. Latex allergy is becoming an increasingly recognized problem that requires strict adherence to hospital policies to avoid serious adverse reactions.

Routine preoperative investigations are unnecessary in healthy children and should be performed only if indicated. Blood should be cross-matched or serum group-and-saved if the surgery warrants it.

IMPORTANT COMORBIDITIES AND ANAESTHESIA

Upper respiratory tract infection

General anaesthesia in the presence of acute or recent upper respiratory tract infection (URTI) has been associated with hypoxaemia, laryngospasm, bronchospasm and death.

> **Box 8.3 Factors indicating that elective surgery should be postponed in a child presenting with an upper respiratory tract infection**
>
> Systemically unwell
> Fever >38 °C
> Mucopurulent nasal secretions
> Lower respiratory symptoms or signs
>
> Have a lower threshold for postponing surgery if the patient is under 12 months of age or if surgery requires tracheal intubation.

Factors that are of greatest concern are listed in Box 8.3. If the URTI is mild in nature, i.e. the child is well and has clear nasal secretions and a clear chest to auscultation, then surgery, if minor, need not necessarily be postponed. Patients under 12 months of age and older children for whom tracheal intubation will be necessary probably should have surgery deferred, even if the URTI is only mild.

Asthma

A careful history to determine severity and frequency of episodes is of most value. Assessment of the adequacy of bronchodilator medication is important. Objective assessment of pulmonary function such as measurement of peak flow rate is not normally possible until the child is more than seven years of age. It is unwise to perform elective surgery within four weeks of a major exacerbation of asthma.

Apnoea

Ex-premature infants and, rarely, term neonates are at risk of postoperative apnoea. The risk decreases with post-conceptual age (PCA). Although consensus is lacking, it is common practice to admit all babies less than 56 weeks PCA for postoperative overnight apnoea and oxygen-saturation monitoring. Spinal anaesthesia may be associated with a lower incidence of postoperative complications, although the patient will still require an overnight stay.

Detection of a previously unsuspected heart murmur

Heart murmur is a relatively common problem. Its importance lies in distinguishing an innocent or flow murmur from a pathological or structural murmur. Any child under the age of one year should be referred for expert assessment before elective surgery. A child with any murmur other than a soft early systolic murmur should also be referred for investigation. In a child with an soft early systolic murmur and no other symptoms or signs and a normal electrocardiogram (ECG),

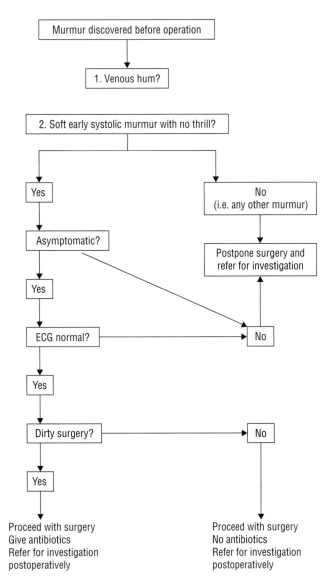

Figure 8.1 *Algorithm for the preoperative management of a child over the age of one year with a heart murmur. From McEwan AI, Birch M, Bingham R. The preoperative management of the child with a heart murmur.* Paediatric Anaesthesia *1995;* **5***: 151–6. With permission. ECG, electrocardiogram.*

surgery may proceed (Figure 8.1). Critical aortic stenosis and hypertrophic obstructive cardiomyopathy, both of which may be asymptomatic, are the two serious conditions that must be ruled out. In both conditions, the ECG will show signs of left ventricular hypertrophy. Appropriate antibiotic prophylaxis against endocarditis should be administered to all patients who have structural lesions.

PREOPERATIVE PREPARATION

Anxiety felt by parents is transmitted to the child, and although the patient should be the focus of attention, the entire family requires care. Preoperative information is vital

Table 8.4 *Preoperative fasting times in hours for elective surgery*

Oral intake	Duration of fasting required (h)
Clear fluids	2
Breast milk	4
Formula or cows' milk	6
Solid food	6

to allay anxiety; leaflets explaining the procedure and pre-admission programmes are very useful. The medical assessment of the patient as outlined above is only part of the function of the preoperative visit. Gaining the confidence of both the patient and the family by providing simple explanations in a manner that the child can understand is essential.

Parental presence at induction and premedication

Although not universally practised, parental presence at induction of anaesthesia may be of benefit in reducing the child's anxiety and distress at induction. Age under 12 months, emergency surgery and marked parental anxiety are relative contraindications to parental accompaniment. Additional nursing resources are required to provide an escort. Pharmacological sedation occasionally may be required, and the benzodiazepines are now most commonly used, either orally or nasally. Local anaesthetic creams have improved the acceptability of intravenous cannulation for the induction of anaesthesia.

Starvation policies

Fasting before induction of anaesthesia is important to minimize the risk of pulmonary aspiration, and instructions should be simple and easy to follow (Table 8.4). Free intake of clear fluids up to two hours before surgery in otherwise healthy children undergoing elective surgery is usually permitted, as both gastric acidity and the volume of gastric contents do not appear to be any greater than after longer periods of starvation.

Stomach emptying is delayed in injured and ill patients. It is prudent to wait six hours from the last oral intake before surgery, although the time between the last intake and the injury is probably more important than the total fasting time. A reduced period of fasting may be acceptable if surgery is considered urgent. The risk of pulmonary aspiration is minimized by performing a rapid-sequence induction. This consists of pre-oxygenation of the patient, intravenous induction and rapid-onset neuromuscular blockade, the application of cricoid pressure by a skilled assistant, and tracheal intubation.

CONSENT

In the UK at present, it is not necessary to obtain separate consent for anaesthesia and surgery. However, it is advisable to record a brief summary of the discussions about the

Table 8.5 *Anaesthesia-related complication rates for patients classified as American Society of Anesthesiologists (ASA) I or II*

Complication	Approximate incidence
Nausea and vomiting	1/4
Sore throat	1/10
Muscle pains	1/20
Headache	1/20
Serious drug reaction	1/5000
Death solely from anaesthesia	1/500 000–1/100 000

Box 8.4 Anaesthetic management considerations

Have instructions about fasting been given?

Is premedication necessary?

Will a parent be accompanying the child to the anaesthetic room?

Will induction of anaesthesia be intravenous or inhalational?

Will tracheal intubation be required?

Will muscle relaxation be required, either for the purposes of tracheal intubation or for surgical reasons?

What form of analgesia will be required intraoperatively and postoperatively (local or regional techniques or systemic analgesics)?

What special postoperative facilities will be required?

---

anaesthetic technique and the anticipated risks, where appropriate. The incidence and severity of anaesthesia-related complications (Table 8.5) are influenced by the patient's age, the patient's general physical status (ASA classification), the surgical procedure and the anaesthetic technique employed. A correlation between ASA grading and postoperative mortality has been demonstrated, although there is a considerable margin for error in the assessment of a patient's ASA grade. It is worth noting that death attributable solely to anaesthesia is extremely rare in otherwise healthy patients.

CONDUCT OF ANAESTHESIA

It is beyond the scope of this chapter to discuss detailed anaesthetic management. However, when formulating an anaesthetic plan, the considerations shown in Box 8.4 are important.

INTRAOPERATIVE FLUID MANAGEMENT

Intravenous fluids should be administered to patients undergoing intermediate and major surgery. Intraoperative fluid management includes the administration of the hourly maintenance requirements, the replacement of any deficit

Table 8.6 *Maintenance fluid requirements*

Body weight (kg)	Fluid requirements
0–10	4 mL/kg/h
10–20	40 mL/h + 2 mL/kg/h for each kilogram over 10 kg
21–70	60 mL/h + 1 ml/kg/h for each kilogram over 20 kg

Table 8.7 *Nerves at risk from damage as a result of poor positioning during surgery*

Nerve injury	Risk factor
Ulna	Pressure on elbow
Radial	Pressure on medial aspect of upper arm
Common peroneal	Lithotomy, lateral position
Supraorbital	Prone position
Nerves of the brachial plexus	Arm abducted, lateral position

from preoperative starvation or any other cause such as diarrhoea or vomiting, and the replacement of intraoperative losses. Normal maintenance requirements are shown in Table 8.6. Intraoperative fluid loss relates mainly to third-space loss and blood loss. It should be replaced with isotonic fluid such as normal saline or Ringer-lactate. The sequestration of fluid in the non-functional third space increases according to the degree of surgical trauma and may exceed 12 mL/kg/h. Blood loss should be replaced with crystalloid in a ratio of three to one or with colloid or blood in a ratio of one to one. Once blood loss exceeds ten per cent of the circulating blood volume, consideration should be given to the transfusion of blood.

POSITIONING OF PATIENT

Responsibility for the positioning of the patient on the operating theatre table is shared between the anaesthetist, the surgeon and the theatre staff. Skin damage or peripheral nerve injury can occur during the movement and positioning of the patient (Table 8.7). The skin over bony prominences is especially vulnerable, and padding of all pressure areas is essential.

Particular care should be taken with patients in the prone position. Direct pressure to the abdomen can cause obstruction to venous return and a reduction in cardiac output. Chest-wall movement is restricted in the prone position, and controlled ventilation is mandatory. The eyes should always be closed and protected during anaesthesia and padded carefully in patients who are to be placed prone.

THERMOREGULATION

A large surface area/body weight ratio makes children particularly vulnerable to heat loss during anaesthesia. Body heat may be preserved by vasoconstriction and generated by shivering.

Infants under three months of age cannot shiver but increase heat production by non-shivering thermogenesis (NST). Both shivering and NST increase oxygen consumption, which may predispose to hypoxaemia, particularly in the presence of cardiac or lung disease. Other deleterious effects of hypothermia (temperature $< 35\,^{\circ}\text{C}$) include myocardial depression, poor peripheral perfusion and acidosis, impaired coagulation and poor wound healing. Anaesthetic agents and regional techniques cause peripheral vasodilation, encouraging heat loss by redistributing heat from the core to periphery. Continuous monitoring of temperature is almost routine. Thermometer probes are available to measure skin and core temperatures. Core temperature may be measured reliably in the nasopharynx or lower oesophagus. Passive insulation or active warming devices, or both, are used routinely. Circulating water mattresses, although still in common use, are being superseded by more effective forced air-warming devices. Intravenous fluids should be warmed, particularly if they are to be administered rapidly or in large quantities, and inspired gases should be humidified.

STRESS RESPONSE TO SURGERY

Surgery or major trauma produces a systemic reaction involving a wide range of endocrine, immunological and haematological effects. There is increased secretion of pituitary hormones and activation of the sympathetic nervous system. Increased catabolism leads to the mobilization of substrates to provide energy sources. Retention of salt and water also occurs in order to maintain circulating volume. The stress response may have a useful role in helping the injured animal survive, but it may not be beneficial during the controlled circumstances of surgery. Indeed, it may delay recovery and have other adverse sequelae. For example, hyperglycaemia resulting from the release of catabolic hormones may increase the incidence of wound infection.

Opioids suppress the adverse haemodynamic effects of surgery and, in high dosages, suppress the stress response to major abdominal surgery, with possible improvements in postoperative recovery. However, this technique necessitates postoperative ventilation. General anaesthesia combined with epidural analgesia also reduces the stress response to major abdominal surgery but is technically challenging, particularly in neonates and infants, and it is not without the potential for morbidity. To maximize the attenuation of the stress response, blockade from dermatomal segments T4–S5 is required. There is limited objective evidence that epidural analgesia is more effective than intravenous opioid analgesia in children.

ANALGESIA

Pain assessment is fundamental to the good provision of pain relief. A variety of pain rating scales have been devised, depending on the age and cognitive ability of the child. Self-reporting scales and observer-based scales are available. The latter involve an assessment of behavioural changes such as crying, facial grimacing, motor activity, posture and sleep, and physiological variables such as sweating, heart rate and blood pressure. The importance of a pain-management plan employing a multimodal approach cannot be overemphasized. This includes the routine use of local or regional anaesthetic techniques unless there are contraindications, the use of opioids and the regular use of non-steroidal anti-inflammatory drugs (NSAIDs) and paracetamol. Other strategies that address the emotional aspects of pain perception, such as comforting measures, the provision of a child-friendly environment and the use of distraction techniques, are important.

POSTOPERATIVE RECOVERY

Following surgery, patients require a period of physiological stabilization in the recovery room. Staffing ratios should enable close observation of the patient and monitoring of vital signs. Oxygen should be administered routinely to maintain oxygen saturations greater than or equal to 94 per cent. For patients who have undergone major surgery, oxygen saturation monitoring should be continued on the ward. Oxygen administration may be necessary for several days, particularly for patients receiving opioid infusions, who are at risk from hypoxaemic episodes during sleep. Before discharge from the recovery room, the patient should have full return of protective reflexes, good airway control, and an easy and relaxed respiratory pattern and should be able to cough well. Blood pressure and pulse should be stable. There should be no bleeding, and intravenous fluids should be prescribed where indicated. All intravenous cannulae, catheters and drains should be secured carefully. Pain should be under control and nausea or vomiting should be treated appropriately. The patient should be awake and able to move all extremities voluntarily. Efforts to maintain body temperature should continue throughout the postoperative recovery phase.

Respiratory complications

Clinically significant hypoventilation resulting in hypoxaemia or hypercarbia may occur postoperatively. Treatment should be directed at reversing the primary cause (Table 8.8). It should be noted that the administration of supplementary oxygen to a patient who is hypoventilating can provide an adequate arterial oxygen saturation but will not reverse hypercarbia. Clinically, carbon dioxide retention leads to warm peripheries, a bounding pulse and, eventually, central nervous system depression (CO_2 narcosis). If suspected, arterial blood gases should be measured. Hypoventilation due to residual neuromuscular blockade needs urgent treatment, whereas hypoventilation due to opioid overdose can be reversed with the pure opioid antagonist naloxone. If the dose is titrated carefully, then the respiratory depressant effects can be reversed without significantly affecting analgesic efficacy.

Table 8.8 *Some causes of postoperative hypoxaemia*

Problem	Cause
Hypoventilation	*Adverse effects of drugs:* Opioids Inhalational anaesthetic agents Residual neuromuscular blockade Apnoea Pain Upper airway obstruction Tracheal oedema Pneumothorax Inadvertent high epidural blockade
Pulmonary shunting	Atelectasis Pneumonia Pulmonary aspiration Pulmonary oedema
Increased oxygen expenditure	Shivering
Anaemia*	Blood loss
Decreased cardiac output*	Residual effect of anaesthetic agents Hypovolaemia Regional blockade

* A decrease in oxygen content or oxygen delivery rather than hypoxaemia is the effect here. Measurements of oxygen saturation will usually be normal.

Cardiovascular complications

Postoperative hypotension is usually the result of hypovolaemia or vasodilation. The latter may be caused by the residual effects of general anaesthetic drugs or by epidural or subarachnoid blockade, although children under five years of age show little change in blood pressure or heart rate following regional blockade. Volume expansion is generally the first step in the resolution of hypotension in the recovery room, although vasopressor agents may also have a role.

FURTHER READING

Great Ormond Street Hospital. www.ich.ucl.ac.uk/clinserv/anaesthetics/index.html

Hatch D, Sumner E, Hellmann J. *The Surgical Neonate: Anaesthesia and Intensive Care.* London: Arnold, 1994.

Hughes DG, Mather SJ, Wolf AR. *Handbook of Neonatal Anaesthesia.* London: WB Saunders, 1996.

Mather SJ, Hughes DG. *Handbook of Paediatric Anaesthesia.* Oxford: Oxford University Press, 1996.

Royal College of Paediatrics and Child Health. *Prevention and Control of Pain in Children: A Manual for Health Care Professionals.* London: BMJ Publishing Group, 1997.

Steward D, Lerman J. *Manual of Paediatric Anaesthesia*, 5th edn. New York: Churchill Livingstone, 2001.

9

Homeostasis: fluid and electrolyte balance

EVELYN GP ONG AND AGOSTINO PIERRO

Learning objectives

- To understand the normal homeostatic mechanisms.
- To understand the hormonal and metabolic responses to surgical stress.
- To understand the theories underlying normal fluid maintenance and appropriate application of fluid regimens to different clinical scenarios.

INTRODUCTION

The concept of homeostasis (*homeo* = same, *stasis* = stop) was introduced by a nineteenth-century French physiologist, Claude Bernard, who described it as 'the fixity of the *milieu interieur*'. In current terms, homeostasis is the maintenance of a steady internal environment in the presence of changing conditions. Parameters maintained are temperature, glucose, electrolytes, acid–base balance, fluids, metabolic rate, respiration and haemodynamics. Due to the unique nature of neonatal physiology, a large proportion of this chapter will focus on neonates.

NEONATAL PHYSIOLOGY

Thermoregulation

Heat generated from muscles, food and catabolism is balanced by heat loss from evaporation (sweat), conduction (direct skin contact with cool surfaces), convection (air currents), radiation and excretion. Thermoneutrality, the optimal thermal environment, is between 32 and 34 °C in neonates and between 36.3 and 37.1 °C in young adults.

Thermoregulation is particularly difficult for neonates, as they lose relatively higher amounts of heat due to a larger surface area to volume ratio. They compensate by utilizing brown adipose tissue for non-shivering thermogenesis. This highly specialized fat contains an abundance of mitochondria and is capable of uncoupling metabolism and production of adenosine 5'-triphosphate (ATP), thus generating more heat. Brown fat is also innervated by sympathetic nerve fibres, which, when stimulated, increase lipolysis, fatty-acid oxidation and blood flow to brown adipocytes. This sympathetic stimulus may be integral to the stimulus to feed.

Glucose metabolism

Fetal serum glucose levels are slightly higher than maternal levels, but levels fall rapidly within the first hour to 2.5 mmol/L postpartum as glycogen stores accumulated antenatally are consumed (Hoseth *et al.* 2000). Increased insulin secretion results in mobilization of glucose and fat and stimulates gluconeogenesis, thereby increasing endogenous production of glucose and stabilizing serum glucose between 2.5 and 7.2 mmol/L.

Hypoglycaemia

Clinical signs of hypoglycaemia (serum glucose less than 2–2.5 mmol/L) are non-specific and include tremors, lethargy, irritability, pallor, poor feeding, apnoea or tachypnoea, cyanosis, temperature instability, tachycardia, convulsions, coma and death. Premature and low-birth-weight infants have limited hepatic glycogen stores and a lower capacity to mobilize glucose, which results in an increased risk of hypoglycaemia. These stores are also depleted rapidly following catecholamine release stimulated by perinatal stress. Infants of diabetic mothers frequently have larger fat and glycogen stores, but these can be depleted by reactive hyperinsulinism, and therefore these neonates can still become hypoglycaemic. Other contributing causes of hypoglycaemia are vomiting, inadequate exogenous glucose, prematurity, sepsis and hypothermia.

Treatment is by increasing the percentage of dextrose in intravenous infusions up to a maximum of 50% dextrose solution if a central venous line is used. Peripheral veins tolerate infusions of up to 12.5% dextrose solution. Occasionally, persistent hypoglycaemia is treated using steroids, glucagon or somatostatin analogues.

Hyperglycaemia

Hyperglycaemia (serum glucose above 14 mmol/L) may be asymptomatic or manifest as glucosuria with an osmotic diuresis and dehydration. The rise in plasma osmosis increases the risk of intracranial haemorrhage. Insulin-secreting pancreatic cells of infants are less sensitive to rising glucose concentrations, and hyperglycaemia can result from stress and catecholamine-stimulated glucose mobilization. Preterm infants are particularly prone to labile serum glucose levels. Insulin insensitivity is greater in the preterm infant than in the term infant, and the preterm infant may become hyperglycaemic while receiving a glucose infusion.

Treatment is by reducing exogenous dextrose administration, e.g. intravenous 10% dextrose solution reduced to 5% dextrose solution. Occasionally, insulin infusions are required.

Body water composition

Total body water (TBW) is divided into two compartments, intracellular water and extracellular water. During the first trimester, 92 per cent of body mass is TBW, but this declines to 80 per cent by 32 weeks' gestation and is approximately 75 per cent by term. This is mirrored by contraction of the extracellular compartment from 65 per cent of body mass at 20 weeks' gestation to 40 per cent at term (Friis-Hansen 1983).

There is an initial oliguria during the first day postpartum. Over the following one to two days, there are dramatic shifts in fluid from the intracellular to the extracellular compartment, with a resultant diuresis and natriuresis. The resultant loss of weight during the first week of life is five to ten per cent in the term neonate and 10–20 per cent in the premature infant. This diuresis occurs regardless of fluid intake or insensible losses. However, by the fifth day postpartum, excretion begins to reflect the fluid status of the infant.

Renal function

Neonatal renal blood flow and plasma flow are low, but renovascular resistance is high, resulting in a reduced glomerular filtration rate (GFR). During the first 24 hours postpartum, distribution of cortical perfusion alters, with increased perfusion of the outer cortex. The GFR rises rapidly during this time despite total renal blood flow being the same. Gradually, total renal blood flow increases and renovascular resistance decreases. As a result, GFR rises rapidly during the first three months of life and then undergoes a slower rise to adult levels by 12–24 months of age. Premature and low-birth-weight infants may have a lower GFR than term infants, and the subsequent rise may be delayed. All these changes make the monitoring of renal function using serum creatinine in the first few days postpartum difficult.

The counter-current system of the loop of Henlé depends on the osmolality of the medullary interstitium to function. In neonates, the low osmolality in the renal medulla means that the urine concentration capacity is only 50–600 mosmol/kg compared with 1200 mosmol/kg in adults. Antidiuretic hormone (ADH) release regulates serum osmolality in the term infant between 275 and 280 mosmol/kg and is secreted at almost adult levels. However, compared with adults, neonatal renal tubules are relatively insensitive to ADH.

Sodium

Serum sodium levels are maintained at 135–140 mmol/L mainly by the kidneys and are the major determinant of osmolality and, therefore, extracellular fluid volume. Urinary sodium excretion is dependent on the GFR and therefore is low in neonates compared with adults. In addition, neonates have a limited tubular capacity to reabsorb sodium and therefore have greater urinary sodium losses (more so in preterm than term infants). Normal maintenance sodium requirement is 2–4 mmol/kg/day.

HYPONATRAEMIA

Serum sodium concentrations of less than 135 mmol/L can occur in a state of hypovolaemia, euvolaemia and hypervolaemia (Table 9.1). Symptoms often are not apparent until serum sodium falls below 120 mmol/L and manifests as the effects of cerebral oedema: apathy, nausea, vomiting, headache, fits and coma. The severity of symptoms is related directly to the rapidity of onset and magnitude of hyponatraemia.

Table 9.1 *Causes of sodium balance derangement in infants and children*

	Hypovolaemic	Euvolaemic	Hypervolaemic
Hyponatraemia	Gastrointestinal losses, e.g. vomiting, diarrhoea, small-bowel fistula, ileostomy Congestive cardiac failure	Syndrome of inappropriate secretion of ADH	
	Intake of hypotonic solutions	Diuretics	Liver cirrhosis
	Renal disease		Nephrotic syndrome
	Cerebral salt wasting disease		Renal failure
	Perspiration, e.g. cystic fibrosis, adrenal insufficiency		
Hypernatraemia	Diabetes insipidus Excessive sweating Increased insensible losses	ADH insufficiency	Excess sodium intake

ADH, antidiuretic hormone.

The kidneys respond to a fall in serum sodium by excreting more dilute urine, but the secretion of ADH in response to hypovolaemia affects this. We can therefore use urinary sodium to help determine the underlying cause of hyponatraemia. Urine sodium concentrations below 10 mmol/L indicate an appropriate renal response to euvolaemic hyponatraemia. However, if the urinary sodium concentration is above 20 mmol/L, then this can indicate either sodium leak from damaged renal tubules or hypervolaemia.

HYPERNATRAEMIA

Hypernatraemia (serum sodium > 145 mmol/L) can occur in varying states of hydration (Table 9.1). This occurs in children most commonly secondary to hypotonic fluid losses, e.g. diarrhoea. Clinical signs include dry mucous membranes, loss of skin turgidity, drowsiness, irritability, hypertonicity, fits and coma. Fluid loss from the cerebral tissues can result in tearing blood vessels and cerebral haemorrhage. Cerebral tissues respond by retaining intracellular taurine to increase return of water from the extracellular compartment. Be aware that hypocalcaemia can often accompany hypernatraemia.

Potassium

Potassium is the most abundant intracellular cation and is essential for maintaining the cellular transmural ion gradient. A maintenance intake of 1–3 mmol/kg/day is required to maintain serum potassium at normal levels (3.5–5.8 mmol/L). In the 24–72 hours postpartum, a large shift of potassium from intracellular to extracellular compartments occurs, resulting in a rise in plasma potassium. This is compounded by the diuresis phase, which limits the amount of tubular excretion of potassium by limiting the availability of water and sodium. This effect is related directly to the degree of prematurity and can cause significant morbidity. However, potassium falls eventually as the diuresis phase ends and potassium excretion rises.

HYPOKALAEMIA

This is most commonly iatrogenic, due to either inadequate potassium intake or use of diuretics, but it can also be caused by vomiting, diarrhoea, alkalosis (which drives potassium intracellularly) or polyuric renal failure. Insulin and sympathetic system stimulation also drive potassium into cells and can exaggerate pre-existing hypokalaemia. The normal ion gradient is disrupted and predisposes to muscle current conduction abnormalities, e.g. cardiac arrhythmias, paralytic ileus, urinary retention and respiratory muscle paralysis.

HYPERKALAEMIA

This can occur secondary to sever metabolic acidosis, cell necrosis with release of intracellular potassium, e.g. severe crush injuries, acute renal failure, iatrogenic excessive intake, adrenal insufficiency, insulin-dependent diabetes mellitus and severe haemolysis. Hyperkalaemia can deteriorate further in the presence of hypoxia, metabolic acidosis, catabolic stress and oliguria. Preterm infants may also suffer from hyperkalaemia, with high insensible fluid losses. As in hypokalaemia, hyperkalaemia alters the electrical gradient of cell membranes, and patients are vulnerable to cardiac arrhythmias, including asystole.

Calcium

Calcium plays important roles in enzyme activity, muscle contraction and relaxation, the blood coagulation cascade, bone metabolism and nerve conduction. Calcium is maintained at a total serum concentration of 1.8–2.1 mmol/L in neonates and 2–2.5 mmol/L in term infants and is divided into three fractions. Between 30 and 50 per cent is protein-bound; 5–15 per cent is complexed with citrate, lactate, bicarbonate and inorganic ions; and the remaining free calcium ions are metabolically active, and concentrations fluctuate with serum albumin levels. Hydrogen ions compete reversibly with calcium for albumin binding sites and, therefore, free calcium concentrations increase in acidosis.

Calcium metabolism is under the control of many hormones, but primarily 1,25-dihydroxycholecalciferol (gastrointestinal absorption of calcium, bone resorption, increased renal calcium reabsorption), parathyroid hormone (bone resorption, decreased urinary excretion) and calcitonin (bone formation and increases urinary excretion). Calcium is actively transported from maternal to fetal circulation against the concentration gradient, resulting in peripartum hypercalcaemia. There is a transient fall in calcium postpartum to 1.8–2.1 mmol/L and a gradual rise to normal infant levels over 24–48 hours.

HYPOCALCAEMIA

In addition to the physiological hypocalcaemia of neonates, which is usually asymptomatic, other causes of hypocalcaemia are hypoparathyroidism, including Di George syndrome, and parathyroid hormone insensitivity in infants of diabetic mothers, which may also be related to hypomagnesaemia. Clinical manifestations are tremor, seizures and a prolonged QT interval on the electrocardiogram (ECG).

HYPERCALCAEMIA

This is less common than hypocalcaemia, but it can result from inborn errors of metabolism such as familial hypercalcaemic hypocalcuria and primary hyperparathyroidism. Iatrogenic causes include vitamin A overdose and deficient dietary phosphate intake. Less common causes in children are tertiary hyperparathyroidism, paraneoplastic syndromes and metastatic bone disease.

Magnesium

As an important enzyme cofactor, magnesium affects ATP metabolism and glycolysis. Only 20 per cent of total body magnesium is exchangeable with the biologically active free ion form. The remainder is bound in bone or to intracellular protein, ribonucleic acid (RNA) or ATP, mostly in muscle and liver. Gastrointestinal absorption of magnesium is controlled by vitamin D, parathyroid hormone and sodium reabsorption. Hypomagnesaemia is often related to hypocalcaemia and should be considered.

Acid–base balance

Acid–base balance is achieved using three systems: (i) a buffer system, e.g. carbonic anhydrase, (ii) respiration and (iii) renal function. Conditions that can upset this balance are listed in Table 9.2. Arterial blood gases are used to help identify the cause. Acid–base state is given by the pH, while high or low bicarbonate and carbon dioxide partial pressures indicate whether the source is metabolic or respiratory. The priority is to treat any underlying cause, e.g. metabolic acidosis caused by dehydration or sepsis. The slow infusion of buffers such as sodium bicarbonate and tris-hydroxymethylaminomethane

Table 9.2 *Causes of acid–base balance disturbance in surgical infants and children*

	Acidosis	Alkalosis
Metabolic	Hypovolaemia Lactic acidosis Renal failure	Prolonged vomiting Gastric aspiration Diuretic use
Respiratory	Respiratory depression, e.g. opiates Underexpansion of lungs Airway obstruction	Hyperventilation Acute hypoxia, e.g. pneumonia

(THAM; a sodium-free buffer) should be used as therapeutic adjuncts. The amount of sodium bicarbonate required can be calculated using the following equation:

$$NaHCO_2 \text{ in millimoles} = \frac{(\text{base excess} \times \text{body weight in kilograms})}{3}$$

RESPONSE TO SURGICAL STRESS

Injury to tissues provides stimulus to nociceptors, baroreceptors and chemoreceptors, thus initiating a neuroendocrine reflex. Evidence of the ability to respond to pain has been found in the fetus as early as 20 weeks' gestation. The efferent arc of the reflex originates in the hypothalamus, which communicates with the autonomic nervous system and the pituitary gland. Catecholamines are released from the adrenal glands by stimulation of the sympathetic system. Corticotrophin releasing hormone is produced by the hypothalamus and stimulates the release of adrenocorticotrophic hormone from the anterior pituitary, resulting in an increase in cortisol. Growth hormone is released from the anterior pituitary and ADH is released from the posterior pituitary.

The hormonal and metabolic responses to surgery are well documented in adults, but we are only now elucidating the responses in infants and children. Essential differences are children's lower endogenous energy reserves and the energy-consuming demands of growth and development in neonates: protein turnover in neonates is 6.7 g/kg/day compared with 3.5 g/kg/day in adults. Adult studies demonstrate that a prolonged negative nitrogen balance is associated with poorer clinical outcome, and therefore adequate nutritional support is essential.

In contrast with adults, the energy requirement of infants and children undergoing major operations seems to be modified minimally by the actual operative trauma. In adults, trauma or surgery causes a brief 'ebb period' of a depressed metabolic rate followed by a 'flow phase' characterized by an increase in oxygen consumption to support the massive exchanges of substrate between organs (Cuthbertson et al. 2001) (Figure 9.1). In newborn infants, major abdominal

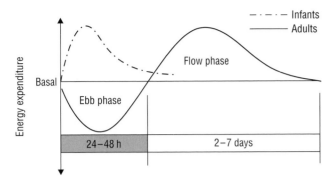

Figure 9.1 *Variations in postoperative energy expenditure in adults and infants. Note the contrast between the 'ebb' and 'flow' phases in adults compared with the monophasic changes in infants.*

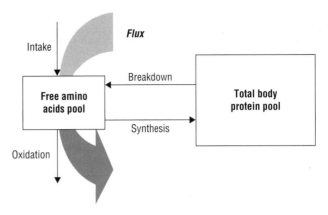

Figure 9.2 *Simplified model of whole-body protein dynamics (after Pierro 2002).*

surgery causes a moderate (15 per cent) and immediate (peak at four hours) elevation of oxygen consumption and resting energy expenditure and a rapid return to baseline 12–24 hours postoperatively (Pierro 2002) (Figure 9.1). There is no further increase in energy expenditure in the first five to seven days following an operation. The timing of these changes corresponds with the postoperative increase in catecholamine levels. The maximum endocrine and biochemical changes are observed immediately after the operation and gradually return to normal over the next 24 hours (Pierro 2002). Resting energy expenditure is directly proportional to growth rate in healthy infants, and growth is retarded during acute metabolic stress. It is possible that energy is utilized for growth recovery following the resolution of the acute injury response in surgical infants (Pierro 2002).

Recently, there has been considerable interest in the cytokines tumour necrosis factor (TNF) and interleukins (IL) as mediators and markers of the stress response in adults. Cytokines bond to specific membrane receptors of target organs. Their actions in the acute stress response include (i) changes in gene expression and proliferation, thereby affecting wound healing and immunocompetence; (ii) release of counter-regulatory hormones; and (iii) facilitation of cell-to-cell communication. Substrate utilization is also affected by cytokine release. However, systemic cytokine release cannot account for all the metabolic changes seen after injury, since cytokines are not found consistently in the bloodstream of injured patients, and systemic cytokine administration does not produce all of the metabolic effects observed in injured adult individuals.

Whole-body protein metabolism kinetics can now be investigated non-invasively with the use of stable isotope-turnover techniques. Protein turnover can be calculated using the simplified model of protein dynamics shown in Figure 9.2. This assumes that there is a plasma free amino acid pool that is in constant equilibrium with the intracellular pool, which together comprise a single homogeneous body protein pool. Amino acids enter the free amino acid pool from dietary intake and from the breakdown of body protein

(catabolism), and leave by protein synthesis and oxidation. Thus, in the steady state:

Amino acids flux = intake + breakdown = synthesis + oxidation

After infusion of a labelled amino acid, e.g. ^{13}C-leucine, flux can be calculated from the plateau isotopic enrichment of the amino acid in plasma, and oxidation can be calculated from the plateau isotopic enrichment of expired CO_2. If intake is known, then synthesis and breakdown can be derived from the above equation.

Studies in adult surgical patients have shown that operative stress causes marked changes in protein metabolism characterized by a postoperative increase in protein degradation, a negative nitrogen balance, and a decrease in muscle protein synthesis. The protein metabolism kinetics of infants and young children who have undergone major operations have been investigated and shown that children do not increase their whole-body protein turnover after major operations. It is possible that infants and children are able to convert energy expended on growth to energy directed to wound repair and healing, thereby avoiding the overall increase in energy expenditure and catabolism seen in adults.

FLUID AND ELECTROLYTE MANAGEMENT

Maintenance regimes

The principle of any fluid maintenance regime is to replace volume and electrolyte losses with fluids of like volume and composition. These include quantifiable (e.g. urine, faeces, stoma losses, vomitus or nasogastric aspirates) and insensible (e.g. sweat, gastrointestinal secretions, breath condensate) losses. The volume of insensible losses varies depending on the condition of the patient and the environment (Table 9.3). The lower the birth weight, the higher the insensible water loss tends to be (60–80 mL/kg/day < 1000 g versus

Table 9.3 *Factors affecting insensible water loss in neonates*

Increased insensible water loss	Strategies to prevent water loss
Increased respiratory rate	Humidification of ventilatory gases
Skin injury or loss	Use of transparent plastic barriers, e.g. clear plastic wrap, bubble wrap
Congenital body-wall defects, e.g. gastroschisis, exomphalos, neural tube defects	Use of incubators
Increased body temperature: 30% increase per degree Celsius	Use of heat shields
Increased environmental temperature: 30% increase per degree Celsius	Humidification of ambient air
Use of radiant heater or phototherapy lights	
Decreased environmental humidity	
Increased motor activity or crying	

Table 9.4 *Calculation of fluid requirement*

Age range	Weight	Fluid requirement/24 h
Premature infants	1000 g	200 mL/kg
	1500 g	175 mL/kg
	2500 g	150 mL/kg
Term neonates, infants	2–10 kg	100 mL/kg for first 10 kg
Infants, children	10–20 kg	1000 mL + 50 mL/kg over 10 kg
Children	>20 kg	1500 mL + 25 mL/kg over 20 kg

20 mL/kg/day > 1500 g). Transepithelial water loss accounts for up to 70 per cent of insensible water loss, with the remainder being lost largely from respiration, and can be prevented using different measures.

Day one of the fluid regimen of a neonate consists of 10% dextrose solution 80 mL/kg/day if body weight is less than 1500 g or 60 mL/kg/day if body weight is over 1500 kg. Additional adjustments are made for use of radiant heaters and phototherapy lights (add a further 20 mL/kg/day per light or heater used). After day one, provided urine is passed, sodium and potassium may be added, and the total fluid volume administered is increased gradually over a week up to 150–180 mL/kg/day of 10% dextrose solution plus electrolytes. Daily fluid requirements for older children are also based on body mass (Table 9.4).

Monitoring fluid and electrolyte balance

Assessment and reassessment are the key to effective fluid management. Clinical assessment of a child's fluid status differs from that in adults. Poor skin turgor, hypotension, poor peripheral perfusion, a sunken fontanelle and sunken eyes usually manifest only after ten per cent of TBW is lost. Blood pressure and heart rate are also well maintained until 15–20 per cent dehydration. The first sign of dehydration may therefore be oliguria. Normal urine output is 2 mL/kg/hour in neonates and children and >1 mL/kg/hour in adolescents.

Daily weights help assessment of fluid status. Neonates would be expected to lose up to ten per cent of their birth weight during the first week of life. Any excessive loss may indicate dehydration. Likewise, oedema and failure to lose any weight would merit fluid restriction. Other indications for fluid restriction include the immediate postoperative period (due to physiological fluid retention) and a clinically significant patent ductus arteriosis.

Creatinine and electrolyte measurement during the first 24 hours reflects maternal renal function. Subsequent rapid changes in GFR and fluid compartment shifts mean that a steady state is not achieved. Creatinine falls rapidly in the first few days postpartum (more so in prematurity) and therefore is not a reliable indicator of renal function (Lorenz 1997). Measurement of serum and urinary electrolytes and osmolality after the first 24 hours postpartum is helpful in adjusting electrolyte replacement.

Correction of electrolyte imbalance

SODIUM

Hyponatraemia must be corrected gradually over 24–48 hours. Cerebral tissues compensate for the hypotonicity of surrounding fluid by losing intracellular potassium and amino acids, thereby decreasing the potential for oedema. However, if hyponatraemia is corrected too rapidly, then the ensuing net shift in fluid from the intracellular compartment could lead to central pontine myelinolysis. Severe symptomatic hyponatraemia of less than 120 mmol/L can be corrected by administering hypertonic saline solution over four hours to 125 mmol/L, and then more slowly. Hypovolaemia can be corrected with isotonic solutions. Estimates of the amount of sodium required to resolve a deficiency can be made using the formula

$$\text{sodium in millimoles} = \text{desired [sodium]} - \text{actual [sodium]} \times 0.6 \times \text{mass in kilograms}$$

Hypovolaemic hypernatraemia should be treated with correction of dehydration. This should be gradual to prevent cerebral oedema and potential permanent brain injury. Hypervolaemic hypernatraemia should be treated by a combination of sodium and fluid restriction. In central diabetes insipidus, vasopressin can be used as an adjunct to fluid management.

POTASSIUM

Hypokalaemia can be prevented by anticipating potential gastrointestinal losses and replacement with the same volume of normal saline supplemented with potassium chloride (20 mmol per litre of saline), to be given in addition to daily maintenance fluids. Mild hypokalaemia may not require treatment in asymptomatic patients. Severe hypokalaemia should be treated by two- to three-hour infusions of 20 mmol potassium chloride in 500 mL normal saline. It is difficult to calculate the precise amount of potassium required because the majority of body potassium is intracellular and the serum levels do not necessarily reflect this; therefore, patients must be cardiac-monitored throughout and serum potassium levels must be checked regularly. In patients with hypochloraemic alkalosis, hypokalaemia may be difficult to treat without correcting the chloride deficiency as well.

Hyperkalaemia is treated by omitting all exogenous sources of potassium, including less overt sources, e.g. potassium-sparing diuretics such as spironolactone and amiloride. This is usually enough to treat mild hyperkalaemia. Severe hyperkalaemia with ECG changes should be treated with an immediate 10 per cent calcium gluconate (1 mL/kg) infusion to stabilize the myocardium. Insulin and dextrose infusions are then used to drive potassium into the intracellular compartment. Any metabolic acidosis should be treated. In addition, cation-exchange resins, e.g. calcium polystyrene sulphonate (0.5–1 g/kg in divided doses), can be given orally or rectally to bind potassium. In patients with renal failure, dialysis may be required.

CALCIUM

Asymptomatic mild hypocalcaemia may not need treatment. Oral supplements can be used if tolerated. However, aggressive treatment of hypocalcaemia in the sick neonate can be hazardous as well as ineffective. Symptomatic hypocalcaemia can be treated with slow infusions of calcium gluconate. Keep in mind that hypocalcaemia may be resistant unless any hypomagnesaemia is treated simultaneously.

Hypercalcaemia is treated by rehydration. Any drugs that contribute to calcium retention and mobilization, e.g. thiazides and vitamin D, should be stopped. The use of chelators such as trisodium edetate is no longer recommended.

MAGNESIUM

Symptomatic hypomagnesaemia can be treated either parenterally or intramuscularly using 50 per cent magnesium sulphate (0.5 mmol/kg two to three times per day). Note that the injections are painful. Oral preparations for maintenance are available.

SEPSIS AND SHOCK

Sepsis occurs in up to five in 1000 infants and accounts for significant morbidity and mortality. Local inflammation and endotoxins released from the infecting organism initiate a cascade of cytokine-mediated reactions, resulting in loss of systemic vascular resistance, depression of the myocardium, fall in tissue perfusion and, ultimately, multiorgan failure. Increased vasodilation and vascular leakage leads to shift of fluid from the circulation to the interstitium. Therefore, despite fluid retention and an increase in TBW, the circulating volume is effectively reduced.

Acute management is by rapid rehydration using a bolus of either 0.9% saline or colloid (10–20 mL/kg). Inotropic agents can be infused to help cardiac output. Dopamine used at a dose of <5 μg/kg/minute increases renal and intestinal blood flow and at higher doses (5–20 μg/kg/minute) is a positive inotrope. Dobutamine is also a positive inotrope with peripheral vasodilator effects. Adrenaline and noradrenaline can also be used to treat profound hypotension but have the effect of peripheral vasoconstriction. Hyperkalaemia can be caused by oliguria and cell injury. Hyponatraemia can result from an increase in TBW due to inappropriate ADH secretion. Both should be corrected as described previously. Blood gases will demonstrate any acid–base imbalance that requires correction, and lactate can indicate the degree of hypoperfusion present. The patient should be monitored closely. The underlying source of sepsis must be identified and treated.

Metabolic response to sepsis

Nutritional integrity should be maintained regardless of the severity of the illness or organ failure, particularly in neonates, due to their limited energy and protein stores (Pierro 2002). Infants and children require nutrition for maintenance of protein status as well as for growth and wound healing. A considerable challenge in paediatrics is nutrition support during critical illness and sepsis.

Sepsis is an intriguing pathological condition associated with many complex metabolic and physiological alterations. Studies in adults have shown that the metabolic response to sepsis is characterized by hypermetabolism, as documented by an increase in resting energy expenditure up to 49 per cent above that predicted. In addition, increased tissue catabolism, gluconeogenesis and hepatic release of glucose have been described. Energy is derived largely from endogenous fat, and the increased protein catabolism provides precursors for enhanced hepatic gluconeogenesis. In adult patients with sepsis, it has been shown that: (i) during the first ten days from the onset of sepsis, 67 per cent of the protein loss is from skeletal muscle; after this time protein loss is predominantly from viscera; and (ii) fat mobilization is far greater than fat oxidation, implying considerable cycling. At a later stage in sepsis, impaired oxidative metabolism and major metabolic abnormalities develop, and exogenous fat utilization may become impaired. The interaction between exogenous lipid administration, immune response and tissue catabolism deserves further investigation.

The existing knowledge of the metabolic response to sepsis in infants is limited. A recent metabolic study in septic neonates with necrotizing enterocolitis failed to show any increase in whole-body protein turnover, synthesis and catabolism. The metabolic rate and hormonal response to stress and sepsis in infants may be different from those of adults and, therefore, it is not possible to adapt recommendations made for adults to the neonatal population. It has been speculated that neonates divert the products of protein synthesis and breakdown from growth into tissue repair (Pierro 2002). This may explain the lack of growth commonly observed in infants with critical illness or sepsis.

REFERENCES

Cuthbertson DP, Angeles Valero Zanuy MA, Leon Sanz ML. Post-shock metabolic response. 1942. *Nutricion Hospitalaria* 2001; **16**: 176–82.

Friis-Hansen B. Water distribution in the foetus and newborn infant. *Acta Paediatrica Scandinavica Supplement* 1983; **305**: 7–11.

Hoseth E, Joergensen A, Ebbesen F, Moeller M. Blood glucose levels in a population of healthy, breast fed, term infants of appropriate size for gestational age. *Archives of Disease in Childhood: Fetal and Neonatal Edition* 2000; **83**: F117–19.

Lorenz JM. Assessing fluid and electrolyte status in the newborn. National Academy of Clinical Biochemistry. *Clinical Chemistry* 1997; **43**: 205–10.

Pierro A. Metabolism and nutritional support in the surgical neonate. *Journal of Pediatric Surgery* 2002; **37**: 811–22.

FURTHER READING

Denne SC, Kalhan SC. Leucine metabolism in human newborns. *American Journal of Physiology* 1987; **253**: E608–15.

Singhi S. Effect of maternal intrapartum glucose therapy on neonatal blood glucose levels and neurobehavioral status of hypoglycemic term newborn infants. *Journal of Perinatal Medicine* 1988; **16**: 217–24.

Vanhatalo S, van Nieuwenhuizen O. Fetal pain? *Brain Development* 2000; **22**: 145–50.

Ward Platt MP, Tarbit MJ, Aynsley-Green A. The effects of anesthesia and surgery on metabolic homeostasis in infancy and childhood. *Journal of Pediatric Surgery* 1990; **25**: 472–8

Nutrition

MARK BEATTIE

Learning objectives

- To understand the basic physiology of the gastrointestinal tract.
- To understand the importance of nutrition in health and disease and the principles of nutritional assessment.
- To understand nutritional requirements.
- To understand the basic principles of nutritional support, including feed type and methods of feed delivery, the importance of the nutrition team, and the basics of parenteral nutrition, including potential problems.
- To appreciate specific conditions of relevance, e.g. short bowel syndrome.

INTRODUCTION

Nutrition is a fundamental part of the assessment of any child. It is relevant to all aspects of medical practice, with impaired nutrition being a significant risk factor for ill health and a major concern in hospitalized patients. Poor nutrition is associated with increased morbidity and mortality, including delayed recovery from surgery and, as a consequence, longer hospital stays. Nutrition can be impaired as a consequence of poor intake or impaired absorption or because needs exceed intake in the child with increased requirements. This is negative energy balance. There are many pathological, psychological and social factors that contribute to this, and the key to effective intervention is multidisciplinary input using a sound knowledge base of the underlying mechanisms and different interventions available. It is important also to be aware of the emerging problem of over-nutrition, with childhood obesity now reaching epidemic proportions with implications for the short and long term.

Nutritional status reflects:

- what you are;
- what you eat;
- what you do.

BACKGROUND INFORMATION

Basic physiology of the gastrointestinal tract

STOMACH

The stomach is lined by columnar epithelium. Chief cells produce pepsin; parietal cells produce gastric acid and intrinsic factor. Gastric-acid secretion is stimulated by vagal stimulation, gastrin and histamine via histamine H_2 receptors on parietal cells. Secretion is inhibited by sympathetic stimulation, nausea, gastric acidity and small-intestinal peptides. Three litres of gastric secretions are produced per day in adults.

SMALL INTESTINE

The main function of the small intestine is absorption, which occurs mostly in the duodenum and jejunum, apart from bile salts and vitamin B12, which are absorbed in the terminal ileum. The length of the small bowel is 2–3 m in adults and 250 cm at birth in term infants.

COLON

The primary function of the colon is salt and water reabsorption. Its length is approximately 1 m in adults.
Sites of absorption are as follows:

* *Duodenum and jejunum*: fluids, carbohydrates, proteins, fat, iron, calcium, zinc, folate, most vitamins.
* *Terminal ileum*: vitamin B12, bile salts, vitamin K, vitamin C.
* *Colon*: water and sodium, fermented carbohydrates.

CARBOHYDRATE DIGESTION

Carbohydrates are consumed as monosaccharides (glucose, fructose, galactose), disaccharides (lactose, sucrose, maltose, isomaltose) and polysaccharides (starch, dextrins, glycogen). Salivary and pancreatic amylases break down starch into oligosaccharides and disaccharides. Disaccharidases (maltase, sucrase, lactase) in the microvilli hydrolyse oligosaccharides and disaccharides into monosaccharides, i.e. maltose into glucose, isomaltose into glucose, sucrose into glucose and fructose, and lactose into glucose and galactose. Glucose and galactose are then absorbed by an active transport mechanism, and fructose is absorbed by facilitated diffusion.

PROTEIN DIGESTION

In the stomach, gastric acid denatures protein and facilitates the conversion of pepsinogen into pepsin. Trypsin, chymotrypsin and elastase, secreted as their inactive precursors, are produced by the exocrine pancreas. Enterokinase (secreted in the proximal duodenum) activates trypsin; trypsin further activates trypsin, chymotrypsin and elastase. These proteases convert proteins into oligopeptides and amino acids in the duodenum. The small intestine absorbs, by active transport, free amino acids and peptides, which then enter the portal vein and are carried to the liver.

FAT DIGESTION

Entry of fats into the duodenum causes release of cholecystokinin-pancreozymin, which stimulates the gallbladder to contract. Pancreatic lipase hydrolyses triglycerides. Free fatty acids, glycerol and monoglycerides are emulsified by bile salts to form micelles, which are then absorbed along the brush border of mucosal cells. Short-chain fatty acids enter the portal circulation bound to albumin. Long-chain fats are re-esterified within the mucosal cells into triglycerides, which combine with lesser amounts of protein, phospholipid and cholesterol to create chylomicrons. Chylomicrons enter the lymphatic system and are transported via the thoracic duct into the bloodstream.

PANCREATIC FUNCTION

The pancreas secretes more than 1 L of pancreatic juices per day in adults. These juices are bicarbonate-rich and contain enzymes for the absorption of carbohydrate, fat and protein. Faecal elastase, which can be measured in the stool, is a useful test of pancreatic function.

GUT HORMONES

The main gut hormones are:

* *Gastrin*: stimulated by vagal stimulation and distension of the stomach. Increases gastric acid, pepsin and intrinsic factor release, promoting gastric emptying and pancreatic secretion.
* *Secretin*: stimulated by intraluminal acid. Increases pancreatic bicarbonate secretion; inhibits gastric acid and pepsin secretion and delays gastric emptying.
* *Cholecystokinin-pancreozymin*: stimulated by intraluminal food. Promotes pancreatic bicarbonate and enzyme secretion and gallbladder contraction; inhibits gastric emptying and gut motility.
* *Gastric inhibitory peptide*: stimulated by glucose, fats and amino acids. Inhibits gastric acid secretion; stimulates insulin secretion and reduces gut motility.
* *Motilin*: stimulated by acid in the small bowel. Increases gut motility.
* *Pancreatic polypeptide*: stimulated by protein-rich meals. Inhibits gastric and pancreatic secretion.
* *Vasoactive intestinal peptide (VIP)*: released by neural stimulation. Inhibits gastric acid and pepsin secretion; stimulates insulin secretion; reduces gut motility.

ENTEROHEPATIC CIRCULATION

Bile is produced by the liver and stored in the gallbladder. It is secreted into the duodenum following gallbladder contraction, stimulated by the release of cholecystokinin-pancreozymin. Bile acids, formed from cholesterol, aid fat digestion. Primary bile acids are produced in the liver. Secondary bile acids are formed from primary bile acids through conjugation with amino acids by the action of intestinal bacteria. Primary and secondary bile acids are deconjugated in the intestine, reabsorbed in the terminal ileum, and transported back to the liver bound to albumin for recirculation.

Nutritional requirements

Nutritional requirements are age-dependent. Standard reference tables are available (reference nutrient intake, RNI). Energy needs per kilogram of body weight in infants are higher than those in older children (Table 10.1).

Energy requirements list calories, but nutrient and micronutrient requirements are also important to ensure that intake is balanced. It is essential, for example, to have an appropriate balance of fat, carbohydrate and protein. Calcium is essential for bone growth. Iron is required to prevent anaemia.

Table 10.1 *Comparison of daily nutritional requirements in an infant and a 12-year-old boy*

	Fluid (mL/kg)	Calories (kcal/kg)	Protein (g/kg)	Sodium (mmol/kg)	Potassium (mmol/kg)
Infant 0–3 months	150	100	2.1	1.5	3
12-year-old boy	55	50	1	2	2

Physical status (metabolic condition, bedridden, physical activity level) will impact on requirements. Energy requirements include resting energy expenditure (basal metabolic rate), which represents 60–70 per cent of requirements and the component that arises as a consequence of physical activity. Energy requirements increase significantly if there are increased needs, and then 100–150 per cent of standard reference requirements may be needed. Requirements in disease are generally greater than in health.

NORMAL GROWTH

It is important to remember that during childhood, there is a large surface area to body mass area and increased basal metabolic rate, and sufficient intake is required to maintain a positive energy balance in order to allow for growth. The energy needs for growth during childhood are at their highest during the first year, with a further energy boost required later to help facilitate the onset of puberty and the pubertal growth spurt.

Remember, birth weight triples by age 12 months, quadruples by age three years, and has increased ten-fold by age ten years.

Nutrients and micronutrients

Nutrients and micronutrients are an essential part of good nutrition. Only some can be measured.

IRON

Iron is absorbed from the proximal small bowel. Five to ten per cent of dietary iron is absorbed. Deficiency causes hypochromic microcytic anaemia. Common causes of deficiency include poor diet, chronic blood loss and malabsorption. Treatment is directed against the underlying cause. Dietary advice and iron supplements, of which numerous commercial preparations are available, are indicated in most patients. Side effects of iron supplements include abdominal discomfort and constipation.

Caution is advised in the interpretation of tests of iron status. Low serum iron and a high transferrin suggests deficiency. Low iron with low transferrin suggests chronic disease and not necessarily iron deficiency. Ferritin is an indicator of total body stores but is also an acute-phase reactant.

FOLATE

Folate is absorbed from the proximal small bowel. Deficiency causes megaloblastic anaemia, irritability, poor weight gain and chronic diarrhoea. Treatment of deficiency is with oral folic acid. Folate levels are not affected by the acute-phase response.

The serum folate level reflects recent changes in folate status. Red-cell folate is an indicator of total body stores.

VITAMIN B12

Vitamin B12 is absorbed from the terminal ileum, facilitated by gastric intrinsic factor. Deficiency causes megaloblastic anaemia (raised mean cell volume, MCV) and increased methylmalonic acid in the urine. Causes of deficiency include pernicious anaemia (rare in childhood), poor intake, e.g. from a vegan diet, and malabsorption, e.g. blind-loop post-terminal ileal resection (post-neonatal surgical resection, Crohn's disease). Treatment is with vitamin B12, usually given intramuscularly initially once or twice a week and then every three months. Folic acid is also needed.

ZINC

Zinc deficiency occurs secondary to poor absorption rather than poor intake. Deficiency responds well to oral zinc.

FAT-SOLUBLE VITAMINS

Vitamins A, D, E and K are fat-soluble. Deficiency occurs particularly in fat malabsorption, e.g. cystic fibrosis, intestinal failure (particularly short-bowel syndrome) and liver disease. Deficiency responds to oral or, in children on total parenteral nutrition (TPN), intravenous replacement.

NUTRITIONAL ASSESSMENT

Nutritional assessment is essential, particularly in patients at high risk, e.g. with chronic disease or before major surgery. It is important to take a careful history, assess intake, consider requirements and weigh the patient. This is particularly important in chronically hospitalized patients. Dietetic input is essential in children underweight for height. Body mass index (BMI) is a useful marker of 'fatness', measured as (weight in kilograms)/(height in metres)^2. BMI values need to be plotted against age on standard charts. Other methods of assessing nutritional state include skin-fold thickness as an estimate of fat mass and mid-arm circumference as an estimate of lean body mass. Standard age-matched reference values are available. Bio-impedance and indirect calorimetry as research tools are also used, although less is known about the normal ranges.

Patients with chronic illness and patients at risk for malnutrition should have detailed nutritional assessments undertaken. Consider:

- conditions that interfere with intake;
- conditions that interfere with absorption, e.g. intestinal resection;
- conditions associated with increased losses, e.g. diarrhoea, vomiting;
- condition associated with increased needs, e.g. fever, sepsis, tissue injury;
- conditions that restrict intake, e.g. cardiac disease, renal disease, food intolerance;
- gastrointestinal conditions, e.g. gastro-oesophageal reflux, constipation.

Constipation, particularly if severe, can have a very major impact on nutritional intake. It is common in children with nutritional impairment from any cause.

Ensure that you understand relevant social and family factors that may impact on the child's nutrition.

Nutritional impairment

ENERGY BALANCE

A positive energy balance implies that intake exceeds requirements, while a negative energy balance implies that intake is less than requirements. It is important to remember that requirements during childhood include those needed for growth.

PATHOGENESIS OF MALNUTRITION

It is essential to think about the pathogenesis of malnutrition when assessing nutritional status and looking at nutritional supplementation. Malnutrition can result only from:

- inadequate intake or excessive losses;
- increased metabolic demand without increased intake;
- malabsorption.

One or all of these may contribute to malnutrition in an individual. A good example is cystic fibrosis:

- Pancreatic malabsorption results in increased losses.
- Increased metabolic demand due to the following results in increased needs:
  - chronic cough
  - dyspnoea
  - recurrent infection
  - inflammation.
- Reduced intake due to the following results in reduced intake:
  - anorexia
  - vomiting
  - psychological problems.

Together, these factors result in an energy deficit. All these factors need to be considered when nutritional supplementation is considered. The child with cystic fibrosis has the unfortunate scenario of needing more food but being unable to take it.

FALTERING GROWTH

Faltering growth, known previously as failure to thrive, refers to the failure to gain weight at an adequate rate. It is common in infancy. It occurs as a result of one or more of the following:

- failure of the carer to offer adequate calories;
- failure of the child to take in sufficient calories;
- failure of the child to retain adequate calories.

Faltering growth can be organic or non-organic. Insufficient calories may be offered as a consequence of parental neglect or because of a failure of the carer to appreciate the calorie requirements of the child. Insufficient calories may be taken in as a consequence of feeding difficulties, e.g. cerebral palsy. Calories may not be retained because of absorptive defects or may be lost because of vomiting or diarrhoea. The investigation of failure to thrive generally is fruitful only when specific pointers to organic problems are elucidated in the history. The management of severe non-organic failure to thrive requires dietary assessment, often accompanied by hospital admission for evaluation and to ensure an adequate weight gain can be obtained if sufficient calories are given.

DISEASE-RELATED MALNUTRITION

There are many causes of disease-related malnutrition, including:

- *decreased intake*: anorexia, fatigue and muscle weakness, fasting, pain, difficulty swallowing, inability to eat independently;
- *increased requirements*: metabolic response to disease, impaired organ function, catch-up growth;
- *increased losses*: impaired absorption, impaired digestion, excess losses.

Nutritional status often deteriorates in hospital; the most common causes include disease- and treatment-associated factors, prolonged periods of fasting for tests and operations, inadequate provision of nutrition, and lack of awareness among staff.

Scoring systems are available to help calculate the patients at risk of malnutrition or worsening of malnutrition during a hospital stay. Factors such as poor weight or BMI centile and severity of disease on admission are key.

Some of the consequences of nutritional impairment are listed in Box 10.1.

PRACTICAL MANAGEMENT

Nutritional supplementation

Nutritional supplementation requires the help of a dietician. It is important, however, for doctors to understand the basic

Box 10.1 Some of the consequences of nutritional impairment

Impaired gastrointestinal function
Impaired immune function
Reduced muscle mass/strength
Reduced respiratory function
Poor/delayed wound healing
Increased operative/perioperative morbidity and
  mortality
Altered behaviour, poor mental function, apathy
Micronutrient and nutrient deficiency
Osteoporosis
Growth failure

principles. In the management of any child with a nutritional deficit, it is essential first to optimize treatment of the underlying pathology. An assessment of the child's requirements is then needed. These requirements may be in excess of standard reference values for the child's age. Additional calories can be given either by increasing the calorie density of feed or by feeding via a different route, e.g. nasogastric tube, gastrostomy tube or parenterally.

GENERAL PRINCIPLES OF MANAGEMENT

1 Treat underlying pathology.
2 Assess requirements.
3 Increase calories by increasing feed volume or calorie density.
4 If necessary, give calories by another route, e.g. gastrostomy.

CASE 1

A six-month-old infant with congenital heart disease is failing to thrive. Comment on the infant's nutritional status. What nutritional supplementation would you recommend?

In this infant, the poor nutritional state will be a consequence of increased metabolic demands (heart failure causing increased resting energy expenditure) and poor intake secondary to breathlessness. Supplementation would involve increasing the calorie density of feeds and consideration of other methods of administration, such as via a nasogastric tube. It is also important to maximize medical therapy of the heart disease.

CASE 2

A six-month-old infant has bronchopulmonary dysplasia and severe failure to thrive. Comment on the possible causes.

There will be increased metabolic demands as in the first scenario. In addition, other factors may be relevant, such as chronic respiratory symptoms, gastro-oesophageal reflux and neurodevelopmental issues. Supplementation would involve increasing the calorie density and considering using a nasogastric tube or gastrostomy. In addition, investigation for problems such as gastro-oesophageal reflux may be considered.

CASE 3

A three-month-old infant born at 29 weeks' gestation and who had a massive resection for volvulus in the neonatal period has poor feed tolerance, TPN dependence and severe liver disease. What strategies are required in this child's subsequent management?

This child has intestinal failure with persistent TPN dependency and liver disease. The priority is to maximize enteral intake, which will reduce the likelihood of progression of the liver disease. A hydrolysed feed given by continuous infusion will probably be tolerated best. TPN should be weaned only when the feed is tolerated and absorbed. Loperamide may reduce transit. Bacterial overgrowth is likely and should be managed with antibiotics given cyclically, e.g. gentamicin, metronidazole. Macro- and micronutrients should be checked to ensure they are adequate. Attention should be given to promoting the child's oral feeding skills.

CASE 4

A 13-year-old boy has cerebral palsy. Comment on his nutritional status. What strategies could be used to improve his nutrition? Why do you think his nutritional status is so poor?

This child's principal problem is likely to be with intake, either because of reflux or secondary to bulbar problems, or both. In addition to nutritional supplements, this child may benefit from help with feeding practices, including the involvement of a dietician, a speech and language therapist, an occupational therapist and a neurodevelopmental paediatrician. Other medical problems may also be relevant, such as recurrent chest infections secondary to aspiration, constipation and intractable fits. Consideration needs to be given to nasogastric or gastrostomy tube feeding if appropriate. In some instances, a fundoplication will be required for gastro-oesophageal reflux.

Nutritional supplementation

Nutritional supplementation needs to be done in conjunction with a paediatric dietician. Normal infant feeds or milk contain 0.7 kcal/mL. There are many commercially available products.

- Feeds can be concentrated, e.g. by 15 per cent by using four scoops in 100 mL (normal concentration: one scoop in 30 mL).
- Carbohydrate supplements can be used, usually as a glucose polymer in powder form to add to feeds.
- Combined carbohydrate and fat supplements can be used.
- Feeds with a higher calorie density can be used, e.g. 1 kcal/mL, 1.5 kcal/mL.

- Special feeds can be used, e.g. hydrolysed protein formula feeds, soya-based feeds, lactose-free feeds, medium-chain triglyceride (MCT)-based feeds.
- Milk- or juice-based supplements can be given.

Enteral nutrition

Enteral feeding strictly refers to enteral feed given directly into the gastrointestinal tract. For the purpose of this chapter, however, we will consider an enteral feed as a supplementary feed, i.e. not including foods normally taken by mouth, and therefore refer principally to feeds given by either nasogastric or gastrostomy tube or, in rare cases, via a jejunostomy.

INDICATIONS FOR ENTERAL TUBE FEEDING

- insufficient energy intake by mouth
- wasting
- stunting.

Diseases for which enteral nutrition may be indicated are listed in Box 10.2.

CHOICE OF FEED TYPE

There is a wide range of feeds available. The decision about which to use should be based on the child's needs. Factors that are of relevance include whether the enteral feed will be the sole source of feeding, in which case the feed needs to be nutritionally complete, or whether the feed is going to be given as a supplement. Feed tolerance and calorie requirements are relevant. A modified feed may be required, e.g. a lactose-free feed in a child with carbohydrate intolerance. Factors such as fibre content and calorie density are also important, particularly if supplementary feeding is going to be a long-term requirement.

A hydrolysed protein is a protein that is broken down into oligopeptides and peptides. A hydrolysed-protein milk formula is therefore a milk formula that does not contain whole protein (e.g. Pregestemil®, Nutramigen®, Prejomin®, Pepti-Junior®). An elemental formula is a hydrolysed protein formula in which the protein is broken down into amino acids (e.g. Neocate®, E028®).

Hydrolysed protein formula feeds are used in children with cows' milk allergy and in enteropathies, e.g. post-gastroenteritis, post-necrotizing enterocolitis, short gut syndrome, severe eczema and Crohn's disease.

CHOICE OF FEED REGIMEN

This will depend on a combination of requirements, tolerance and factors such as gastric emptying. Options include bolus feeding and continuous feeding, or a combination of the two.

In a severely malnourished child, the volume and calorie density of a new feed regime may need to be increased slowly as tolerated over a few days. This avoids metabolic upset (refeeding syndrome) in the vulnerable child, e.g. severe postoperative weight loss, anorexia nervosa.

Box 10.2 Diseases for which enteral nutrition may be indicated

Gastrointestinal:
- Short bowel syndrome
- Inflammatory bowel disease
- Pseudo-obstruction
- Chronic liver disease
- Gastro-oesophageal reflux
- Glycogen storage disease types I and III
- Fatty acid oxidation defects

Neuromuscular disease:
- Coma, severe facial and head injury
- Severe mental retardation, cerebral palsy
- Dysphagia secondary to cranial nerve dysfunction, muscular dystrophy or myasthenia gravis

Malignant disease:
- Obstructing disease: head and neck, oesophagus, stomach
- Abnormality of deglutition following surgical intervention
- Gastrointestinal side effects from chemotherapy and/or radiotherapy
- Terminal supportive care

Pulmonary disease:
- Bronchopulmonary dysplasia
- Cystic fibrosis
- Chronic lung disease

Congenital abnormalities:
- Oesophageal atresia
- Cleft palate
- Pierre Robin syndrome

Other:
- Anorexia nervosa
- Cardiac cachexia
- Chronic renal disease
- Severe burns
- Severe sepsis
- Severe trauma

DYSMOTILITY

The motility of the gut is a key factor in feed tolerance. Preterm infants and children with cerebral palsy have delayed gastric emptying, which impacts significantly on the ability to feed, particularly if nutrition is dependent upon nasogastric or gastrostomy feeding. Gut motility will be reduced in the postoperative period. Abdominal pain, bloating and constipation are common features of gut dysmotility. Therapeutic strategies include the recognition of the problem, prokinetic agent such as domperidone, laxatives and, occasionally, if there is a need for distal gut deflation, suppositories. It may be necessary to give feeds by continuous infusion. Milk-free diets can be used. In difficult cases, full gastrointestinal investigation, including upper- and lower-gastrointestinal endoscopy, barium radiology, pH studies and scintography, may be indicated. A number of children, particularly those with cerebral palsy, respond to milk exclusion, using a hydrolysed protein formula feed as an alternative.

BACTERIAL OVERGROWTH (SMALL BOWEL)

This can be a significant problem, particularly in children with underlying dysmotility. The use of repeated courses of antibiotics is a risk factor. Stasis causes bacterial proliferation, with the emergence of resistant strains. Malabsorption results with steatorrhoea and fat-soluble vitamin deficiency. Diagnosis is by a high index of suspicion, particularly in patients with risk factors, e.g. previous gastrointestinal surgery and short bowel syndrome. Hydrogen breath testing may be useful. Radioisotope-labelled breath testing may also have a role. Barium radiology should be performed if obstruction is suspected, e.g. at the site of an anastomosis. Treatment involves appropriate management of the underlying cause. Metronidazole, which is effective orally and intravenously, is the antibiotic of first choice. Probiotics have been used, although their role is as yet unproven.

METHODS OF FEED DELIVERY

Nasogastric tube feeding

This is the most commonly used route for short-term enteral feeding given either by bolus or continuously. There is a risk of reflux and aspiration pneumonia. Nasal irritation and inhibition of oral feeding sometimes occur. Most infants will not tolerate long-term nasogastric feeding.

Nasojejunal feeding

This is indicated when nasogastric feeding is not tolerated due to delayed gastric emptying or gross gastro-oesophageal reflux. Feed usually needs to be given continuously to avoid dumping. If nasojejunal feeding is required long term, then a jejunostomy can be fashioned.

Gastrostomy tube feeding

Gastrostomy is probably the best route for long-term feeding. Gastrostomy tubes are generally inserted endoscopically (percutaneous endoscopic gastrostomy). There are few complications.

Indications for gastrostomy tube placement include:

- chronic disease with nutritional impairment, e.g. cystic fibrosis, bronchopulmonary dysplasia;
- nutritional therapy, e.g. Crohn's disease;
- difficulties with feeding, e.g. cerebral palsy, particularly with an associated bulbar palsy. Some of these children may also have severe gastro-oesophageal reflux requiring fundoplication;
- children long-term dependent upon nasogastric feeding for any other reason.

Box 10.3 Indications for total parenteral nutrition (TPN)

Neonates

- *Absolute indications*:
  - Intestinal failure (short gut, functional immaturity, pseudo-obstruction)
  - Necrotizing enterocolitis
- *Relative indications*:
  - Hyaline membrane disease
  - Promotion of growth in preterm infants
  - Possible prevention of necrotizing enterocolitis

Older infants and children

- *Intestinal failure*:
  - Short gut
  - Protracted diarrhoea
  - Chronic intestinal pseudo-obstruction
  - Postoperative abdominal or cardiothoracic surgery
  - Radiation/cytotoxic therapy
- *Exclusion of luminal nutrients*:
  - Crohn's disease
- *Organ failure*:
  - Acute renal failure, acute liver failure
- *Hypercatabolism*:
  - Extensive burns
  - Severe trauma

Total parenteral nutrition

There are many indications for TPN (Box 10.3). However, it is important to use the gut where possible. The complete exclusion of luminal nutrients is associated with atrophic changes in the gut, reduced pancreatic function, biliary stasis and bacterial overgrowth. It is not usually necessary to use TPN for less than five days, except in the extremely preterm infant. There is no indication to start TPN as an emergency, although the addition of even small amounts of nitrogen as amino acids can reverse catabolism of muscle mass.

Benefits of minimal enteral nutrition in children who are fed by TPN include:

- stimulation of mucosal adaptation (trophic feeding);
- protection against sepsis (normalize flora);
- improved bile flow, with decreased risk of cholestasis;
- reduced time to establish enteral feeds.

GENERAL PRINCIPLES

There are differences between children and adults, particularly in terms of nutritional reserve:

- An adult can survive for 90 days without food.
- A preterm infant weighing 1 kg can survive for four days without food.

- A preterm infant weighing 2 kg can survive for 12 days without food.
- A term infant weighing 3.5 kg can survive for 32 days without food.
- A one-year-old can survive for 44 days without food.

TOTAL PARENTERAL NUTRITION PRESCRIBING

There are standard regimens for TPN prescribing. This will include the starter regimen, which then increases in nutrient density over the first few days. Protein is supplied as amino acid, carbohydrate as glucose and fat as a lipid emulsion. Electrolyte, calcium and phosphate content needs to be controlled carefully. Fat- and water-soluble vitamins and trace elements are added to the mix. Calorie density is increased through increasing carbohydrate and lipid, as tolerated. It is important to use standard regimens adjusted according to fluid balance, electrolyte status and tolerance of, e.g., increases in glucose. It is important not to push up the calorie density too much without seeking expert advice, as this may result in poor tolerance and toxicity, with a net reduction in metabolized energy intake. The input of a TPN pharmacist in conjunction with a nutrition team is essential in difficult cases.

It is important that continuing losses, e.g. from a stoma, are taken into account in the child's fluid regimen or TPN prescription. Generally, stoma losses are high in sodium, and half or complete replacement of losses with normal saline incorporated into the overall fluid regimen is required. This requires careful monitoring of fluid and electrolyte balance and plasma and urinary electrolytes.

NUTRITION TEAM

Most large units will have a nutrition team, which enables a multidisciplinary approach to difficult feeding problems. Different team members can contribute their expertise to ensure that the TPN regimen is optimum, that oral feeding occurs where possible, and that there is a smooth transition to discharge on supplementary feeding if appropriate. The team will also develop policies and procedures and indications for referral.

The precise makeup of the team and the responsibilities of the different team members will vary between units, depending on the individual unit's needs and available personnel.

VENOUS ACCESS AND COMPLICATIONS OF CENTRAL CATHETER INSERTION

See Chapter 11.

LINE INFECTION

Infection is one of the potentially life-threatening hazards of TPN. Coagulase-negative staphylococcal infection is the most common. Children on long-term TPN are at significant risk of life-threatening bacterial sepsis. Therefore, there should be

in place a local protocol to ensure that cultures are taken and antibiotics started promptly in any child on TPN and with a high fever. Children with short gut/enteropathy are at highest risk because of bacterial translocation; such children should have regular gut decontamination, particularly if infections are frequent. It is important that appropriate procedures are in place to ensure that lines are dealt with aseptically and only by trained personnel. Long-term feeding lines should not be used for blood-letting.

MONITORING

There should be a local protocol for monitoring. The initial frequency of monitoring will depend on the degree of electrolyte impairment and other factors, e.g. sepsis, liver disease. It is generally necessary in the acute situation to do at least routine biochemistry (including blood glucose and urine reagent strips) daily until the patient is stable, and then twice weekly. Urine biochemistry should be monitored twice weekly initially. Liver function, calcium and phosphate should be tested weekly. Trace metals (copper, zinc, selenium, magnesium) should be checked monthly. In children on long-term TPN, iron, vitamin B12, red cell folate, fat-soluble vitamins, aluminium and chromium should be measured every six months. Chest X-ray, liver ultrasound and cardiac echo should be done every 6–12 months.

Blood glucose should be monitored frequently during periods of increasing carbohydrate load.

Complications of TPN are listed in Box 10.4.

TOTAL PARENTERAL NUTRITION-INDUCED LIVER DISEASE

TPN-induced liver disease develops in 40–60 per cent of infants who require long-term TPN for intestinal failure. The clinical spectrum includes cholestasis, cholelithiasis, hepatic

---

Box 10.4 Complications of total parenteral nutrition (TPN)

Phlebitis
Infection
Hypo-/hyperglycaemia
Electrolyte disturbance
Fluid overload
Hypophosphataemia
Anaemia
Thrombocyte and neutrophil dysfunction
Trace-element deficiencies/excesses
Vitamin deficiencies
Hyperammonaemia
Essential fatty-acid deficiency
Cholestasis, hepatic dysfunction
Metabolic acidosis
Hypercholesterolaemia/hypertriglyceridaemia
Metabolic bone disease

fibrosis with progression to biliary cirrhosis, and the development of portal hypertension and liver failure. The pathogenesis is multifactorial and is related to prematurity, low birth weight and duration of TPN. The degree and severity of the liver disease are related to recurrent sepsis, including catheter sepsis, bacterial translocation and cholangitis. Lack of enteral feeding leading to reduced gut hormone secretion, reduction of bile flow and biliary stasis are important mechanisms in the development of cholestasis, biliary sludge and cholelithiasis. The management strategies for the prevention of TPN-induced liver disease include early enteral feeding, a multidisciplinary approach to the management of parenteral nutrition, and the use of aseptic catheter techniques to reduce sepsis. The administration of ursodeoxycholic acid may improve bile flow and reduce gallbladder and intestinal stasis. Fat-soluble vitamin replacement must be via the intravenous route when the child is being fed parenterally but may be given orally with regular monitoring during the transition to oral/enteral feeding.

The surgical patient

PREOPERATIVE ASSESSMENT

Patients with chronic illness and patients at risk for malnutrition should have detailed nutritional assessments undertaken. It is well known that nutritional status is a very important factor in the recovery process from all kinds of surgical interventions. Patients at significant risk include people underweight for height and people with a current (chronic illness) or predicted (major gut resection) high metabolic demand. Preoperative awareness and joint multidisciplinary input can impact significantly on progress during the postoperative period.

POSTOPERATIVE NUTRITION

It is important to get nutrition into the patient as soon as possible postoperatively, particularly if nutrition is an issue in the preoperative period. If there is a prolonged ileus, then TPN may have to be considered. The enteral route, however, is preferable. Issues such as nausea and pain need to be managed appropriately if food intake is going to be established rapidly.

Specific advice regarding how early to feed postoperatively is dependent on the procedure performed and the preferences of the surgeon, and thus specific guidelines cannot be set. Most patients will not require specific nutritional input in the postoperative period, particularly if surgery is straightforward.

GUT RESECTION

Significant nutritional problems are possible after gut resection. It is important when thinking about this to remember the specific functions of specific parts of the gut (see earlier). Management also depends on the presence or absence of a stoma, as a stoma will increase fluid and electrolyte loss.

Potential problems of gut resection include:

- bacterial overgrowth;
- rapid transit;
- dysmotility: mechanical (resection with anastomosis, microcolon), functional (interruption of peristaltic complexes).

Careful postoperative fluid and electrolyte balance must be carried out, particularly if a stoma is present. If there is going to be a delay in establishing full enteral feeds, then a period of TPN should be considered. It is important to introduce enteral feeding early and wean TPN as soon as possible. Continuous feeding or frequent small-bolus feeds may be required, particularly in infants. Consider using hydrolysed or lactose-free feeds if there is a delay in establishing feeds or significant feed intolerance. Metronidazole may help if bacterial overgrowth is suspected.

SHORT BOWEL SYNDROME

This is defined as intestinal failure secondary to massive resection. Aetiologies include the following:

- *Neonate*: necrotizing enterocolitis, intestinal atresia, volvulus.
- *Older child*: trauma, inflammatory bowel disease, vascular abnormalities.

Factors determining outcome include the following:

- Length of bowel resected and remaining bowel length: preterm bowel is likely to undergo further growth (bowel length increases by 100 per cent in the third trimester).
- Quality of bowel remaining: ischaemic, distended, ileum greater potential to adapt than jejunum.
- Presence of ileocaecal valve: loss of ileocaecal valve results in faster transit. Backflow (loss of the one-way valve) makes bacterial overgrowth more likely. There is a need for vitamin B12 replacement in the longer term.
- Improved outcome if colon is still present, which facilitates salt and water reabsorption.
- Coexistent disease, e.g. enteropathy, is an adverse risk factor.
- Presence of liver disease is an adverse risk factor.
- Less than 40 cm of small bowel is usually associated with the need for long-term nutritional support.

There are three phases of intestinal adaptation: acute (TPN-dependent, postoperative ileus), adaptive (increasing enteral nutrition can take months to years) and chronic. The priority is to maintain normal growth and development through adequate calorie, nutrient and micronutrient intake during these phases. The early introduction of enteral feeds promotes intestinal adaptation and will improve subsequent feed tolerance. Feeds usually are best given as a continuous infusion in the first instance and should be increased only if tolerated, i.e. no diarrhoea (or no excess stoma output, if present). Explosive stools imply feed intolerance, which will increase the risk of metabolic upset and bacterial translocation, leading to sepsis.

TPN should not be weaned until feed is tolerated and absorbed. Body weight must be monitored carefully during weaning of TPN. Artificial feeds (e.g. hydrolysed feeds) are often tolerated better than standard formulas, although osmolality is higher. Liver disease is a serious complication of TPN and may lead to death from liver failure; it may be reduced by maximizing the amount given per feed, avoidance of sepsis, artificial bile salts (e.g. ursodeoxycholic acid) and vitamin supplementation. Bacterial overgrowth, with the risks of malabsorption and bacterial translocation, is common and requires treatment with oral antibiotics (metronidazole either alone or in combination with gentamicin) given in cycles. Loperamide may help reduce gut transit and thus increase absorption. Monitoring of micronutrients and fat-soluble vitamins is essential during long-term TPN. Bowel-lengthening surgery may reduce stasis and, thus, translocation. In severe cases, isolated liver transplant or intestinal transplantation may be considered. Multidisciplinary management, including paying attention to the child's oral skills and social and psychological development and the needs of the family, is essential.

SPECIFIC CONDITIONS OF RELEVANCE

Cerebral palsy

Children with cerebral palsy are difficult to assess with respect to nutrition. Feeding difficulties may be secondary to bulbar weakness, with oesophageal incoordination, primary or secondary aspiration or reflux oesophagitis. Additional factors, including the child's mobility, the degree of spasticity, the nutritional state and the presence of other conditions, such as gut dysmotility and constipation, are also relevant. Such children require careful multidisciplinary assessment by a feeding team, including dietetics, speech and language therapy, occupational therapy and a neurodevelopmental paediatrician. Attention to nutrition is of key importance, and many children benefit from a feeding gastrostomy. Insertion of a gastrostomy does not need to be accompanied by an anti-reflux procedure unless there is proven gastro-oesophageal reflux unresponsive to medical treatment. These children benefit from assessment in a joint paediatric gastroenterology/surgical clinic, particularly if fundoplication is being considered.

Idiopathic constipation

Childhood constipation is common, and it is often an underappreciated but highly important issue in the undernourished patient. Risk factors of relevance to the paediatric surgeon include perianal pathology, poor intake, e.g. following an acute illness or postoperatively, and gut dysmotility. Constipation also is often a factor in children referred to the acute unit with abdominal pain.

Most children with constipation do not have an underlying cause and their constipation is functional (idiopathic). Most constipation is short-term and is treated readily with bulk and/or stimulant laxatives. Commonly used laxatives include lactulose, docusate sodium, senna and sodium picosulfate. Enemas are required rarely.

FURTHER READING

Ball PA, Booth IW, Holden CE, Puntis JW. *Paediatric Parenteral Nutrition*, 3rd edn. Milton Keynes: Pharmacia and Upjohn Nutrition, 1998.

British Association for Parenteral and Enteral Nutrition. www.bapen.org.uk

British Society of Gastroenterology. www.bsg.org.uk

British Society of Paediatric Gastroenterology, Hepatology and Nutrition. www.bspghan.org.uk

Goulet O, Ruemmele F, Lacaille F, Colomb V. Irreversible intestinal failure. *Journal of Paediatric Gastroenterology and Nutrition* 2004; **38**: 250–69.

Preedy V, Grimble G, Watson R. *Nutrition in the Infant: Problems and Practical Procedures*. London: Greenwich Medical Media, 2001.

Shaw V, Lawson M. *Clinical Paediatric Dietetics*, 2nd edn. Oxford: Blackwell Science, 2001.

Shulman R, Phillips S. Parenteral nutrition in infants and children. *Journal of Paediatric Gastroenterology and Nutrition* 2003; **36**: 587–607.

Warner BW, Vanderhoof JA, Reyes JD. What's new in the management of short bowel syndrome. *Journal of the American College of Surgeons* 2000; **190**: 725–36.

11

Vascular access

SIMON PHELPS AND ROBERT A WHEELER

Learning objectives

- To understand the indications for vascular access.
- To understand the types of device available for vascular access.
- To understand the methods and routes of insertion of vascular-access devices.
- To understand the complications of vascular-access devices.

INTRODUCTION

The acquisition of short- and long-term access to the venous circulation is essential to the successful management of acute and chronic conditions in infants and children. It is a task undertaken by most clinicians in many subspecialties, but it is a mandatory skill that should fall within the remit of all paediatric surgeons. Although considered to be a straightforward procedure in adult medicine, gaining vascular access is often the rate-limiting step in paediatric practice and perhaps one of the most potentially distressing events for child and parent alike.

HISTORY

Access to the circulation was first proposed by Andreas Libavius (1546–1616), who suggested that a silver conduit could be used to transfer arterial blood of an elder to the vein of a youth. It was not until after his death that the first vascular-access device was invented by Francesco Folli (1624–85), using an animal vessel to connect a silver cannula in a donor to a bone cylinder inserted into the recipient.

The cholera pandemic of the 1830s prompted the pioneering work of Thomas Latta, who successfully administered intravenous water and salt (half normal saline) through a silver needle. The administration of such fluids was facilitated by the first steel needle and syringe manufactured by Alexander Wood in 1855.

Despite improved survival rates of, for example, cholera patients, intravenous infusions did not gain universal acceptance until the early twentieth century because of the complications of air embolism and sepsis. By 1911, the usual infusate was normal saline; glucose was not added routinely until 1925.

Intraosseous puncture was first proposed in 1922. By the 1940s, this was a well-accepted route for fluid administration in children and is currently a recommended means of paediatric emergency circulatory access.

The use of the standard metal hypodermic needle for venous access was superseded in 1950 by the 'Rochester needle'. This consisted of a plastic cannula with a central removable metal stylet and a separate cannula hub and was the true predecessor of all modern intravenous cannula-over-needle devices.

The first central venous catheterization was performed by Hale, who, in 1733, inserted a glass tube into the internal jugular vein of a horse and measured the venous pressure. Bleichroder in 1912 described the placement of a ureteric catheter in the inferior vena cava in four human subjects via the femoral vein, and in 1929 Forssmann placed a similar device in his own right atrium from the antecubital fossa.

The first purpose-built central venous catheter was made from varnished silk and used by Cournand in 1941 for cardiac catheterization. A central venous catheter utilizing silicone elastomer (silastic) was first produced in 1961. With the advent of total parenteral nutrition in children, Dudrick in 1968 described the insertion of silastic, polyethylene or polytetra-fluoroethylene central lines into the superior vena cava of nine newborn infants. Broviac in 1973 and Hickman in 1979 both designed silastic catheters for placement in the right atrium.

PERIPHERAL VENOUS ACCESS

General considerations

The placement of intravenous cannulae in infants and children is difficult, as infants and children differ physiologically and psychologically from adults. Subcutaneous fat in infants makes the veins less visible and impalpable, and vasoconstriction is promoted by the tendency of infants to lose heat rapidly due to a relatively large surface area/weight ratio. In non-emergency situations, planning and preparation may facilitate the procedure, with attention being paid to the following points:

- appropriately experienced assistance;
- age-appropriate explanation of the procedure to the patient and the parents;
- early application of topical local anaesthetic agents;
- presence of the parents;
- adequate lighting and a warm environment away from the child's bed;
- tapes/dressings to secure the cannula;
- availability of containers for blood samples.

The administration of oral sucrose to neonates has been shown to reduce procedural pain. Distraction techniques and the input of play therapists are often invaluable for infants and children. Practical manoeuvres such as the application of local heat and the use of cold light transillumination may also increase the possibility of successful venous puncture.

Sites of peripheral venous access

The common sites for peripheral venous access are shown in Table 11.1 in order of preference of use, with their individual advantages and disadvantages. All of these sites may be cannulated percutaneously, but an open approach is not recommended in all sites.

Emergency access

In an emergency situation with hypovolaemia, respiratory arrest or circulatory arrest, the priority of resuscitation after

Table 11.1 *Common sites for peripheral venous access*

Vein	Advantages	Disadvantages	Open
Dorsum hand/foot	Visible, straight	Limits mobility/dexterity	Yes
Antecubital fossa, cephalic/basilic	Large calibre, constant anatomy	Kinks with elbow flexion, adjacent brachial artery/median nerve	Yes
Saphenous vein at ankle	Constant anatomy, large calibre	Not always visible	Yes
External jugular	Large, visible	Difficult to cannulate, difficult to fix cannula, infusions often intermittent from angle of entry into subclavian vein	No
Scalp	Large calibre	Neonates only, difficult to secure cannula	No
Ventral aspect of wrist	None	Small veins, difficult to thread cannula	No

securing the airway and ensuring adequate ventilation is to gain venous access. However, it should not be forgotten that the airway provides some access to the circulation, and some drugs, such as atropine, adrenaline and lidocaine (lignocaine), may be instilled down an endotracheal tube followed by a saline flush.

When access to the circulation is required urgently, current recommendations are that this should be achieved with two short wide-bore peripheral cannulae. This optimizes infusion rates, as flow through a cannula is proportional to the fourth power of the radius and has an inverse relationship to its length (Poiseuille's law).

Traditionally, venous cut-down provided circulatory access when percutaneous means had failed. Even in expert hands, this procedure may be time-consuming, and the rapid intraosseous route is preferred. The latter approach should be used if, after 90 seconds, access has not been attained with an intravenous cannula.

Intraosseous infusion

The intraosseous route relies on the presence of a non-collapsible venous network of sinusoids within the medullary cavity of bones. These drain from a central venous sinus into central veins via emissary or nutrient veins. The safest site for this technique is the flat anteromedial surface of the tibia 2–3 cm distal to the tibial tuberosity, as there are no adjacent vital structures and the bone cortex is close to the skin surface. Alternative insertion sites are the iliac crest and the lateral

---

Box 11.1 Contraindications to intraosseous infusion

Previous failed attempt
Bone fracture
Older children
Use as long-term or non-emergency access

Box 11.2 Potential complications of intraosseous infusion

Local:
Subcutaneous extravasation
Subperiosteal infiltration
Epiphyseal damage
Osteomyelitis
Cellulitis
Displacement of needle
Systemic:
Fat embolism

Box 11.3 Relative contraindications of femoral vein cannulation

Ipsilateral lower-limb trauma
Pelvic or abdominal trauma
Inferior vena cava injury

Box 11.4 Complications of umbilical venous catheters

Infective:
Septicaemia
Malposition:
Arrhythmias
Erosion of atrial wall
Left atrial via foramen ovale
Superior vena cava
Thromboembolic:
Portal venous thrombosis
Hepatic infarction

---

femoral surface 3 cm above the condyle. Contraindications to its use are listed in Box 11.1. A commercially made device or a bone-marrow needle may be used. Intravenous fluids need to be infused by pump or syringe, and all drugs must be followed by a saline flush.

Intraosseous infusion has a high successful insertion rate (98 per cent), with a complication rate of 0.9 per cent; complications are summarized in Box 11.2.

Once cardiac output has been restored in the emergency situation, by drugs or fluids administered by this route, conventional peripheral or central venous access should then be achieved. The preferred site for the latter is the femoral vein.

Femoral venous access

With ongoing cardiopulmonary resuscitation, the femoral vein offers the safest route to the central circulation. Its advantages are a constant anatomical position medial to the femoral artery (4–6 mm), distance from the chest when cardiac massage is in progress, and a non-existent risk of pneumothorax compared with jugular or subclavian puncture.

Cannulation of the femoral vein is performed with the Seldinger technique. This consists of venous puncture with a needle, through which a guide wire is passed. Having removed the needle, the skin is incised at the wire and a dilator is advanced with a twisting movement over the wire into the vein. The dilator is then removed and replaced by the catheter.

In children, femoral vein cannulation has a 90 per cent success rate. The main complication is puncture of the femoral artery. Relative contraindications are shown in Box 11.3.

Umbilical venous catheterization

Venous access in the first one to two weeks of life can be can be achieved by catheterization of the umbilical vein, even in an apparently desiccated cord.

In an emergency situation, the catheter is advanced approximately 5 cm in the preterm infant and 10 cm in the term infant. Ideally, the tip of the catheter should lie within the inferior vena cava rather than the liver. Nomograms based on the infant's weight give a more precise measurement of the length of catheter to be inserted.

Umbilical venous catheters may be used for emergency venous access, exchange transfusion and central venous pressure measurements. Complications of such catheters are listed in Box 11.4.

ELECTIVE VENOUS ACCESS

Elective venous access may be peripheral or central. The former has already been discussed above in the emergency setting; sites of access and equipment are no different in the elective situation, although the use of veins over joints (e.g. antecubital fossa) where a cannula may be occluded by kinking should be avoided. One of the factors influencing the process of thrombophlebitis is the relative diameter of the catheter to that of the vein. A larger cannula will touch venous endothelium more often than a small cannula, with a proportionately more rapid onset of an inflammatory reaction.

In contrast to the emergency situation, where the ideal cannula has as large a diameter as possible to enable rapid infusion, the electively placed cannula should have as small a gauge as is feasible.

A peripherally sited venous cannula gains short-term access to the circulation and, ideally, should be used for only 48–72 hours before being re-sited. Removal of the cannula before thrombophlebitis and venous occlusion have occurred will preserve that vein as a potential site of access. Furthermore, an infected cannula is a potential source of bacteraemia and septicaemia.

Maintenance fluids, blood products, drugs and peripheral parenteral nutrition may be administered peripherally in infants and children. Hypertonic fluids (i.e. more than five per cent dextrose) and fluids containing calcium must be infused carefully, as they are irritant to venous endothelium and can cause necrosis upon extravasation into subcutaneous tissues, particularly in neonates. Prompt irrigation with saline and hyaluronidase may minimize tissue damage from such an event. Considerable scarring may result over the dorsum of the hands and feet in neonates, where there is little subcutaneous fat.

CENTRAL VENOUS ACCESS

A central venous catheter is one in which the tip lies in a vein draining directly into the right side of the heart or the right atrium itself. It may be inserted directly into the central vein or advanced to that position from a peripheral venous site (peripheral inserted central venous catheter, PICC).

The indications for insertion (see Box 11.5) and the anticipated duration of usage govern the type of device used.

Duration of use

Central venous catheters may be inserted for short-, medium- and long-term use.

SHORT-TERM USE

Central venous catheters are placed when the anticipated duration of usage is short (one to two weeks). They are non-cuffed, not tunnelled and inserted percutaneously via the Seldinger technique into the subclavian, internal jugular or femoral vein. They are manufactured in different lengths and diameters and usually with either two or three lumens. Such a line might be placed in the operating theatre or intensive care unit in situations where peripheral access might be inadequate for the required infusion rates or multiple drug infusions or where venous pressure monitoring is needed.

MEDIUM-TERM USE

In the medium term (up to four weeks) for parenteral nutrition or drug administration, a PICC could be used. These are fine (2 F) silastic catheters placed in a peripheral upper limb

---

Box 11.5 Indications for insertion of central venous catheter

Drug administration:
Cytotoxic chemotherapy
Antibiotics
Parenteral nutrition
Blood products
High-flow access:
Haemodialysis
Plasmapheresis
Monitoring:
Central venous pressure
Blood sampling

---

vein through either a metal needle or a splittable cannula system. They are secured at the exit site to the skin with a transparent adhesive dressing. They do not have a Dacron® cuff and their usual exit site does not lend itself to tunnelling. The thin wall and narrow lumen renders such catheters prone to fracture and thrombosis. Patency is not guaranteed by 'locking off' with heparinized saline and must be maintained by a constant infusion (1 mL/h). Furthermore, catheter rupture and embolization may occur from the very high intraluminal pressures generated by flushing an occluded catheter with a small volume syringe (<5 mL). In most neonatal studies, their median duration of use is three weeks.

LONG-TERM USE

A tunnelled cuffed catheter is used in situations where access to the central circulation is anticipated for months or years.

Integral catheter and hub
Such devices are silastic Broviac or Hickman lines. A Broviac line has a single lumen, is of either 2.7 or 4.2 F diameter and is appropriate for neonates and infants. With their larger diameter (7–12 F), Hickman lines are suitable for older infants and children; they may be single- or double-lumen. Both types of catheter are usually tunnelled from the lateral chest wall to the neck (antegrade direction) and placed under direct vision into the internal jugular vein, which has been controlled between two vascular slings. Hickman lines also have the facility of percutaneous insertion into the subclavian vein using the Seldinger technique and a peel-away sheath. Whichever catheter or method of insertion is used, the integral Dacron cuff is sited halfway between the skin entry and the vein.

Separate hub and catheter
An alternative to silastic lines is a device such as the Leader Cuff™. This consists of a cuffed polyurethane catheter on to which a hub can be screwed. This feature enables the catheter to be tunnelled retrogradely from the venous entry point to the exit site on the chest wall.

Implantable devices

These consist of a subcutaneous port (metal or plastic with a silastic diaphragm) to which is attached a tunnelled central venous catheter. The port is usually anchored in a subcutaneous pocket on the lateral chest wall and accessed percutaneously with a Huber needle. This type of needle has a side rather than an end hole, thus preventing a core being taken from the port's diaphragm on puncture.

This type of device is easier to care for and places fewer restrictions upon activities compared with externally exiting devices. The necessity for percutaneous needle access remains, which is a significant problem in needle-phobic children. Ports are being developed with multiple lumens, although the single-lumen port is still the most common type currently available. Preoperative siting is essential in older girls to avoid placement of the port beneath bra straps.

Methods of insertion of central lines

PREOPERATIVE ASSESSMENT

Some of the complications of central venous catheter insertion may be avoided by careful preoperative assessment.

Inability to access an adequate or patent vein may be due to venous stenosis or obliteration from previous catheters. A history of multiple central lines or difficulty in gaining access at a previous attempt would be an indication for preoperative ultrasound to identify venous patency. If ultrasound does not provide this information, then more detailed venous anatomy could be obtained from standard or magnetic resonance imaging (MRI) angiography.

Haemorrhage is one of the more immediate problems encountered during insertion of a central line, whether by open or percutaneous methods, particularly in the presence of thrombocytopenia from cytotoxic chemotherapy. Significant bleeding may occur from needle venepuncture, open venotomy or catheter tunnelling, and thus preoperative measurement of platelet count and coagulation (international normalized ratio (INR), prothrombin time (PT), activated partial prothrombin time (APPT)) is mandatory. If an unexpected coagulopathy or thrombocytopenia is identified, then haematological advice should be sought. Coagulation factors or platelets must be readily available for intraoperative administration.

Access to the site of insertion may be gained by either percutaneous methods or an open technique, with the exceptions shown in the classification of the common sites in Table 11.2. The open route should be avoided with peripherally inserted central lines, as these are more likely to become infected. Detailed descriptions of these methods may be found in the texts listed under Further reading.

INTRAOPERATIVE IMAGING

Ultrasound has become a useful adjunct to the percutaneous insertion of central venous catheters. It may identify venous patency or the presence of an appropriate collateral vein if

Table 11.2 *Classification of common sites of central line insertion*

	Percutaneous	Open
PICC		
Cephalic/basilic	Yes	Yes/No
Saphenous	Yes	Yes/No
Scalp	Yes	No
Central		
Internal jugular	Yes	Yes
Subclavian	Yes	No
Femoral	Yes	Yes

PICC, peripheral inserted central venous catheter.

venous occlusion has occurred; compressibility of a vessel distinguishes vein from artery. Thus, in comparison with the use of anatomical landmarks (blind cannulation), real-time imaging should reduce both the number of attempts required to access a central vein and inadvertent arterial puncture.

Studies investigating the use of intraoperative ultrasound for central venous catheter placement show a beneficial reduction in number of attempts and complications for successful internal jugular and femoral vein puncture, but not the subclavian approach. In the UK, the National Institute for Clinical Excellence (NICE 2002) has used such evidence to recommend that ultrasound guidance is used in the insertion of central venous catheters into the internal jugular vein in all age groups.

CATHETER TIP POSITION

A number of methods are available to determine the position of the central venous catheter tip:

- electrocardiogram (ECG)
- plain X-ray
- fluoroscopy.

The ECG method consists of the catheter (saline-filled) acting as an ECG lead. When the tip of the catheter passes the sinoatrial node, the P wave becomes biphasic and then inverted. However, radiological confirmation of the exact tip position is still required.

Fluoroscopy is the method of choice in the operating theatre, as it provides static and dynamic images. It may also be used to screen the guide wire during a percutaneous approach.

Intravenous contrast should be used to opacify a catheter if its position is at all unclear and particularly with the virtually radiolucent peripherally inserted catheters (2–3 F). If, after screening, there is any suspicion that the catheter is not in the venous system, then connection to a simple manometer or pressure transducer will rule out arterial placement.

The optimum site for the tip of a central venous catheter remains controversial. The thrombotic risk of placement in the superior or inferior vena cava has to be balanced against the rarer, though potentially fatal, complication of cardiac perforation from a right atrial catheter. Conversely, a central venous catheter in the latter position is less likely to malfunction. In the UK, the current recommendation from the Medical

Devices Agency is that, for the purpose of parenteral feeding, the tip of a central venous catheter in a neonate should be positioned at the junction of the superior or inferior vena cava and the right atrium.

SECURING THE CATHETER

A cuffed device remains at risk of being pulled out until its cuff becomes incorporated with fibrous tissue from the subcutaneous tunnel. The corollary of this is that such a catheter may be removed by traction until about four weeks after insertion; beyond that time, the cuff can be detached from the surrounding tissues only by sharp dissection.

A variety of methods are used alone or in combination to reduce the chance of a central line falling out:

- suture at exit site to catheter;
- purse-string suture at exit site;
- subcutaneous purse-string suture to narrow tunnel below cuff ('cuff stitch');
- retrograde tunnelling of catheter (see above);
- dressings.

Complications of central venous catheters

Complications resulting from a central venous catheter may be categorized as early or late. The former consist of those occurring during catheter insertion, may be underreported and potentially may be reduced by intraoperative imaging techniques such as ultrasound guidance. Late complications largely comprise infective and occlusive events throughout the catheter's lifespan.

EARLY COMPLICATIONS

The overall early complication rate is around four per cent. The complications resulting from percutaneous puncture of the subclavian or jugular veins, and their approximate incidences, are listed in Table 11.3.

Vascular injuries

Inadvertent arterial puncture may result in a haematoma, haemothorax or a haemomediastinum if more medial arterial structures are injured. Haemothorax or haemomediastinum would present with signs of hypovolaemic shock. Haemothorax would require drainage with an intercostal drain. In only a very few cases where there is persistent blood loss from the drain or haemodynamic instability would a thoracotomy be necessary in these instances. Injuries to the subclavian vein, subclavian artery or superior vena cava are found to be responsible.

Carotid puncture may create a haematoma with the potential for airway obstruction.

Passage of a guide wire, dilator or catheter into an artery may create an intimal flap with the potential for thrombus formation and embolization, or vessel occlusion. In this situation, removal of the device usually restores distal flow and, therefore, arteriography and arterial exploration are required rarely.

Table 11.3 *Complications resulting from percutaneous puncture of subclavian and jugular veins*

Complication	Incidence (%)
Vascular injury, arterial	0.2–7
Vascular injury, venous	–
Pneumothorax	0.1–3.1
Air embolus	0.5
Malposition	–
Bleeding from subcutaneous tunnel	–
Thoracic duct injury	–
Arrhythmia (requiring DC cardioversion)	0.1

Injury to the internal jugular vein during an open approach may result in profound blood loss. This may be avoided by gaining adequate control of the vessel. An incision too low in the neck or only just above the clavicle precludes safe distal control, particularly in very young patients, where the innominate vein can lie above the upper sternal edge. In such an emergency situation, exposure of vessels at this level can be achieved by splitting the upper sternum – the 'trapdoor incision', in which such a vertical sternal incision is taken laterally through the third intercostal space and combined with sternomastoid division.

Pneumothorax

This is most common with left-sided subclavian venous access and may be simple or under tension. Small pleural air collections may be asymptomatic and may not be detected if fluoroscopy rather than a plain chest X-ray is used to determine the catheter tip position. The risk of this complication can be minimized by using as small a needle as possible for placement of the guide wire.

Air embolism

Air embolism is most likely to occur when the obturator/dilator is removed from the peel-away sheath before catheter insertion. It is avoided by always ensuring that the patient is placed in the most head-down position that does not compromise ventilation.

Catheter malposition

Internal jugular catheters may pass into the ipsilateral subclavian vein. Equally, subclavian catheters may pass into the opposite upper limb or up into the jugular system. This problem is usually overcome by partially withdrawing the catheter and repassing it. Abduction of the ipsilateral upper limb or stiffening it with a guide wire may direct the catheter into the correct site.

Bleeding from subcutaneous tunnel

Subcutaneous vessels may be torn whilst tunnelling the catheter. In the long term, this may increase the possibility of line infection. Correction of coagulopathy or thrombocytopenia and the use of a blunt tunnelling instrument will reduce the frequency of this complication.

Box 11.6 Long-term complications of central venous catheters

Occlusion, extrinsic
Occlusion, luminal
Infection
Fracture
Malposition/displacement

Thoracic duct injury

Damage to this structure may occur because of its position in the angle between the subclavian and internal jugular veins. Injury may result in a chylothorax or, rarely, a lymphocutaneous fistula.

LATE COMPLICATIONS

Review of the literature describing different centres' experiences of central venous catheters shows long-term complication rates of up to 50 per cent (Box 11.6).

Catheter occlusion

Central venous catheter occlusion initially may present with difficulty upon attempted aspiration. Latterly, both this and infusion may be difficult; ultimately, both may be impossible.

Extrinsic causes of occlusion should be sought first, including:

- closed clamps;
- tight anchoring sutures;
- external kinks (within dressings);
- 'pinch-off syndrome' (compression or kinking of a subclavian catheter in the angle between the first rib and the clavicle);
- internal kinks.

The first three of these may be eliminated by removing any dressings and doing an external inspection of the catheter. Pinch-off syndrome should be suspected if aspiration or infusion is possible only when the patient is recumbent, with the shoulders braced back or the upper limb abducted. Once these have been excluded, a plain chest X-ray must be obtained to display any kinks in the course of the catheter from the skin exit site to its tip; this investigation may also demonstrate that a catheter is extravascular.

Correction of external causes of catheter occlusion is straightforward. Internal kinks or an extravascular position may entail complete revision of the line, although an initial attempt should be made to preserve the existing track by passage of a guide wire.

Once extrinsic causes of occlusion have been excluded, the following luminal problems should be considered:

- drug precipitates
- thrombus
- fibrin sheath around catheter.

Table 11.4 *Substances that may block lines and their appropriate dissolving agents*

Precipitate	Dissolving agent
Lipid/protein	70% ethanol, 0.1-N NaOH
Phenytoin	$NaHCO_3$ 1 mmol/L
Calcium phosphate, heparin	0.1-N HCl

Whatever the cause, passage of a guide wire may be sufficient to both unblock the catheter lumen and disrupt the fibrin sheath covering its end. Intraluminal brushes are also available for the same purpose and for providing material for microbiological culture. If this manoeuvre is not possible or only partially relieves the obstruction, and drug precipitates are thought to be the cause, then the agents listed in Table 11.4 can be used.

Intraluminal catheter thrombus may be lysed using the thrombolytic agents urokinase or tissue plasminogen activator (tPA). If the catheter will flush, then it is filled with a volume of the thrombolytic drug equal to the catheter volume. If the catheter is completely occluded, then a three-way tap is attached to the end and one port aspirated to generate negative pressure in the lumen. A syringe containing the thrombolytic agent is attached to the remaining port and the tap is opened to allow it to be drawn into the catheter. After 30 minutes, the catheter is aspirated to retrieve the drug; if the lumen is still occluded, the treatment can be repeated twice. Most series investigating the efficacy of this treatment suggest that patency can be restored in 90 per cent of occluded catheters with one to three thrombolytic doses.

A sheath forms around the intravascular portion of every catheter within 24 hours of placement. This sheath consists of fibrin, to which platelets and bacteria adhere. It may completely encase the device; thus, infusate can track retrogradely to extravasate into subcutaneous tissues or appear at the catheter skin exit site. However, sheaths often are incomplete, with perforations at the end and more proximally; in this case, catheter flow may be reduced or aspiration may fail because the sheath is sucked into the tip. A fibrin sheath can be disrupted with a guide wire or thrombolytic agents, but usually the catheter requires replacement if these methods fail. Interventional radiological techniques such as stripping the sheath with a snare-type catheter passed via the femoral vein have also been described.

Catheter infection

As many as 60 per cent of catheters become infected, and half of these require removal. The infection rate is five episodes per 1000 catheter days. At least two-thirds of catheter infections are due to *Staphylococcus aureus*, *S. epidermidis* or *Candida* species. Gram-negative infections are more prevalent in neutropenic and immunosuppressed patients.

Infection occurring within two weeks of catheter insertion usually was introduced at the time of the procedure. Sepsis occurring more than two weeks after catheter insertion usually originates from poor accessing techniques.

Colonization of central venous catheters arises from four sources:

- skin at exit site
- catheter hub
- seeding from bloodstream
- contaminated infusion fluids.

The first two of these are the most significant sources in terms of preventive measures against infection.

Predisposing factors to catheter infection may be patient- or device-related. Device factors include the following:

- *Number of lumens*: the incidence of infection rises with multiple lumen catheters.
- *Cuffs*: a Dacron cuff reduces the incidence of infection by preventing ingress of bacteria along the external surface of the catheter.
- *Ease of insertion*: an increased number of passes to achieve access correlates with infection, as does bleeding from the subcutaneous tunnel.
- *Subcutaneous port volumes*: these often contain a sludge of blood or drug residue, which acts as a culture medium for bacteria.
- *Fibrin sheath and catheter thrombus*: both of these favour the adhesion of bacteria.

Patient-related factors include the following:

- *Disease process*: haematological malignancies carry a greater risk than solid tumours of catheter sepsis.
- *Catheter care*: Scrupulous care by trained individuals when accessing the catheter reduces the risk of infection.

Central venous catheter infection may be classified in the following ways:

- *Local*:
  - pus at or within 2 cm of the exit site;
  - port pocket infection;
  - cellutitis along track of a tunnelled line.
- *Systemic*:
  - uncomplicated: the same organism is identified from both the catheter and peripheral cultures taken simultaneously, and the ratio of colony-forming units (cfu) of the catheter compared with that of the peripheral sample is ten to one;
  - complicated: associated with infected venous thrombosis.

The use of antibiotic-coated catheters, catheter hubs containing iodinated alcohol and exit-site antiseptic dressings/topical antibiotics have been advocated in the reduction of central venous catheter infection (Mermel 2001).

Displacement/malposition

Central venous catheters may migrate in either direction. In some series, 30 per cent of catheters fell out. Catheters that have moved inwards may be detected either because they malfunction or from the direct consequence of their new extravascular

Table 11.5 *Possible consequences of catheter migration*

Original site	Extravascular position	Clinical consequence
Right atrium	Pericardial sac	Cardiac tamponade
Iliac vein	Retroperitoneum	Acute abdomen
Inferior vena cava	Via lumbar vein to extradural space	Spinal cord necrosis
Inferior vena cava	Via renal vein to renal pelvis	TPN in urine
Right atrium	Via pulmonary artery to lung parenchyma	TPN in endotracheal aspirate/lung oedema

TPN, total parenteral nutrition.

site. Peripherally inserted catheters in neonates are prone to this complication through a process of intimal ulceration and, ultimately, perforation; clinical examples are given in Table 11.5.

Displacement is virtually eliminated if catheters with detachable hubs are tunnelled retrogradely. Subcutaneous ports may rotate around the axis of the catheter, and three to five per cent erode through the overlying skin.

Catheter fracture

Silastic catheters eventually will fracture because of the incursion of serum lipids into the infrastructure of the silicone matrix, which is weakened by this molecular disruption. Polyurethane catheters are immune from this problem, but consequently they tend to be stiffer and more prone to kinking.

Central venous catheters may fracture at any point from the hub to the tip. Specific points of weakness are at the joint of the hub and the catheter and where clamps are applied.

The catheter of a subcutaneous port may be severed inadvertently with an access needle. All types of device may be ruptured by force-flushing with a small (<5 mL) syringe.

Intravascular parts of a catheter that have fractured and embolized to the right ventricle or pulmonary artery may be retrieved percutaneously via the femoral vein.

Long-term outcomes of central venous catheters

Venograms in children at time of catheter removal suggest that up to 50 per cent will have deep venous thrombosis, of which three-quarters will be asymptomatic. A substantial percentage of children with long-term central venous catheters will have demonstrable perfusion defects on V/Q scanning.

Longer-term follow-up shows that in the order of 12 per cent have 'permanent' venous occlusions but only four per cent will be clinically significant.

Conclusion

Central venous access in children is a necessary evil. The disadvantages should not be underestimated, and these should be reflected by the issues disclosed when consent for placement of a catheter is sought. However, the advantages of secure venous access for the child are also obvious and will usually outweigh the risks involved.

REFERENCES

Mermel L. New technologies to prevent intravascular catheter-related bloodstream infections. *Emerging Infectious Diseases* 2001; **7**: 197–9.

National Institute for Clinical Evidence. Central venous catheters: ultrasound locating devices. Technology Appraisal Guidance No. 49. London: NICE, 2002.

FURTHER READING

Advanced Life Support Group. *Advanced Paediatric Life Support: The Practical Approach*, 2nd edn. London: Royal College of Surgeons, 2000. [Description of routes and techniques of central line insertion.]

Central Venous Access. www.venousaccess.com

Raad I, Bodey G. Infectious complications of indwelling vascular catheters. *Clinical Infectious Diseases* 1992; **15**: 197–208.

Wheeler R, Griffiths D, Burge D. Retrograde tunnel: a method for the fixation of long-term pediatric central venous catheters. *Journal of Parenteral and Enteral Nutrition* 1991; **15**: 114–15.

12

Communication skills

CATHERINE HILL AND VICTORIA McGRIGOR

Learning objectives

- To understand the importance of communication skills in paediatric practice.
- To recognize the child as an active participant in his or her healthcare.
- To understand how a child's development influences participation in his or her care.
- To review an approach for children with special needs.
- To review basic principles of good communication in difficult situations.

WHY READ THIS CHAPTER?

Communication, with both children and their parents, forms an essential component of paediatric surgical practice. It is assessed formally in higher surgical exams, including the intercollegiate Fellow of the Royal College of Surgeons (FRCS) examination in the UK. This chapter illustrates why it is so important to communicate effectively and describes some of the problems that may be encountered.

Doctors are often poor communicators

There is a wealth of evidence to show that doctors do not communicate as effectively as they could and arguably should (Maguire and Pitceathly 2002). The reasons for this are complex. However, the paternalistic tradition of medicine ('doctor knows best'), the ever-present pressures of time and the fear of upsetting the patient with difficult news are all powerful antagonists to ideal communication. Most doctors will be familiar with these obstacles.

Doing it well improves clinical care

There is no doubt that in adult practice, effective doctor–patient communication reaps benefits in terms of improved diagnosis, patient satisfaction, treatment adherence, reduction of patient distress and, not least, the doctor's sense of wellbeing. There is a growing body of research showing that children's satisfaction with care and adherence to treatment benefits from improved communication. Evidence that good communication improves children's health status is emerging (Holzheimer *et al.* 1998), although biomedical parameters are rarely studied in outcome research on communication skills interventions. In short, effective communication reaps dividends for doctor and patient alike.

Doing it badly is dangerous

In the litigious world of twenty-first-century clinical practice, we need skills to protect ourselves from the stress of unjustified complaints. A significant proportion of complaints about medical practice relate to poor communication. The Bristol Royal Infirmary enquiry highlighted improved communication between healthcare professionals, children and their parents as a key recommendation in the care of children.

Lord Laming's inquiry into the murder of eight-year-old Victoria Climbié at the hands of her aunt in 2003 highlighted poor communication between health professionals and lack of communication with the child as failures in basic clinical practice.

Like a stethoscope or scalpel, competent communication is an essential tool in the doctor's armoury. Practise without it at your peril!

THE TIMES THEY ARE A-CHANGING ...

Social trends

Over the past 30 years, public expectations of doctor–patient communication have changed. The traditional doctor-centred approach to the medical consultation (doctor 'knows best' and controls discussion) has shifted to a patient-centred approach as patients have become more active in their health decisions. Real-life practice does not always conform to sociological trends, and patients differ in their expectations of their doctors. Each encounter requires an assessment of how the patient would like to participate and the patient's expectations of the doctor.

Passive or participant child, or 'Whose operation is it anyway?'

Children are citizens with rights. Nowadays, adult–child interactions are characterized by greater openness and parenting is less repressive. The participation of the child in healthcare decisions is now recognized as good practice. Internationally, the United Nations (UN) Convention on the Rights of the Child recommends specifically that children's wishes and views about their healthcare be respected. The Child Friendly Healthcare Initiative has translated this principle into standards expected of hospitals worldwide; for example, Standard 5 states:

All staff should approach children as individual people with their own needs and rights to privacy and dignity, involving them in decisions affecting their care.

Research and rhetoric promote the child as an active participant rather than a passive recipient of healthcare. Applying the principles of participation to children in practice requires a quantum leap for many doctors. Many of us still make powerful assumptions about children's incompetence and vulnerability. Furthermore, adults may misguidedly protect a child from knowledge of his or her condition. We know that when shielded from information, children acquire their own knowledge. Children dying from leukaemia acquire knowledge

of their fate through their own observation and interpretations of adult behaviour.

Therefore, if we pause for thought, intuitively it is crucial to involve the child. A parent, no matter how empathetic, cannot feel their child's pain. The child's concept of his or her illness, and his or her experiences of hospitalization, are likely to differ significantly from those of the parent. The child needs not only to be listened to but also to hear. Whatever the seriousness of the problem, whether it is constipation or cancer, treatment adherence requires the understanding and support of the child. We know that when children understand their condition, treatment and prognosis, they are more likely to cooperate, tolerate painful treatments and recover effectively. Communicating with the child is not only politically correct – it also works!

THE BASICS

Good communication skills are both the foundation stones of clinical practice and a vehicle for the expression of our humanity as doctors. Traditional clinical methods rely upon communication at each step (Box 12.1) to achieve:

- a good interpersonal relationship with the child and their parents;
- the exchange of information;
- clinical decision-making.

Think critically about your own practice. Most doctors are trained in the requisite skills for steps 1 and 2 in Box 12.1, which are crucial to reach a diagnosis, but how many have equal training in steps 3–6?

Box 12.1 Key tasks in communication with patients (adapted from Maguire and Pitceathly 2002)

1   History: eliciting the child's main problems, the child's perception (and that of the parents) of these, and the impact of the problem on the child's family and school life.
2   Examination: eliciting the child's (and the parents') consent and cooperation to examination.
3   Tailoring diagnostic information to what the child and the parents want to know, and checking their understanding of this.
4   Determining how much the child and the parents want/are able to participate in decision-making about treatment options.
5   Discussing treatment options so that the child and the parents understand the implications.
6   Maximizing the chances that the child and the parents will follow agreed decisions about treatment and advice about changes in lifestyle.

HOW ARE WE DOING SO FAR?

How good are doctors in practice at involving children in discussion about their healthcare?

The doctor–parent–child triad in the paediatric consultation has been subject to only limited research. However, a number of consistent patterns emerge:

- A child's total conversational contribution is limited to only 2–14 per cent and is correlated positively with age.
- A doctor's total contribution is consistently around 60 per cent, with any involvement of the child occurring at the expense of parental contribution, i.e. involving the child does not prolong consultations.
- Parents often will answer questions directed to their child, and children's control is limited. In one study, parents interfered in more than half of questions directed to their children.
- A doctor's conversation with the child comprises mostly two areas. First, 'affective' social or joking talk predominates. This clearly plays an important role in developing a relationship with the child to gain his or trust for physical examination. Second is factual questioning. It is striking that although children are considered capable of providing information – 'Tell me where it hurts' – they are rarely considered capable of receiving information. In the context of the conventional clinical method (Box 12.1), there is fallout in the child's involvement as the consultation develops. The parent is frequently left with the responsibility of interpreting diagnostic and treatment information for the child.

TRANSLATING PRINCIPLES TO PRACTICE

Developing age

Children once they grow out of infancy are acute observers of the mood and body language of others. It is impossible to avoid communicating with them. For this reason, good practice is now founded on the principles of truthfulness, clarity and awareness of the child's age. (Bristol Royal Infirmary Inquiry)

Knowledge of a child's cognitive and language abilities is a prerequisite for any communication. This does not require complex developmental knowledge, although a basic framework and experience clearly help. The most helpful clue can be to observe the child and parent communicating. Pitching your communication at too high a developmental level will alienate a child. Most children tend to 'switch off' to language that is complex or beyond their developmental understanding.

For all children, establish the child's preferred name and the name he or she uses for his parent. Just as the newly qualified FRCS will resent being titled 'Doctor', so the 'Toms' of this world may feel uncomfortable with 'Thomas'. Referring to 'Mum' as 'Mummy' may patronize a 'streetwise' child and may inadvertently cause offence.

INFANTS AND TODDLERS

Most adults intuitively adopt child-directed speech, characteristically high-pitched, slow, simplified, and with exaggerated vowel sounds, when addressing infants and toddlers. For prelinguistic infants and toddlers, participation in their healthcare will be limited by both their communicative and cognitive development. They will be sensitive to the moods and reactions of their parents. Clear explanations to the parents of what to expect and how they can best support their child are helpful. Ask the parent what the child's previous experience and past behaviour has been in medical encounters. Remember that a child's comprehension is more advanced than his or her expressive language skills. Parents should be discouraged from vocalizing their fears and anxieties in the child's presence. Avoid approaching the child immediately – allow them to get used to you first. A calm unhurried approach, if possible preceded by play, is likely to yield more information.

PRESCHOOLERS

From three years upwards, children have a vocabulary of 1000 words and can express emotion and concepts such as past, present and future. Children, just like adults, will come to any clinical encounter with their own fears and fantasies about their problem. Ascertain the child's presenting complaint: he or she may have quite a different interpretation from that of the parents. When directing information-seeking questions to the child, first check what term the child is familiar with and try to adjust your language accordingly. 'I'm just going to examine your testicles' is likely to leave any preschool child confused. If unsure, ask the parent to help in making your request understood. Young children will have a limited vocabulary for body parts. They rarely distinguish 'chest', instead recognizing neck to thigh as 'tummy'. Explanations of examination are better addressed gently but assertively. Asking a three- to five-year-old 'Can I look at your ears?' is likely to elicit 'No', whereas 'I would like to look at your ears – shall I look in this one or that one?' allows the child a choice and is more likely to elicit cooperation as the child has a sense of control.

Children may appear disinterested in adult discussion but 'listen in' and misinterpret what they hear. Their misinterpretation becomes translated into a personal fantasy; thus, 'oedema' may become 'demon in my belly' (Perrin and Gerrity 1980). It is important, therefore, that information is given directly to the child in words and, ideally, images that they can understand.

Even when information is given carefully to a child in an appropriate format, it may be misinterpreted or exaggerated. At our own hospital, children undergoing myringotomy attend a preadmission visit, where play therapists explain what will happen to them. Despite this, one five-year-old child fantasized about the intravenous cannula as a huge hypodermic in her abdomen (Figure 12.1).

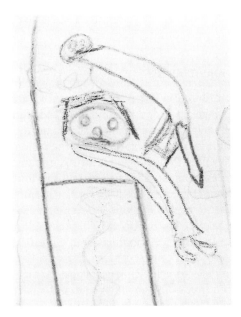

Figure 12.1 *Drawing by a five-year-old child, who fantasized that the intravenous cannula would be a huge hypodermic in her abdomen.*

Another child understood the anaesthetic induction but totally misinterpreted the operative procedure: 'They are going to put a needle in my hand and the magic cream on and the injection and they are going to poke a hole in your bum …'

It is useful, therefore, to ask the child to explain what they have understood of your diagnosis and proposed treatment and give them permission to ask questions.

SCHOOL-AGE CHILDREN

Communication becomes easier as children's verbal skills improve, although inevitably they will regress when distressed or in pain. It is important to remember that up to the age of seven years, children may still ascribe causality of disease to their own thoughts or actions – this is also a reflection of the egocentric nature of young children: 'I forgot to wash my hands after the toilet and now I've got a bad tummy pain.' These ideas may not be expressed, reinforcing the importance of checking the child's perception of his or her problem. From the age of seven years, children retain a rather magical understanding of disease and tend to relate disease states to 'germ' concepts. In middle-childhood, children can take more responsibility for decisions about their treatment.

ADOLESCENTS

By the teenage years, a more mature understanding of health and disease can be expected. Adolescents can engage in hypothetical deductive reasoning. Their ability to participate will be impaired not by cognitive level but rather by the tendency for emotion to override rational thinking. This presents different challenges to the doctor who may be faced with anger, embarrassment, resentment and rebellion. Where possible, this can be defused by seeing the adolescent without the parents present for part of the consultation to encourage a sense of control and independence. This also allows discussion of lifestyle issues relevant to the presenting problem that may not be disclosed in the presence of the parents. While the temptation may be to avoid communication, 'difficult' adolescents will require more of your time to achieve compliance and informed consent.

Children with special needs

Children with physical, intellectual or sensory difficulties form an important and vulnerable group. Prior knowledge of a child's abilities, particularly his or her understanding, is vital. The disparity between comprehension and expressive speech may be more marked; for example, a child with athetoid cerebral palsy, and with perhaps little or no speech, may have normal cognitive abilities masked by a severe motor disorder. Beware a misappreciation of a child's skills and level of functioning. Many inexperienced doctors are uncertain how to approach and include a disabled child in a consultation. If you are unclear of a child's understanding, then do not be afraid to ask the child's parents how best to include the child in the consultation. Whatever you do, do not ignore the child.

Children with disabilities are highly susceptible to low self-esteem. This in turn requires patience, understanding and encouragement on the part of the health team to enable the child's views on treatment to be sought. Parents quite rightly feel that they are the 'experts' on their child's complex needs, but, as mentioned already, the child's agenda may differ from that of his or her parents. It is necessary to explore this – often a time-consuming exercise, but time that must not be overlooked.

The use of body language and tone of voice are essential in any consultation but are brought sharply into focus when a child cannot participate readily. Be wary of unspoken communication. It is easy to forget that the child may nonetheless 'read' these important signals. The child's awareness of the parental response to the doctor will be heightened and is a powerful influence on the child's understanding and subsequent involvement in treatment. Try to find out in advance whether the child uses an alternative method of communication, e.g. signing, so that you are as prepared as possible to talk to the child.

Difficult situations

There is a wealth of information to suggest that the sharing of difficult news with parents and children is not handled well and that many parents are supported poorly at such a time. However, there is growing evidence that this need not necessarily be the case. This is a critical time for families that may influence their view of their child from this time on and permanently influence their relationship with health professionals.

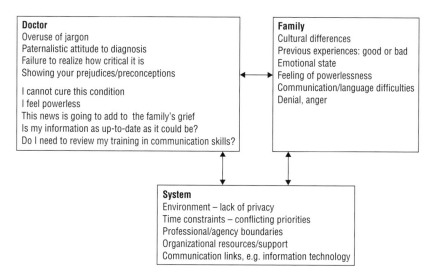

Figure 12.2 *Barriers to good practice.*

In order to change things, it is helpful to explore and understand the barriers to good practice in ourselves, the child and family, and the system. You may identify with many of these (Figure 12.2).

HOW TO IMPROVE THINGS: TRANSLATING THE BARRIERS INTO PRACTICAL ADVICE

There is a need for flexibility and sensitivity, and no 'model' is correct, but the following points are key (SCOPE 2003). This list was written concerning the disclosure of news of a disability, but the principles can be applied equally to other settings, e.g. when a lump initially thought to be innocent is found to be malignant:

- Parents' suspicions should be taken seriously and responded to.
- The need for privacy at the time of disclosure should be recognized.
- If at all possible, parents generally need to be together when told.
- Plenty of time should be made available, including opportunities to ask questions at the time of disclosure and subsequently.
- Written material is helpful as a supplement to, but in no circumstances as a substitute for, direct face-to-face communication.
- All information should be given in understandable language.
- Always value the child – remember that children with disabilities are children first.
- Adopt a whole-team approach – the family must be a part of this team.
- Sharing the information is a process, not an event.
- Always consider the perspectives and feelings of the family.
- Take into account the needs and perspectives of other professionals and agencies.
- Listen to what the family is saying.
- Share power and information appropriately.

KEY POINTERS IN DIFFICULT SITUATIONS

- Have another healthcare professional with you.
- Use a calm, unhurried manner (bleep must be turned off!).
- Think about body language, including seating arrangements, e.g. sit forward, face the parents and child directly.
- Maintain good eye contact.
- Avoid negative phrases, especially without meaning, e.g. 'I'm afraid it doesn't look good.'
- Use a positive approach without providing false reassurance, e.g. 'It is important that the diagnosis has been made swiftly.'
- Use simple explanations and keep jargon to a minimum.
- Repeat information at least twice.
- Check at intervals what the parents and the child have understood.
- Allow time for news to 'sink in'.
- Arrange contact with you, or another member of the team, within a very short time.

MOVING ON UP: IMPROVING YOUR COMMUNICATION SKILLS

Remember that communication is a series of skills that can be both learned and retained. It is not just a personality trait. Finally, a quote from Dr Rob Buckman who has written extensively on doctor's communication skills:

> Expectations of the general public and our patients are high. Based on what they see on television and read, most people have high expectations of our medical prowess and our communications. We will never meet everyone's expectations, but the skill and effort that we put into our clinical communication does make an indelible impression on our patients, their families, and their friends. If we do it badly, they may never forgive us; if we do it well they may never forget us.

REFERENCES

Holzheimer L, Mohay H, Masters IB. Educating young children about asthma: comparing the effectiveness of developmentally appropriate asthma education video tape and picture book. *Child: Care, Health and Development* 1998; **24**: 85–99.

Maguire P, Pitceathly C. Key communication skills and how to acquire them. *British Medical Journal* 2002; **325**: 697–700.

Perrin EC, Gerrity PS. There's a demon in your belly: children's understanding of illness. *Pediatrics* 1980; **67**: 841–9.

SCOPE. *Right From the Start Template*. London: SCOPE, 2003.

FURTHER READING

Butler R, Green D. *Children and Illness: The Child Within*. Oxford: Butterworth-Heinemann, 1998.

Silverman J, Curtz S, Draper J. *Skills for Communicating with Patients*. Abingdon: Radcliffe Medical, 1998.

13

The child and the law

VIVIEN McNAMARA AND ROBERT A WHEELER

Learning objectives

- To understand the concepts of capacity and disclosure.
- To understand who has the right to give consent for a child's treatment, and how that right might be acquired.
- To understand the process of consent, and what to do if it is not available or if it is refused.
- To understand the framework within which decisions to withdraw or withhold treatment are made.

CAPACITY

The differences in legal terms between adult and paediatric practice flow from the fact that children have not reached the age of majority (18 years). It is only at this age that the law treats individuals as having full rights and responsibilities. Lacking these, issues flowing from how the child's rights and duties initially handled are represented by their parents.

However, the law recognizes that children may acquire the relevant skills, i.e. have the capacity, to make decisions for themselves before the age of 18 years. The difficulty for the legislators is where to draw the line. Some flexibility has already been recognized by statute, whereby 16- and 17-year-olds have been given the right of consent, although their parents retain a parallel right should their child become incapacitated. This parallel arrangement ends at 18 years.

We have all encountered eight-year-olds who seem to have achieved capacity, but eight years would seem, intuitively, too young to draw a legal line that would acknowledge capacity in all eight-year-olds. The legal approach is to apply a legal test, the Gillick test, which attempts to identify those children who

have adequate capacity to make medical decisions, which, in terms of surgery, is translated as giving consent to treatment.

There is no prescribed lower age limit for use of the test, although common sense should give a clue as to likely candidates. The child will need to demonstrate that he or she can understand the nature of the proposed procedure when it is explained in suitable language. The benefits that the procedure confers, the associated risks and the alternatives must also be discussed. The doctor must be satisfied that the child can understand and retain these issues, at least for long enough to consider them and reach a decision. If the child is able to complete this process, then he or she has passed the Gillick test and is said to possess capacity.

The courts do not view the capacity to agree to treatment in the same light as the capacity to refuse. Relying on the doctors' intention to act in the best interest of the child, the courts have found little difficulty with Gillick competent children of any age agreeing to treatment and signing their consent. For the most major procedures, it would seem to be a prudent precaution to have a parent countersign the consent document, but this is not mandatory.

Dissent is a different matter. Courts, once again, assume that proffered treatment is in the child's best interests. If a Gillick competent child refuses this treatment, then the gravity of the underlying condition must be considered. If the condition were relatively innocuous, then it would be prudent to postpone the procedure and have further discussions with the parents and child. If the procedure is necessary to avoid permanent harm that will otherwise result from the disease, then the consent of the parents will override the refusal of the Gillick competent child. However, if such a rare event occurs, then consultation with colleagues or the local clinical ethics committee would be prudent.

Whether the inequality of weight given to assent and refusal by the Gillick competent child will survive the Human Rights Act 1998 remains to be seen. For the time being, recent judgments make it clear that the courts would rather ignore the newly acquired autonomy of a child, in order to give the emergent adult the right to exercise autonomy in the longer term.

DISCLOSURE

In gaining consent for any procedure, what should be discussed? The paternalist would suggest that as little as possible should be revealed to the patient, saving them from unnecessary anxiety. At the opposite end of the spectrum, it could be argued that each patient must decide what they wish to be told, setting individualized wholly subjective standards of disclosure. The doctrine of informed consent falls just short of this, advocating that every patient should receive the same, exhaustively detailed disclosure package, to furnish them with the same knowledge as the consenting doctor.

Although adopted in a minority of American states, the UK courts have not accepted the doctrine of informed consent, but it has greatly influenced our consenting process. There is evidence that patients (and parents) suffer anxiety as a result of detailed disclosure but would still prefer to receive it. It is now settled law that a fear of causing upset to the patient is not a sufficient reason to withhold information. How much detail should be given?

Originally, disclosure came under the auspices of the Bolam test, asking courts to consider whether a reasonably competent practitioner would have provided similar disclosure. The problem is that this test left it to the medical establishment to determine the appropriate standard of disclosure. The courts were anxious to make it clear that the standard setting was a matter for the courts, not the doctors.

Although this area of law is changing constantly, a widely accepted maxim is to disclose whatever information a reasonable patient might wish to know. This fictitious 'reasonable person' provides an objective standard, for if there is consensus concerning what their attitudes is likely to be, then the information disclosed during consent should become more consistent. It is important to note that this information should cover the proposed treatment, complications and alternatives.

WHO HAS PARENTAL RESPONSIBILITY, AND WHO CAN ACQUIRE IT?

Only people with parental responsibility can give consent on a child's behalf. Parental responsibility will be held by the mother, and by the father provided he is married to the mother at the time of giving consent. For children born after 1 December 2003, if the father and mother register the birth together, then the father acquires parental responsibility, irrespective of marital status. In children born before this date, unmarried fathers can gain parental responsibility only by marrying the mother, by signing an official agreement with the mother or by getting a court order. We are therefore all obliged to enquire from a father who proposes to sign the consent form whether he is married to the child's mother. Divorce does not sever this responsibility.

If the mother remarries, then the stepfather does not automatically acquire parental responsibility. There is a complete lack of legal recognition of step-parenthood in this respect, and a step-parent would have to apply to the court for a variety of legal orders to obtain parental responsibility. This may even involve adoption of the stepchild, although such proceedings will remove parental responsibility from the natural parent. Adoptions in these circumstances are unusual.

Courts can give local authorities or guardians a share of the parental responsibility for a child on a temporary basis, although this does not remove the ability of the natural married parents to consent on the child's behalf. Parental responsibility for an adopted child is transferred fully to the adoptive parents, with the natural parents retaining no rights. In the situation of disagreement between parents, only one consent is required. However, in these circumstances, advice should be sought before proceeding with surgery.

PROCESS OF CONSENT

Following several well-publicized scandals, political focus has sharpened upon the process of consent. This has resulted in several very useful publications, notably the British Medical Association's (2001) Consent Toolkit, which is widely available and is mandatory reading. The advent of the new Department of Health consent form reinforces many of the points made but represents a significant challenge, demanding substantial detail to be entered on the form itself and raising questions about where the threshold for written consent should be drawn.

There is no legal requirement for written consent. However, writing provides a record that a conversation has taken place, in which all the elements for proper consent have been addressed. Given the complexity of the process, a form may well be the best-organized structure in which to present the written record. For elective surgery, the decision to operate is usually made in the outpatient setting. Ideally, the first part of the consent form is filled in during this consultation. The surgeon who is going to undertake the procedure should record the issues addressed during the process of disclosure and those brought up by the patient and parents. The family is given a copy of this partly completed form to take home, allowing them to consider the issues further. The family also should be given a procedure-specific information sheet to take home, acting as a prompt for any further questions.

On their presentation for surgery, the consent is reaffirmed by any member of the team competent to answer outstanding questions. From this description, it can be seen why consent is described as a 'process'.

In an emergency situation, the consent procedure is inevitably truncated. The parents are denied a period of reflection, and the urgency of the situation will probably reduce the available alternatives. This is understood well by the courts, which demand simply that the consent, in an emergency, is taken in such a way as to correspond with how any reasonable paediatric surgeon, in identical circumstances, would handle the situation.

NO CONSENT AVAILABLE

Consent has been likened to a shield. You need only one consent to protect yourself from the arrows of criticism. However, it may not be available in an emergency situation. A doctor is under a duty to help the patient in an emergency, and it is clearly in the public interest for doctors to act in this manner. As long as the proposed treatment is in a child's best interests, then a surgeon may provide the treatment without parental permission.

The typical situation is in a desperately ill child who lacks capacity, because of either age or illness. Although the parents are unavailable to give oral or written consent, emergency surgery is required. To operate without consent is clearly a very major step, and 'best interests' requires definition. In this context, 'best interests' means medical treatment that is immediately necessary to save life or avoid significant and permanent harm.

NO CONSENT AGREED

Circumstances can arise when both the parents and the child steadfastly refuse to give consent for necessary treatment. Where there is such a clear disagreement between doctors and patients, a colleague's opinion and reference to the clinical ethics committee should be the first step. This is a very unusual situation and arises most commonly in the context of blood transfusions in Jehovah's Witnesses. Although it is understood clearly that people over the age of 18 years can exercise their right to refuse treatment, the courts will rarely countenance this before majority is reached.

In an emergency situation, the court can make a care order if it is satisfied that, without it, the child may suffer significant

harm. This enables the local authority to share parental responsibility and, thus, provide the shield of consent. However, this has the great disadvantage of passing far more responsibility to the court than either party may wish. A more precise instrument would be a specific issue order, enabling blood to be used (blood use being the 'specific issue' referred to in this particular example) without removing the other aspects of parental responsibility from the parents. Specific issue orders can be applied equally to any particular aspect of medical treatment and are available from the court, if necessary by telephone.

WITHDRAWAL/WITHHOLDING OF TREATMENT

It is within neonatal surgery that the decisions of whether to withdraw or withhold treatment are most commonly made. There is no effective difference between them. Both are onerous for parents, nurses and doctors, and both require a similar pattern of questioning and reasoning, but there is no basis for the argument that it is more difficult to withdraw treatment once it is commenced. Babies in whom complex support has started will inevitably be receiving a mixture of ventilatory, circulatory and systemic support, together with hydration, nutrition and antibiotics.

It is tempting to organize these into a hierarchy of supportive elements, with ventilation and inotropes at one end and mere hydration and nutrition at the other. If the hierarchy is accepted, then the issue of where the line is drawn has to be addressed.

The basic position is that hydration and nutrition are given as a matter of right to all patients. The only situation where courts have accepted withdrawal of these is the persistent vegetative state.

A second opinion, whether from a local colleague or the clinical ethics committee, will address all the relevant issues. The diagnoses of the child will be reviewed and the prognosis from each separate diagnosis considered, as well as the overall effect of the combination on the child's present and future function. The implications for the siblings and the parents also have to be considered. Clarification should be sought over any uncertain issues of fact. Detailed discussions should involve the parents, nurses and doctors who are looking after then child, with differing weight being given to individuals according to their proximity to the child and their experience. During all of this fact-finding, the information gained should serve to define which of the treatment options will best serve the child's overall welfare.

These can be described broadly in the language of ethics. What are the prospects for this child exercising his or her rights of self-determination or autonomy? To what extent will the child be able to influence his or her own path through life? Will the child be able to take his or her own decisions, and act upon them? Will function as a thoughtful human be possible?

What are the prospects for beneficence and for doing good? Will a prolonged life be seen as a source of pleasure and fulfilment by this child? Will there be the chance to derive happiness and benefit from living?

Will the act of living be a source of pain or of continued and repeated harm if this child's life is prolonged? Will prolongation be consistent with the principle of non-maleficence?

Are there issues of justice that must be addressed? In the healthcare setting, this is generally construed to be a question about the availability of resources and is not yet discussed widely in the field of neonatal surgery. Given time, it may come: will the occupancy of this child (with a hopeless prognosis) in the nursery prevent the admission of a more deserving (very sick but completely remediable) child?

At first sight, this set of ethical questions seems totally unhelpful. How can many of these be answered? How can the doctor (or the judge) take a view about whether a child with bilateral grade 4 intraventricular haemorrhage will survive in any event? Or, if the child does survive, how can we predict how the child will feel about the quality of his or her life?

This is a fair point, but the law provides an answer using the so-called substituted judgment. The deciders simply ask themselves how they would feel in the circumstances that we are guessing our patient will end up in if the patient's life is to be prolonged. Placing themselves in this position, the deciders then answer these quality-of-life issues as though from the patient's point of view.

In normal circumstances, the essence of the decision to withdraw has often been taken before the second opinion is requested. The treating clinicians and parents have lived with the problems of their child for days or weeks, and the realization has dawned that continued treatment may be more burdensome than the benefits that it is likely to confer.

Following a second confirmatory opinion, treatment is withdrawn in a carefully planned fashion. In this phase of palliative care, the duty of care changes radically. While a patient is being treated in a non-palliative fashion, the doctor's duty is to make the patient better, by whatever means are necessary. Once palliation commences, the duty shifts to require doctors to relieve symptoms, to make the patient comfortable and to preserve the patient's dignity. Thus, palliative care is a highly active clinical activity, but it is different from the usual normative approach.

If there is any form of disagreement among the clinical team, or with the parents, about the propriety of withdrawal, then either an external second opinion or a court judgment should be sought. This is for guidance and should not, in any circumstances, be presented as an adversarial option. Parents are understandably reluctant to let go; their distress occasionally becomes translated into a demand for treatment. Parents do not have the right to demand treatment, and doctors can reasonably decline to treat if they think it is not in their patient's best interests. Nonetheless, such conflicts can only add to the parents' distress, and the correct action is to take the matter, for direction, on to neutral territory in the courts. The case of Charlotte Wyatt confirms the court's role in resolving disputes concerning treatment withdrawal.

The law acknowledges just how difficult it is to withdraw treatment, if only by the reluctance of the courts to take these decisions out of doctors' hands. There is no appetite for legislation in this area. Although we are encouraged to ask the court for guidance in the difficult cases, the answer from the court is rarely a surprise. The court will be anxious to ensure that full consultation has taken place.

It can be seen from the ethical framework that a poor prognosis for brain development will be a significant determinant during the overall judicial consideration of the child's condition. However, the potential ensuing disability will still have to be very severe before it is considered that the prognosis warrants withdrawal. It is settled law that the educational disabilities associated with Down syndrome were absolutely not an indication to withdraw treatment.

The court will obtain expert opinions from senior doctors and will listen to the views of the parents and all relevant parties. However, the most solid facts that they will consider concerning the current situation and the prognosis inevitably come from the doctors. All the courts can do, using the doctrine of substituted judgment, is to ask how they would feel in the patient's position, and the answer is very likely to depend on the picture painted by doctor. This is not undesirable and allows for the doctor to reaffirm in a public forum that, given all the circumstances, the decision to withdraw treatment is the most appropriate one available to them, because it is in the best interests of the child.

CLINICAL SCENARIO

A father brings his 14-year-old insulin-dependent son to hospital for surgery. The proposed operation is excision of an ingrowing toenail under general anaesthetic. The toenail bed is not currently infected. The boy, now nil by mouth, has been admitted to hospital for routine diabetic stabilization, which is under way. He now refuses to have the procedure, but his father urges you to continue and signs a consent form. They have travelled 200 miles by aeroplane and taxi and stayed in a local hotel overnight to ensure that they were here in time for the procedure.

1 What questions would you like to ask?
2 What are your options?
3 What is your preferred option?

Answer 1

- Is the father married to the mother? (If so, then his consent is valid.)
- Does the father have a court order giving him parental responsibility? (If so, then his consent is valid.)
- Was a consent form signed previously by the mother in the outpatient setting? (It should have been, as consent is a process.)

- Is the surgery definable as being in the child's best interests?
- Is the child Gillick competent?

Answer 2

- Postpone surgery if no consent is available. This surgery will not come under the definition of best interests, and further negotiations are needed.
- If the father is married to the mother, or if the father has been given parental responsibility by the court, or if the mother has signed the form previously, then consider forcing the surgery through. (Not a favoured position.)
- As above, but postpone and ask the court's advice.
- Cancel in any event, commence prophylactic antibiotics and review in the outpatient setting in three months.

Answer 3

There is a good chance that this boy is Gillick competent. Given that his surgery is clearly relevant to his diabetes, a case may be made for a best-interests defence if you decide to force surgery. Frankly, however, the defence looks pretty thin.

If there is no parental consent, then it is much safer to postpone the procedure and have a family discussion once the parental responsibility issue is settled. Given the drive to support autonomy, and the low immediate risks to the patient's life and health, it would seem unlikely that a court would approve of forcing treatment on this boy. A safer and more pragmatic course might be to give low-dose antibiotics until he gets so disenchanted that he relents and consents.

REFERENCE

British Medical Association. *Report of the Consent Working Party: Incorporating Consent Toolkit.* London: British Medical Association, 2001.

FURTHER READING

Bainham A. *Children: The Modern Law.* Bristol: Jordan Publishing, 1998.
Montgomery J. *Health Care Law.* Oxford: Oxford University Press, 2003.
Royal College of Paediatrics and Child Health. *Withholding or Withdrawing Life Saving Treatment in Children: A Framework for Practice.* London: Royal College of Paediatrics and Child Health, 1997.

14

Principles of minimally invasive surgery

AZAD NAJMALDIN

Learning objectives

- To understand the meaning and scope of minimally invasive surgery.
- To appreciate the basic changes and potential risks that might follow the creation of a working space.
- To be able to describe the basic techniques in certain aspects of minimally invasive surgery.

INTRODUCTION

Minimally invasive surgery (MIS) is the application of established or new surgical procedures in a fashion that leads to the reduction of the trauma of access and thereby minimizes tissue trauma and accelerates recovery of the patient. Surgical operations are conducted by remote manipulation within the closed confines of body cavities, lumens of hollow organs and body planes under visual control via telescopes, cameras and screens.

The ability to perform safe and successful minimally invasive procedures relies greatly on the understanding of sound surgical principles and appropriate application of the equipment and instruments. Failure to do this produces unnecessary complications and puts patients at risk.

SCOPE

Endoluminal surgery

Endoluminal surgery is applicable to the upper and lower gastrointestinal tracts, biliary tree, ear, nose and throat (ENT) passages, upper airways, cardiovascular tree, upper and lower urinary tracts, and vaginal and uterine lumens. The indications are:

- inspection and assessment of the lumen of hollow organs;
- tissue and fluid sampling;
- removal of foreign bodies;
- insertion and removal of stents/drainage tubes and stoma devices;
- treatment of stones;
- haemostasis by injection, cautery or banding;
- dilation or release of strictures;
- excision of small, usually benign, lesions;
- vascular embolization.

Percutaneous approaches in vascular, cardiac, biliary, gastric and urological procedures are usually embraced by those who are surgically untrained, such as radiologists and physicians.

Transperitoneal laparoscopy

Laparoscopy is the inspection of the peritoneal contents and execution of largely established surgical procedures by means of camera and instruments introduced through the abdominal wall after creation of a safe access and pneumoperitoneum. Although most abdominal procedures can be executed laparoscopically, diagnostic laparoscopy, anti-reflux surgery, appendicectomy and intestinal pull-through are the most commonly performed laparoscopic procedures in children.

Transpleural thoracoscopy

The application of thoracoscopy in paediatric surgery is becoming increasingly fashionable. The benefits accruing from the avoidance of thoracotomy by the thoracoscopic procedures are even greater than those given by laparoscopic surgery. The various operations that are currently performed by this route are diagnostic thoracoscopy, sympathectomy, treatment of effusion/empyema, resection of lung and duplication lesions, repair of tracheo-oesophageal fistula and oesophageal atresia, and ligation of patent ductus arteriosus.

Body–plane endoscopy

Body planes can be accessed in the absence of a natural cavity. Loose connective tissue planes are accessed, insufflated and visualized. Structures within these created spaces are then dissected as necessary. Examples are retroperitoneoscopy for kidney, adrenal gland and urinary tract surgery, and mediastineoscopy for thymectomy.

Arthroscopy

Orthopaedic surgeons have long used the arthroscopic approach to the knee and other joints. Other examples include spinal discectomy and fusion.

Neuroendoscopy

The indications for neuroendoscopy include treatment of obstructive hydrocephalus, biopsy and resection of intraventricular lesions, deroofing of cysts, and placement of shunt and evacuation of abscess and haematoma.

Minimally invasive surgery in oncology

The treatment of paediatric malignant conditions increasingly is being supplemented by the use of MIS. Endoluminal endoscopy, thoracoscopy and laparoscopy are available to help in the diagnosis, staging and treatment of various benign and malignant conditions. The role of MIS in cancer resection has remained highly controversial. There are fears of inadequate access for complete resection and the possibility of malignant seeding, and concerns regarding the histological integrity of specimens taken for examination. In children who are undergoing chemotherapy and who are neutropenic,

the technique of MIS avoids the morbidity that may be associated with open conventional surgery.

Combined minimally invasive surgery and open surgery

This approach combines the inherent nature of MIS and the speed and simplicity of open surgery in situations when MIS alone may prove technically difficult or when the two approaches complement each other. Examples include an inexperienced surgeon, lack of adequate facilities, the use of endoscopy/laparoscopy as a preliminary measure to diagnose and localize pathology, the abdominoperineal approach to intestinal surgery, the abdominothoracocervical approach to gastro-oesophageal surgery, percutaneous vascular embolization before open organ resection, and complex urinary-stone surgery.

ADVANTAGES

In addition to avoiding large and painful access wounds of conventional surgery, MIS allows the operation to be carried out with minimal parietal trauma, avoiding unnecessary exposure and tissue dissection, cooling, desiccation, handling and forced manipulation, retraction and even destruction of tissue and organs. Thus, the overall assault on the patient is reduced drastically (Barkun *et al.* 1992; Sfez *et al.* 1995). As a result of this:

- postoperative pain, tissue destruction, adhesion formation and wound complications are reduced;
- postoperative chest complications secondary to pain, immobilization and anaesthesia are reduced;
- the patient's recovery and return to normal activities are accelerated;
- cosmetic results are greatly improved;
- repeat surgery, if necessary, becomes less complicated.

Other advantages of MIS include:

- improved exposure in places such as intracranial spaces inside hollow organs and chest and pelvic cavities;
- visual enhancement by the magnifying effect of the telescope;
- greatly reduced contact with the patient's blood and body fluids. This has important implications for both the patient and the surgeon, in relation to the transmission of viral diseases.

DISADVANTAGES

The main difficulties with MIS emanate from access to the space/plane via a needle and trocar or endoscope, the necessity to insufflate or maintain fluid irrigation and the remote nature of the manipulation (Deziel *et al.* 1993). With the correct conditions for safe MIS, morbidity can be contained well. Disadvantages of MIS include the following:

- Potential injury to the hollow organs, vessels and nearby structures as a result of needle/cannula insertion and inappropriate instrumentation and diathermy or laser burns.
- Creation of a working space may cause problems, albeit rarely:
  - in neurosurgery, large-volume/high-pressure and inappropriately cold or electrolytically imbalanced fluid may cause an increased intracranial pressure;
  - in intraluminal surgery (gastrointestinal, urological), large-volume/high-pressure gas or fluid distension may cause perforation;
  - in laparoscopy/thoracoscopy and tissue plane surgery, gas insufflation may cause deranged cardiovascular and respiratory function or gas embolus.
- Eye and hand coordination, loss of direct hand manipulation and tactile feedback, and the two-dimensional image provided by the current camera system cause potential difficulties, at least initially.
- Intact organ retrieval, particularly of cancer-containing organs, is significantly limited.

CONTRAINDICATIONS

- Lack of facilities or trained operators.
- Inability of patient to tolerate general anaesthesia or surgery in general.
- Inability of patient to tolerate CO_2 insufflation (laparoscopy, thoracoscopy), e.g. in major cardiovascular disease.
- Major haemorrhage requiring life-saving procedures expeditiously.
- Inability to create space, e.g. major adhesions in laparoscopy or thoracoscopy, perforated hollow organs in gastrointestinal endoscopy and urology.
- Thromboembolic diseases (vascular procedures).

Although bleeding is technically more difficult to control endoscopically than in open surgery, the presence of a reasonably well-controlled coagulopathy is not a contraindication for the MIS approach. The role of endoscopic surgery in oncology remains controversial.

PHYSIOLOGICAL CHANGES

Some physiological changes are common to both MIS and open surgery. These are secondary to:

- administration of drugs, sedation and general anaesthesia;
- trauma of surgery;
- cardiopulmonary and intestinal dysfunction from handling or exposure;
- postural changes required for optimal surgical access;
- hypothermia from internal and external exposure;
- complications of surgery, e.g. bleeding, use of electrocoagulation or other energy.

Specific physiological changes that may occur in relation to MIS include:

- changes related to the speed of administration and the volume and pressure of gas insufflation or fluid irrigation;
- changes related to the nature of gas used for insufflation or irrigation fluid.

In neurosurgery, prolonged use of saline irrigation can lead to a washout of ventricular electrolytes. A sudden rise of intracranial pressure secondary to high-pressure irrigation may cause tentorial herniation or sudden cardiac arrest. Therefore, the use of warm Ringer's solution by gentle two-way manual flushing or a specifically designed pedal-operated irrigation pump is preferred.

All laparoscopic and thoracoscopic surgery requires that the peritoneal and pleural cavities and tissue planes are turned into a space to enable diagnostic or therapeutic procedures to be performed. This space is created by distension with gas insufflation. Oxygen and air support combustion and have a higher risk of gas embolism. Nitrous oxide has an unpredictable rapid absorption, carries a risk of gas embolism and is an occupational health hazard to the theatre staff. Carbon dioxide is the most commonly used gas. It is safe, is cleared rapidly by the lungs, has no optical distortion, suppresses combustion and is readily available and inexpensive.

Surgical emphysema may occur from gas tracking along the tissue planes or surgically traumatized barriers. Gas may diffuse through the gastrointestinal wall and pleura and peritoneal membranes.

Direct insufflation pressure on the main intrathoracic and/or intra-abdominal veins reduces venous return, and consequently causes a fall in cardiac output. An increase in systemic vascular resistance by mechanical compression of the aorta and splanchnic vessels and the release of humoral factors are noted. Diaphragmatic displacement and splinting causes a reduced functional residual capacity of the lungs and a rise in peak airway pressure. These, in turn, lead to airway collapse, shunting and hypoxia.

These cardiovascular and respiratory changes are of no clinical significance (Sfez et al. 1995; Lister et al. 1994) provided that the insufflation pressure is kept below 15–18 mmHg for laparoscopy (usual requirement 8–10 mmHg in newborns and young children, 10–12 mmHg in older children) and below 8–12 mmHg for thoracoscopy (usual requirement 4–6 mmHg).

Clinical gas embolus, a potentially lethal event, is exceptionally rare. It is usually caused by accidental intravascular injection and insufflation of gas through a misplaced needle/cannula, forcing gas into a vein splinted open or air from a cooled laser tip. The physiological effects will depend on the rate and volume of gas introduced: 3 mL/kg may cause an air lock in the right atrium. A patent cardiac fraenum or shunt may allow coronary and cerebral gas embolism. Gas embolism may be a delayed phenomenon as the result of trapping in the portal circulation.

Arrhythmia or cardiovascular collapse as the result of vagal response to rapid peritoneal or pleural distension and tension pneumothorax due to an unrecognized congenital defect of the diaphragm or accidental perforation of the diaphragm are exceedingly rare phenomena.

ANAESTHETIC CONSIDERATIONS

General anaesthesia with intubation and controlled ventilation is the preferred anaesthetic technique for all paediatric MIS procedures. In healthy and cooperative very young infants and old children, an appropriate level of sedation with or without topical/local anaesthetic agents may be considered for:

- upper-airway endoscopy;
- upper- and lower-gastrointestinal endoscopy;
- percutaneous nephrostomy;
- percutaneous vascular intervention.

In thoracoscopy, endotracheal intubation with or without lung retraction and/or low-pressure CO_2 (4–6 mmHg) insufflation provides good exposure to all hemithoracic compartments, including the mediastinum. Double-lumen intubation, which is an ideal technique, is not suitable in children weighing less than 30 kg. Selective bronchial intubation, with or without contralateral bronchial occlusion with a balloon catheter, is technically demanding and may prove helpful in certain circumstances.

In thoracoscopy and laparoscopy, postoperative analgesia is provided effectively with local anaesthetic infiltration of the trocar, sites with or without 12–24 hours of opiate infusion or epidural analgesia. In intraluminal surgery and percutaneous procedures, postoperative analgesia usually is not required.

ANATOMICAL CONSIDERATIONS FOR ENDOSCOPIC SURGERY

The principle of endoscopic anatomy is that structures and their relations are viewed across the television screen in two dimensions instead of the normal three dimensions, with the quality and size altered in accordance with the distance from the telescope as well as the character of the camera, light source and monitor in use. Anatomical landmarks and colour variations are used to identify structures. Inappropriately placed telescopes, technical problems with imaging, adhesions, unexpected enlarged structures and bleeding can greatly hinder the endoscopic access and views of the anatomical structures. It is important to recognize that in infants and small children, the surface area for access is small, the body wall and hollow organs are thin and highly compliant, the liver margin is below the ribcage, the bladder is largely an intra-abdominal structure, the viscera and major vessels are close to the body surface, and the working spaces are small. In small infants, only 200–400 mL of CO_2 may be required to establish a pneumoperitoneum/pneumothorax. Stressed by insufflation or irrigation fluid and endoscope, hollow organs such as the gastrointestinal tract and genitourinary tract form acute bends, which make the passage of instruments difficult and hazardous. It is important, therefore, to distend as little as possible, consistent with vision and instrumentation.

These anatomical characteristics make access and manipulation in the younger age group more demanding and difficult tasks compared with in older children and adults.

OPERATIVE CONSIDERATIONS

Before starting any procedure:

- Informed consent must be available for both MIS and conventional open approaches. In all cases of thoracoscopic and laparoscopic surgery, as well as intraluminal endoscopic and percutaneous surgery, a set of conventional instruments should be available for emergency use or conversion to an open procedure.
- Check that all the required equipment and instruments are available, functioning and compatible. The electrocoagulation power or other sources of energy such as laser and ultrasound must be set at the minimal effective level.
- Consider bladder catheterization:
  - if the bladder is palpable and cannot be emptied by expression;
  - in cases of major lower-abdominal procedures;
  - if monitoring of renal function is thought to be necessary during the procedure;
  - in specific urological procedures.
- Consider insertion of a nasogastric tube to:
  - ensure safe anaesthesia;
  - drain a full or inadvertently insufflated stomach;
  - facilitate certain gastric procedures, such as anti-reflux surgery.
- Consider preoperative bowel preparation in:
  - colonoscopy;
  - laparoscopic colonic procedures.

TRANSPERITONEAL LAPAROSCOPY

A pneumoperitoneum may be created by two methods: the closed method using a Veress needle and the open method using a cut-down technique (Humphrey and Najmaldin 1994). The blind insertion of a Veress needle may cause, albeit very rarely, injury to the viscera and vessels, but usually it causes little damage (Deziel *et al.* 1993). Open-technique laparoscopy is the preferred method of insertion of the primary cannula (telescope) and creation of a pneumoperitoneum in children. In an unscarred abdomen, an incision to fit the size of the primary cannula is usually made at the umbilical region. An insufflation pressure of 6–8 mmHg at a CO_2 flow of 0.1–0.5 L/min in neonates and infants, and 8–10 mmHg at a CO_2 flow of 0.5–1 L/min in older children, is adequate for all procedures. The placement of working cannulae under direct telescopic vision should be modified according to the type of surgical procedure to be executed, individual anatomy and size of the patient. Blind insertion of working cannulae rarely may cause serious intra-abdominal, vascular or visceral injury (Deziel *et al.* 1993).

RETROPERITONEAL LAPAROSCOPY

In paediatric surgery, the routine use of the extraperitoneal approach is confined largely to renal and ureteric procedures. The technique avoids the morbidity that may be associated with traversing the peritoneal cavity. The patient is usually positioned lateral, semilateral or prone. Extraperitoneoscopy may be performed effectively within a space created by breaking up the connective tissue binding the extraperitoneal space with either a combination of blunt dissection through a small incision, using the tip of the telescope and CO_2 insufflation, or a homemade or (not) specifically designed balloon dissector. The technique is contraindicated in patients with major bleeding disorders, malignant lesions and major scarring. An accidental peritoneal tear and extension pneumoperitoneum can make extraperitoneal surgery difficult.

THORACOSCOPY

The position of the patient depends largely on the operation to be performed. Gravity is an important mode of lung retraction.

The decubitus position is the most versatile position. Tilting towards supine for operations in the anterior mediastinum and towards prone for posterior mediastinum is usually necessary. Positioning of trocars depends upon the nature of the operation to be executed; the open (cut-down) technique is the preferred method for insertion of the primary cannula (telescope). Thoracic insufflation is not required when a double-lumen endotracheal tube is used or if there is selective bronchial intubation and contralateral bronchial occlusion or unguarded (valveless) cannulae are in place. Adequate working space may be achieved with gravity and low-pressure insufflation (4–6 mmHg) and low CO_2 flow (0.1–0.5 L/min).

REFERENCES

Barkun JS, Barkun AN, Sampalis JS, *et al.* Randomised controlled trial of laparoscopic versus minilaparotomy cholecystectomy. *Lancet* 1992; **340**: 116–19.

Deziel DJ, Millikan KW, Economou SG, *et al.* Complications of laparoscopic cholecystectomy: a national survey of 4,292 hospitals and an analysis of 77,604 cases. *American Journal of Surgery* 1993; **165**: 9–14.

Humphrey GM, Najmaldin A. Modification of the Hasson technique in paediatric laparoscopy. *British Journal of Surgery* 1994; **81**: 1320–23.

Lister DR, Rudston-Brown B, Warriner CB, *et al.* Carbon dioxide absorption is not linearly related to intraperitoneal carbon dioxide insufflation pressure in pigs. *Anaesthesiology* 1994; **80**: 129–36.

Sfez M, Guerard A, Desruelle P. Cardiorespiratory changes during laparoscopic fundoplication in children. *Paediatric Anaesthesia* 1995; **5**: 89–95.

FURTHER READING

Najmaldin A, Guillou P. *A Guide to Laparoscopic Surgery*. Oxford: Blackwell Science, 1998.

Najmaldin A, Rothenberg S, Crabbe D, Beasley S. *Operative Endoscopy and Endoscopic Surgery in Infants and Children*. London: Arnold, 2005.

Part 2

Gastrointestinal surgery

15

Oesophageal atresia and tracheo-oesophageal fistula

SPENCER W BEASLEY

Learning objectives

- To understand how the various anatomical types of oesophageal atresia may be distinguished on investigation.
- To identify associated congenital abnormalities in infants born with oesophageal atresia.
- To describe the surgical technique of repair of oesophageal atresia with distal tracheo-oesophageal fistula.
- To list the sequence of surgical steps to overcome a long gap in oesophageal atresia.

INTRODUCTION

Oesophageal atresia is a congenital abnormality that occurs in approximately one in 4000 live births, in which a variable length of the mid-portion of the oesophagus is missing. Most affected infants have a blind-ending upper-oesophageal pouch and an abnormal communication between the trachea and distal oesophagus called a distal tracheo-oesophageal fistula.

RELEVANT BASIC SCIENCE

A large number of anatomical variations of oesophageal atresia and tracheo-oesophageal fistula have been described (Kluth 1976). However, oesophageal atresia with a distal tracheo-oesophageal fistula is by far the most common variant, occurring in about 85 per cent of cases in most large series.

The five most common anatomical variants are shown in Figure 15.1.

Where there is a distal tracheo-oesophageal fistula, air will pass through the fistula and enter the stomach below the diaphragm within minutes of birth. If there is no gas in the abdomen, i.e. below the level of the diaphragm, for more than a few minutes after birth, then it is reasonable to assume that the infant does not have a distal tracheo-oesophageal fistula, although about 20 per cent of these infants will have a proximal tracheo-oesophageal fistula.

There is accumulating evidence that the oesophagus in oesophageal atresia is inherently abnormal. Oesophageal dysmotility and consequent delayed oesophageal emptying increase the duration of exposure of the oesophageal mucosa to gastric acid in those infants who have gastro-oesophageal reflux. Many infants also have an abnormally soft trachea (tracheomalacia). When the tracheomalacia is severe, the trachea tends to collapse and may cause obstruction on expiration.

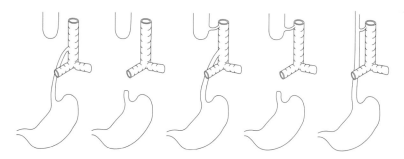

Figure 15.1 *The five most common variants of oesophageal atresia and/or tracheo-oesophageal fistula.*

Box 15.1 When to suspect oesophageal atresia after birth

Baby is excessively 'mucusy' or drooling saliva

Cyanotic episodes (due to aspiration of saliva, which has accumulated in the blind upper-oesophageal pouch) and/or respiratory distress shortly after birth

History of maternal polyhydramnios

Other abnormalities (e.g. imperforate anus, radial dysplasia) that are known to occur in association with oesophageal atresia

---

PRESENTATION

Occasionally, oesophageal atresia is diagnosed on antenatal ultrasonography by the observation of maternal polyhydramnios, a small stomach and an upper-oesophageal pouch (Shulman *et al.* 2002). The observation of other abnormalities known to be associated with oesophageal atresia (e.g. congenital heart disease, urinary-tract abnormalities) may increase the suspicion of oesophageal atresia.

After birth, the infant is noted to be abnormally 'mucusy', with drooling of excessive saliva. A history of maternal polyhydramnios during pregnancy in an infant born slightly prematurely heightens the suspicion of oesophageal atresia. The infant may have other congenital abnormalities known to be associated with oesophageal atresia (Box 15.1).

Where possible, the diagnosis should be made before feeding. If a feed is given, explosive rejection of the milk will occur, usually with cyanosis, choking and respiratory distress. This should alert the clinician immediately to the correct diagnosis. Sometimes, the infant may suffer cyanotic attacks without feeding. Milk entering an obstructed oesophagus has a high chance of being aspirated into the lungs and causing an aspiration pneumonia.

INVESTIGATION

The diagnosis of oesophageal atresia is confirmed by the inability to pass a 10-gauge catheter through the mouth into the stomach; the catheter becomes arrested at 9–13 cm from the gums (Figure 15.2). A relatively stiff 10-gauge catheter is used because smaller catheters tend to curl up in the upper-oesophageal pouch, giving a false impression of oesophageal continuity. Litmus paper can be used to confirm that the fluid aspirated is saliva and not acidic (gastric acid). Introduction of the tube through the nose should not be attempted because it may injure the nasal passages, which are relatively small in newborn infants.

Confirmation that there is a distal tracheo-oesophageal fistula is obtained by performing a plain X-ray of the torso (i.e. chest and abdomen), showing that there is gas below the level of the diaphragm. Contrast studies are not required when there is intra-abdominal gas on X-ray. Some centres perform routine bronchoscopy to identify the point at which the distal fistula enters the airways and to exclude an upper pouch fistula (Pigna *et al.* 2002).

If the plain X-ray shows no evidence of gas in the stomach or beyond, then it implies that there is no distal tracheo-oesophageal fistula, and further investigation is required (Figure 15.3). First, it is necessary to exclude an upper-pouch fistula; this is done either by introducing contrast into the mid-oesophagus under continuous fluoroscopic control or by performing bronchoscopy. If there is a fistula, then it will be evident as an obvious opening in the posterior wall of the trachea, a variable distance above the carina.

The next step is to determine the distance between the two oesophageal ends, as the gap is often extensive in patients who have no distal tracheo-oesophageal fistula. This is done under general anaesthesia at the time of gastrostomy by simultaneously inserting a radio-opaque tube into the upper pouch from above whilst introducing a metal bougie through the gastrostomy opening and into the lower oesophageal segment from below, under fluoroscopic control. Often, it may not be possible to overcome a long gap at birth, and a delayed primary repair is performed one to three months later (see below).

ASSOCIATED ABNORMALITIES

Major associated congenital anomalies are present in about 50 per cent of babies with oesophageal atresia. When a baby is diagnosed at birth as having oesophageal atresia, it is necessary to examine the infant for one or more associated anomalies (Table 15.1). The most common anomalies belong to

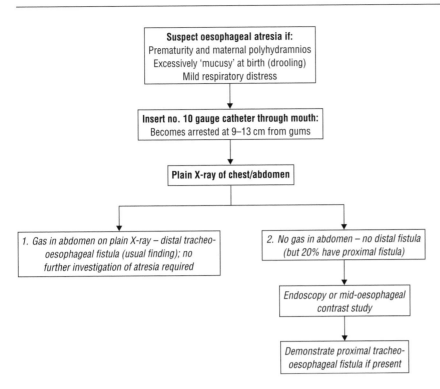

Figure 15.2 *Confirmation of diagnosis of oesophageal atresia, and determination of the anatomical type.*

the VATER or VACTERL (vertebral, anorectal, tracheo-oesophageal and renal anomalies and radial aplasia) association. Major chromosomal abnormalities, e.g. trisomy 18 or 21, and the CHARGE (coloboma, congenital heart disease, choanal atresia, genital anomalies and ear abnormality) association are encountered frequently.

Associated congenital abnormalities are the main determinant of survival in infants born with oesophageal atresia. For example, infants born with severe congenital heart disease (e.g. hypoplastic left ventricle), bilateral renal agenesis or trisomy 18 have an extremely poor prognosis. In these infants, active treatment of the oesophageal atresia is not justified. The overall mortality rate of oesophageal atresia in infants who have no chromosomal abnormality is about seven per cent, but the mortality in those with an identifiable chromosomal abnormality is 70 per cent (Beasley *et al.* 1997).

In addition, it is important to identify infants with a duct-dependent cardiac lesion before repair of the oesophageal atresia; this allows a prostaglandin E1 infusion to be commenced. The timing of surgery is determined by the infant's stability (Mee *et al.* 1992). Those with duodenal atresia and imperforate anus will require surgery for these abnormalities as well, usually under the same anaesthetic. The oesophageal atresia is repaired first, followed by a duodenoduodenostomy and finally a colostomy (usually) for the anorectal anomaly.

MANAGEMENT

General considerations

Handling should be keep to a minimum because excessive disturbance increases the infant's oxygen consumption, exposes the infant to cold stress and, if the infant is unstable, may cause dramatic cardiovascular responses. Care must be exercised to avoid excessive cooling in the delivery room and during subsequent stabilization and transport.

Oxygen therapy

A number of infants with oesophageal atresia will have respiratory distress because of prematurity, aspiration pneumonia or diaphragmatic splinting caused by excessive escape of air through the distal fistula into the stomach. If no blood-gas monitoring facilities are available, then the infant must be kept pink at all times. It is preferable to have several hours of hyperoxia than a short period of hypoxia.

Posture

In general, the infant in transport should be nursed in the right lateral position with maintenance of a clear airway if fluid, i.e. excessive saliva, enters the pharynx. This will also minimize regurgitation of gastric contents up the distal tracheo-oesophageal fistula and will decrease the work of breathing and improve oxygenation. The neonate depends on contraction of the diaphragm for effective ventilation, which is more accomplished easily in this position.

Care of the upper pouch

The upper oesophagus should be suctioned intermittently to remove accumulating saliva. This should be done at least every 10–15 minutes, irrespective of whether there appear to be excessive secretions, and more often if necessary. Saliva may accumulate in large volumes in the upper pouch, regurgitate suddenly and be aspirated into the lungs if it is not sucked out. Occasionally, a distended upper pouch may compress the trachea from behind, particularly if tracheomalacia is marked. A suction catheter should be firm but soft, such

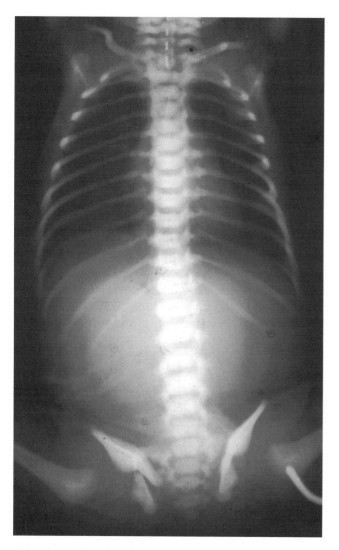

Figure 15.3 *A gasless abdomen implies that there is no distal tracheo-oesophageal fistula.*

as an 8- or 10-gauge tube. Y-suction catheters are preferred because they enable pressure adjustments to minimize oesophageal mucosal damage. Replogle tubes require constant nursing care but do keep the oesophagus empty.

Gentle handling

The infant should be handled gently to minimize crying, since crying tends to fill the stomach with air. This, in turn, increases the likelihood of regurgitation of gastric contents into the trachea, increases abdominal distension and impedes ventilation.

Care of associated medical problems

One-third of infants with oesophageal atresia are premature and require specific attention to temperature control, oxygen therapy, and early fluid and dextrose solution resuscitation to limit the problems of apnoea, respiratory distress and hypoglycaemia. The majority of infants with oesophageal atresia and respiratory distress can be managed with increased ambient oxygen concentration, but about five per cent will require assisted ventilation. This presents problems if the ventilation pressures are high, since gastric distension and rupture may develop, making ventilation more difficult. This problem can be reduced by placing the tip of the endotracheal tube just proximal to the carina but distal to the fistula. Infants with intrauterine growth retardation are at risk of hypoglycaemia, which must be corrected.

Care of the family

The parents should be given an honest appraisal of the situation. Provided there are no associated severe congenital abnormalities, then the prognosis for survival is excellent. An outline of the nature of oesophageal atresia should be given, and the parents should be informed of the transport planned and of what to expect at the tertiary institution, with details of the receiving unit, including names (if known) of the personnel who will be caring for their infant. The transfer of their infant

Table 15.1 *Diagnosis of associated abnormalities in oesophageal atresia (OA)*

Clinical inspection	Plain X–ray	Urine passed before surgery?	Echocardiograph: ?duct-dependent cardiac lesion
Look for features of VATER association, e.g. imperforate anus, radial aplasia, syndactyly	Vertebral, e.g. hemi-vertebrae	Yes: proceed to surgery	No: repair OA
Look for features of chromosomal abnormality, e.g. rocker-bottom feet, Down syndrome; if suspected, consult geneticist and chromosomal studies	Rib, e.g. supernumerary, bifid or absent	No: do renal ultrasound to confirm presence of renal tissue	Yes: commence PGE infusion
	Duodenal atresia: 'double bubble'	MCU with or without other tests, as indicated after OA repair	Repair OA when infant stable

MCU, micturating cystourethrogram; PGE, prostaglandin E1; VATER, vertebral, anorectal, tracheo-oesophageal, radial/renal abnormalities.

can leave an enormous sense of loss in parents: it is thus of great importance for them to view and, if practicable, touch, stroke and cuddle their infant before transfer. It may be helpful to give the parents a photograph of their infant. Parents may require advice on their own travel and accommodation if they live far from the neonatal receiving unit. In the receiving institution, the surgeon will explain to the parents what the surgery involves, the likely postoperative course and the potential complications. Informed consent must be obtained.

INVESTIGATION OF ASSOCIATED ABNORMALITIES

Before surgery, renal ultrasonography is obtained if the infant has not passed urine, because in about three per cent of cases there is inadequate renal tissue for long-term survival (e.g. bilateral severely dysplastic kidneys or bilateral renal agenesis), in which case no surgery is justified. An echocardiogram is obtained because 25 per cent of infants with oesophageal atresia have congenital heart disease. It is important to identify duct-dependent cardiac lesions preoperatively so that a prostaglandin E1 infusion can be commenced before repair of the oesophagus (Mee *et al.* 1992). In most babies, congenital heart disease does not delay the oesophageal surgery, and oesophageal repair usually takes precedence when surgery to the heart is required. An echocardiogram may be used to identify a right aortic arch and influence the surgical approach to the oesophagus.

OPERATIVE MANAGEMENT

Timing of surgery

Complete correction of the abnormality is performed as a single operation shortly after birth, following the renal ultrasound examination and echocardiogram.

Operative procedure

The infant is placed in the full lateral position, with the right side uppermost and the right arm raised over the head to facilitate the thoracic approach. A transverse incision is centred just below the inferior angle of the scapula. After division of the latissimus dorsi in the line of the incision, the posterior fibres of the serratus inferior are retracted anteriorly. If, for reasons of exposure, they need to be divided, then this is done near their origin on the chest wall, as low as possible, thus preserving the muscle's innervation (long thoracic nerve). The chest is entered through the fourth intercostal space and the pleura swept off the chest wall. The oesophagus is approached in this extrapleural plane. The azygos vein is ligated and divided. After incision of the fine endothoracic

fascia of the posterior mediastinum, the lower oesophagus can be found immediately anterior to the aorta and is recognized by the vagal fibres running along its surface. The connection between the distal oesophagus and the trachea is identified and exposed. A vessel loop may be passed around the fistula where the upper part of the lower oesophageal segment joins the trachea, once the angle between the oesophagus and trachea has been dissected clear. Care is taken to avoid damage to the vagus nerves and its branches and the segmental blood supply of the oesophagus. The tracheo-oesophageal fistula is closed with 4/0 or 5/0 absorbable transfixion sutures and divided.

The upper-oesophageal segment can be identified readily within the chest once the anaesthetist introduces a catheter into it. A stay suture, passed through its lowest part, may assist in its mobilization and avoids unnecessary handling of (and trauma to) the oesophagus. The upper-oesophageal pouch may seem to be adherent to the trachea initially; this part of the dissection must be performed carefully to avoid injury to the trachea and to allow recognition of a proximal fistula in the (relatively unlikely) event that one is present. The upper oesophagus may be mobilized as far as the cricopharyngeus muscle, should that be necessary to make the oesophageal anastomosis without excessive tension. Once the upper segment has been mobilized adequately, its most dependent part is opened. In many instances, the gap between the oesophagus ends is minimal, such that little mobilization is required.

The end-to-end oesophago-oesophageal anastomosis is constructed by inserting three or four interrupted 5/0 absorbable sutures in the back wall of each oesophageal end. Special care must be taken to ensure that the mucosal layer of the oesophagus is included, as the mucosa of the upper pouch in particular tends to retract upwards out of view when it is opened. When the 'posterior' sutures have been placed, the oesophageal ends are gently apposed and the sutures tied on the mucosal surface. An orogastric or nasogastric tube can be passed through the upper oesophagus into the lower segment before completion of the anastomosis with a further four to six interrupted sutures including all layers (mucosa and muscle), with the knots tied on the outside.

Before closure of the chest, the tube is removed (unless tube feeding is planned, as in the premature infant) and the thoracic cavity is irrigated with warm saline solution. This fluid allows confirmation that there is no air leakage with ventilation from the closed fistula. A chest drain is not normally required unless there is concern about the integrity of the anastomosis. The intercostal spaces are infiltrated with 0.25 per cent plain bupivacaine. The ribs are approximated with 2/0 or 3/0 absorbable suture, the muscles with 3/0 and 4/0 absorbable suture, and the skin with 5/0 subcuticular suture. Postoperative feeds can be commenced on about the third postoperative day.

The exact role of thoracoscopic repair of oesophageal atresia is yet to be determined (Bax and van Der Zee 2002).

Intraoperative difficulties

RIGHT AORTIC ARCH

This may be suspected on the plain film of the chest or by preoperative echocardiogram. If diagnosed preoperatively, the operation is best performed through a left thoracotomy. If the right arch is first recognized during a right thoracotomy, then it is often possible to achieve an anastomosis from this side. An anastomosis to the right of a right arch does not usually cause compression of the oesophagus and has the advantage of being relatively easy to perform when the arch would otherwise obscure the level of the anastomosis and almost guarantees no recurrent fistula. When an anastomosis is difficult to construct from the right, then the right thoracotomy can be closed, the infant repositioned and a left thoracotomy performed.

IDENTIFICATION OF LOWER OESOPHAGUS

The location of the lower oesophagus may not be immediately apparent, particularly if there is no distal fistula. In this case, the vagus nerves may act as a guide to its location. The vagus nerves can be recognized as fine white fibres leaving the posterolateral aspect of the trachea to sweep downwards and encompass the lower oesophagus. These fibres should not be divided or have traction applied to them during dissection of the tracheo-oesophageal junction or mobilization of the oesophagus.

CONTINUOUS OESOPHAGUS

Apparent continuity of the oesophagus at thoracotomy may lead the surgeon to believe the preoperative diagnosis to be incorrect. However, the lumen may be obstructed even though it appears intact externally, i.e. the two ends overlap. Advancement of the catheter in the upper oesophagus peroperatively by the anaesthetist will clarify the level of obstruction.

DOUBLE FISTULA

The surgeon should be aware of the possibility of a second (upper pouch) fistula, which may extend upwards from the oesophagus to the trachea. A proximal fistula is rare when there is a distal fistula. Clues to its presence include distension of the upper oesophagus during ventilatory inspiration, difficulty in separating the oesophagus from the trachea during upper pouch mobilization, and an upper pouch that is less hypertrophied than usual. Where routine preoperative endoscopy is performed, it may be diagnosed during bronchoscopy immediately before surgery.

COMPLICATIONS

A number of problems may occur following repair of oesophageal atresia. Some, such as anastomotic leak, recurrent tracheo-oesophageal fistula and a shelf at the site of the anastomosis, are, in large part, the result of technical inadequacies. Others, such as poor oesophageal clearance and gastro-oesophageal reflux causing the late development of a stricture, reflect abnormalities related more directly to the oesophageal atresia itself or to gastro-oesophageal reflux.

Anastomotic leak

Major leakage from an oesophageal anastomosis represents a rare but potentially serious complication of repair of oesophageal atresia. The likelihood of an anastomotic leak occurring depends on the type of anastomosis employed and the extent of mobilization of the oesophagus. An interrupted, all-layers, end-to-end oesophageal anastomosis using an absorbable suture appears to have the lowest leakage and stricture rate, making it the anastomosis of choice. Leakage from an anastomosis may vary enormously in significance, from a minor radiological leak in an otherwise well infant, for which no treatment is required, to complete anastomotic disruption with mediastinitis, empyema, pneumothorax and septicaemia. Factors that contribute to anastomotic leakage include tension at the anastomosis, ischaemia of the oesophageal ends, and sepsis. The extent of oesophageal dissection undertaken is determined by the balance between the dissection required to gain adequate length to avoid excessive tension at the anastomosis and damage to the blood supply of both oesophageal ends, which may occur when the oesophagus is mobilized extensively or oesophageal myotomy is performed. There is a relationship between leakage and subsequent stricture formation and recurrent tracheo-oesophageal fistula.

In most infants, an anastomotic leak can be managed non-operatively. Safe total parenteral nutrition enables oral feeds to be ceased. Antibiotics are commenced, and the leak will usually close spontaneously. Cervical oesophagostomy is necessary only rarely, when supportive therapy has been unsuccessful and there is ongoing difficult-to-control sepsis. A long-standing leak may require gastrostomy to allow continuation of enteral feeds.

Recurrent tracheo–oesophageal fistula

A recurrent tracheo-oesophageal fistula is a severe and potentially dangerous complication. Failure to close the fistula adequately at the time of surgery and subsequent anastomotic leak with local infection increases the chance of developing a recurrent fistula. The use of silk as the suture material may be another predisposing factor.

The development of coughing, gagging, choking, cyanosis, apnoea, dying spells and recurrent chest infections suggests that a recurrent tracheo-oesophageal fistula has developed. The typical presentation is that of an infant who coughs and splutters with each feed. The most reliable method of confirming the diagnosis is cine-radiographic tube oesophagography, with the patient in the prone position. Barium is introduced through a nasogastric tube positioned in the oesophagus as the tube is gradually withdrawn. Bronchoscopy is an alternative method.

Spontaneous closure of recurrent fistulae is unusual. Most surgeons wait about four weeks from the first operation before closing a recurrent fistula, although the best time for reoperation has not been established with certainty. A thoracotomy is performed through the original incision when the child is in optimal respiratory and general condition following a period of intravenous nutrition. The fistula is divided via a transpleural approach. Some surgeons pass a fine ureteric catheter through the fistula endoscopically to facilitate its localization; others place mediastinal tissue or pericardium between the ends of the divided fistula to reduce the likelihood of further recurrence. Numerous other techniques to close a recurrent fistula by endoscopic ablation have been described, but there are no studies to provide evidence of their relative efficacy.

Anastomotic stricture

Anastomotic stricture is the most common reason for further surgery to the oesophagus being required after repair of oesophageal atresia. Factors that influence the development of an oesophageal stricture include rough handling of the oesophagus at the time of repair, ischaemia of the oesophageal ends, excessive tension of the oesophageal anastomosis, the choice of suture material (e.g. silk), anastomotic leak or dehiscence, the use of a two-layer anastomosis and gastro-oesophageal reflux. Gastro-oesophageal reflux is the most common cause of late stricture development.

Patients with strictures develop feeding difficulties and dysphagia, the onset of which may be insidious. The first symptom in infants is often the infant being slow to feed and having excessive regurgitation, with or without cyanotic episodes. Older children present with foreign-body impaction of food in the oesophagus. Diagnosis is confirmed by barium-swallow or endoscopy.

In patients with mild or moderate narrowing of the oesophagus, one or two dilations may be all that is required. The technique of radial balloon dilation under continuous fluoroscopic control is probably the most effective and least traumatic method of achieving oesophageal dilation. However, in patients with associated gastro-oesophageal reflux, it will usually be necessary to perform an anti-reflux operation (e.g. Nissen fundoplication), after which the stricture tends to resolve spontaneously.

Motility problems

Oesophageal motility is abnormal both before and after repair of oesophageal atresia. It is likely that vagal fibres are injured during mobilization of the oesophagus, worsening the already abnormal oesophageal motility. Oesophageal motility tends to improve gradually with age, but older children with repaired

oesophageal atresia often need to drink with their meals. Abnormal oesophageal motility can contribute to oesophagitis and oesophageal stricture formation in the presence of gastro-oesophageal reflux; the fact that the oesophagus does not empty normally allows acidic gastric juice to sit in the lower oesophagus for a longer period than in patients with normal oesophageal muscular function.

Oesophageal diverticulum and shelf

A pseudo-diverticulum may occur following leakage from the oesophageal anastomosis. Ballooning at the site of a circular myotomy is common and may result in a diverticulum. A shelf at the site of the oesophageal anastomosis occurs when the upper-oesophageal pouch has been opened eccentrically or when the end-to-end oesophageal anastomosis has not been performed with sufficient precision.

OESOPHAGEAL ATRESIA WITHOUT FISTULA

When no tracheo-oesophageal fistula is present, there is almost always a substantial gap between the oesophageal ends (Beasley 1991). Sometimes, there is virtually no lower oesophageal segment above the level of the diaphragm. Box 15.2 provides guidelines for the management of long-gap oesophageal atresia. The absence of a fistula and long-gap oesophageal atresia may produce a number of specific surgical problems, which are described below.

Small stomach

Where there is no distal tracheo-oesophageal fistula, the stomach is small as a result of the inability of the fetus to swallow amniotic fluid or for fluid to enter the stomach through the distal fistula. The significance of this relates to the problems created by a small stomach when a gastrostomy is being fashioned so as not to compromise later gastric interposition or greater curvature tube (if required) or a subsequent anti-reflux operation.

Assessment of length of gap

The length of the upper segment of the oesophagus can be demonstrated by a contrast study performed to exclude a proximal fistula and confirmed at operation by the passage of a radio-opaque flexible catheter through the mouth into the upper oesophagus by the anaesthetist.

The lower segment is evaluated at the time of gastrostomy by introducing a metal bougie into the stomach through the gastrostomy opening and through the gastro-oesophageal junction into the lower oesophageal segment. Simultaneous pressure exerted on the catheter from above and on the bougie from below can be used to assess how closely the

---

Box 15.2 Management of long-gap oesophageal atresia

- Suspect long-gap oesophageal atresia if:
  - gasless abdomen on plain X-ray;
  - proximal tracheo-oesophageal fistula;
  - oesophageal atresia and cleft palate;
  - short (i.e. high) upper pouch on plain X-ray.
- Assessment of length of cap (under general anaesthetic, using image intensifier):
  - Gastrostomy and pass metal bougie through gastro-oesophageal junction upwards into lower-oesophageal segment.
  - Anaesthetist simultaneously passes radio-opaque tube into upper-oesophageal segment.
- Decision on appropriateness of immediate repair:
  - Immediate repair if it is thought that the oesophageal ends can be anastomosed.
  - Delayed repair (two to three months) if ends are too far apart.
- Manoeuvres to achieve oesophageal anastomosis:
  - full upper pouch mobilization;
  - dissection of lower segment to (or through) oesophageal hiatus;
  - myotomy: circular (spiral), usually of upper pouch;
  - mobilization of stomach into chest: through oesophageal hiatus, division of lesser curve (Scharli 1992).
- If anastomosis fails:
  - Cervical oesophagostomy (or regular upper pouch suction) and gastrostomy; later, oesophageal replacement at body weight 10 kg or one year (or earlier if infant well).
  - Options:
    greater curvature tube: isoperistaltic gastric tube, reversed gastric tube
    gastric transposition (Spitz 1998; Hirschl *et al.* 2002)
    jejunal interposition
    oesophagocoloplasty.

---

oesophageal segments can be approximated and provides an indication of whether early successful oesophageal anastomosis is possible (Figure 15.3)

Timing of definitive repair

In infants in whom early primary repair is not possible because of the gap, definitive surgery is delayed. Primary anastomosis is attempted as soon as the gap appears small enough to achieve oesophageal continuity – as judged on serial contrast studies – or at about three months of age.

Technique of repair

The following manoeuvres may be undertaken to overcome a long gap between oesophageal ends:

- The upper pouch is identified and mobilized fully, avoiding damage to the trachea. The mobilization can be extended superiorly as far as the cricopharyngeus without compromising the blood supply to the upper oesophagus. This should always be the first manoeuvre.
- Mobilization of the distal segment. The lower oesophagus can be identified by following the fine white fibres of the vagus nerve as they run down the posterior mediastinum. Mobilization of the lower segment can be achieved without complete disruption of the segmental vascular supply (Farkash *et al.* 2002), which appears as a small leash of vessels from the aorta. Care is taken to avoid excessive handling of the oesophagus.
- If the above manoeuvres still do not allow the oesophageal ends to be anastomosed, then more extensive mobilization of the oesophagus through the oesophageal hiatus can be employed to allow the intra-abdominal oesophagus to ride up into the thorax. This may come at the cost of worsening gastro-oesophageal reflux, which may require surgical correction at a later date.
- A circular or spiral myotomy of the upper oesophagus can be performed, but this will cause significant damage to the motility and vascular supply of the upper pouch and may result in later diverticulum formation. Preferably, it should be done more than 2 cm from the end, which may be difficult when the upper-oesophageal segment is short, as is usually the case when a myotomy is required.
- An anterior mucomuscular flap can be fashioned using the upper-oesophageal segment. Viability of the flap relies on the fact that the upper oesophagus has an excellent longitudinal blood supply and is somewhat wider (more dilated) than the lower oesophagus. The results of this technique have been very disappointing.
- If all of these measures fail, then a cervical oesophagostomy (Box 15.3) as a prelude to a subsequent oesophageal replacement (Box 15.4) may be required. A number of methods are available for achieving oesophageal replacement (Table 15.2).

EXTREME PREMATURITY

In the extremely premature infant who is likely to develop or is developing severe hyaline membrane disease (HMD), early ligation or division of the tracheo-oesophageal fistula by a thoracotomy (usually without simultaneous oesophageal anastomosis, depending on the condition of the infant at the time of operation) is important. The greater the difficulty in achieving adequate gaseous exchange, the more urgent is the

Box 15.3 Indications for cervical oesophagostomy

No distal oesophagus or the gap between the oesophageal ends is extensive, making oesophageal anastomosis impossible

Life-threatening anastomotic complications

Long-gap oesophageal atresia, with inadequate facilities for prolonged upper-pouch care (regular suction)

Cervical oesophagostomy is required very rarely in a patient with oesophageal atresia and a distal fistula

Box 15.4 Indications for oesophageal replacement

Oesophageal atresia without fistula, with minimal or no intrathoracic component to the lower oesophageal segment

Attempted oesophageal anastomosis at thoracotomy proves impossible (a rare event)

Total anastomotic disruption with sepsis has required a cervical oesophagostomy; even in this situation, in some infants it may still be possible to salvage the oesophagus

Table 15.2 *Selection of method of oesophageal replacement*

Viscus	Stomach	Antegrade tube
		Retrograde tube
		Transposition of stomach
	Colon	
	Small bowel (jejunum)	
Route	Retrosternal	
	Transpleural	
	Posterior mediastinal	

need to close the fistula. Ideally, this is done in the first 12 hours of life and before the HMD becomes fully established. Attempts to ventilate the infant until the HMD resolves before closing the fistula tend to be hazardous. High ventilatory pressures may be required over a prolonged period to achieve adequate ventilation in the presence of severe HMD and are effective only if the airway resistance is lower than that of the fistula. If the fistula acts as a low-resistance vent, then ventilation becomes ineffective and the stomach distends with air, leading to gastric perforation, pneumoperitoneum and elevation of the diaphragm, with splinting, hypoxia, cardiac arrest and death. Placement of a gastrostomy may encourage preferential passage of air through the fistula, thus preventing satisfactory ventilation.

Administration of surfactant increases the safety by which the ligation or division of the fistula in the extremely premature infant with HMD can be achieved.

Delayed primary repair can be performed at seven to ten days of age, when the HMD is settling.

TRACHEO-OESOPHAGEAL FISTULA (THE 'H' FISTULA)

Tracheo-oesophageal fistula without oesophageal atresia presents a different clinical spectrum because the oesophagus is intact and patent. It is usually included in discussion of oesophageal atresia because of its presumed common embryological origin. A fistula passes obliquely from the trachea in a caudal direction to enter the oesophagus at a slightly lower level. Air may pass through the fistula from the trachea to the oesophagus, and oesophageal contents, e.g. saliva and gastric juices, may enter the trachea.

Presentation

Maternal polyhydramnios and prematurity are uncommon, unlike in oesophageal atresia. Symptoms result from the passage of air or liquid through the fistula and include choking and cyanotic attacks with feeds, usually relieved by nasogastric tube feeding. The infant may present with recurrent bouts of pneumonia or unexplained abdominal distension. Excessive drooling is sometimes seen, secondary to irritation of the respiratory tract from the passage of saliva and milk through the fistula. Vomiting, a hoarse cry and failure to thrive are less common features.

Investigation

The purpose of further investigation is to confirm the presence of a tracheo-oesophageal fistula and to establish the level of that fistula. The two methods used are radiology and endoscopy. A properly performed contrast study requires meticulous attention to detail, including recording the entire study on video. Contrast introduced through a catheter placed in the mid-oesophagus will identify a fistula in a high percentage of cases. Should diagnostic doubt persist despite an adequate mid-oesophageal radiological study, then bronchoscopy should be performed. Alternatively, bronchoscopy may be the initial investigation. There is no role for oesophagoscopy, as the fistula is difficult to find, or for the introduction of dyes such as methylene blue. Both contrast radiology and endoscopy have a place in the diagnosis of tracheo-oesophageal fistulae; with appropriate expertise, neither is clearly superior to the other.

Operative management

A summary of the management of the 'H' fistula is provided in Table 15.3. The best surgical approach is usually through a supraclavicular incision on the right side to reduce the

Table 15.3 *Summary of management of 'H' fistula*

Preoperative management	Surgical ablation of fistula	Postoperative management
Cessation of feeds	Cervical approach	Inspection of the vocal cords
Commencement of antibiotics	Division of the fistula	Commencement of oral feeds on day two
Observation and monitoring of vital signs, particularly respiratory rate and temperature		

likelihood of injury to the thoracic duct. An incision 2–3 cm in length above and parallel to the clavicle, deepened through the platysma, will usually allow access to the fistula without the need for division of the sternomastoid muscle. The strap muscles are retracted medially and the dissection is continued anteromedial to the carotid sheath. Introduction of a naso-oesophageal tube by the anaesthetist may help to determine the exact position of the oesophagus. The trachea can be recognized by its rings. The fistula will be found in the groove between the trachea and the oesophagus; it is short, runs obliquely and is surprisingly broad. Damage to the recurrent laryngeal nerves, which also run between the oesophagus and trachea, must be avoided. The placement of catheter slings around the oesophagus above and below the fistula is not necessary and increases the risk of damage to the recurrent laryngeal nerves. However, a sling placed around the fistula itself may help to control it during division. Each end of the fistula is closed using 4/0 or 5/0 absorbable sutures. Drainage of the wound is not normally required; nor is a routine gastrostomy. The anaesthetist should inspect the vocal cords at the completion of the operation.

Complications

Recurrent laryngeal nerve palsy (unilateral or bilateral) and recurrence of the fistula may occur. Leakage at the site of closure may result in mediastinitis, a recurrent fistula or oeosphagocutaneous fistula. Pneumothorax, tracheal obstruction, pneumonia and postoperative aspiration have also been reported. Good surgical technique reduces the likelihood of these complications.

LONG-TERM OUTCOMES AFTER REPAIR OF OESOPHAGEAL ATRESIA

The majority of adults with repaired oesophageal atresia lead relatively normal lives. Ongoing minor dysphagia is common, and many routinely drink water with their meals. Food impaction of the oesophagus is rare in adult life. The oldest survivors of oesophageal atresia are now in their fifties. Since 1989, there have been sporadic reports of oesophageal malignancy in these patients, raising concerns that they may be at

increased risk of malignant degeneration of the oesophagus. A high incidence of gastro-oesophageal reflux, disordered oesophageal propulsion and delayed oesophageal clearance may be contributing factors. Malignancy also has been reported in the oesophageal remnant after oesophageal replacement, e.g. colonic conduit, and in antethoracic skin-tube oesophageal conduits. Initiatives to minimize the risk of malignancy include routine excision of the oesophageal remnant during oesophageal replacement, ongoing monitoring of gastro-oesophageal reflux, early surgical control of persisting gastro-oesophageal reflux, and routine endoscopic surveillance of the oesophagus in adults.

CLINICAL SCENARIO

A 3.2-kg term baby is born with normal antenatal scans, except for polyhydramnios. Initial examination reveals a baby boy who is salivating excessively despite suction, and who has an absent anus, marked by a large triangular skin tag with meconium visible beneath. A 10-F nasogastric tube cannot be passed to the stomach, and X-rays show gas below the diaphragm and clear lung fields. A Replogle tube is passed orally and managed carefully to prevent inhalation of saliva. Echocardiography demonstrates a structurally normal heart and the renal ultrasound is normal. At operation, the lower oesophageal pouch is of good calibre and almost overlaps the thick-walled upper pouch. The tracheo-oesophageal fistula is transfixed and divided. A straightforward primary anastomosis is performed using eight interrupted sutures. Finally, a cut-back anoplasty is performed. Postoperatively, the baby is allowed to breathe spontaneously. At 48 hours, the child is well and allowed to breastfeed. Subsequent spinal X-rays and ultrasound of the back are normal.

Before surgery, the parents were told the diagnosis and the likely results of the surgery. Later, they are told in more detail the potential oesophageal and tracheal complications together with the management of the bowel following the anal cut-back procedure.

Once the baby is established on full breastfeeds and the parents have been trained in resuscitation, they are allowed to take the baby home.

REFERENCES

Bax KM, van Der Zee DC. Feasibility of thoracoscopic repair of oesophageal atresia with distal fistula. *Journal of Pediatric Surgery* 2002; **37**; 192–6.

Beasley SW. Oesophageal atresia without fistula. In: Beasley SW, Myers NA, Auldist AW (eds). *Oesophageal Atresia*. London: Chapman & Hall, 1991; pp. 137–9.

Beasley SW, Allen M, Myers NA. The effect of Down syndrome and other chromosomal abnormalities on survival and management in oesophageal atresia. *Pediatric Surgery International* 1997; **12**: 550–51.

Farkash U, Lazar L, Erez I, Gutermacher M, Freud E. The distal pouch in oesophageal atresia: to dissect or not to dissect, that is the question. *European Journal of Pediatric Surgery* 2002; **12**: 19–23.

Hirschl RB, Yardeni D, Oldham K, *et al.* Gastric transposition for oesophageal replacement in children: experience with 41 consecutive cases with special emphasis on oesophageal atresia. *Annals of Surgery* 2002; **236**: 531–9.

Kluth D. Atlas of esophageal atresia. *Journal of Pediatric Surgery* 1976; **11**: 901–19.

Mee RBB, Beasley SW, Myers NA, Auldist AW. Influence of congenital heart disease on the management of oesophageal atresia. *Pediatric Surgery International* 1992; **7**: 90–93.

Pigna A, Gentili A, Landuzzi V, Lima M, Baroncini S. Bronchoscopy in newborns with oesophageal atresia. *Pediatria Medica e Chirurgica* 2002; **24**: 297–301.

Scharli AF. Esophageal reconstruction in very long atresia by elongation of the lesser curvature. *Pediatric Surgery International* 1992; **7**: 101–7.

Shulman A, Mazkereth R, Zalel Y, *et al.* Prenatal identification of oesophageal atresia: the role of ultrasonography for evaluation of functional anatomy. *Prenatal Diagnosis* 2002; **22**: 669–74.

Spitz L. Gastric replacement of the oesophagus. In: Spitz LV, Nixon HH (eds). *Rob and Smith's Operative Surgery: Paediatric Surgery*, 4th edn. London: Butterworths, 1998; pp. 142–5.

16

Neonatal gastrointestinal obstruction

TOLGA E DAGLI

Learning objectives

- To understand the types and aetiology of neonatal gastrointestinal obstruction.
- To learn how to approach the neonate with potential gastrointestinal obstruction.
- To be able to recognize the clinical manifestations and the imaging features of various types of neonatal gastrointestinal obstruction.
- To be able to describe the surgical techniques required to treat the various types of neonatal gastrointestinal obstruction.

INTRODUCTION

Neonatal gastrointestinal (NGI) obstruction is one of the most common surgical emergencies in the neonatal period. Classically, it presents with bilious (green) vomiting, abdominal distension and no or delayed passage of meconium. The diagnosis must be established as early as possible to prevent clinical deterioration, aspiration pneumonia, sepsis and biochemical and haematological derangements. Early consideration of the need for surgical intervention may mean the difference between intestinal salvage and catastrophe.

Many causes of bowel obstruction in the newborn can be diagnosed easily with physical examination and simple radiographic studies. However, the surgeon's approach to a newborn with a potential bowel obstruction is to rule out the worst possibility first.

The previously high mortality of NGI obstruction has been reduced by perinatal diagnosis of pathology, improved paediatric intensive care, safer anaesthesia and refined surgical techniques. Prematurity, associated congenital anomalies and intercurrent infections are the major causes of death in neonates with NGI obstruction.

TYPES OF NEONATAL GASTROINTESTINAL OBSTRUCTION

Intestinal obstructions are either intrinsic or extrinsic and may be divided morphologically into atresia and stenosis. The term 'atresia' denotes complete intrinsic occlusion of the intestinal lumen, while the term 'stenosis' refers to localized narrowing of the bowel or a diaphragm with a small perforation, which causes incomplete obstruction. Extrinsic obstructions may be caused by, for example, malrotation with volvulus, peritoneal bands and annular pancreas.

Table 16.1 *Types of neonatal gastrointestinal obstruction*

(a) High obstruction

Gastric outlet	Duodenal	Jejunal
Pyloric atresia	Duodenal atresia	Jejunal atresia
Antral web	Duodenal stenosis	Jejunal stenosis
	Annular pancreas	
	Preduodenal portal vein	
	Malrotation	

(b) Low obstruction

Distal small bowel	Colonic	Uncommon causes
Ileal atresia	Colonic atresia	Intussusception
Meconium ileus, uncomplicated	*Dysmotility states:*	Meckel's diverticulum
Meconium ileus, complicated	Meconium plug	
	Small left colon syndrome	
	Hirschsprung disease	

Approximately 30 per cent of infants presenting with neonatal intestinal obstruction have atresia or stenosis. Duodenal atresia is the most frequent type of intestinal obstruction, followed by jejunal atresia and ileal atresia.

NGI obstruction can also be grouped as high or low obstructions, which in turn simplifies the understanding of the clinical findings (Table 16.1).

RELEVANT BASIC SCIENCE

NGI obstruction occurs in approximately one in 1500–2000 live births. It may result from:

- intrinsic developmental defects;
- insults acquired *in utero*, after the formation of normal bowel;
- abnormalities of peristalsis and/or abnormal intestinal contents.

The main pathological features of intestinal atresia or stenosis are marked dilation of the proximal segment and collapse of the distal segment beyond the obstruction.

Pyloric atresia is a rare (one in one million live births) autosomal genetic defect and has an association with epidermolysis bullosa. It is unknown whether this association is due to a genetic linkage or whether there is a causative effect on the antropyloric mucosa.

Duodenal obstruction is believed to be the result of an error of development occurring in the early weeks of gestation. During the third week of gestation, the duodenum is a solid core of epithelium, which undergoes vacuolization followed by recanalization. Tandler (1902) proposed that failure of recanalization of the duodenal lumen produces stenosis or

atresia. At the same time, there may be anomalies of the extrahepatic pancreaticobiliary ductal system and the pancreas. Approximately 50 per cent of babies with duodenal atresia have one or more cardiac, renal, central nervous or musculoskeletal system anomalies, and up to 30 per cent have trisomy 21. Congenital heart disease is found in about 20 per cent of all infants with duodenal atresia (Grosfeld *et al.* 1979).

Most jejunoileal obstructions are caused by late intrauterine mesenteric vascular accidents such as volvulus, intussusception, internal hernia, and bowel incarceration in an omphalocele or gastroschisis. The late occurrence of such events accounts for the relatively low incidence of associated anomalies in jejunoileal obstructions in the newborn. The ischaemic insult also affects the function of the markedly dilated proximal end and distal atretic segments. The disparity in lumen diameter varies from a two- to five-fold difference between the proximal and distal segments. There is a deficiency in coordinated peristalsis of the bulbous end of the proximal segment. This may be explained by hyperplasia of ganglion cells in the dilated proximal segment and absent acetylcholinesterase activity at the ends of the blind proximal and distal atretic segments.

The pathophysiology of colonic atresia parallels that of jejunoileal atresia, in that it results from an intrauterine mesenteric vascular impairment or intrauterine volvulus. Colonic atresia has many similarities with jejunoileal atresia but is much less common. Associated anomalies are uncommon, and its rarity may result from better protection of the colon from segmental ischaemia afforded by the well-developed vascular arcade that runs immediately adjacent to it. Colonic atresia may be associated with cloacal extrophy, vesicointestinal fissure and abdominal-wall defects.

Malrotation results from a failure of the gastrointestinal tract to complete its normal rotation and fixation as it returns to the abdominal cavity in the eighth to tenth weeks of gestation. As first recognized, the intestinal tract is a straight tube from the stomach to the rectum. Active growth of the midgut and hindgut begins during the fifth week of development, peaks during the eighth week and slows around the tenth week. During the fifth to eighth weeks, the bowel develops outside of the abdominal cavity as a single long loop of bowel forming a temporary physiological hernia. The axis of this primary midgut loop is the superior mesenteric vessels (Figure 16.1a). While the developing midgut and hindgut are lying in the physiological hernia, there is a rotation of 90 degrees anticlockwise. The duodenum curves downward and to the right of the superior mesenteric artery (Figure 16.1b). Meanwhile, the caecocolic loop moves to the left of the superior mesenteric artery from its starting position inferior to the artery (Figure 16.2a,b). A further 90-degree rotation occurs before the midgut moves out of the umbilical hernia. The duodenum comes to lie beneath the superior mesenteric artery. This increases the rotation of the duodenojejunal loop to 180 degrees (Figure 16.1c). By the tenth week of gestation, the bowel returns to the abdominal cavity. As the bowel

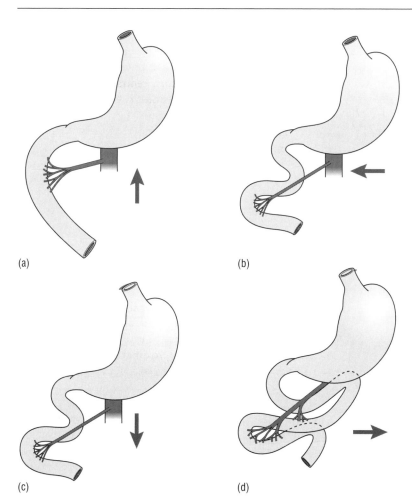

(a)

(b)

(c)

(d)

Figure 16.1   *Normal rotation of the duodenojejunal loop. (a) The primary midgut loop (PML); note the axis of the loop is the superior mesenteric vessels (SMV). (b) The duodenojejunal loop has rotated 90 degrees anticlockwise from its starting position to the right of the SMV. (c) Further rotation of the duodenojejunal loop to a position below the SMV. (d) Final rotation of the duodenojejunal loop to a position to the left of the SMV.*

returns to the abdomen, the proximal small bowel returns first, and the duodenum rotates underneath the superior mesenteric vessels towards the left side, where the future ligament of Treitz will be located (Figure 16.1d). This additional 90-degree anticlockwise rotation results in a total rotation of the midgut of 270 degrees. The caecum and ascending colon reduce last and come to lie in the right upper quadrant (Figure 16.2c). Further growth of the colon pushes the caecum into the right loin (Figure 16.2d). The final step in the normal midgut positioning process is the fixation of the intestine. The ascending and descending colon and the duodenum (excluding the first part) become fixed to the posterior abdominal wall. The terminal ileum has followed the caecum into the right lower abdomen. Therefore, the small-bowel mesenteric attachment is a diagonal line from the ligament of Treitz ligament to the right iliac fossa. This broad-based anchoring of the small-bowel mesentery prevents rotation.

If the rotation of the bowel does not occur, then the normal mesenteric attachments are absent and abnormal peritoneal bands, known as Ladd's bands, may develop. These bands may obstruct the duodenum. The malrotated bowel itself does not cause any significant problem. Most concerning in malrotation is the lack of peritoneal attachments of the bowel. The unfixed small bowel may twist around its narrow base, perhaps

triggered by peristaltic action, and compromise the blood supply of the superior mesenteric pedicle. Unusual distension of the intestine by fluid or meconium may also initiate the volvulus. The specific condition of midgut volvulus refers to a twisting of the entire midgut from the duodenum to the transverse colon about the axis of the superior mesenteric artery. Acute onset of volvulus is a true surgical emergency. Unless it is treated in a timely manner, bowel strangulation results in an ischaemic loss of extensive bowel, causing short gut syndrome.

Meconium ileus is an intraluminal obstruction characterized by retention of thick tenacious meconium in the bowel and comprises approximately 20 per cent of cases of neonatal intestinal obstruction. Between 90 and 95 per cent of patients with meconium ileus have cystic fibrosis. Only 15 per cent of patients with cystic fibrosis present with meconium ileus in the neonatal period. Meconium ileus appears to be the result mainly of abnormal intestinal secretions. Excessively viscous mucus secretion causes the meconium to stick to the intestinal wall, and the involved bowel is distended by meconium retention during fetal life. The distal ileum is small and contracted and contains firm, greyish putty-like secretions of meconium. The mid-ileum becomes dilated and hypertrophied and contains black material with a thick, tar-like consistency. The small, unused microcolon is poorly developed and contains inspissated meconium pellets.

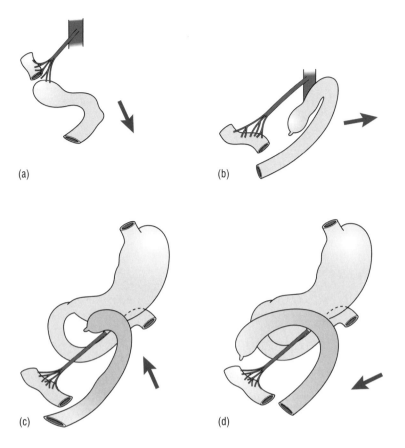

(a)

(b)

(c)

(d)

Figure 16.2   *Normal rotation of the caecocolic loop. (a) Caecocolic loop lies inferior to the superior mesenteric vessels (SMV) before the rotation of 90 degrees anticlockwise takes place. (b) Note the position of the caecocolic loop at the left of the SMV. The caecocolic loop has rotated 90 degrees anticlockwise. (c) Rotation of the caecocolic loop to a position superior to the SMV. (d) Final position of the caecocolic loop to the right of the SMV.*

Meconium ileus can be either simple or complicated. Simple meconium ileus occurs with distal small-bowel obstruction alone in approximately 60–80 per cent of infants with meconium ileus. Complicated meconium ileus results from an intrauterine volvulus, producing atresia, a bowel perforation with generalized meconium peritonitis or giant cystic meconium peritonitis. Meconium-filled bowel proximal to the obstruction may become twisted causing volvulus. Ischaemia of the base of the volvulus may lead to bowel perforation or atresia. When bowel perforation occurs, the extruded bowel contents provoke an intense peritoneal inflammatory reaction, leading to the formation of dense fibrotic tissue. This tissue often calcifies, resulting in the characteristic intraperitoneal calcifications. Extravasation and liquefaction of the meconium may result in giant cystic meconium peritonitis (Murshed *et al.* 1997).

Meconium plug syndrome typically presents as colonic obstruction caused by a plug of inspissated and dehydrated meconium in the distal colon and rectum. Diminished colonic motility is the key feature in this condition. The aetiology is unknown. However, it may occur in infants of diabetic mothers, hypothyroid babies and premature infants with intestinal dysmotility. Meconium plug syndrome is often associated with Hirschsprung's disease and cystic fibrosis. Suction rectal biopsy is needed to rule out Hirschsprung's disease, and a diagnostic sweat test may be appropriate to exclude cystic fibrosis. In patients with simple meconium plug syndrome, evacuation of the plug results is complete cure. Generally, these infants have normal bowel function afterwards.

CLASSIFICATION OF INTESTINAL ATRESIA

In pyloric atresia, the pyloric lumen is completely obliterated by a diaphragm or a solid core of tissue, or there is a complete absence of pylorus.

Duodenal atresia may be seen with an intact web with duodenal wall continuity (type 1), with a fibrous tissue that connects the two ends of atretic duodenum (type 2), or with complete separation (type 3). Usually, the gap is filled in with pancreatic tissue. In type 1 duodenal atresia, the web may stretch out distally in the lumen of the duodenum and is referred to as a 'windsock anomaly'. Intrinsic duodenal stenosis may be due to an incomplete web or a diaphragm with a small central opening.

Atresia and stenosis of the jejunum and ileum are distributed equally from the ligament of Treitz to the caecum. The proximal jejunum is the site of atresia in 30 per cent of cases, the distal jejunum in 20 per cent, the proximal ileum in ten per cent, and the distal ileum in 40 per cent. Five different types of atresia are described by Grosfeld *et al.* (1979) (Table 16.2).

Colonic atresia can occur at any level. The various types of atresia described for the jejunum and the ileum also occur in

Table 16.2 *Classification of intestinal atresia*

Atresia type	Prevalence (%)	Description
1	20	Thin mucosal membrane with intact bowel; bowel is normal in length
2	30	Blinds ends joined by a fibrous band; corresponding defect in the mesentery is rare
3a	46	Disconnected blind ends; single gap in the mesentery; subnormal bowel length
3b		Apple-peel or Christmas-tree atresia: gross defect in mesentery; extensive loss of bowel length
4	4	Multiple atresias: string of sausages; considerable shortening of bowel

the colon, with the exception of multiple atresias, which are extremely rare.

PRENATAL DIAGNOSIS

Prenatal imaging, especially with ultrasound, can be effective in detecting bowel obstruction. A fetus with proximal bowel obstruction may present with polyhydramnios. Approximately 50 per cent of newborns with duodenal atresia and proximal jejunal atresia have polyhydramnios. The finding of polyhydramnios is a clear indication for obtaining a fetal ultrasound.

Prenatal diagnosis of duodenal obstruction is based on the demonstration of the characteristic 'double-bubble' appearance of the dilated stomach and proximal duodenum. Although the characteristic 'double bubble' can be seen as early as 20 weeks' gestation, it is usually not diagnosed until after 25 weeks' gestation. The fetus is unable to swallow a sufficient volume of amniotic fluid for bowel dilation to occur before the end of the second trimester of pregnancy.

Sonographic diagnosis of small-bowel obstruction relies on demonstrating multiple interconnecting overdistended bowel loops. The number of dilated loops depends on the level of obstruction: the lower the level of obstruction, the greater the number of dilated loops. The abdomen is usually distended, and active peristalsis may be observed. Polyhydramnios is more common in high obstruction. Thus, more distal atresias may not be associated with polyhydramnios. If bowel perforation occurs, then transient ascites, meconium peritonitis and meconium pseudo-cysts may ensue.

A variety of abnormal findings in fetuses with meconium ileus can be identified with prenatal sonography, including calcification, dilated loops of bowel, meconium pseudo-cyst, polyhydramnios and fetal ascites. In the typical case, the association of intra-abdominal echogenic areas, dilated bowel loops and ascites suggests meconium peritonitis. The diagnosis should be considered if the fetal bowel is observed to be dilated or if intra-abdominal hyperechogenicity is detected. However, these findings can be extremely difficult to interpret.

Phelps and colleagues (1997) reported that only 42 per cent of prenatally diagnosed gastrointestinal malformations were confirmed postnatally, and only 16 per cent of gastrointestinal malformations observed at birth were detected by prenatal ultrasound. Although prenatal ultrasound is reliable in the detection of gastrointestinal obstructions, suspected fetal gastrointestinal abnormalities should be interpreted with caution.

APPROACH TO THE NEONATE SUSPECTED OF HAVING GASTROINTESTINAL OBSTRUCTION

When a neonate develops bilious vomiting, a surgical condition should be suspected. Bilious gastric aspirates or emesis suggests an obstruction distal to the ampulla of Vater. As a rule, any neonate with bilious vomiting must be considered to have a bowel obstruction until proven otherwise and demands immediate evaluation. Abdominal distension or tenderness may indicate bowel obstruction or bowel compromise from other causes, e.g. septic ileus or necrotizing enterocolitis. The degree of abdominal distension is related directly to the site of the obstruction. Proximal obstructions produce epigastric distension, and distal obstructions produce more dramatic abdominal distension. Scaphoid abdomen is also possible for high obstructions. Infants with abdominal distension and bilious vomiting usually fail to pass meconium. Rectal examination is necessary in all of these newborns. Partial obstructions may produce minimal or no physical findings.

Remember that extra-gastrointestinal conditions such as neonatal sepsis, birth trauma, prematurity and transplacental transfer of maternal medication can closely mimic mechanical intestinal obstruction in the newborn.

After a focused physical examination, a nasogastric or orogastric catheter (e.g. 8F) should be placed immediately for gastric decompression to prevent vomiting, further gaseous distension of the obstructed intestine, and aspiration. This should be done before any diagnostic or therapeutic manoeuvres are performed, because aspiration is a significant complication and should be avoided. An adequate intravenous route is established. Estimated losses from vomiting and fluid sequestered into the third space must be replaced. Infants who are dehydrated may receive fluids equivalent to one per cent of their body weight per hour until adequate urine output has been restored. If there is clinical evidence of pneumonia, or if peritonitis or sepsis is suspected, then pre-operative antibiotics should be needed. Once the patient is haemodynamically stabilized, appropriate imaging studies of the abdomen should be performed.

RADIOLOGICAL DIAGNOSIS

Radiography is the most valuable means of determining whether NGI obstruction is present. If NGI obstruction is not present, then radiography may help to determine the next most useful diagnostic procedure. An abnormal gas pattern visualized on an abdominal radiograph often leads to the diagnosis of bowel obstruction (Hernanz-Schulmann 1999).

Swallowed air can usually be detected in the stomach within the first minute after birth. Within three hours, the entire small bowel usually contains gas, and after eight to nine hours, neonates demonstrate sigmoid gas. The diagnosis of obstruction is based on some interruption in the dispersion of air. The pattern of bowel gas on a plain film can differentiate between proximal and distal bowel obstruction.

In cases of proximal or high obstruction, a few loops are identified on a plain radiograph (Figure 16.3). Neonates with complete high intestinal obstruction do not usually require further radiological evaluation other than plain X-rays. However, an upper-gastrointestinal series must be performed in patients with incomplete high obstruction. When plain films suggest a high small-bowel obstruction but there is gas in the distal small bowel, then upper-gastrointestinal contrast study is the procedure of choice to demonstrate the level and nature of the obstruction.

Low intestinal obstruction is defined as an obstruction that occurs in the distal ileum or colon. Abdominal distension is typically marked, regardless of whether the loops are filled with fluid, meconium or air. The diagnosis of low obstruction is usually apparent on abdominal radiography because of the presence of many dilated intestinal loops (Figure 16.4). However, the differentiation between ileal and colonic obstruction is difficult. This distinction can be made readily with a contrast enema. Demonstration of an unused colon on contrast enema is usually diagnostic of a distal small-bowel obstruction.

Plain abdominal films of patients with simple meconium ileus demonstrate a distal obstruction. The abdomen is filled with gas-distended loops and there are few or no air–fluid levels, due to abnormally thick intraluminal meconium. (This is in contradistinction to the findings in patients with ileal atresia.) The admixture of gas with meconium may give rise to a 'soap-bubble' or 'ground-glass' appearance. The soap-bubble appearance depends on the viscosity of the meconium and is not a constant finding. However, its presence is pathognomonic. Meconium ileus may be complicated by volvulus of a distal intestinal loop, perforation, atresia or peritonitis. The plain abdominal films need to be viewed carefully for the presence of calcification, which indicates an intrauterine bowel perforation and meconium peritonitis (Hernanz-Schulmann 1999).

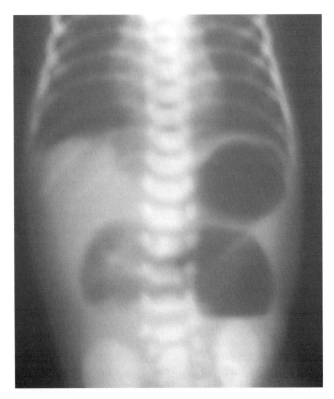

Figure 16.3 *Jejunal atresia. Upright radiograph, showing air–fluid levels in the stomach and the first part of the small bowel. No distal gas is seen.*

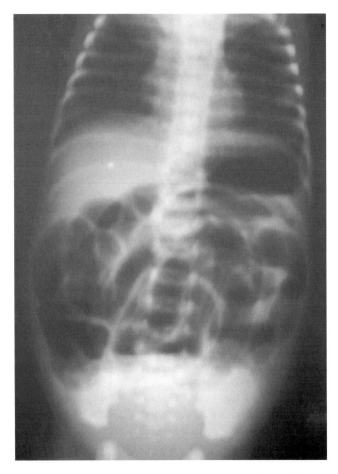

Figure 16.4 *Low intestinal obstruction. Upright abdominal film, showing distension of the bowel with multiple air–fluid levels.*

The radiographic findings of colonic atresia are those of a distal obstruction and are often indistinguishable from obstruction of the distal ileum, especially when the atresia is located in the ascending colon. In some patients, however, a hugely and disproportionately dilated loop of bowel may be present, and a mottled pattern of gas and faeces may be identified. The diagnosis is confirmed by contrast enema, which reveals an unused colon terminating at the point of atresia.

In meconium plug syndrome, diagnosis is made through contrast enema revealing the outline of meconium plug within an otherwise normal-appearing colon. Contrast enema can also be therapeutic in stimulating passage of the meconium.

COMMON CAUSES OF NEONATAL GASTROINTESTINAL OBSTRUCTION

Duodenal obstruction

INCIDENCE

Duodenal obstruction occurs in one in 10 000 to one in 5000 live births. Thirty per cent have Down syndrome.

PRESENTATIONS

There are several causes of duodenal obstruction: duodenal stenosis, atresia and malrotation. Polyhydramnios is present in up to 50 per cent of neonates with duodenal obstruction. Neonates with duodenal atresia usually present with bilious vomiting, and more than half of neonates with duodenal obstruction are born prematurely. If the atresia is proximal to the ampulla of Vater, then the vomit is non-bilious. Bilious or clear vomiting starts a few hours after birth. Distension may not be present. There may be fullness in the epigastrium. Approximately one-third of patients have malrotation or annular pancreas associated with duodenal atresia, although volvulus in the collapsed bowel has not been described.

DIAGNOSTIC PROCEDURES

An abdominal film with a classic 'double-bubble' sign is sufficient to confirm the diagnosis of duodenal atresia. A dilated stomach and obstructed duodenum, indented at the waist by the pylorus, gives this characteristic appearance (Figure 16.5). An upper gastrointestinal series might be necessary to distinguish between malrotation and duodenal stenosis. Intestinal gas beyond the duodenum indicates incomplete obstruction. Contrast studies demonstrate passage of a small amount of contrast and the site of stenosis. Partial obstruction may be caused by annular pancreas, aberrant pancreatic tissue in the duodenal wall, perforate web or a preduodenal portal vein. The diagnosis of incomplete obstruction is usually delayed.

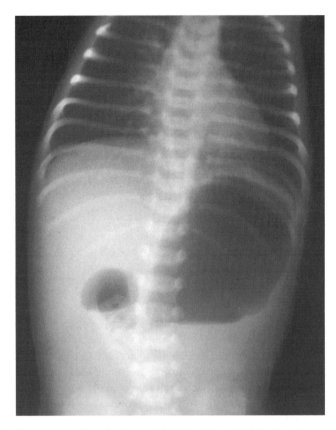

Figure 16.5 *Duodenal atresia. Upright abdominal film, showing the characteristic 'double bubble' sign. Note the dilated stomach and the dilated proximal duodenum.*

PREOPERATIVE MANAGEMENT

Gastric decompression by nasogastric suction and intravenous fluid administration should be started. Associated anomalies should be excluded. A cardiac consultation with echocardiogram may be helpful.

TREATMENT

A diamond-shaped or side-to-side duodenoduodenostomy through a supraumbilical transverse abdominal incision is preferred. Ladd's procedure should be performed if it is needed. The membranous-type lesion can be treated simply by excision of the obstructing membrane. The duodenum is opened and the web is excised carefully, paying attention to the papilla in order not to cut the common bile duct close to papilla. The papilla of Vater is located by observing bile flow, facilitated by gentle compression of the gallbladder.

POSTOPERATIVE MANAGEMENT

The stomach is emptied using a nasogastric tube. When upright abdominal films show that gas has passed into the distal intestine, the nasogastric tube is clamped and opened intermittently to measure the gastric aspirates. When the gastric residual is less than 20 mL, gradually increasing feeds are offered as tolerated, until sufficient calorific intake and weight gain are achieved. During this time (up to six weeks), nutritional support is provided by total parenteral nutrition (TPN).

OUTCOME

The outcome is good unless associated with serious cardiac anomaly or chromosomal disorder. A megaduodenum may be seen in long-term follow-up, and reoperation with tapering duodenoplasty may be needed.

Malrotation with midgut volvulus

INCIDENCE

The incidence of rotational abnormalities is difficult to determine, but the incidence of symptoms leading to clinical discovery is estimated at one in 6000 live births.

PRESENTATION

A midgut volvulus is the most common cause of symptoms in patients with malrotation. Thirty per cent occur at three to seven days of life, and 50–75 per cent occur before one month of age. Acute onset of volvulus is a true emergency and must be diagnosed quickly. Bilious vomiting starts in an infant who has not been ill previously. These infants usually have passed meconium or have had normal stools. Soon there is rapid deterioration with abdominal distress. Rectal bleeding may occur. Abdominal distension typically is not present initially. With progressive midgut ischaemia and injury, small-bowel distension may develop. Intestinal necrosis may lead to hypotension, respiratory failure, systemic acidosis and sepsis.

Associated congenital anomalies are common, occurring in 70 per cent of children with intestinal malrotation. Duodenal abnormalities, including atresia, stenosis and web, occur in 11 per cent of patients (Rescorla *et al.* 1990).

DIAGNOSTIC PROCEDURES

A patient with midgut volvulus may have the double-bubble sign and some air beyond the double bubble on a normal plain radiograph. A relatively airless abdomen is highly suggestive of volvulus with malrotation. If malrotation is a concern, then an immediate upper-gastrointestinal contrast study must be done to determine the position of duodenojejunal junction. Incomplete obstruction of the duodenum, with the appearance of extrinsic compression and torsion (corkscrew, coiled or bird's beak sign), may be seen. Ultrasonography is a useful screening device for infants suspected of having midgut volvulus. The whirlpool sign of midgut volvulus can be demonstrated with colour Doppler ultrasound.

PREOPERATIVE MANAGEMENT

Neonates with malrotation and midgut volvulus with the findings of acute abdomen require emergency laparotomy to correct the volvulus. As the operating room is prepared, nasogastric suction should be started, intravenous fluids must be given rapidly and broad-spectrum antibiotics should be infused. Operation should not be delayed for resuscitation.

TREATMENT

The abdomen is usually entered through an upper-abdominal transverse incision. The ischaemic bowel is de-rotated anticlockwise and observed for reperfusion. A period of intraoperative warming is often necessary. If the midgut is viable, then Ladd's procedure is performed. The abnormal peritoneal attachments from the caecum crossing to the first and second portions of the duodenum (Ladd's bands) are divided. This allows maximal separation between the duodenum and the caecum and widens the base of the small bowel mesentery. Then the bowel is returned to the abdomen by placing the small bowel on the right and the caecum in the left upper quadrant. It is unnecessary to fix the bowel. Finally, an incidental inversion appendectomy is performed.

If necrotic bowel is encountered at surgery, then the infarcted intestine is resected. The length of necrosis is a predictor of survival. Patients with 50 per cent necrosis have a 90 per cent survival rate. However, patients with 75 per cent necrosis have only a 35 per cent survival rate. If extensive bowel is ischaemic, then the bowel is reduced into the abdominal cavity, and the abdomen is re-explored 24 hours later for a second look. At this time, a demarcation may be visible between the necrotic and the viable bowel, allowing the surgeon to resect the necrotic bowel and create a stoma at the distal end of the normal bowel. This approach can avoid development of short gut syndrome. The difficult situation is to encounter complete necrosis of the midgut. Some surgeons resect the bowel, create stomas and start TPN. Others close without resection and discuss terminal care with the family (Rescorla *et al.* 1990).

POSTOPERATIVE MANAGEMENT

Postoperative management is similar to that associated with any abdominal surgery. Return of intestinal function depends on the duration of obstruction. TPN is essential for infants with massive intestinal loss.

OUTCOME

Results after surgical correction of malrotation are generally good without bowel resection, but gastrointestinal motility disturbances are common. The mortality rate for the operative correction of malrotation ranges from three to nine per cent overall. The mortality rate is increased with intestinal necrosis, bowel resection and short gut syndrome. Long-term sequelae include short gut syndrome, feeding difficulties and sepsis from intravenous catheters.

Jejunoileal atresia and stenosis

INCIDENCE

The incidence of jejunoileal atresia and stenosis is one in 1000 live births.

PRESENTATION

Abdominal distension and bilious vomiting is observed within 24 hours of birth. The degree of abdominal distension is related directly to the site of obstruction. Abdominal distension is more pronounced with distal small-bowel obstruction. Most infants fail to pass meconium. Jaundice is present occasionally. Polyhydramnios is more common in instances of jejunal obstruction.

DIAGNOSTIC PROCEDURES

Air–fluid levels on the abdominal film and abdominal distension are diagnostic. High jejunal atresia may show a few air–fluid levels, which is more than would be seen in duodenal atresia and fewer than in ileal atresia or other causes of low bowel obstruction. There is no further gas beyond that point (Figure 16.3). In cases of ileal obstruction, erect abdominal radiographs often demonstrate many dilated loops of intestine, with air–fluid levels. Ileal atresia may be more difficult to diagnose preoperatively because of conditions such as meconium ileus and Hirschsprung's disease. A contrast enema will exclude meconium ileus and confirm the diagnosis of small bowel obstruction.

PREOPERATIVE MANAGEMENT

Nasogastric suction and intravenous hydration are essential. Dehydration and acid–base and electrolyte imbalances should be corrected. Intravenous fluid is given at a rate of 10–20 mL/kg/h until the patient's condition is stabilized. Antibiotics are given routinely.

TREATMENT

The aim is to establish intestinal continuity and preserve as much normal bowel as possible. The proximal bowel is dilated and a limited resection is usually needed. This resection also facilitates an end-to-end or end-to-oblique anastomosis. A single-layer, end-to-oblique anastomosis is simple and efficacious. If proximal resection is not possible, then tapering or plication of the dilated bowel is indicated. The distal bowel should be evaluated for additional atresias or stenosis by an intraluminal injection of 0.9% saline. If multiple atresias are present, then many anastomoses may be required (see case study).

POSTOPERATIVE MANAGEMENT

TPN should begin as soon as a stable postoperative state has been reached. Nasogastric suction is necessary during the period of intestinal dysfunction. When the gastric aspirates are reduced, oral feedings must be started in small quantities and increased slowly in order to avoid aspiration.

OUTCOME

In most infants with jejunoileal atresia, the prognosis is good unless there is excessive loss of bowel.

Meconium ileus

INCIDENCE

Meconium ileus occurs in approximately 15 per cent of newborns with cystic fibrosis. There is an incidence of one in 10 000 to one in 5000 live births. The disease is much rarer in Asian births.

PRESENTATION

In the newborn with simple meconium ileus, abdominal distension and bilious vomiting occur immediately after birth. There is no passage of meconium. Often, dilated loops of bowel become visible on physical examination. The rectum and anus are narrow.

In the newborn with complicated meconium ileus, the presentation is more dramatic. At birth, an erythematous and oedematous distended abdomen may be present. Signs of peritonitis may be noted. A mass may be palpated in the abdomen, indicating pseudo-cyst formation. The abdominal distension leads to respiratory compromise, and hypovolaemia may be noted secondary to third-space losses.

DIAGNOSTIC PROCEDURES

X-ray studies are essential. Dilated loops of intestine with absent or few air–fluid levels and 'ground-glass' or 'soap-bubble' signs are seen on plain X-rays in simple meconium ileus. A contrast enema is diagnostic and also may be therapeutic. Perforation with meconium peritonitis or pseudo-cyst formation, usually with calcification, may be noted in complicated meconium ileus. Decubitus radiographs to determine the presence or absence of free air may be helpful. A sweat test (quantitative measurement of chloride) is the only reliable test for the definitive diagnosis of cystic fibrosis. Confirmation of the diagnosis is by analysis of sweat: sodium and chloride should exceed 60 mEq/L on a sample weighing over 100 mg. Genetic markers of cystic fibrosis (e.g. ΔF508) should be performed.

PREOPERATIVE MANAGEMENT

Both simple and complicated meconium ileus should be managed as NGI obstruction. For simple meconium ileus, treatment with meglumine diatrizoate containing 0.1% polysorbate 80 and 37% organically bound iodine (Gastrografin™) or a water-soluble contrast enema is recommended. If hyperosmolar solutions are used, then the patient must be prepared well with fluid and electrolyte replacement, and intravenous antibiotics should be administered. The aim is to reflux the enema into the terminal ileum and, by softening and hydrating the meconium mass, to remove the abnormal meconium (Figure 16.6). The flow of the contrast through the thick meconium is slow, and usually more than one enema is needed. Complications of therapeutic enema include hypovolaemic shock and acute or late

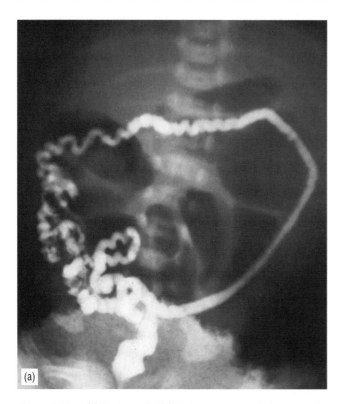
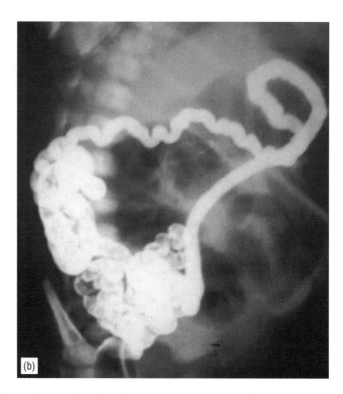

Figure 16.6   *(a) Gastrografin™ (diatrizoate meglumine) enema of a patient with meconium ileus. A microcolon is observed, indicating that the level of obstruction is in the small bowel. (b) Note the inspissated pellets in the terminal ileum.*

perforation between 12 and 96 hours. If enemas are not successful, then open laparotomy is necessary.

TREATMENT

Only 60–70 per cent of simple meconium ileus patients are cured with enema. The remaining cases need operative treatment. The goal of operative treatment is to evacuate the meconium from the intestine and to preserve the maximum length of bowel. This goal may require simple enterotomy, with irrigation or resection with or without a stoma. After confirming the diagnosis at laparotomy, an enterotomy is made in the dilated segment of the ileum. With the help of an irrigating catheter, saline or 1–4% *N*-acetylcysteine (a mucolytic agent) is instilled into the bowel lumen to emulsify the abnormal meconium. This can also be managed via T-tube enterostomy (Bishop–Koop, Santulli or Mikulicz types).

In complicated meconium ileus, surgery is always needed. Persistent abdominal distension, bowel obstruction, meconium cyst formation, perforation, enlarging abdominal mass, volvulus or intestinal atresias are complications necessitating surgical management. Bowel resection is often necessary, and temporary stomas are almost always required.

POSTOPERATIVE MANAGEMENT

Postoperatively, nasogastric decompression is continued and the patient receives antibiotics. Normal bowel function returns usually within five to ten days. Neonates with complicated surgical courses require either TPN or continued enteral feedings with predigested infant formulas. Ostomies should be reversed as soon as possible. Once oral feeds are started, pancreatic enzymes may need to be given orally.

OUTCOME

Improvement in neonatal support has increased five-year survival rates to 85–100 per cent in the past decade. Once infants are discharged from the hospital, they do well. However, the long-term outcome depends on the systemic problems, which will be managed by the cystic fibrosis team.

CLINICAL SCENARIOS

Case 1

A full-term infant presented at the age of two days with persistent bilious vomiting beginning at one day of age. The typical stigmata of Down syndrome were present. A plain erect film of the abdominal film revealed two air–fluid levels, 'double-bubble sign' and no distal air. There were increased vascular markings and an enlarged cardiac silhouette on the chest film. Further evaluation revealed findings consistent with congenital heart disease. Surgery verified type 1 duodenal atresia in the second part of the duodenum. Patency of the distal bowel segments was established by injection of air and saline. A diamond-shaped duodenoduodenostomy was performed. The postoperative course was uneventful. The boy was doing well six months after the operation, with normal psychomotor development and no intestinal problems.

Case 2

A girl weighing 2500 g was born at 36 weeks' gestation after an uncomplicated pregnancy. At six hours of age, the baby developed abdominal distension and bilious vomiting. An abdominal radiograph showed a few markedly dilated loops of bowel without distal bowel gas. A contrast enema was performed, which showed a microcolon. At surgery, the proximal jejunum was markedly dilated, with 15 cm of bowel from the ligament of Treitz to the first atresia. The proximal atretic segment was separated with a mesenteric gap from the distal bowel. At the distal end, multiple atresias were noted as a 'string of sausages'. This led into the mid-ileum. The 18 cm of multiple segmental jejunoileal atresias were resected. This left 45 cm of ileum from the ileocaecal valve. A tapering enteroplasty was performed on the dilated segment of the proximal jejunum, and an end-to-oblique jejunoileal anastomosis was constructed. TPN was begun on the third postoperative day and enteral nutrition was started on day ten. The patient was discharged on day 19 on full enteral feeding. At one-year follow-up, there were no problems with malabsorption and growth was normal.

Case 3

A three-day-old girl weighing 2950 g at birth, and with an Apgar score of 9, was transferred with a history of bilious vomiting and abdominal distension. She had not passed meconium since birth. A distended abdomen with hyperactive peristalsis was noted on admission. A plain erect film of the abdomen showed distended loops of small bowel of similar size without air–fluid levels. A water-soluble contrast enema was performed. An unused colon was observed, indicating that the level of obstruction was in the small bowel. Reflux of contrast material into the distal small bowel showed obstructive concretions in the distal ileum. A Gastrografin™ enema was done, and subsequently abnormal meconium was passed. The abdominal distension subsided and the bowel sounds became normal, and she improved clinically. Later, a diagnosis of cystic fibrosis was confirmed.

REFERENCES

Grosfeld JL, Ballantine TVN, Shoemaker R. Operative management of intestinal atresia and stenosis based on pathologic findings. *Journal of Pediatric Surgery* 1979; **14**: 368–75.

Hernanz-Schulmann M. Imaging of neonatal gastrointestinal obstruction. *Radiological Clinics of North America* 1999; **37**: 1163–86.

Murshed R, Spitz L, Kiely E, Drake D. Meconium ileus: a ten year review of thirty-six patients. *European Journal of Pediatric Surgery* 1997; **7**: 275–7.

Phelps S, Fisher R, Partington A, Dykes E. Prenatal ultrasound diagnosis of gastrointestinal malformations. *Journal of Pediatric Surgery* 1997; **32**: 438–40.

Rescorla FJ, Shedd JL, Grosfeld JL, Vane DW, West KW. Anomalies of intestinal rotation in childhood: analysis of 447 cases. *Surgery* 1990; **108**: 710–15.

Tandler J. Zur Entwicklungsgeschichte des menschlichen. *Duodenums Morphologisches Jahrbuch* 1902; **29**: 187–216.

FURTHER READING

Ashcraft KW, Murphy JP, Sharp RJ, Sigalet DL, Synder CL. *Pediatric Surgery*, 3rd edn. Philadelphia, PA: WB Saunders, 2000.

Lister J, Irving IM. *Neonatal Surgery*, 3rd edn. London; Butterworths, 1990.

Oldham KT, Colombani PM, Foglia RP. *Surgery of Infants and Children: Scientific Principles and Practice*. Philadelphia, PA: Lippincott-Raven, 1997.

O'Neill JA, Rowe MI, Grosfeld JL, Fonkalsrud EW, Coran AG. *Pediatric Surgery*, 5th edn. St Louis, MO: Mosby, 1998.

Hirschsprung's disease

ELIZABETH B WHAN

Learning objectives

- To understand the pathological and genetic basis of Hirschsprung's disease.
- To recognize the modes of presentation of Hirschsprung's disease and its complications.
- To be able to formulate a plan of investigation required to confirm the diagnosis of Hirschsprung's disease.
- To be able to describe the surgical and long-term management of Hirschsprung's disease.

INTRODUCTION

Hirschsprung's disease (HD), or congenital aganglionic megacolon, is characterized by the absence of ganglia and the presence of hypertrophic nerve bundles in the bowel wall, beginning at the internal sphincter of the anus and extending proximally for a variable distance (Table 17.1).

Harald Hirschsprung described the clinical entity of congenital megacolon in 1887, in a post-mortem report of two cases. However, it was not until the 1940s that the underlying pathology was discovered and the first successful operation was performed.

Further developments in the understanding of the disease have led to reliable investigations for diagnosis, a variety of surgical options for its treatment, and an ongoing investigation of the underlying genetic and embryological mechanisms of its pathogenesis.

BASIC SCIENCE

Embryology

The enteric ganglion cells are derived primarily from vagal neural crest cells. These migrate from the neural crest to the developing bowel and along it in a craniocaudal direction. HD is postulated to occur when this migration fails; the earlier the arrest of migration, the longer the aganglionic segment.

In the human, neural crest-derived neuroblasts migrate between the oesophagus and the anus between the fifth and twelfth weeks of gestation, forming the myenteric plexus on

Table 17.1 *Extent of bowel involvement in Hirschsprung's disease*

Extent of bowel involvement	Proportion of patients (%)
Rectosigmoid (short segment)	75
Ascending or transverse colon (long segment)	17
Total colonic (may involve distal few centimetres of ileum)	8
Total intestinal aganglionosis	Rare

the outside of the circular muscle layer first. They then migrate through the muscle, again progressing in a craniocaudal direction, to form the submucous plexus between the twelfth and sixteenth weeks.

This migration and subsequent differentiation require not only normal cells but also the correct microenvironment. Cell–cell and cell–matrix adhesion molecules must be balanced correctly to allow cell migration. Neural cell-adhesion molecule (NCAM) is an example of such a protein. It is expressed transiently during smooth-muscle development, and it appears to be involved in the development of initial contact between nerve and muscle cells. Abnormally high levels of NCAM have been shown in smooth muscle and nerve fibres in aganglionic bowel.

Extracellular matrix proteins are also critically important for cell signalling, differentiation, adhesion and movement. For example, fibronectin and hyaluronic acid provide a migration pathway, and laminin and collagen type IV promote growth and maturation of neural crest-derived cells.

Neurotropic factors playing an important role in enteric neuron development include nerve growth factor (NGF), neurotropic factor 3 (NT-3) and glial cell line-derived neurotropic factor (GDNF). Low levels of these neurotropic proteins have been found in aganglionic bowel compared with normal bowel.

Genetics

HD occurs in about one in 5000 births. It is four times more common in boys than girls, although the sex ratio drops to 1.5–2 to one for long-segment disease. Although 80–90 per cent of cases are sporadic, the remainder are familial or associated with a familial syndrome. Reported incidence of familial HD varies between 3.6 and 7.8 per cent for short-segment disease and between 15 and 20 per cent for long-segment disease. It may be as high as 50 per cent for total colonic aganglionosis.

About ten per cent of non-familial cases and 25 per cent of familial cases will have another associated abnormality (Box 17.1). Between 1.5 and 17.6 per cent of siblings and offspring of familial cases are affected, the risk varying with sex and length of affected colon; the highest risk is in a male child of a mother with long-segment HD.

The complex mode of inheritance and variety of associated conditions points to more than one gene being involved in

the aetiology of HD. Familial examples with autosomal dominant or recessive inheritance have been found, with variable or incomplete penetrance. Generally, however, Mendelian inheritance patterns are not seen. Both long- and short-segment disease may be found within some families, but in other families there is no crossover of types. It is not entirely clear from observed inheritance patterns whether long- and short-segment disease are in fact separate disorders or degrees of severity of the same condition.

A number of chromosomal syndromes are associated with HD. By far the most common is trisomy 21 (Down syndrome): between three and 16 per cent of children with HD also have Down syndrome. Other syndromes, such as 13q deletion, partial 2p deletion and trisomy 18 mosaic, have also been associated with HD.

Other associated syndromes mostly involve other parts of the autonomic nervous system – 'neurocristopathies' – or other neural crest derivatives, such as melanocytes (Table 17.2).

The *RET* proto-oncogene has been found to be involved in both sporadic and familial/syndromic HD. Mutations of the *RET* tyrosine kinase receptor account for 50 per cent of

---

Box 17.1 Commonly associated malformations in Hirschsprung's disease

Cardiac malformations
Cataract, coloboma, microphthalmia
Cleft palate
Craniofacial malformations
Gastrointestinal atresias
Imperforate anus
Meconium plug, meconium ileus
Polydactyly

Table 17.2 *Syndromes and implicated genetic defects in Hirschsprung's disease (HD)*

Gene	Locus	Function	Syndromes
RET	10q11.2	Tyrosine kinase receptor	Sporadic HD
			Familial HDMEN2A, 2B, familial medullary thyroid cancer
			Central hypoventilation syndrome (Ondine's curse)
GDNF	5p12–13.1	Glial cell-derived neurotropic factor	Sporadic HD
			Central hypoventilation syndrome
EDN3	20q13	Endothelin-B	Sporadic HD
EDNRB	13q22	Endothelin-B-receptor	Familial HD
			Waardenburg–Shah
			Central hypoventilation syndrome
NTN	19q13.3	Neurturin (*RET* ligand)	Sporadic HD
			Familial HD
SOX10	22q13.1	Transcription factor	Waardenburg–Shah
Phox2b	4p12	Transcription factor	Sporadic HD
			Familial HD

familial cases and 15–20 per cent of sporadic cases. *RET* knockout mice have total intestinal aganglionosis. *RET* ligands include GDNF, an important neurotropic factor for the normal development of intestinal ganglia.

Other genes known to be implicated in HD include *EDNRB*, *EDN-3* and *SOX10*. Mutations of these genes have also been found in the various syndromes that may include HD.

Currently, routine gene testing is not generally recommended in HD, as the finding of a known mutation does not reliably predict the occurrence or severity of disease. Also, failure to detect a known mutation cannot exclude the likelihood of genetic transmission of HD, as there are likely to be many other mutations that are, as yet, unknown. Multiple endocrine neoplasia syndrome mutations might be worth looking for in familial cases of HD, as early diagnosis and thyroidectomy can alter the course significantly and other at-risk family members may be identified.

As genetic testing becomes easier and more commonly performed, further patterns of gene mutation are likely to emerge. Ultimately, the interaction of the mutations, gene products and neural development will become clearer.

Pathophysiology

AGANGLIONOSIS

The gross pathological feature of HD is dilated and hypertrophic proximal bowel, a cone-shaped transition zone, and narrow distal bowel. On histological examination, the affected distal bowel has no ganglionic cells in either the submucous or myenteric plexi, and hypertrophied non-myelinated nerve trunks are present. The hypoganglionic transition zone is of variable length, and the distribution of ganglia around the bowel circumference may not be regular. This must be considered when siting the biopsies for determining the resection level of the bowel; ganglia need to be confirmed around the full circumference of the margin.

The physiological effect of the absence of ganglia is tonic contraction of the bowel, with no ability to propagate peristaltic waves. However, the lack of the coordinating effect of the ganglia does not, on its own, explain the spasticity of the aganglionic segment. Abnormalities of both the adrenergic and cholinergic innervation have been shown. Most convincingly, the spasm may be due to excess acetylcholine release, with a resultant abundance of acetylcholinesterase activity, which can be demonstrated in the hypertrophic nerve fibres. The smooth-muscle cells may also have increased sensitivity to acetylcholine.

Abnormalities of the peptidergic nerves, nitergic nerves, nerve-supporting cells and interstitial cells of Cajal have all been demonstrated in the aganglionic segment in HD but are not described fully.

The bowel proximal to the aganglionic section, whilst appearing normal on histology with the currently widely used stains, may not function normally. The relative hypoganglionosis of the transition zone may extend some distance proximally, without being histologically obvious on isolated biopsies taken at surgery, resulting in hypomotility of the remaining bowel following pull-through.

The immune function of the bowel in HD also may be abnormal, conferring a risk of enterocolitis in some individuals. As it may occur postoperatively once the aganglionic bowel has been removed, the underlying abnormality must also involve the more proximal bowel. Enterocolitis is a serious complication of HD and the leading cause of death, both pre- and postoperatively. Faecal stasis with mucosal ischaemia and bacterial invasion/translocation produces the clinical picture; however, the precise pathogenesis of HD-associated enterocolitis is not known. Abnormalities of intestinal mucin, mucosal defence mechanisms (immunoglobulin A, IgA), alteration in intestinal neuroendocrine cell populations, increased prostaglandin E1 activity, *Clostridium difficile* infection and rotavirus infection have been implicated.

ABNORMAL MUCUS

The mucosal barrier of the colon is a deterrent to both microbial adherence and toxin absorption and plays a part in controlling the colonic faecal flora. In HD, the mucin precursors have a very reduced turnover in both ganglionated and aganglionic bowel. This abnormality in mucin production is especially noticeable in the 'normal ganglionated' bowel post-pull-through in children who are prone to enterocolitis, suggesting that the mucus-defensive barrier is defective, even in bowel that has ganglion cells.

Many children with HD have socially unacceptable flatus, which is produced by the metabolic activity of their faecal flora. This flora can be modified by courses of metronidazole or probiotics.

PRESENTATION

HD most commonly presents in the neonatal period (90 per cent) as bowel obstruction or severe constipation. Classically, there is failure to pass meconium in the first 24 hours in an otherwise well infant. (This is often quoted as 90 per cent, although 43 per cent of neonates subsequently diagnosed with HD in one series had in fact passed meconium in the first 24 hours (Singh *et al.* 2003).) This is associated with the development of abdominal distension and green, bile-stained vomiting. The presence of well-known associated conditions such as trisomy 21 or a strong family history should heighten suspicion of the diagnosis of HD. Examination at this stage will usually reveal a well baby with a distended but non-tender abdomen. Anal examination sometimes releases a rush of air and meconium, or a meconium plug may be passed. There will be multiple distended bowel loops on plain abdominal radiography, classically with little or no gas in the rectum, and lacking the signs suggestive of other common causes of neonatal distal small-bowel obstruction, such as ileal atresia or meconium peritonitis.

Alternatively, HD-associated enterocolitis may develop in the neonate before the diagnosis is made. This presents with foul-smelling explosive diarrhoea, progressing to fever, dehydration, mucosal ulceration, generalized sepsis, toxic megacolon and shock in the most severe cases.

In some children, the constipation is less severe in the first few weeks of life but tends to worsen with changes in feeding, e.g. weaning from breast milk to formula or solids. This group of children present in subsequent months or years with prolonged severe constipation, marked abdominal distension, anorexia and malnutrition/failure to thrive, or with an episode of enterocolitis. All children with HD, except for a very few purely breastfed infants, have significant 'bowel problems' – usually failure to open their bowels – within the first four weeks. The children's mothers remember this early difficulty very clearly.

INVESTIGATION

Once HD is suspected on clinical grounds, the diagnosis is established using a range of investigations. Which of these are performed, and in what order, will be determined by the age and mode of presentation, availability and local preferences.

Radiology

Plain abdominal X-rays showing markedly distended bowel, with air–fluid levels in the colon in the older child, are suggestive of HD.

A contrast enema classically shows a normal-calibre rectum and a narrow distal segment, with a funnel-shaped transition zone and markedly dilated proximal bowel. In total colonic HD, the colon may appear of normal calibre, with reflux of contrast into a markedly dilated ileum. In the neonate, a contrast enema is more sensitive if performed before anal examination or colonic washout; a false-negative enema is more likely if the bowel has been decompressed.

Whilst not diagnostic in ten per cent of cases subsequently confirmed with HD, the main use of contrast enema in the neonate may be in showing the level of the transition zone. This may be of use in surgical planning, once confirmed, if not in the definitive diagnosis of the condition.

In cases of suspected meconium plug, water-soluble rectal contrast is used; this may be therapeutic as well as diagnostic. Where a meconium plug is passed during or after the enema, the diagnosis of HD needs to be confirmed or excluded by rectal biopsy.

In children outside of the neonatal period, retention of barium for more than 24 hours post-enema may be suggestive of HD, or colonic transit studies may be used to distinguish HD from other causes of constipation.

Anorectal manometry

In HD, the normal reflex relaxation of the internal anal sphincter with rectal distension is absent, and this may be demonstrable on anorectal manometry. The reflex is not developed fully in infants under 12 days of age or 39 weeks' gestational age and therefore may be misleading in neonates.

Manometry is of most use as a screening test in older children, where it may distinguish HD from other causes of chronic constipation without performing a rectal biopsy.

Rectal biopsy

The gold-standard diagnostic test for HD is a rectal biopsy. Histological examination of paraffin (haematoxylin and eosin, H&E) sections for ganglia, and frozen sections for immunohistochemical staining for acetylcholinesterase, are the most widely used diagnostic tests. NADPH diaphorase histochemistry is also used in some centres.

A variety of methods may be used to take the biopsy. In neonates and infants up to six months of age, suction rectal biopsy may be performed. The biopsy is performed without general anaesthesia, but it carries a small risk of bleeding or perforation. The specimen obtained must include submucosa. Both H&E and acetylcholinesterase staining are performed for the reliable diagnosis of HD. Full-thickness rectal 'strip' biopsy is used in older infants and children. This has the advantage of providing a larger, more robust specimen including the intermuscular plexus, and allows for direct control of any bleeding. It does, however, require a general anaesthetic, and the scarring produced may interfere with definitive surgery.

At laparoscopy/laparotomy, seromuscular biopsies are taken, usually to determine the level of aganglionosis. This technique avoids peritoneal contamination and provides specimens that include the intermuscular plexus and are amenable to frozen-section examination.

SURGICAL MANAGEMENT

Initial management

Once the diagnosis of HD is confirmed, definitive surgical management can be planned. The essential final aim of the various available approaches is to bring ganglionated bowel to the anus.

Before the definitive surgery is performed, some form of management must be instituted to decompress the bowel because of the risk of enterocolitis. In most neonates, and in some infants diagnosed beyond the neonatal period, regular colonic lavage with 100–400 mL of physiological saline will produce sufficient decompression to allow enteral feeding and safely staged operative management. This lavage needs to be performed expertly by an appropriately trained person;

whether this is one of the parents after education on the ward or a member of the community nursing staff may depend on parental preference and factors such as geography and locally available resources.

The role of colostomy is controversial. In some centres, primary pull-through without enterostomy is performed in the majority of cases. In other centres, colostomy or ileostomy formation is routine. Levelling (end) colostomy or loop ileostomy/colostomy may be used; ganglionated bowel must be confirmed at the stoma site. The stoma may be placed proximally (e.g. terminal ileum or hepatic flexure) to allow pull-through without taking it down, or it may be placed just proximal to the transition zone and then taken down at pull-through (which is then unprotected by a stoma).

If colostomy formation is not done routinely, then there are clinical situations in which it may become necessary:

- If it is not possible to adequately decompress the bowel with washouts: this is more likely to occur with long-segment or total colonic HD.
- If the child is unwell at presentation, with enterocolitis, sepsis or dehydration, then surgical decompression may be life-saving.
- If severe associated abnormalities (e.g. cardiac) are going to require staged treatment, then initial colostomy may be the preferred option, allowing definitive surgery to be deferred safely.

In most cases diagnosed outside the neonatal period, the proximal bowel is very distended and unsuitable for immediate pull-through, and washouts may not be successful. A period of time between colostomy formation and definitive surgery will allow the colon to return to a more normal diameter.

Primary pull-through

Traditionally, the surgery for HD was performed in two or three stages: colostomy, definitive pull-through after six months of age, and, if covered by an enterostomy, subsequent stomal closure. Over the past 20 years however, one-stage pull-through, performed in the neonatal period, has become the common way of managing HD. Provided that all conditions are favourable, there are low morbidity and mortality. The results, at least in the moderately short term, have been shown to be just as good as the more traditional staged procedures (Teitelbaum and Coran 2003), although there are no large randomized trials comparing outcomes.

Techniques

The operations commonly used include the Duhamel, Swenson, Rehbein and Soave pull-throughs, with many variations and modifications. The common features of all are as follows:

- Biopsies (frozen section) to confirm the level of ganglionated bowel: normal ganglia should be shown

around the circumference of the bowel in order to avoid an anastomosis to the transition zone.
- Mobilization of the colon from within the abdomen, to allow the ganglionated bowel to reach the anal margin without tension (with the exception of the transanal endorectal pull-through, in which mobilization can be performed from below).
- Open laparotomy or the laparoscopic approach may be used to perform the intra-abdominal portion of each operation.
- Delivery of the mobilized colon via the anus.
- A form of anastomosis at or above the dentate line.

The main difference between the operations is how the anastomosis is done.

DUHAMEL PROCEDURE

After biopsies are taken and the colon has been mobilized, the retro-rectal space is developed down to the pelvic floor. The rectum is divided just above the peritoneal reflection. An incision is made in the posterior wall of the rectal stump, just at the dentate line, and the proximal bowel is passed through. It is divided and anastomosed to the posterior wall of the rectum. The side-to-side rectum-to-colon anastomosis is performed with a long gastrointestinal anastomosis (GIA) stapling device, opening the posterior wall up to the apex of the rectal stump. The colon-to-apex of rectal stump defect is finally closed.

SWENSON PROCEDURE

The rectum is fully mobilized, staying close to the wall, down to the pelvic floor. It is divided at the lowest point, the rectal stump is everted via the anus, and the proximal colon is pulled through and divided at the level identified by the biopsies. A colo-anal anastomosis is made with interrupted sutures about 1 cm above the dentate line. Then the anastomosis is replaced into the pelvis.

REHBEIN ANTERIOR RESECTION

This differs from the Swenson operation in that the anastomosis is further above the dentate line (up to 5 cm in a child) and the anastomosis is either stapled or sewn from inside the pelvis. The internal sphincter is dilated at the time of operation and regularly from ten days postoperatively.

SOAVE ENDORECTAL PULL-THROUGH

When this was first described, the technique was developed in order to avoid a primary anastomosis and to protect the pelvic nerves by dissecting down to the pelvic floor within the rectal muscle. When performed via open laparotomy with the original technique, the rectal muscle is incised circumferentially 2 cm below the peritoneal reflection, and the dissection is carried to the pelvic floor outside the intact mucosal tube. The mucosa is incised 1 cm above the dentate line, and the proximal colon is pulled through. The free edge of the muscle cuff is anchored to the serosa of the proximal colon by suturing within the abdomen. From the perineum, the serosa is anchored to the everted anal mucosa. The protruding colonic stump is left in place for ten days, by which time the serosa is adherent to the muscle cuff. It is then amputated and the mucosa-to-mucosa anastomosis is completed.

Commonly, the anastomosis is now completed at the initial operation. Other variations include a posterior rectal myotomy to avoid subsequent rectal obstruction from compression by the muscle cuff.

TRANSANAL ENDORECTAL PULL-THROUGH

The Soave technique may be modified further by performing the dissection of the muscle cuff via the anus. This allows colonic biopsies and mobilization to be done via open laparotomy or laparoscopically or, for short-segment HD (demonstrated on contrast enema), via the anus.

The perianal skin is retracted and the mucosa incised 5 mm above the dentate line. The proximal edge is held with stay sutures, and the plane between the muscle and submucosa is developed. When the peritoneal reflection is reached, the muscle is divided circumferentially, and the full-thickness rectum and sigmoid are mobilized out through the anus. If no mobilization has been performed from within the abdomen, then the posterior vessels are divided as the colon is brought through.

When the transitional zone is reached, biopsies are taken above it to confirm the presence of ganglia. The muscle cuff is divided longitudinally, and the ganglionated colon is divided and anastomosed to the anal mucosa.

OUTCOME

Immediate postoperative complications

Apart from the general complications of any laparotomy/laparoscopy, such as bleeding and wound infection, each technique has complications specific to that procedure.

Anastomotic leaks are the most common early complication of the Duhamel, Swenson and Rehbein techniques, at a rate of up to 11 per cent for the Swenson technique. The management of a leak is usually to form an enterostomy and then allow the anastomosis to heal. Depending on the degree of anastomotic disruption, and subsequent stricturing, redo pull-through ultimately may be required.

Cuff abscess or retraction of the proximal bowel may occur with the Soave technique and increase the chance of long-term stricturing.

Voiding dysfunction may occur postoperatively with any of these operations. Bladder innervation may be disrupted partly at the time of surgery, rather than it being a congenital problem. This is more common in older children and with the extensive pelvic dissection of the Swenson technique.

Long-term results

Long-term complications include anastomotic stricture, recurrent enterocolitis, constipation and faecal incontinence.

Anal dilations may be required for some time postoperatively, most commonly following the Soave and Rehbein procedures. Stricture is very rare after the Duhamel operation, where, alternatively, a rectal spur or diverticulum may be left or may develop with time.

Enterocolitis may occur at any time, although the incidence does decrease with age. Maturation of the gut mucosal immune defences may account for this decrease. Whether a degree of obstruction contributes to the probability of developing enterocolitis in susceptible individuals is unclear. Some series have found that there is a slightly increased rate of enterocolitis after transanal pull-through (Teitelbaum and Coran 2003).

Postoperative constipation tends to improve with time, being much more common in the first months following surgery. Chronic constipation may occur as a result of incomplete resection, abnormal motility of the proximal colon or internal anal sphincter achalasia. In addition, the aganglionic rectal stump after the Duhamel operation may allow faeculoma formation. In the case of anal sphincter achalasia, dilations, botulinum toxin injections or sphincteromyectomy may be required. If incomplete resection is suspected, then biopsy and even redo pull-through may be necessary. Redo surgery may be considered for stricture and the pull-though of aganglionic bowel. A stricture, especially after the Soave procedure, is best treated by a posterior anorectal myomectomy. An aganglionic pull-though sometimes can work adequately and need no revision. If this is not the case, then opinions differ about the optimal redo surgery, but surgeons who prefer a Soave approach report good results with a Soave-type redo. Most others think that a Duhamel approach, either posteriorly or laterally, is easier from a technical point of view.

Faecal incontinence occurs either because of constipation with overflow or because of dysmotility and sphincter dysfunction. Nocturnal incontinence is more common when the internal sphincter is inadequate. Some soiling is a common outcome, but more significant incontinence is less common. The actual incidence of either is poorly quantified, as definitions vary and patients may underreport symptoms unless they are asked specifically. The long-term outcomes for the newer operative techniques have not yet been reported in large numbers.

Late mortality as a direct consequence of HD is rare, except in total colonic or intestinal involvement, most deaths being related to associated conditions such as cardiac abnormalities.

CLINICAL SCENARIOS

Case 1

A term male neonate was referred to the surgeons at 36 hours of age, with progressive abdominal distension and bilious vomiting. He had not yet passed meconium. Examination revealed a distended non-tender abdomen. Anal examination confirmed a normal-sized patent anus, and some meconium and a rush of gas were passed. Plain abdominal X-ray showed distended bowel loops throughout the abdomen but no gas in the rectum. Colonic lavage via a rectal tube successfully decompressed the abdomen, and suction rectal biopsy confirmed a diagnosis of HD. The infant was recommenced on feeds and discharged home on daily colonic washouts to be performed by a trained community nurse. Four weeks later, he was electively re-admitted and underwent primary laparoscopically assisted transanal endorectal pull-through.

Case 2

A seven-month-old girl was brought to the emergency department, unwell, with fever, abdominal distension and watery diarrhoea. She had a history of constipation and abdominal distension since the second week of life, but she had passed meconium in her first 24 hours. The constipation had worsened with the introduction of solids, and she had not gained any weight in the past month. Examination revealed dehydration, gross distension of the abdomen and foul-smelling explosive diarrhoea. HD-related enterocolitis was suspected, and brisk resuscitation with intravenous fluids and antibiotics was commenced. At subsequent laparotomy, the colon was found to be dilated down to the mid-sigmoid, with biopsies confirming aganglionosis of the distal sigmoid colon. A split sigmoid colostomy was formed in bowel confirmed to contain ganglia, and a definitive pull-through was performed three months later.

Case 3

A three-year-old boy with a history of Duhamel pull-through for HD at four weeks of age was brought to the emergency department after collapsing at home. His mother gave a history that the child and his normal five-year-old brother had both had acute gastroenteritis five days earlier.

The older boy had recovered within 24 hours, but the diarrhoea had continued in the boy with HD. The diarrhoea had changed from green to grey and become increasingly offensive and explosive. Over the 12 hours before collapsing, his abdomen had become distended and he had refused all oral intake. Examination showed a pale dehydrated boy with a pulse rate of 148 beats/minute, a capillary refill time greater than five seconds and a temperature of 38.7 °C. His abdomen was grossly distended and tender. Rectal examination released a jet of foul-smelling diarrhoea and gas. Rapid intravenous resuscitation was commenced immediately. A plain abdominal film was obtained, showing distended bowel with some wall thickening but no sign of perforation. Intravenous antibiotics including Gram-negative and anaerobic cover were commenced, and intravenous fluids were continued. Regular colonic lavage successfully decompressed the bowel, and laparotomy was avoided.

REFERENCES

Singh SJ, Croaker GD, Manglick P, et al. Hirschsprung's disease: the Australian Paediatric Surveillance Unit's experience. *Pediatric Surgery International* 2003; **19**: 247–50.

Teitelbaum DH, Coran AG. Primary pull-through for Hirschsprung's disease. *Seminars in Neonatology* 2003; **8**: 233–41.

FURTHER READING

Bates MD. Development of the enteric nervous system. *Clinical Perinatology* 2002; **29**: 97–114.

Holschneider A, Ure B. Hirschsprung's disease. In: Ashcraft KW (ed.). *Pediatric Surgery*. Philadelphia, PA: WB Saunders, 2000; pp. 453–72.

Puri P. Hirschsprung's disease. In: Puri P (ed.). *Newborn Surgery*. London: Arnold, 2003; pp. 513–33.

Puri P, Shinkai T. Pathogenesis of Hirschsprung's disease and its variants: recent progress. *Seminars in Pediatric Surgery* 2004; **13**: 18–24.

Stewart DR, von Allmen D. The genetics of Hirschsprung disease. *Gastroenterology Clinics of North America* 2003; **32**: 819–37.

18

Congenital anorectal anomalies

RISTO J RINTALA

Learning objectives

- To understand the types of anorectal malformation.
- To understand the types of associated malformation that frequently accompany anorectal anomalies.
- To be able to diagnose clinically different types of anorectal malformation.
- To be able to describe the appropriate imaging required to diagnose anorectal anomalies and associated malformations.
- To be able to describe the planning of surgical treatment for different types of anorectal malformation.
- To be able to organize appropriate postoperative therapy and follow-up.
- To able to describe the treatment modalities for faecal incontinence in patients with anorectal malformations.

INTRODUCTION

Malformations of the anorectum include a series of congenital lesions, ranging from a slight malposition of the anus to complex anomalies of the hindgut and urogenital organs. The reported incidence of anorectal anomalies ranges between one in 5000 and one in 3300 live births. In Western communities, there is a male preponderance: 55–70 per cent of the patients in larger series have been males. The more severe malformations tend to be more common in male patients.

In most cases, anorectal malformations present as an absence of an anus in its normal position. In mild forms of anal anomalies, the bowel outlet opens in the perineal region outside the usually well-developed voluntary sphincter complex. In more severe anomalies, the bowel outlet opens in an ectopic position in the urogenital tract in males or the genital tract in females. Neonatal recognition of the type of the malformation is essential for the planning of the surgical management of anorectal anomalies.

Despite advancements in basic embryological, anatomical and physiological knowledge, modern surgical methods cannot offer normal anorectal function in many unfortunate children who were born with anorectal anomalies. A significant number of these children suffer from faecal incontinence or severe constipation. Some have urinary incontinence and some have poor sexual function as adults.

RELEVANT BASIC SCIENCE

The aetiology of anorectal anomalies is not known. Genetically determined syndromes with anorectal malformations are relatively uncommon. However, anorectal anomalies occur commonly in multi-anomaly sequences, such as the VACTERL

Table 18.1 *Associated malformations*

Malformation	Incidence (%)
Urogenital anomalies	45
Skeletal anomalies (excluding coccyx)	30
Gastrointestinal anomalies	20
Cardiovascular anomalies	15
Chromosomal anomalies	10
Central nervous system anomalies	5
Others	15

Overall incidence of associated anomalies 65%.

(vertebral, anorectal, cardiac, tracheo-oesophageal, renal and limb (radius)) and CHARGE (colobomata, heart disease, atresia choanae, retarded growth, genital anomalies (in males) and ear) associations. The overall incidence of associated anomalies in patients with anorectal malformations is over 60 per cent (Table 18.1). This suggests that the stimuli that induce abnormal development of the anorectum operate throughout the developing fetus and may cause maldevelopment of several organ systems.

The pathogenesis of anorectal malformations has been much clarified by modern embryological studies using experimental models of anorectal anomalies. Anorectal anomalies occur spontaneously in some animal models (SD-mouse) and can be induced by several substances, such as ethinylthiourea, retinoic acid derivatives and doxorubicin. The spectrum of malformations following administration of these substances is variable, but they are valuable tools for embryological studies. The most significant findings in these embryological models are abnormalities and absence of the cloacal membrane. An abnormal cloacal membrane does not allow normal breakdown of the bowel into the perineum. In animal models, a clinically important discovery has been the character of the recto-urogenital or perineal communication: a fistulous communication is actually an ectopic anus. This ectopic anus has the characteristics of a normal anal canal, including a distal zone of transitional epithelium, anal glands and the internal anal sphincter, which is a thickening of the circular muscle layer around the bowel outlet. The voluntary external sphincter complex, including the levator ani muscle, develops separately in a normal position. The voluntary sphincters are always hypoplastic; the degree of the hypoplasia is dependent on the distance of the rectal pouch from the perineum and the severity of the commonly associated sacral deformity.

Rectal atresia

Rectal atresia is a separate and rare entity among anorectal malformations and has a different pathogenesis. The cause of rectal atresia has been suggested to be a local vascular incident such as in atresias of more proximal bowel. The patient usually has a patent distal anal canal that ends in a short septum of fibrous tissue, which separates the anal canal from the blind-ending rectal pouch.

Table 18.2 *Wingspread international classification*

Classification	Female	Male
High	Anorectal agenesis Rectovaginal fistula No fistula Rectal atresia	Anorectal agenesis Rectoprostatic fistula No fistula Rectal atresia
Intermediate	Rectovaginal fistula Rectovestibular fistula Anal agenesis	Bulbar fistula Anal agenesis
Low	Anovestibular fistula Anocutaneous fistula Anal stenosis	Anocutaneous fistula Anal stenosis
Rare	Cloaca	Rare malformations

Table 18.3 *Pena classification*

Male	Female
Perineal fistula	Perineal fistula
Recto-urethral fistula:	Vestibular fistula
Bulbar	*Persistent cloaca:*
Prostatic	<3 cm common channel
Rectovesical fistula	>3 cm common channel
Imperforate anus without fistula	Imperforate anus without fistula
Rectal atresia	Rectal atresia

CLINICAL FEATURES AND INVESTIGATIONS IN A NEWBORN WITH AN ANORECTAL ANOMALY

A provisional diagnosis of the severity of an anorectal malformation is usually made easily in a newborn. In most patients, the type of anomaly can be determined by careful clinical examination and simple laboratory tests such as urinalysis. The most important issue is to ascertain the level of the anomaly, because this determines the operative treatment in the neonatal period. There is rarely any urgency: most patients tolerate a low bowel obstruction without symptoms for more than 24 hours if the upper gastrointestinal tract is decompressed by a nasogastric tube.

There are a number of classifications for anorectal malformations (Tables 18.2 and 18.3). Classifications have been based on the level of bowel termination in relation to the perineum and descriptively on the site of the fistulous bowel outlet. A practical classification in terms of the definitive treatment of anorectal anomalies is to classify the defect as a low anomaly or an intermediate or high anomaly.

Low anomalies

If the patient has an ectopic anal opening in the perineum, then the anomaly is low. The opening may be very small, but usually some meconium will be seen coming out of it during the first day of life. Clinical examination of an apparently low

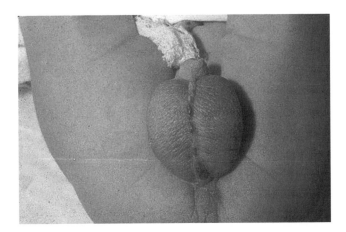

Figure 18.1 *Anocutaneous fistula. Newborn boy with a fistula extending from the rectal blind pouch to the midline raphe of the scrotum.*

anomaly should always include gentle probing of the ectopic anal opening. Free access into the rectum usually extends down very close to the perineal skin, which confirms the diagnosis.

The most common type of low anomaly in males is an anocutaneous fistula (Figure 18.1). In this anomaly, a fleshy median bar covers the anal site. The anus is often slightly displaced anteriorly, but the voluntary sphincter complex surrounds the main part of the anal canal. From the bowel termination, a narrow fistula runs anteriorly for a variable distance within the median bar. Another common low anomaly in males is a 'covered' anal stenosis: the anal site is covered with a median bar and there is a tiny opening leading to a normal anal canal on either side of the bar. In females, a perineal fistula is usually not associated with a median bar. The anal canal is also clearly anterior to the sphincter funnel. Anterior perineal anus, which is a normal-looking anus situated just behind the vestibule, is an abnormality that is seen exclusively in females. In about half of the cases, the anterior anus is stenotic, and normal voluntary sphincters surround the posterior half of the anus but are very thin between the anal opening and the vestibular fourchette. Female perineal fistula and anterior ectopic anus are associated quite commonly with a perineal groove, a superficial 'ditch', lined by transitional epithelium, between the vestibular fourchette and the anus (Figure 18.2).

Intermediate and high anomalies

In females, the most common anorectal malformation is a vestibular fistula. The ectopic anus opens to the posterior vestibular fourchette, and the urethra and the vagina have normal appearances. The opening is usually difficult to see because of its small size and position under the vestibular fourchette. Meconium staining of the vulva during the first day of life gives a helpful hint in making the correct diagnosis (Figure 18.3). The diagnosis in this type of anomaly is

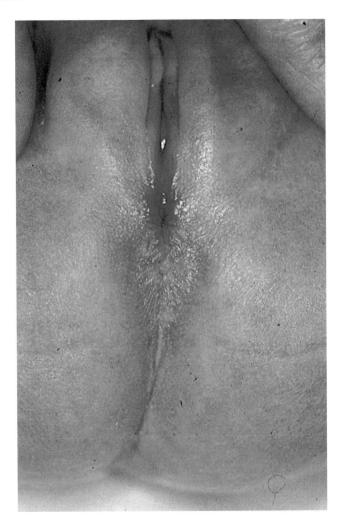

Figure 18.2 *Perineal fistula with groove. Newborn girl with a rectoperineal fistula anterior to the sphincter complex and an associated mucous groove between the vestibule and fistula opening.*

confirmed by gentle probing of the anal opening. Sometimes, the posterior fourchette opening is almost the same size as a normal anus. In a vestibular fistula, the anal canal is situated completely outside the sphincter funnel, so its classification as an intermediate anomaly is justified.

Male patients who have no detectable opening in the perineum usually have a fistulous communication between the high-ending anorectum and the urethra (Figure 18.4). The urethral opening of the communication is usually at or below the level of the prostate. In rectoprostatic fistula, the rectal pouch lies above the level of the levator plate. In rectobulbar fistula, the rectal pouch is located within the proximal part of the sphincter funnel. The voluntary sphincter complex is always hypoplastic, and the degree of hypoplasia is related to the severity of the sacral deformities, which are common in these patients. Examination of the perineum can give a clue to the degree of sphincter hypoplasia. If the patient has a well-developed natal cleft and a shallow pit at the anal site, then the sphincters usually are well developed. A flat bottom

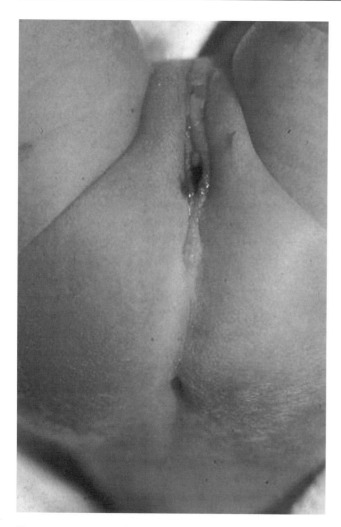

Figure 18.3 *Vestibular fistula. Newborn girl with a fistula from the rectum to the vaginal vestibule. Meconium is pouring from the fistula. The sphincter centre is shown clearly as a thickening of the median raphe.*

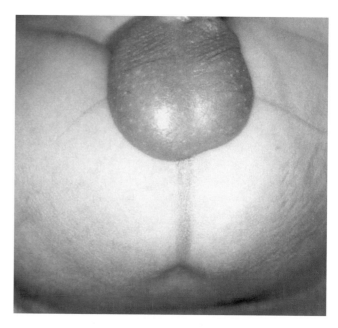

Figure 18.4 *Recto-urethral fistula. Newborn boy with a relatively blank perineum. There is a fistula from the rectum to the prostatic urethra.*

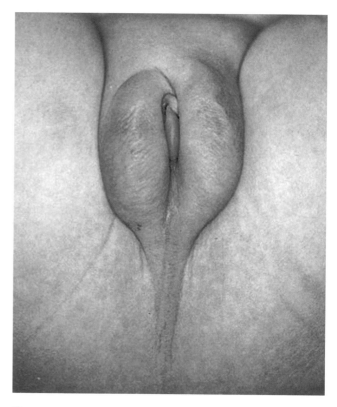

Figure 18.5 *Cloaca. Female with a single opening in the perineum. The cloacal common channel opens behind the tip of the clitoris.*

suggests that the voluntary sphincters are very hypoplastic. Often, these patients pass meconium-stained urine per urethram, which confirms the diagnosis of a recto-urethral communication.

A female patient with only one external opening in the perineum has a cloacal malformation (*cloaca*: Latin sewer) (Figure 18.5). In cloacal defects, the rectum, vagina and urethra join in a common recto-urogenital channel, which opens at the perineum with a single opening. The opening may be anywhere between the anal site and the base or tip of the clitoris; in most cases, the common channel opens between the normal vaginal site and the clitoris. The length of the common channel is variable; an anterior location of the external opening usually suggests a long common channel. The anatomical relationships between the rectum, vagina and urethra are highly variable. Abnormalities of the internal genital organs, such as duplication of the Müllerian structure, are common.

Currarino triad

The Currarino triad is a hereditary disorder that was described originally as a sacral bony defect, presacral mass and anorectal malformation. In most cases, it is caused by an autosomal dominant genetic defect linked to the chromosomal region 7q36. The triad is complete when all three anomalies are present. Incomplete cases also occur, with only one or two defects present. The main stigma, the scimitar-shaped sacral bony defect, must be present if the diagnosis of Currarino triad is to be made. Currarino patients may have other anomalies, such as urogenital tract abnormalities and tethered cord.

The typical anorectal malformation in patients with Currarino triad is an anorectal stenosis, which is often associated with a funnel-shaped, skin-lined anal canal. The severity of the stenosis varies from mild to almost complete anorectal dissociation, which in females may be associated with high vaginal fistula.

The presacral mass is usually a mature teratoma or anterior meningocele, or a combination of both. Presacral dermoid cyst occurs sometimes in Currarino patients.

The symptoms associated with the triad vary significantly. Constipation is present almost uniformly; its severity depends on the severity of the anorectal stenosis. Occasionally, patients are asymptomatic and present only following family screening for the condition.

Treatment of Currarino patients is focused on the management of the, often intractable, constipation. Treatment includes dilation of the anorectal stenosis and very often anterior resection of the hugely dilated rectosigmoid. The presacral mass is usually resected. In the long term, many Currarino patients have reduced anal continence. Some also suffer from urinary incontinence problems, because of the partially neurogenic bladder associated with the sacral defect.

Radiology

Radiological methods may be helpful if the height and the type of the anomaly cannot be determined by clinical examination. Ultrasound, computed tomography (CT) or magnetic resonance imaging (MRI) may be used to assess the distance of the rectal pouch from the perineal skin. There is no evidence that these would be better than the classic cross-table lateral plain radiograph with raised buttocks, which shows the terminal gas shadow and hence allows the distance between the terminal bowel and skin to be determined. The reliability of all imaging is increased if the study is performed after 24 hours of age. However, all radiological methods are relatively inaccurate, and in practice performing a colostomy is safer if the presence of a low anomaly cannot be verified definitely.

Associated malformations

Before any treatment for the anorectal malformation is carried out, associated life-threatening malformations should be ruled out. A nasogastric tube should be passed in all patients to rule out oesophageal atresia and to decompress the gastrointestinal tract. A plain abdominal X-ray should be obtained to evaluate the dilation of the bowel and to exclude upper-bowel obstruction, especially duodenal atresia. Careful auscultation and clinical examination of the chest, a chest X-ray and echo should be undertaken to detect congenital cardiac defects. Ultrasound examination of the urinary tract is mandatory in all cases, because urogenital tract abnormalities occur in at least 40 per cent of patients, especially in patients with high malformations. If the findings on ultrasound examination show dilation of the upper urinary tract, then a micturating cystogram should be performed to detect severe vesicoureteral reflux. The cystogram may also reveal the level of recto-urethral communication in male patients with high anomalies.

After the neonatal management of the anorectal malformation, some additional investigations for associated anomalies should be performed. A spinal X-ray should be obtained to rule out significant vertebral anomalies. Intraspinal pathology such as lipomas and conal anomalies in the lumbosacral region are common in patients with anorectal malformations, especially those with high anomalies. Spinal-cord imaging by ultrasonogram or MRI is indicated in all patients. If a cardiac defect is detected in the neonatal period, then more detailed cardiological evaluation may be required.

OPERATIVE MANAGEMENT

Recent developments in our understanding of the pathophysiology of anorectal malformations have had a significant impact on the treatment of these anomalies. The voluntary external sphincter anatomy in different types of anomalies has been delineated clearly by Pena (1988) and Pena and de Vries (1982). The embryological and clinical findings have suggested that the internal anal sphincter is present in the region of the rectal termination, regardless of whether the connection is to the perineal skin or the urogenital tract. These findings have led to surgical techniques that try to preserve as much as possible of the distal bowel.

Low anomalies

In males, low anomalies with a perineal fistula can be treated safely with a neonatal repair. Because the anal canal is at least partly within the voluntary external sphincter complex, the operation may be limited to a simple opening of a passageway for the bowel contents. In anocutaneous fistula, this can be accomplished by cutback of the fistula. The incision is extended from the fistula opening to the posterior margin of the voluntary sphincter funnel, which is identified by muscle stimulation. The mucosal edges of the bowel termination are sutured to the perianal skin. No formal skin-flap anoplasties are required; in fact, these can be harmful because fibres of the subcutaneous part of the external sphincter may be severed during the operation. The anal opening is dilated gradually with Hegar dilators to normal size. The size of the dilator is increased at weekly intervals. Some surgeons use anal transposition by limited posterior sagittal anorectoplasty (PSARP) for anocutaneous fistula. This procedure is more extensive and more prone to operative complications than cutback. There is no evidence that PSARP would give a better functional outcome than simple fistula cutback in low anom-alies. Covered anal stenoses can be treated primarily by simple dilations; however, the median bar should be excised at some time.

Females with perineal fistula usually require more extensive surgery, as the anal canal is less contained within the sphincter complex than in males. Today, the most commonly used approach for female perineal fistula is limited PSARP. The timing of the operation is critical; it is safest to proceed with surgery during the first two or three days of life, because meconium is then less likely to be colonized by pathogenic bacteria. If the operation is delayed or the surgeon is not experienced in the neonatal repair of these anomalies, then it may be safer to perform a colostomy before the definitive repair.

An anterior perineal anus requires treatment only if it is stenotic. The treatment is gradual dilation using the same principles as for postoperative dilations in males with low anomalies.

High and intermediate anomalies

In males, all anorectal anomalies without an anal opening in the perineal region require an initial colostomy to relieve the obstruction. Some surgeons have advocated one-stage reconstruction in the neonatal period without a protective colostomy for high anomalies, but such an approach has not gained popularity. A major problem associated with a neonatal single-stage repair without a colostomy is that it involves a more or less blind dissection of the rectal termination and recto-urinary fistula in a meconium-stained field, without precise radiological information of the exact anatomy of the defect. A one-stage reconstruction also precludes the possibility of tapering the dilated distal rectum; tapering is necessary sometimes to accommodate the pulled-through neo-anal canal within the narrow external sphincter complex funnel.

The preferred site of colostomy is the proximal sigmoid colon, because the risk of stoma prolapse is less than in a transverse colostomy. The stool from a sigmoid colostomy is also more solid than from a transverse colostomy, which makes stoma-bag management easier. The only exception requiring a more proximal diversion is a cloacal anomaly, because the sigmoid colon may be required for vaginal reconstruction. The colostomy should be fashioned to divert the faecal stream completely; a faecal collection in the diverted distal bowel may complicate the reconstruction and may be a source of urinary tract infection. Before the definitive repair of a high or intermediate malformation is performed, a detailed evaluation of the anatomy of the recto-urogenital communication is produced by a contrast distal loopogram via the colostomy. Any faecal accumulations in the rectal pouch can also be detected by this investigation and should be washed out.

Today, the most widely used operation for repairing high and intermediate anorectal malformations is a PSARP, originally developed by de Vries and Pena. The unique feature of this operation compared with earlier ones is that all steps of the procedure are performed under direct vision. Of the earlier techniques, the sacroperineal operation of Stephens and modifications of the anterior perineal approach described originally by Mollard are still used by some surgeons. The timing of the definitive anorectal repair by PSARP has changed since the introduction of the operation. Many surgeons prefer to do the operation at one month instead of one year of age, which was once the standard age. There is some evidence that the functional results are better if the repair is performed as early as possible. The operation is technically more demanding in a young infant, because of the patient's small size. However, the postoperative treatment is easier and the total period with a colostomy is shorter. An infant also tolerates the necessary postoperative anal dilation regime better than an older child. After the operation, the neo-anus is dilated gradually with increasing sizes of Hegar dilators, which are changed weekly. The diverting colostomy is closed when the anus has been dilated to an age-appropriate size, usually two to three months after reconstruction.

Recently, some surgeons have advocated laparoscopic repair of high anorectal malformations. The operation entails laparoscopic mobilization of the rectal termination and fistula closure and subsequent pull-through of the fistula to the anal site through the sphincter funnel, which has been identified by muscle stimulation. The experience from this sort of procedure is still very preliminary, and follow-up results are lacking. Theoretically, laparoscopically assisted pull-through involves less manipulation of the voluntary sphincter complex than the PSARP procedure. This may be associated with a decrease in operative scar-related fibrosis formation and may preserve sphincter function better than the PSARP procedure.

Treatment of the most common anorectal anomaly in females, the vestibular fistula, is still controversial. Patients with a vestibular fistula have a potential to full bowel control. Therefore, surgical complications that may jeopardize this are unacceptable. Many surgeons advocate colostomy for patients with vestibular fistula to minimize the risk of potentially deleterious infectious complications. Others perform a neonatal operation without a covering stoma. Currently, there are no scientific data that would clearly support either approach. For less experienced surgeons, neonatal colostomy followed by a reconstruction later is probably the safest way to proceed.

The time-honoured treatment for vestibular fistula has been a simple neonatal cut-back procedure to make the anal opening wide enough for passage of stool. The cosmetic appearance of the perineum is not very satisfactory following a cut-back, but the function in terms of faecal continence usually has been relatively good. The faecal continence of adult patients who have undergone simple cut-back may worsen due to ageing and pregnancies. A traditional alternative to a cut-back has been anal transposition to the normal anal site. This operation usually was performed later during infancy or childhood; the passage of stools was maintained by initial dilations of the fistula. However, the long-term functional results after this operation, despite better cosmesis, have not been better than those after a cut-back procedure. The main late complication has been severe constipation. Today, the preferred method for repairing a rectovestibular fistula is limited PSARP. The advantage of this method when compared with a blind transposition is that the preservation and reconstruction of all sphincter structures are accomplished under direct vision. For the limited PSARP procedure for a vestibular fistula, the patient can be positioned either prone or in a lithotomy position. The most difficult and meticulous part of the operation is the separation of the rectum from the vagina.

A specific and complex group among female patients with anorectal anomalies are those with persistent cloaca. The spectrum of cloacal anomalies is highly variable. Bizarre arrangements of the urogenital and rectal anatomy are possible, so there is no standard operation for a cloaca. A neonate with a cloacal anomaly requires special attention compared with more straightforward types of anorectal anomalies. Of vital importance is the status of the upper urinary tract. Obstructive uropathy is common and has to be ruled out before any surgical treatment is undertaken. Hydrometrocolpos in association with a cloaca is not uncommon. The status of both the urinary tract and the genital organs in a neonate may be imaged by ultrasound. The length of the common channel should be assessed, preferably by neonatal endoscopy. Neonatal surgical management of a cloaca entails colostomy formation, accompanied by drainage of the urinary tract and hydrometrocolpos when indicated. If future vaginal reconstruction requires augmentation by a sigmoid loop, then a transverse colostomy is the best choice for bowel diversion. Proximal sigmoidostomy is the preferred procedure if pull-through of the native vagina is considered possible. A large hydrometrocolpos should be drained by a tube colpostomy; drainage through the common channel is often unreliable and may not prevent infection of the hydrometrocolpos, which may destroy the uterus and vagina. In patients with poor bladder-emptying, intermittent catheterization can be tried primarily, but urinary diversion should be performed without delay if reliable bladder decompression cannot be achieved.

The planning of reconstructive surgery for a cloacal anomaly requires exact information about the anatomy of the defect. A distal loopogram is essential to determine the anatomy of the rectocloacal communication. Delineation of the vaginal anatomy may require repeated endoscopy if neonatal assessment is not conclusive. The most important anatomical issue is the length of the common channel. This dictates the type of approach that is necessary for full reconstruction.

Cloaca patients require not only anorectal reconstruction but also simultaneous reconstruction of the vagina and urethra. The operative approach is similar to other types of high anomalies; however, many patients require an additional laparotomy to mobilize the vagina and uterus. Many patients have a duplicated and/or dilated genital tract, which may require tapering, resection of the vaginal septum or refashioning to gain enough length for a tension-free pull-through to the perineum. Sometimes the Müllerian structures are absent or the vaginal length is insufficient to reach the perineal skin. The best solution in this situation is vaginal replacement or augmentation using a bowel flap, usually fashioned from a segment of the sigmoid colon. The use of bowel in vaginal reconstruction minimizes the risk of postoperative necrosis and stenosis.

If the patient has a short common channel (less than 3 cm long) and a well-developed vagina, then the urogenital reconstruction may be performed by using total urogenital mobilization. The common channel, urethra and distal vagina are mobilized *en bloc*. This requires extensive dissection between the urethra and the pubic symphysis up to the bladder neck anteriorly. The rectum is dissected free from the vagina before urogenital mobilization is commenced. After full urogenital mobilization, the native urethral and vaginal openings are sutured behind the clitoris to form a mucosa-lined vulva. This can be augmented further by bivalving the cloacal common channel. The anorectal reconstruction is performed as was described for other high and intermediate anomalies.

If total urogenital mobilization is not feasible, then the vagina has to be separated from the urethra and bladder neck. This is the most tedious and difficult part of cloaca reconstruction and is much more difficult than the separation of the rectum from the vagina. The surgeon has to keep in mind that the vagina surrounds about the half of the urethral circumference. Innervation of the bladder neck may suffer from the dissection between urinary tact and vagina. Operative damage to the urethra and vagina may cause urethrovaginal fistula formation, even if operative defects are repaired. The common recto-urogenital channel is preserved for a neo-urethra, provided that the channel is narrow. A wide common channel needs to be tapered to a normal urethral calibre.

In some patients, the high or intermediate anorectal anomaly is not accompanied by a fistula. Patients with Down syndrome have no fistula. The rectal termination is often situated very near the urethra, so the surgical procedure is very similar to a routine PSARP for a high anomaly with fistula.

Repair of a rectal atresia by end-to-end anastomosis can be accomplished through a posterior sagittal approach.

POSTOPERATIVE CARE

Postoperative management following anorectal repair is usually uncomplicated. If the operation has been completed without laparotomy, then the patient has remarkably little postoperative pain and tolerates oral feeding usually during the first 24 hours. Antibiotic prophylaxis is advisable in patients with high or intermediate malformation and an indwelling urethral catheter. Patients who have undergone neonatal perineal repair without dissection in the vicinity of urethra do not need a transurethral catheter. In males with a recto-urinary fistula, the catheter can be removed on the third postoperative day and the patient can be discharged. Cloaca patients require a longer catheter time, often up to two weeks, because bladder emptying is often affected by the extensive dissection behind the bladder neck. If the indwelling catheter falls out prematurely, then it is advisable not to recatheterize. Recatheterization may damage the urethral repair; therefore, suprapubic urinary drainage is a safer alternative.

Anal dilations with Hegar metal dilators are started two weeks after the repair. The starting size is usually between 7 and 10 mm, depending on the age of the patient. Dilations are performed once or twice daily, and the dilator is changed weekly to a size 1 mm bigger each time. Dilations are continued until the desirable anal size is reached. The author dilates small infants up to Hegar size 14 mm and older infants up to Hegar size 15 mm. In patients with a colostomy, the stoma can be taken down when the dilator is changed to the last definitive size.

Many patients with repaired high or intermediate anorectal malformations have abnormal bowel function following closure of the protecting colostomy. The most common problem is frequent bowel movements, causing perineal skin problems. This stage may last several weeks or months. In low anomalies, many patients resume early bowel function that is comparable to that in their healthy peers. However, constipation, which is the major functional problem in patients with a low malformation, may begin at any time after the operation. A typical onset is when the patient starts having solid foods at the age of four to six months. Constipation is a major problem in patients with high or intermediate anomalies. The onset of constipation in these patients cannot be predicted; several daily loose bowel movements may turn to unrelenting constipation very rapidly, within days. The early follow-up of patients with anorectal anomalies must be regular and frequent. During the first six months following closure of the stoma or neonatal repair, the patient must visit the outpatient clinic every four to six weeks. After the first six months and for up to two years, the interval between clinic visits may be lengthened to three months. Severe constipation has its onset in most cases during the first two postoperative years. After that, the frequency of the follow-up visits can be decreased. The child's parents must be able to contact the team responsible for care at any time during the postoperative period to sort out any problems that may arise.

POSTOPERATIVE COMPLICATIONS

Neonatal colostomy carries a high morbidity. The most common complications are colostomy prolapse and stricture.

Stoma complications may be less common with a completely divided sigmoid colostomy. The reported total incidence of complications in infant colostomies ranges between 17 and 68 per cent. Complications include a few colostomy-related deaths.

Early complications after neonatal treatment of low anomalies are uncommon. However, local complications may occur later; usually they are caused by insufficient long-term follow-up and care. A typical local problem is postoperative anal stenosis, which can be prevented by gradual postoperative dilations and careful follow-up of the patient. Untreated anal stenosis may cause secondary megacolon, which may require operative treatment.

Early complications occur following all commonly used reconstructions for high and intermediate anorectal anomalies. Peritonitis, retraction and dehiscence of the pull-through segment and refistula between the bowel and the urogenital tract are typical severe early complications. The reported incidence of these major complications has ranged between ten and 30 per cent following abdominoperineal or sacroabdominoperineal pull-through operations. Severe complications seem to be less common following posterior sagittal anorectoplasty. In the large series of Pena (1995), serious complications requiring major preoperative surgery occurred in two per cent of cases, mainly following repair of a cloaca. In the author's series of 210 patients, there were five major early complications requiring reoperation: wound dehiscences following repair of a vestibular fistula without a colostomy in two patients, urethrovaginal fistula following cloaca repair in two patients, and dehiscence of the vaginal-vulvar anastomosis, which required re-pull-through of the vagina, in one cloaca patient.

Anal complications have been common following traditional pull-through operations. Anal stenosis and mucosal prolapse have been found in 15–78 per cent of patients. Stenosis usually has been attributed to inadequate anal dilations during the follow-up period. Anal stenosis may respond to dilation, but in refractory cases surgical excision of scar tissue is needed. Mucosal prolapse usually requires operative treatment to reduce mucous soiling and to improve sensation in the neo-anal canal. However, local anal problems have been rare following posterior sagittal anorectoplasty. Pena (1995) reported very few local complications in his series of 792 patients. In the author's series of 210 posterior sagittal anorectoplasties, anal stenosis requiring anoplasty occurred in three patients; in addition, three patients early in the series required local operation for a minor mucosal prolapse. In some cases, the rectal blind pouch is primarily so ectatic that it is symptomatic without any associated anal stricture or stenosis.

Urinary tract complications may arise following surgery for anorectal malformations. Before definite repair, it is essential to minimize the risk of urinary tract infections caused by the recto-urogenital connection if such is present. This is best accomplished by establishing a completely diverting colostomy and by careful washout of the rectal pouch. Infection may cause permanent damage to the kidneys because the upper urinary tract anomalies and neurovesical dysfunction are common in patients with anorectal malformations. Hyperchloraemic acidosis due to intestinal absorption of urine refluxing to the bowel through a recto-urogenital connection is a rare complication and may occur in patients with bladder-neck fistulas or with urethral obstruction distal to the rectourogenital communication. Infection may persist after definitive repair and then is caused in most cases by a urological anomaly, vesicoureteric reflux being the most common. Damage to the pelvic innervation and urethra during dissection of the rectal blind pouch may cause urinary incontinence or urethral stricture. However, many of the anatomical and functional abnormalities attributed previously to surgical intervention are congenital.

Associated anomalies cause significant morbidity in patients with anorectal malformations. Congenital heart disease occurs in more than 15 per cent of patients with anorectal malformations and often requires major cardiac surgery during early childhood. Associated gastrointestinal anomalies are found in almost 20 per cent of patients. Half of these patients have oesophageal atresia, which may require additional surgery such as oesophageal dilations and fundoplication despite successful neonatal repair. Vertebral anomalies occur frequently in patients with anorectal malformations. Hemi-vertebral anomalies may cause scoliosis, which may require operative stabilization or bracing early in childhood. Spinal dysraphism, detected by MRI or ultrasound examination during the neonatal period, has been found to be more common than previously appreciated. Spinal dysraphism occurs in 20–40 per cent of patients and is more common in those with more severe anomalies and bony sacral defects. Normal sacral X-rays during the neonatal period, however, do not exclude the presence of a spinal cord anomaly. Spinal dysraphism may have significant impact on the functional outcome in terms of urinary function and faecal incontinence. Careful neuroradiological and neurological follow-up is warranted in patients with spinal dysraphism.

FUNCTIONAL OUTCOME

In the literature, there is a great variation in the functional results after repair of anorectal malformations. There is no generally agreed method for assessing the bowel function of patients with anorectal malformations, and the main problem in comparing different series is the highly variable criteria used in the evaluation of faecal continence. Evaluation of bowel function during childhood may be biased because the information concerning the functional outcome is derived mainly from the children's parents: parents may not want to report unfavourable results to a surgeon who has been responsible for the treatment of their child. Parents may also ignore minor and moderate defects in continence in a child whose bowel function has been abnormal from birth. With younger children, parents may consider deficient bowel control as a part of normal maturation of defecation. There are several ways of overcoming these difficulties. The evaluation can be performed by an independent person who is not a member of the team responsible for the care of the child. A questionnaire with detailed questions concerning bowel function may give more reliable information than a visit to a busy hospital outpatient clinic. If a questionnaire is used, then validation by a control group of healthy children with similar age and sex distribution as the patients is essential. Ideally, when the above-mentioned methods are used simultaneously, they serve as controls for each other. In any case, the final outcome cannot be assessed until the patients have reached adulthood and, as independent individuals, can evaluate the social consequences of possibly defective bowel control.

Patients with low malformations are usually reported to have a good functional outcome. However, some recent studies have shown that this is not necessarily the case. Abnormal bowel habits or defective bowel control causing social problems have been detected in 20–40 per cent of patients on long-term follow-up. A recent report by the author demonstrated that during childhood, about half of the patients with low anomalies have problems in bowel function. Most suffered from constipation, but frank soiling occurred in ten per cent of patients. These patients had been followed up regularly throughout their early childhood. In another large series by the author, concerning adult patients with low malformations, normal bowel habits were found in only 15 per cent of patients. Good continence with no or minor social problems were found in 60 per cent of patients. This study was performed using a quantitative scoring method to assess continence and sex- and age-matched healthy subjects as controls. These adult patients had had no regular follow-up since the neonatal operation.

The most common long-term functional problem in patients with low malformations is chronic constipation, which occurs in 30–60 per cent of patients. Actual soiling is more common than traditionally is reported in the literature and occurs in a significant percentage of patients. In adult patients, social problems related to deficient anal function, mainly faecal urgency and difficulties in holding back flatus, have been reported in almost 40 per cent of patients. Since the treatment of low anomalies has remained essentially unchanged for decades, these results reported in adults are a relatively reliable reflection of the current functional prognosis for children born with low malformations. The recent reports in the literature largely confirm this. At the moment, there are no reports concerning long-term functional outcome following a limited or mini-PSARP procedure, which is commonly used today for the management of low malformations.

Reports concerning long-term results for high and intermediate anomalies display highly variable results. The long-term outcome usually is graded as good, fair or poor. It has to be kept in mind that in most reported series, a good outcome does not mean that the patient has a normal bowel function.

Patients with good results usually have been considered socially continent, which implies that the possible defects in bowel function do not cause significant social disability. In most series, the evaluation has been performed during childhood, and the age at the assessment has varied significantly, usually between 1.5 and five years. In the era before the PSARP procedure, the percentage of patients with a 'good' result varied between five and 65 per cent, and the percentage of poor results, which means more or less total incontinence, between 15 and 70 per cent of affected patients. The percentage of poor results gives a better indication than the percentage of good results of the actual efficacy of treatment, because a 'good' result does not indicate normal bowel function. In the author's questionnaire-based study of adult patients with high or intermediate anomalies, who responded to the inquiry as independent individuals, none had normal bowel habits. Social continence was reported by 18 per cent of the patients, 54 per cent had a fair continence with marked social limitations, and 28 per cent were totally incontinent or had a permanent colostomy. These grim figures probably reflect the true outcome following the repair of high and intermediate anorectal malformations in the 1950s and 1960s, when the direct perineal approach, abdominoperineal pull-through and sacroperineal techniques were used to repair high anorectal anomalies.

The concept embodied in the PSARP procedure has contributed significantly to the understanding of the sphincter anatomy in patients with anorectal malformations. The voluntary external sphincter muscle complex has been clearly demonstrated to be present in all patients and contributes significantly to faecal continence. This differs from the earlier concept, which stressed that the puborectalis muscle sling is the main factor of faecal continence in these patients. The concept of today is that the puborectalis muscle is an integral part of the external sphincter complex and cannot be separated from it, either anatomically or functionally.

The functional outcome following the PSARP procedure may be better than for conventional reconstructions. This has not been proved, as PSARP has not been compared with traditional surgical techniques in controlled trials. The comparisons have been based on historical case-note material, which makes the evaluation relatively unreliable. Furthermore, there are still few reports concerning long-term functional outcome following PSARP, and the results have been contradictory. Some surgeons report a dismal outcome, with most patients requiring adjunctive measures to maintain social continence. However, in the series of Pena, approximately one-third of patients with high or intermediate anomalies could be considered as totally continent. In the author's series, in which bowel function of the patients was compared with that of healthy children with similar age and sex distribution, 35 per cent of patients had an age-appropriate normal bowel function. Fair outcome, with intermittent soiling requiring frequent change of underwear or protective aids, or poor outcome, with intractable constipation or total incontinence, was found in 30 per cent of patients.

The traditional view has been that one has to wait until adolescence before faecal continence can be assessed finally in patients with anorectal malformations. However, recent reports by Pena and by the author on patients operated on by PSARP have shown that in favourable cases, the patient may gain normal or near-normal bowel function as early as three years of age, provided that the inherent functional complications related to the procedure, especially constipation, are treated early and vigorously. Both of these series demonstrate a high incidence of constipation in operated patients, the cause of which is unknown. It is not associated with an organic stenosis in the bowel outlet. The motility of the colon is impaired in patients with anorectal malformations, and this affects the whole colon, not only the rectum. The nature of this motility disturbance is understood poorly. Poor motility of the rectum may be explained by the extensive mobilization of the anorectum, which may cause partial sensory denervation of the rectum and impair rectal sensation. In many cases, soiling during the early years after definitive repair has been a consequence of severe constipation with overflow incontinence, rather than sphincter insufficiency. The treatment of soiling associated with constipation is much more rewarding than the treatment of soiling related to sphincter insufficiency. Reports have appeared in the literature showing a significant decrease in constipation as patients reach adulthood. This has been accompanied by improved faecal continence. The endpoint of the development of bowel control in patients who have undergone PSARP procedure for a high or intermediate anorectal anomaly is the time when patients go through puberty. It appears that approximately half of them may develop normal bowel function without any need for protective aids or medication.

The poor results following PSARP are in patients with coexisting severe sacral anomalies, very high rectal anomalies (recto-bladder neck fistula, high cloaca), severe constipation and absent postoperative internal sphincter function. The voluntary sphincter complex is hypoplastic in patients with significant sacral anomalies and with very high anomalies, who usually have also sacral defects. The presence of severe sacral defects can be considered the most important negative prognostic factor in terms of later bowel control. A functioning internal sphincter can be preserved in most patients with high and intermediate anorectal anomalies. The presence of a functioning internal sphincter is associated with a higher anal resting tone and better continence outcome.

MANAGEMENT OF LATE FUNCTIONAL PROBLEMS

Although the overall functional outcome of patients with high or intermediate anorectal anomalies undoubtedly has improved since the introduction of the PSARP, many patients still suffer from deficient bowel control during childhood and also as adults. A significant proportion of patients with low malformations have defective bowel function and may need adjunctive measures to maintain faecal control. Minor defects in faecal continence, such as occasional soiling and staining, rarely cause any problems in preschool-age children, but in school-age children even relatively minor soiling may be very embarrassing. According to the author's experience, minor soiling and staining do not cause social problems if the child does not need a change of underwear or protective pads to stay clean during the school day. Any soiling in excess of this requires special treatment, especially if the child has faecal accidents. In addition to social problems, daily soiling causes skin irritation, which increases the discomfort of the child even more. Dietary and medical treatment can be used to modify the consistency of stool. Low-residue diet decreases stool volume and makes the stools more solid. Antipropulsive agents, such as loperamide, increase intestinal transit time and thus facilitate absorption of water from stool. The result is more solid stools and a lower risk of soiling and faecal accidents.

In more severe cases, regular mechanical emptying of the bowel is the only option for achieving social continence. The bowel may be emptied by retrograde enemas or by antegrade washouts through a continent catheterizable caecostomy. A continent caecostomy can be created by using the appendix, a Monti-Yang ileal tube, a caecal button device or a caecal flap. A tube or button into the left colon produces a more physiological washout but may have a higher complication rate. In most cases, antegrade washout is the preferred method. The main indications for this are psychosocial, as school-age children tolerate poorly the daily or regular anal manipulation that is required for retrograde washouts. Retrograde washouts are also difficult to perform without help. Antegrade enemas can be performed without difficulty by a child of six to eight years of age and require very simple instrumentation. The amount of liquid needed for a successful washout is also usually less with an antegrade enema.

In any case of postoperative soiling or staining, overflow incontinence must be ruled out. A typical history suggesting overflow is a late onset of soiling after a period of cleanliness or an increase in the amount of soiling. Faecal impaction can be diagnosed by digital examination or careful abdominal palpation. Overflow soiling usually responds well to faecal disimpaction by enemas and subsequent laxative treatment. These patients usually require prolonged use of stimulant laxatives. Because constipation is the most common functional problem following a successful PSARP procedure, follow-up of patients during the first years of life should be regular and aimed at the early detection of symptoms of constipation. Faecal impaction should be prevented by early treatment, which should be commenced if the child has bowel movements less than every other day.

Biofeedback conditioning has been used to treat faecal incontinence in patients with anorectal malformations. Early results have been encouraging, but in the author's experience most patients with severe incontinence never gain full bowel control. Minor defects in continence are more likely to respond to biofeedback. Limiting factors are that the minimum age for biofeedback is between eight and ten years because it requires the full cooperation of the patient, it is very time-consuming and it requires specially trained personnel and equipment.

Many ingenious secondary surgical methods have been devised to improve faecal continence in patients with anorectal malformations. Gracilis muscle-plasty and levator-plasty are the most commonly used methods to replace or improve the function of the anal sphincters. If the patient is trained properly to use these neosphincters, then voluntary anal control is improved. However, these muscles cannot provide the continuous tone that is typical of anal sphincters, and therefore soiling is not abolished completely. Continuous electrical stimulation of the gracilis muscle has been shown to induce a transition in muscle composition from fatigable type II fibres to fatigue-resistant type I fibres. This finding has been applied in adult patients with anorectal malformations who underwent conventional gracilis-plasty followed by implantation of a muscle stimulator. After a training period, the stimulator was used continuously to maintain constant anal tone. Short-term clinical and manometric results have been promising; more than half of the patients became continent and the high anal pressures were preserved. Stimulated gracilis-plasty may be an alternative for patients who do not comply with washout regimes and have a suitable anatomy. Other recent advances in the treatment of faecal incontinence – direct sacral nerve stimulation and anal sphincter prostheses – have been used in only a few patients with anorectal anomalies. The preliminary results following these procedures have been promising.

Rerouting of the previously pulled-through anorectum has been advocated when the sphincter complex does not properly surround the anal canal. Currently, the most popular method for redo surgery is PSARP, which enables accurate reconstruction of the correct anatomical relationship between the anorectum and the sphincters. However, the long-term outcome following these procedures is highly unpredictable. Some patients gain full control of defecation; these are usually patients with minor sacral defects and a mainly undamaged voluntary sphincter complex. Unfortunately, only a minority of the patients who have had redo PSARP belong to this group. In the long term, most patients require adjunctive measures to stay clean, despite a technically successful operation.

CLINICAL SCENARIOS

Case 1

A boy was born without an apparent anal opening and a relatively flat bottom. Neonatal ultrasonic imaging showed bilateral hydronephrosis. Follow-up micturiting cystogram showed grade IV vesicoureteral reflux and a tiny rectoprostatic fistula. Cardiac echogram displayed a tetralogy of Fallot, and sacral X-ray showed missing distal sacral vertebrae. The child underwent sigmoid colostomy at the age of 24 hours. Posterior sagittal anorectoplasty was performed at the age of three months. After following the anal dilation regime, the stoma was closed at the age of seven months. Follow-up urological imaging at the age of one year showed no remaining vesicoureteral reflux, and prophylactic antibiotics were stopped. Uneventful repair of the cardiac defect was performed at the age of 14 months. The first signs of constipation were detected after cardiac surgery, and medical treatment with stimulant laxatives was commenced. At the age of four years, the child had voluntary bowel movements but daily soiling that required change of underwear but no protective pads; he still used stimulant laxatives for constipation. Micturition function was completely normal. Spinal MRI showed moderate spinal cord tethering with fatty filum, but the patient had no relevant symptoms. Occasional soiling persisted during the early school years, but without any social consequences. He still needed laxatives to maintain bowel function. At the age of 13 years, the need for laxatives ceased completely. The patient has two regular bowel movements per day without any soiling; he is active in sports, playing ice hockey at competitive level. MRI still showed moderate tethering, but as the patient was complete asymptomatic, further neurological follow-up was stopped.

Case 2

A girl was born without an apparent anal opening, but the perineum appeared otherwise normal, with urethral and vaginal openings. At the age of four hours, meconium was detected in the vaginal vestibulum and probing of the vestibular fourchette disclosed a rectovestibular fistula. Ultrasound and X-ray imaging showed no other malformations. A limited PSARP procedure was performed at the age of 36 hours. The postoperative period was uneventful. Postoperative anal dilations were carried out for three months. From the age of six months, the patient required bulk laxatives for moderate constipation. The need for laxatives ceased at the age of three years, when the patient was completely toilet-trained. She had one bowel movement per day without any soiling and no urinary wetting in any circumstances. At the age of 12 years, she had normal urinary and bowel functions. Menstruation had started four months earlier, but she was unable to use regular tampons. Examination under anaesthesia showed a septated vagina and double uteri. The vaginal septum was excised and at follow-up the patient was able to use vaginal tampons.

REFERENCES

Pena A. Surgical management of anorectal malformations: a unified concept. *Pediatric Surgery International* 1988; **3**: 82–93.

Pena A. Anorectal malformations. *Seminars in Pediatric Surgery* 1995; **4**: 35–47.

Pena A, de Vries PA. Posterior sagittal anorectoplasty: important technical considerations and new applications. *Journal of Pediatric Surgery* 1982; **17**: 796–811.

FURTHER READING

Hassink EA, Rieu PN, Severijnen RS, *et al.* Are adults content or continent after repair for high anal atresia? A long-term follow-up study in patients 18 years of age and older. *Annals of Surgery* 1993; **218**: 196–200.

Rintala R, Lindahl H. Is normal bowel function possible after repair of intermediate and high anorectal malformations. *Journal of Pediatric Surgery* 1995; **30**: 491–4.

Rintala RJ, Lindahl HG. Fecal continence in patients having undergone PSARP procedure for a high anorectal malformation improves at adolescence as constipation disappears. *Journal of Pediatric Surgery* 2001; **36**: 1218–21.

Rintala R, Lindahl H, Marttinen E, Sariola H. Constipation is a major functional complication after internal sphincter-saving posterior sagittal anorectoplasty for high and intermediate anorectal malformations. *Journal of Pediatric Surgery* 1993; **28**: 1054–8.

Yeung CK, Kiely EM. Low anorectal anomalies: a critical appraisal. *Pediatric Surgery International* 1991; **6**: 333–5.

19

Necrotizing enterocolitis

VICTOR BOSTON

Learning objectives

- To understand the clinical importance of necrotizing enterocolitis as a cause of neonatal morbidity and mortality.
- To understand the possible causes of necrotizing enterocolitis.
- To be able to describe the various known strategies to reduce the risk of necrotizing enterocolitis.
- To understand the rationale for operative intervention compared with medical management.
- To be able to describe the various surgical approaches to necrotizing enterocolitis.

INTRODUCTION

Necrotizing enterocolitis (NEC) is now recognized as a significant cause of neonatal morbidity and mortality. The pathogenesis of the disease remains poorly understood, although the pathology is now well established.

NEC occurs almost exclusively in neonatal intensive care units (NICU), where its frequency is approximately 12 per cent of all admissions. While NEC is uncommon, approximately six per cent of all neonatal deaths and 15 per cent of infant deaths after the first week of life are caused by NEC.

INCIDENCE

The incidence of NEC is reported to be approximately 0.3 per 1000 live births. Eighty per cent of all affected children are either less than 34 weeks' gestation or weigh less than 2000 g at birth. However, up to 20 per cent are full-term infants. The male/female ratio is two to one. Ninety-five per cent have been fed orally before presentation. Most commonly, the signs of NEC develop on the third day of life, but approximately 15 per cent of cases occur on the day of birth, and the disease has been recognized in children up to three months of age or even older.

RELEVANT BASIC SCIENCE

Of the many risk factors that have been suggested, only prematurity and enteric feeds are proven on multivariant analysis to be associated significantly with NEC. No single mechanism can account for the pathogenesis of NEC in all cases. Pathological and clinical data suggest that the common primary event is a mucosal injury, and this may progress to either mild or fulminant NEC, depending on local circumstances. This initiating mucosal injury probably has many different causes, and in some children more than one mechanism may be at work.

Pathology

NEC is primarily a mucosal disease that extends well into the apparently normal intestine, as viewed from the serosal surface. The most frequently affected parts are the terminal ileum and the ascending and transverse colon. The descending colon and, rarely, the greater part of the small intestine and stomach also can be affected.

The intestinal mucosa is oedematous and haemorrhagic, with ulceration in more severe cases. The capillary bed of the submucosal vascular plexus demonstrates plugging with platelet aggregates, which is associated with engorgement of more proximal vessels and distal venous thrombosis. This process is primarily a micro- rather than a macrovascular disease, and the main mesenteric vessels are usually patent.

There is a notable absence early in the disease of infiltration of the bowel wall with inflammatory cells. However, bacteria can usually be identified at this stage in the mucosa and deeper layers, having migrated from the lumen due to a breakdown of the mucosal barrier.

Macroscopically, in the majority of cases blebs of gas (pneumatosis intestinalis) are visible under the visceral peritoneum. These bubbles often extend into the mesentery. Microscopically, there is gas in the interstitial tissue of the bowel wall, which involves the lymphatics and the smaller branches of the portal vein. This portal-vein gas can often be identified on imaging within the liver (Figure 19.1). Pneumatosis is usually associated with transmural infarction and perforation of the affected gut. Where this has occurred, there are usually signs of generalized peritonitis. Loops of small intestine will often be matted together and associated with local abscess formation at the site of infarction.

After a few days, an inflammatory cell infiltration becomes apparent in the affected segment of the intestine. In most instances, this will resolve without trace, but where there has been significant tissue loss caused by necrosis, repair often results in fibrosis, which may cause a stenosis of the lumen. This process will have occurred in most cases by one month but may take up to three months to become established.

Free radicals

In animal models of NEC, toxic free radicals of oxygen are released in the intestine in response to many different challenges, e.g. reduced intraluminal pH, hypoxia, hypovolaemia, occlusion/reperfusion injury and cold stress. These free radicals cause lipid peroxidation and thus damage cell membranes and increase vascular permeability. In NEC, there is good clinical and laboratory evidence that local production of free radicals then causes the release of cytokines. Complex feedback mechanisms between these factors cause a cascade of events that results eventually in progressive damage to the mucosal intestinal barrier, bacterial translocation from the lumen, and thrombosis of intramural vessels, leading to the transmural infarction that is typical of NEC.

The source of these free radicals is thought to be intestinal macrophages. In normal circumstances, there is 'in-house protection' against these toxic metabolites in the form of 'scavengers', such as superoxide dysmutase/catylase.

The local production of mucosal free radicals probably occurs through several different mechanisms, including direct physical damage to the mucosa by infection or the products of infection, hypoxaemia, decreased perfusion and, perhaps, immune complex formation.

Infective agents and toxins

The neonatal intestine is sterile at birth and becomes colonized with increasing age. The rate and type of colonization will depend on various factors, including the environment in which the child is being nursed, whether antibiotics are being administered, the timing of the introduction of feeds, and the type and volume of feeds that have been employed. Premature and full-term infants colonize differently. This is probably related to differences in immunological status and feeding practices.

Epidemiologically, two different types of NEC are recognized. Eighty per cent are of the sporadic type, compared with the rarer epidemic form, which clusters in both time and space. In the epidemic form, the organism responsible for the outbreak is common to all cases. Nosocomial spread from child to child within the unit therefore can be a problem if there are no appropriate precautions. However, in the vast majority of cases, no specific pathogen will be identified.

Ninety per cent of affected children will have pneumatosis intestinalis. This intramural gas is known to contain hydrogen. Biologically, this can have been derived only from the fermentation of carbohydrate by anaerobic bacteria present within the intestinal wall. These organisms are presumed to contribute to the progression of the disease.

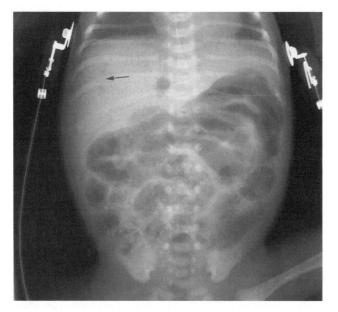

Figure 19.1 *Gas in portal vein (arrowed) in stage III–IV necrotizing enterocolitis. Note also the widespread pneumatosis intestinalis.*

Many species, such as *Clostridia*, produce exotoxins that are cytotoxic. Other less well-known species capable of toxin production also have been implicated, including *Staphylococcus albus*. Exotoxin- or endotoxin-induced NEC is unlikely to be the main cause of mucosal damage, because the vast majority of all cases are not associated with faecal culture of toxin-producing species. Consequently, some other mechanism of pathogenicity must be involved in the majority of cases.

Short-chain fatty acids

Carbohydrate malabsorption occurs in the ileum of all newborn infants. Carbohydrate that reaches the colon can be fermented by normal colonic commensals, with the production of gas and the short-chain fatty acids (SCFAs) acetic, lactic, butyric and propionic acids. Normally, these SCFAs are cleared secondarily from the colon, accounting for up to 30 per cent of carbohydrate absorption. When this process is occurring efficiently, the intraluminal pH rarely drops below 5 and fermentation and absorption can continue to occur. However, the stools of babies who have developed NEC usually contain fatty acids and have a pH below 5, implying that the mechanism for absorption of SCFA has been overwhelmed, either by excessive production or by decreased absorption. Experimental evidence suggests that an intraluminal pH below 5 is associated with mucosal damage. Thus, if absorption of SCFA is impaired, then a cycle of events can occur, which will eventually lead to bacterial translocation through the normally impenetrable mucosal barrier.

Excessive production appears to account for the majority of cases. Increased amounts of carbohydrate reaching the terminal small bowel (which is then available for colonic fermentation) will depend upon not only the total amount of ingested feed but also the degree to which it is malabsorbed.

Decreased absorption can be either primary, due to deficiency of mucosal systems for clearance of SCFA caused by immaturity, or secondary, due to damage to the intestinal mucosa by hypoxia, decreased perfusion, contact with bacterial toxins or decreased intraluminal pH.

Enteral feeds

Babies fed on fresh breast milk are thought to be less likely to develop NEC than their formula-fed counterparts, although this remains to be proven (McGuire and Anthony 2001). If there is a protective effect with fresh breast milk, then this probably has two components. First, breast milk induces colonization of the neonatal intestine with *Bifidobacter*, which reduces the risk of subsequent colonization by pathogens. Second, inappropriate colonization is inhibited by the immunoglobulin and white cell content of fresh breast milk. A similar protection possibly may be conferred by enteral immunoglobulin A (IgA) and immunoglobulin G (IgG), although there is no hard evidence to support this view (Lawrence *et al*. 2001).

In contrast, there is some evidence that suggests that cow's milk formula may increase the risk of NEC in premature infants. This is thought to occur because cow's milk casein creates immune complexes in the gut. The permeability to macromolecules is increased in the immature gut, and these immune complexes are thought to be absorbed, leading to direct damage to the mucosa. This mechanism may be inhibited by prenatal treatment of the fetus using steroids given to the mother. However, the evidence in favour of this prophylactic treatment is controversial (Arroyo Cabrales and Guzman 2000).

Many premature infants cannot physically tolerate the volumes necessary to sustain an adequate calorie intake for growth, due to abnormal function of the intestine. Hyperosmolar feeds therefore have been employed to provide increased calories for a reduced volume load. Clinical and laboratory evidence suggests that this may induce mucosal damage and may be responsible for causing NEC in some cases.

Unfortunately, there are few controlled prospective studies of the various feeding regimens outlined above (McGuire and Anthony 2001). While fresh maternal breast milk may be regarded as theoretically less likely to lead to NEC, it has to be accepted that compared with formula feeds, the calorie value is significantly less and may not provide any overall advantage for the baby. Prospective studies are required urgently to compare the relative benefits and risks of calorie supplementation of breast milk with common formulas designed for premature infants.

Mucosal blood flow

The act of feeding has been shown to increase both the oxygen consumption of the intestine and its blood flow. This is normally controlled to ensure adequate mucosal perfusion during and after feeding. In premature infants, the normal reflex vasodilation of mucosal blood vessels that accompanies feeding does not occur as readily as in more mature babies. In this situation, ischaemic release of free radicals could occur, with subsequent damage.

Hypovolaemia and hypoxaemia cause shunting of blood from the intestine and have been shown to induce experimental NEC. This could occur with congenital heart disease, exchange transfusion, hyperviscosity, umbilical vein catheterization, respiratory distress and low Apgar score at birth, all of which have been suggested, but are unproven, to be risk factors for NEC.

Raised intraluminal pressure

There is evidence that mucosal ischaemia occurs with raised intraluminal pressure. Premature infants often have delay in gastrointestinal transit, and this will cause a degree of intestinal stasis, which will raise intraluminal pressure. Furthermore, there is evidence that there is increased hydrogen production in the intestine just before the onset of NEC. If this is rapid, then the evolved gas may not be cleared adequately. The resultant elevation of intraluminal pressure may contribute to a reduction in mucosal blood flow (Garstin *et al.* 1987).

PRESENTATION

Clinical features

Typically, the patient is a premature baby who has already been established on enteral feeds and who has been making good progress. The child then develops abdominal distension and becomes clinically unwell. There is an increase in the volume of gastric residue, which may be bile-stained, and the baby, who has been defecating normally, becomes constipated or passes a blood-stained stool.

There is a spectrum of clinical disease, from a mild benign disturbance of intestinal function to a rapidly fulminant course characterized by signs of peritonitis, septicaemia and shock. Bell *et al.* (1978) suggested a classification of NEC, which has proven valuable in terms of not only diagnosis but also treatment:

Stage I

These babies will develop a mild systemic illness, associated with temperature instability, apnoea, bradycardia and general lethargy. There may be a minor degree of abdominal distension associated with vomiting and or increased pre-feed gastric residues. Some of these children will demonstrate positive occult blood on stool testing. However, it must be borne in mind that while approximately 40 per cent of NEC patients will have blood in the stool, the majority of positively testing neonates will not have NEC. Stage I has been called 'suspected NEC', and many children who demonstrate these clinical signs will be suffering from the much more common feeding intolerance associated with prematurity or low birth weight. If there is doubt, then an infant who demonstrates these clinical characteristics should be regarded to be at risk of developing more fulminant disease and treated accordingly. These babies usually are not brought to the attention of surgeons.

Stage II

These babies will have a more profound systemic illness, with a mild metabolic acidosis and thrombocytopenia. Abdominal distension is apparent, and bowel sounds cannot be heard. Many will demonstrate abdominal tenderness, and some will have oedema and red/blue discoloration of the abdominal wall, particularly around the umbilicus. There will be definite X-ray findings of NEC.

Stage III

This is associated with severe life-threatening generalized sepsis. In addition to the features of stage II disease, the baby will demonstrate hypotension, metabolic acidosis, hyponatraemia, jaundice and disseminated intravascular coagulation. There will be signs of generalized peritonitis, with marked abdominal tenderness and distension, which will usually be associated with radiological signs of perforation and ascites.

Stages II and III disease therefore represent unequivocal NEC.

INVESTIGATION

X-ray findings

Specific X-ray findings are best demonstrated by sequential examination of at-risk children. In stage I disease, the only finding on abdominal X-ray may be generalized gaseous distension of the intestine.

Pneumatosis intestinalis sometimes can be present in stage I disease. However, this X-ray finding is usually seen in the more severe stages II and III. In less than ten per cent of confirmed cases, this sign will not be present. It appears as crescents or haloes around the gas shadow of the lumen, when viewed in cross-section at right-angles to the luminal axis of the intestine, or a more diffuse 'ground-glass' appearance (Figure 19.2).

When peritonitis and oedema of the intestinal wall become established, the interface between loops of bowel increases in thickness. Persisting distension of a 'fixed loop', apparent on sequential abdominal X-rays, usually indicates necrosis of the affected intestine. Perforation when it occurs often is

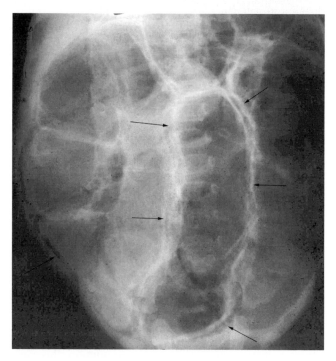

Figure 19.2 *Extensive pneumatosis intestinalis (arrowed).*

associated with a decrease in intraluminal gas, as this escapes into the peritoneal cavity (Figure 19.3). A right-side-up shoot-through X-ray often will demonstrate this free gas, which is particularly evident between the abdominal wall and the liver (Figure 19.4). Gas may also be apparent in the region of the liver in the portal vein (Figure 19.1). Ascites is usually associated with faecal contamination of the peritoneal cavity.

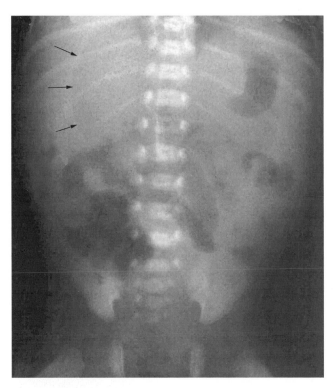

Figure 19.3 *Pneumoperitoneum, with 'football' sign. Gas demonstrated to the right of the falciform ligament in the supine X-ray of abdomen (arrowed).*

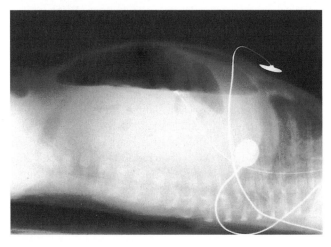

Figure 19.4 *Pneumoperitoneum in lateral decubitus view.*

Abdominal ultrasound scan

Localization of oedema of affected intestine, fluid in the abdominal cavity and gas in the portal vein are simply extensions of conventional X-ray findings. However, in addition, ultrasound offers specific dynamic imaging facilities. Doppler flow techniques can demonstrate opening of the ductus arteriosus and loss or reversal of end-diastolic flow in the superior mesenteric artery (SMA). These latter signs are related to the altered dynamics of septicaemic shock.

Stool-reducing substances

While malabsorption of carbohydrate is a common occurrence, particularly in premature neonates, sequential measurement of stool carbohydrate has been shown to increase significantly before the onset of NEC. This simple test appears to have a positive predicative value of approximately 70 per cent for the development of the condition.

Breath hydrogen

Hydrogen, a product of bacterial fermentation of malabsorbed carbohydrate, is absorbed and can be measured in the expired gas. It is elevated significantly in the period 24–36 hours before the onset of NEC compared with otherwise normal babies. This test is performed easily and non-invasively by sampling air from the oropharynx during the expiratory phase of respiration. A positive test enables proactive observation and treatment of these at-risk babies, many of whom will go on to develop NEC.

Haematological, bacteriological and biochemical screening

These investigations are important in monitoring the baby's general condition and as a guide to treatment, but they do not assist with the diagnosis of NEC. A dropping platelet count and a clotting disorder usually indicate an intravascular coagulopathy associated with bowel infarction and septicaemia. Blood and peritoneal cultures will guide the use of antibiotics.

TREATMENT

Prophylaxis in at-risk babies

Prenatal use of steroids may improve the fetal intestinal mucosal barrier and possibly reduce the risk of development of NEC (Arroyo Cabrales and Guzman 2000).

Postnatally, avoidance of 'stress' situations induced by hypothermia, hypoxaemia, hypercarbia, metabolic acidosis, hypovolaemia or pain will reduce the risk of shunting of blood away from the newborn intestine. Drugs known to have adverse effects on intestinal blood flow, such as methylxanthines and prostaglandin antagonists, should be used with caution.

Strict infection-control measures within the NICU will reduce the risk of nosocomial colonization with pathogens. Unfortunately, there is no evidence that prophylactic antibiotics reduce the risk of NEC developing in premature babies (Bury and Tudehope 2000).

Mothers should be encouraged to provide fresh breast milk. Early introduction of high-volume feeds, particularly with hyperosmolar solutions, should be undertaken with caution. If necessary, total or supplemental parental nutrition should be employed to maintain adequate calorie intake.

After onset

STAGE I DISEASE

Continuing oral feeding is likely to cause progression of the disease in children who have NEC. Therefore, it is important to distinguish those babies who are suffering from NEC from those who are not. This is best undertaken by sequential clinical and radiological assessment as well as routine haematological, biochemical and bacteriological screening. Where possible, expired breath hydrogen and stool carbohydrate should be measured in suspected cases. If there is doubt, then the baby should be treated as though he or she has stage I NEC.

When a firm diagnosis of NEC is established, enteral feeds should be discontinued, gastric drainage instituted and parenteral antibiotics commenced. The exact combination of the latter will be determined by the antibiotic policy of the unit but should include a combination active against both aerobic and anaerobic organisms. Total parenteral nutrition will be necessary to maintain the acute metabolic demands of the infant.

STAGE II DISEASE

Treatment is as with stage I disease, but in addition the systemic effects of sepsis, such as endotoxic shock and disseminated intravascular coagulation, need to be corrected aggressively, if necessary delaying surgical intervention, even if this is indicated.

The main priorities of this resuscitation are as follows:

1 Endotracheal incubation and mechanical ventilation to normalize PO_2 and PCO_2 (partial pressures of oxygen and carbon dioxide, respectively).
2 Maintenance of adequate circulating blood volume. The exact volume to be administered intravenously will be determined by the response of the central venous pressure, which should be maintained between 0 and 0.5 kPa. There is no proven advantage of intravenous colloid compared with crystalloid. Anaemia caused by haemolysis should be treated with a transfusion of fresh whole blood supplemented, if necessary, with platelets.
3 Cardiac output should be maintained if necessary by the use of inotropic agents.
4 The effects of total body fluid overload caused by antidiuretic hormone (ADH) secretion should be treated by the use of diuretics. Intravenous fluid therapy should be used with caution in these circumstances, as fluid overload with subsequent cerebral oedema are real risks.
5 Analgesia should be given as morphine. If this causes significant respiratory depression, then ventilation may be required.

Transmural necrosis of the bowel will usually be present when a distended loop of intestine (fixed loop) is identified on sequential X-rays of the abdomen. This will progress to perforation, which, in most babies, will cause peritonism with erythema or oedema of the anterior abdominal wall. A lateral decubitus radiograph of the abdomen will demonstrate free intraperitoneal gas in most cases when perforation has occurred. Gas in the portal vein is usually associated with fulminant disease with transmural infarction. A fixed loop, perforation and gas in the portal vein are generally regarded as indications for operation.

In the absence of these signs, patients can be treated conservatively, as in stage I.

STAGE III DISEASE

These children are profoundly unwell and usually have extensive transmural infarction and perforation. The disease is usually associated with a high mortality. The same general principles apply as with stage II disease. Intensive cardiopulmonary resuscitation will be required before operative intervention, although in this case the child may be too unwell to tolerate laparotomy initially.

Operation

Approximately half of the recognized cases of NEC will come to surgery. However, there has been much debate as to the appropriate surgical approach in these circumstances.

Peritoneal drainage

For babies who are verging on death, the operative trauma of an open laparotomy may carry a greater risk than simple drainage of the abdominal cavity. Drainage will reduce the source of continuing sepsis, minimize diaphragmatic splinting and improve lung ventilation.

Simple drainage should not be regarded as an alternative to the open surgery that will be required in most cases after the child's general condition improves. Simple peritoneal drainage may be appropriate for children with congenital cyanotic heart disease or where the birth weight is less than 1500 g. Babies of birth weight over 1500 g and who are systemically relatively well may be managed better by immediate laparotomy, with or without resection.

Drainage can usually be performed under local anaesthetic through an incision performed in one or other of the iliac fossae. Under direct vision, a soft French gauge 10 or 12 tube or latex drain is inserted into the peritoneal cavity. The fluid removed from the peritoneal cavity should be sent for culture. If the baby's condition improves, then open laparotomy, if indicated, may be undertaken with relative safety.

Laparotomy

The consequences of operative trauma and the release of endotoxin caused by handling diseased intestine must be taken into account when planning surgery. Expediency in the interests of the child's safety often means that some form of limited primary procedure must be undertaken, with reconstruction being done at a later stage.

Primary resection and direct end-to-end anastomosis can be undertaken safely in some circumstances. It must be remembered that the affected length of the intestine in NEC is greater on the mucosal surface than on the serosal surface. Therefore, in order to obtain a secure primary anastomosis (which might otherwise be of dubious viability and, therefore, at risk of leakage), an extensive resection of potentially viable gut will be necessary. This can be done safely only if there is adequate gut length to avoid intestinal failure.

In most circumstances, if the child is critically unwell, then the duration of surgery should not be prolonged. If a resection is required, then the proximal and distal limbs should be exteriorized at the limits of viability (as judged on the serosal surface), rather than performing an anastomosis.

Alternatively, a proximally based defunctioning enterostomy can be performed without resection, even in the presence of perforation in a sick neonate. This has the added advantage of avoiding unnecessary excision of potentially viable intestine. Peritoneal lavage will be necessary in all cases to remove intestinal contents, including bacterial contamination, from the peritoneal cavity.

Reintroduction of feed

As the general condition of the baby improves, intestinal function will return to normal. Gastric residues and abdominal distension will decrease, and there will be passage of stool, indicating that oral feeds can be reintroduced. It is probably unwise to reintroduce enteral feeds until about seven to ten days after this: if recommended prematurely, there is about a five per cent risk of recurrence of NEC.

Malabsorption can be anticipated in most cases due to the damage to the ileal villi. This damage often takes many weeks to improve after the intestine demonstrates normal peristalsis. A formula containing short-chain carbohydrate, peptones or amino acids and medium-chain triglycerides may be absorbed more readily in these circumstances, and this should be used when feeding is reintroduced. Hyperosmolar feeds may be necessary to promote growth but should be used with caution.

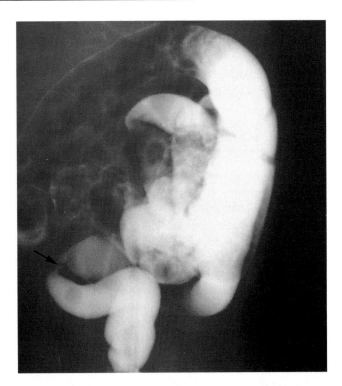

Figure 19.5 *Barium enema approximately one month after necrotizing enterocolitis, demonstrating stricture in mid-sigmoid colon (arrowed). Note also pre-stenotic dilation, indicating subacute intestinal obstruction.*

Closure of the enterostomy

Fluid losses from the stoma may be large and difficult to control. As a consequence, there is a need to restore intestinal continuity as soon as possible. This should be delayed, if circumstances permit, for at least three months, during which time most secondary strictures (which occur in up to 30 per cent of cases), will have developed. Reconstruction should be undertaken only after patency of the distal intestine has been determined by a contrast enema (Figure 19.5).

Outcome

In all affected children, mortality is reported to be between 10 and 40 per cent, increasing to more than 50 per cent in high-risk babies.

Extensive gut resections may result in calorie/protein malabsorption, which may necessitate long-term total or supplemental parental nutrition. While short gut syndrome can occur, many surviving children will compensate and will attain normal growth on normal enteral feeds. With loss of the terminal ileum, selective malabsorption of vitamin B12 and iron can be managed using replacement therapy, but this is not usually necessary long term. Similarly, bile-acid malabsorption in the terminal small intestine, which causes diarrhoea, is usually self-limiting but can be treated in the short term by the use of cholestyramine.

Children who have suffered stage II or III disease are at risk of periventricular and ventricular haemorrhages, secondary hydrocephalus and, as a consequence, psychomotor developmental delay. This has major long-term implications for education and family support.

CLINICAL SCENARIOS

Case 1

A baby who was born at 28 weeks' gestation, of birth weight 850 g, required three days' mechanical ventilation. The child was established on maternal expressed breast milk on the seventh day of life but collapsed suddenly with signs of septicaemia and abdominal distension on the tenth day. Abdominal X-ray confirmed pneumatosis intestinalis and pneumoperitoneum. Resuscitation was commenced with intravenous fluids, antibiotics and endotracheal intubation with ventilation. An abdominal drain was inserted in the right lower quadrant under local anaesthetic, and about 10 mL of brown serosanguinous fluid plus gas was removed.

The baby survived and stabilized and was extubated after four days. Feeds were introduced and tolerated after ten days, and the baby has since thrived without signs of intestinal obstruction and with normal psychomotor development.

Case 2

A baby born at 35 weeks' gestation, of birth weight 1850 g and with normal Apgar scores, was established on full nasogastric feeds by the fourth day of life using expressed maternal breast milk. He was apparently well until the seventh day, when he had a bile-stained vomit, passed a blood-stained stool and developed abdominal tenderness and distension. Investigation showed a dropping haemoglobin and platelet count and typical pneumatosis intestinalis in the right lower quadrant on abdominal X-ray. There was no gas in the portal vein and there was no evidence of intestinal perforation. It was decided to treat the baby conservatively. The child was resuscitated, antibiotics were commenced, oral feeds were discontinued and parenteral nutrition was started. During the next 48 hours, the baby's general condition deteriorated, periumbilical discoloration developed and there was X-ray evidence of pneumoperitoneum. There were signs of septicaemia, with oliguria and cardiovascular instability.

It was decided to perform a laparotomy. At operation, the necrotic terminal ileum and ascending colon were removed and enterostomies were fashioned at the healthy limits of resection, proximally and distally. Despite adequate supportive measures, the baby died three days later from multiple organ failure.

QUESTIONS

1 Is there firm evidence to suggest that in small fragile babies, peritoneal drainage may be a better option than laparotomy?
2 Why should an apparently healthy normal, albeit premature, infant, not survive what appeared to be relatively low-grade NEC?
3 Why should healthy postoperative term babies develop NEC?

REFERENCES

Arroyo Cabrales LM, Guzman BJ. Prenatal steroids for fetal maturation in preterm birth: experience at an institution. *Ginecologia y Obstetricia de Mexico* 2000; **68**: 448–52.

Bell MJ, Ternberg JL, Feigin RD, *et al*. Neonatal necrotizing enterocolitis: therapeutic decisions based on clinical staging. *Annals of Surgery* 1978; **187**: 1–6.

Bury RG, Tudehope D. Enteral antibiotics for preventing necrotising enterocolitis in low birthweight or preterm infants. *Cochrane Database of Systematic Reviews* 2000; (2): CD000405.

Garstin WI, Kenny BD, McAneaney D, Patterson CC, Boston VE. The role of intraluminal tension and pH in the development of necrotizing enterocolitis: an animal model. *Journal of Pediatric Surgery* 1987; **22**: 205–7.

Lawrence G, Tudehope D, Baumann K, *et al*. Enteral human IgG for prevention of necrotising enterocolitis: a placebo-controlled, randomised trial. *Lancet* 2001; **357**: 2090–94.

McGuire W, Anthony MY. Formula milk versus term human milk for feeding preterm or low birth weight infants. *Cochrane Database of Systematic Reviews* 2001; (4): CD002971.

FURTHER READING

Kosloske AM. Necrotizing enterocolitis. In: Puri P (ed.). *Newborn Surgery*. Oxford: Butterworth-Heinemann, 1996; pp. 354–62.

Hepatobiliary disorders

MARK D STRINGER

Learning objectives

- To understand the importance of early diagnosis of biliary atresia and to be aware of the main diagnostic tests, principles of surgery and aftercare.
- To appreciate the presenting features of a choledochal cyst and to understand their complications and the principles of surgical treatment.
- To be able to classify portal hypertension and to be aware of the more common causes and their management.
- To have a working knowledge of the surgical anatomy of the liver and bile ducts.
- To understand the structured approach to a severely injured child and to be able to describe the basic management of blunt liver trauma.

BILIARY ATRESIA

Biliary atresia is an important but rare cause of neonatal jaundice. It is due to an idiopathic obstructive inflammatory process that affects both intra- and extra-hepatic bile ducts. Early diagnosis is essential, since delay in treatment results in irreversible liver damage. If untreated, progressive cholestasis leads to hepatic fibrosis and cirrhosis, and affected infants die from liver failure complicated by portal hypertension and ascites. In the UK, the incidence is approximately one in 16 000 live births. Girls are affected slightly more often than boys.

Aetiology

The aetiology of biliary atresia is unknown. In most cases, obliterative bile-duct malformations are present in the fetus, and the cholangiopathy progresses after birth. Viral infections and abnormal immunologic mechanisms have been suggested as possible causes. About 10–15 per cent of affected children have the biliary atresia splenic malformation syndrome, which can include polysplenia or asplenia, situs inversus, intestinal malrotation, an interrupted inferior vena cava, preduodenal portal vein and congenital cardiac defects. An embryological insult, perhaps associated with a gene defect, is likely in such cases.

Pathogenesis and classification

The lumen of the extra-hepatic bile ducts is obliterated by inflammatory tissue to a variable extent (Figure 20.1):

- *Type 1:* atresia of the common bile duct, with patent proximal ducts (less than ten per cent).

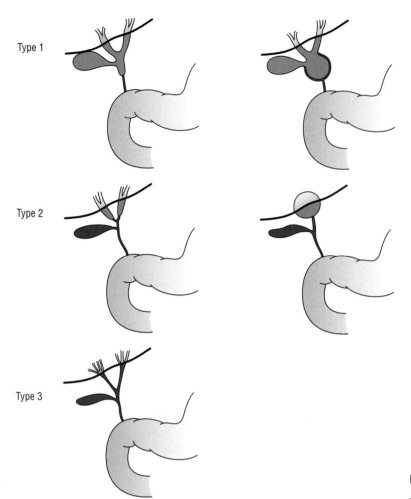

Type 1

Type 2

Type 3

Figure 20.1 *Classification of biliary atresia, after the Japanese Association of Paediatric Surgeons.*

- *Type 2:* atresia of the common hepatic duct, with patent right and left hepatic ducts (very rare).
- *Type 3:* atresia of all proximal extra-hepatic bile ducts (>90 per cent).

In type 3, the gallbladder typically is small and contains clear mucus. Occasionally, a cyst is found proximal or distal to the atretic bile duct, but this should not be confused with a true choledochal cyst.

Basic science: bilirubin metabolism

Bilirubin, a degradation product of haem, is poorly soluble in aqueous phase and is bound to albumin in the circulation for transport to the liver. This is *unconjugated* bilirubin, which is found in raised concentrations in the plasma of neonates with physiological jaundice. Uptake of bilirubin by hepatocytes is followed by conjugation with glucuronic acid, rendering it water-soluble. Under normal circumstances, a small amount of *conjugated* bilirubin diffuses back into the circulation, but most is actively excreted into bile. In the gut, the action of bacterial hydrolysis on bilirubin conjugates leads to the formation of urobilinogens, a small fraction of which are reabsorbed into the enterohepatic circulation.

Clinical features and diagnosis

Babies with biliary atresia present soon after birth with conjugated hyperbilirubinaemia, dark urine and pale stools. Birth weight and gestation are usually normal and most infants initially thrive. Malabsorption of vitamin K may induce a coagulopathy, with a risk of intracranial bleeding. Any infant with a persistent conjugated hyperbilirubinaemia (conjugated fraction >20 per cent of a raised bilirubin) after 14 days of age must be investigated further.

On examination, usually the liver is enlarged and there may be splenomegaly.

The diagnosis of biliary atresia is confirmed at laparotomy, but the following hepatobiliary investigations support the diagnosis:

- *Blood tests:* show a conjugated hyperbilirubinaemia and no evidence of metabolic (e.g. α-1-antitrypsin deficiency, galactosaemia) or infective causes.

- *Ultrasound scan:* can exclude other causes of obstructive jaundice, such as a choledochal cyst or inspissated bile. In biliary atresia, the gallbladder may be absent or small with an irregular outline. Dilated intrahepatic ducts are not seen. Occasionally, a well-defined triangular area of high reflectivity is noted at the porta hepatis, corresponding to fibrotic ductal remnants ('triangular cord sign').
- *Radionuclide scan:* radiolabelled iminodiacetic acid (IDA) derivatives are taken up by the liver but are not excreted into the bowel via the biliary tract.
- *Percutaneous liver biopsy:* early histological appearances consist of expansion of the portal tracts, bile ductular proliferation and a cellular infiltrate.
- *Magnetic resonance cholangiography (MRC):* early experience suggests that this may be a useful method of visualizing the bile ducts in infants.
- *Endoscopic retrograde cholangiography (ERC):* this is technically demanding but is used by some centres to exclude biliary atresia.
- *Mini-laparotomy or laparoscopy and operative cholangiography:* occasionally may be necessary to exclude biliary atresia.

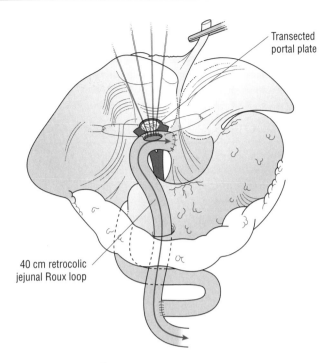

Figure 20.2 *Kasai porto-enterostomy.*

Labels: Transected portal plate; 40 cm retrocolic jejunal Roux loop

Surgery

Early surgical attempts to treat biliary atresia were successful for the so-called 'correctable' types of atresia (types 1 and 2), in which there are patent proximal bile ducts. The majority of affected infants have proximal extra-hepatic bile-duct occlusion (type 3). In 1959, Morio Kasai reported the presence of microscopic biliary channels within tissue at the porta hepatis and showed that radical resection of this tissue could result in bile drainage (Kasai porto-enterostomy).

At laparotomy, the diagnosis of biliary atresia is confirmed. If there is doubt, then cholangiography via a catheter in the gallbladder should clarify ductal patency. The hepatic ligaments are divided and the liver rotated to expose the porta hepatis. The atretic remnants of the biliary tract are dissected free from the underlying portal vein and hepatic artery and transected at the porta hepatis. A jejunal Roux loop is anastomosed to the margins of the transected portal plate (Figure 20.2).

Postoperatively, prophylactic antibiotics are given in an attempt to prevent cholangitis. Choleretic agents (phenobarbital, ursodeoxycholic acid, possibly corticosteroids) may be used to promote bile flow, but their efficacy is unproven. Impaired bile flow causes malabsorption of fat and fat-soluble vitamins, which must be rectified by formula feeds enriched with medium-chain triglycerides and by supplements of fat-soluble vitamins (A, D, E, K).

Successful surgery results in clearance of jaundice and delays or prevents progressive liver disease. About two-thirds of patients achieve normal bilirubin levels, but only a small proportion have completely normal biochemical liver function. Approximately 30–50 per cent of affected children survive to ten years of age with their native liver. In the long term, up to 80 per cent of patients with biliary atresia eventually require a liver transplant. Biliary atresia is the most common indication for liver transplantation during childhood.

Several variables other than the type of atresia influence the success of surgery. Results are better in infants under 90 days of age. The presence of large microscopic bile ductules at the transected portal plate favours bile drainage. Infants with the biliary atresia splenic malformation syndrome generally have a worse prognosis.

Complications

Even after successful Kasai porto-enterostomy, complications may occur:

- *Ascending bacterial cholangitis:* occurs in up to 40 per cent of patients, most often in the first year. Typically, there is worsening jaundice, fever and pale stools. Blood cultures may reveal Gram-negative bacteria. Treatment is with broad-spectrum intravenous antibiotics.
- *Portal hypertension:* this is secondary to hepatic fibrosis and is common. It causes oesophageal varices and bleeding.
- *Nutritional consequences of cholestasis:* this may manifest as impaired growth, coagulopathy (vitamin K deficiency), metabolic bone disease (vitamin D deficiency) or neurological sequelae (vitamin E deficiency).
- *Hepatopulmonary syndrome:* characterized by cyanosis, dyspnoea and finger clubbing secondary to

intrapulmonary shunting. This is usually an indication for liver transplantation.

- *Liver tumour:* rarely, a malignant tumour can develop within the cirrhotic liver of a child with biliary atresia.

CHOLEDOCHAL CYSTS

Choledochal 'cysts' are rare congenital bile duct dilations. More than two-thirds of cases are diagnosed in children under ten years of age, and girls outnumber boys by about three to one. They are more common in East Asian people.

Anatomy and classification

Choledochal cysts are traditionally classified into five types (Figure 20.3). Type I cysts may be cystic or fusiform and account for most cases. Type IVa cysts comprise multiple cystic dilatations of the extra- and intra-hepatic ducts and are the second most frequently found type. Other types are very rare. Choledochal cysts are typically associated with an abnormal junction between the terminal common bile duct and the pancreatic duct; these ducts unite outside the duodenal

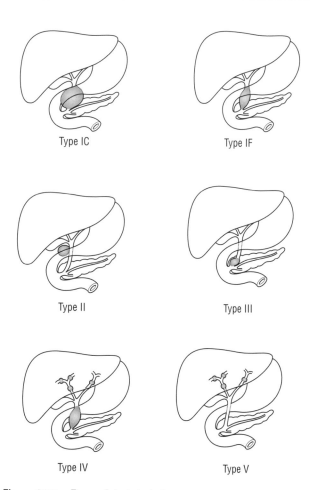

Type IC

Type IF

Type II

Type III

Type IV

Type V

Figure 20.3 *Types of choledochal cyst.*

wall and are not surrounded by the normal sphincter mechanism. This pancreatobiliary malunion forms a common channel, which encourages reflux of pancreatic juice into the biliary tree. High concentrations of pancreatic enzymes are found in the bile. Less frequently, bile refluxes into the pancreatic duct, causing pancreatitis.

Aetiology

Prenatal obstruction of the distal common bile duct may be the cause of type I cysts, but a complex defect in biliary morphogenesis is more likely. Genetic factors may account for the female preponderance and geographical distribution.

Clinical presentation

Most choledochal cysts present in childhood:

- *Prenatal*: choledochal cysts may be detected by prenatal ultrasound scan. Postnatally, affected infants should be treated by early surgery, particularly if they are jaundiced. Some will have a cystic variant of biliary atresia rather than a choledochal cyst. Early treatment reduces the risks of complications.
- *Infants* typically present with obstructive jaundice.
- *Older children* often present with abdominal pain and/or intermittent jaundice.

The classic triad of jaundice, pain and a right hypochondrial mass is uncommon. Abdominal pain is secondary to pancreatitis associated with a common pancreatobiliary channel. A choledochal cyst should always be included in the differential diagnosis of obstructive jaundice and/or pancreatitis.

Complications

Choledochal cysts are prone to complications, including:

- cholangitis;
- rupture: can occur spontaneously in preschool-age children;
- pancreatitis: may be recurrent;
- gallstones;
- portal hypertension: secondary to portal vein compression or liver disease;
- malignant change: this is a possibility in older children and adults; pancreatobiliary ductal malunion is an important predisposing factor.

Investigations

Biochemical liver function tests may be normal or may show obstructive jaundice. A raised serum amylase may be detected during episodes of abdominal pain. A clotting abnormality should be excluded in jaundiced patients.

Ultrasonography is the initial investigation of choice. The cyst and proximal bile ducts can be visualized accurately. Magnetic resonance cholangiopancreatography (MRCP) and endoscopic retrograde cholangiopancreatography (ERCP) define the anatomy in detail. Hepatobiliary scintigraphy is useful in selected cases.

Surgery

Radical cyst excision and hepatico-enterostomy is the optimum treatment for the common types of choledochal cyst. Simple anastomosis of the cyst to a loop of bowel (cystenterostomy) should not be performed, because this is associated with serious long-term morbidity, e.g. cholangitis, cholelithiasis, pancreatitis, biliary cirrhosis and malignancy.

Prophylactic antibiotics are given at the start of surgery. If the anatomy of the choledochal cyst has not been clearly defined preoperatively, then an operative cholangiogram is performed. A sample of bile is aspirated from the cyst for culture and measurement of amylase. The extra-hepatic 'cyst' is excised completely, oversewing the distal common bile duct just above its junction with the pancreatic duct. The common hepatic duct is divided at the level of the bifurcation and a wide hilar bilio-enteric anastomosis constructed with a Roux loop of jejunum. Any dilated proximal intra-hepatic ducts and a dilated common channel should be cleared of debris. A liver biopsy is performed.

Results and complications

Radical cyst excision and hepatico-enterostomy achieves consistently good results (Miyano *et al.* 1996). Early postoperative complications such as anastomotic leakage and bleeding are uncommon. An anastomotic stricture may develop up to ten or more years postoperatively and usually manifests as cholangitis. Pancreatitis may also occur as a late complication in patients with a common channel containing protein plugs or calculi. Malignancy has been reported after choledochal cyst excision but is extremely rare after adequate primary surgery.

SPONTANEOUS PERFORATION OF THE BILE DUCT

This condition may present in infants with rapid-onset abdominal distension, jaundice and acholic stools. Greenish discoloration of hydroceles or the umbilicus may be noted. The perforation occurs at the junction of the cystic and common hepatic ducts. There is usually no obvious cause.

Abdominal ultrasound may show a cystic area at the porta hepatis and free fluid. Hepatobiliary scintigraphy may demonstrate isotope within the peritoneal cavity.

Peritoneal drainage alone is successful sometimes, but usually laparotomy and cholangiography are necessary to exclude distal common bile duct obstruction and to prevent a persistent bile leak. A small T-tube in the common bile duct controls the biliary fistula while the infant recovers from the biliary peritonitis.

INSPISSATED BILE SYNDROME

Bile-duct obstruction by plugs of thickened bile may develop in neonates in association with parenteral nutrition, haemolysis or dehydration. Ultrasound scan typically shows dilated proximal bile ducts and may reveal biliary sludge in the common bile duct. Percutaneous transhepatic cholangiography is diagnostic and occasionally therapeutic if the inspissated bile can be cleared by irrigation. Operative cholangiography and choledochotomy are sometimes required. Early administration of ursodeoxycholic acid and enteral feeding may avoid the need for intervention in infants with biliary sludge complicating prolonged parenteral nutrition.

GALLSTONES

Most studies of cholelithiasis in childhood show a bimodal distribution with a small peak in infancy and a steadily rising incidence from early adolescence onwards. In childhood, boys and girls are affected similarly, but a clear female preponderance emerges during adolescence. The prevalence of gallstones in Western children has increased steadily in recent years.

Basic science: types of gallstone

The dominant factors causing gallstone formation are biliary stasis, excess bilirubin load and lithogenic bile. There are four major types of gallstone: mixed cholesterol, pure cholesterol, black-pigment and brown-pigment stones. Cholesterol stones are the most common variety in adults and are also found in obese adolescent girls. They develop from cholesterol supersaturation of bile in the presence of bile stasis. Black-pigment stones are formed from supersaturation of bile with calcium bilirubinate and typically are found in haemolytic disorders. Brown-pigment stones are associated with biliary stasis and infection and are found more often in the bile ducts than in the gallbladder.

Specific aetiological conditions

- *Haemolysis:* e.g. sickle cell disease and hereditary spherocytosis.
- *Ileal resection/disease:* this disturbs the normal enterohepatic circulation of bile, which is rendered more lithogenic.

- *Fasting and total parenteral nutrition (TPN):* promote biliary stasis.
- *Other risk factors:* adolescents with gallstones typically have adult risk factors, i.e. female gender, obesity and, sometimes, pregnancy. Biliary obstruction, cystic fibrosis, Down syndrome and childhood cancer also predispose to cholelithiasis.

Clinical features

In infants, gallstones are frequently asymptomatic but may cause non-specific symptoms such as poor feeding and vomiting. Rarely, they cause acute cholecystitis, obstructive jaundice or biliary perforation. In older children, symptoms include upper abdominal pain, nausea and vomiting. Occasionally, presentation is with obstructive jaundice or pancreatitis.

Diagnosis

Gallstones are diagnosed readily by abdominal ultrasound scanning. The sensitivity and specificity of ultrasound exceeds 95 per cent for gallbladder cholelithiasis, but only 50–75 per cent of common bile-duct stones are visualized.

Management

Early surgery is unnecessary in the *asymptomatic* infant with gallbladder calculi because spontaneous resolution may occur. Clinical and ultrasound monitoring is appropriate if the infant has no other evidence of biliary tract disease. In older children, the management of asymptomatic gallbladder calculi of non-haemolytic origin is controversial because the natural history is not well defined.

Symptomatic or *complicated* gallstone disease usually requires cholecystectomy. Dissolution therapy for gallstones in children is not successful. In children with gallstones and hereditary spherocytosis, cholecystectomy is superior to cholecystostomy and stone removal.

Common bile duct stones are relatively uncommon but may be complicated by obstructive jaundice, cholangitis or acute pancreatitis. MRC may be helpful in diagnosis, but ERC also offers the opportunity for sphincterotomy and stone retrieval before or after laparoscopic cholecystectomy.

ACALCULOUS CHOLECYSTITIS

Acute acalculous cholecystitis may develop after shock, trauma, burns, systemic sepsis and parenteral nutrition. In the tropics, *Salmonella typhi* infection and ascariasis should be considered. Clinical features include abdominal pain, vomiting, fever, localized tenderness and a palpable right upper quadrant mass. Laboratory investigations reveal leucocytosis, hyperbilirubinaemia and mildly raised serum amylase. Ultrasound scan shows a markedly distended gallbladder.

Initial management is conservative, with antibiotics, intravenous fluids and early enteral feeding. Cholecystectomy or cholecystostomy is indicated if there is progressive clinical deterioration.

PORTAL HYPERTENSION

Portal hypertension is an important cause of serious gastrointestinal haemorrhage in children. Precise diagnosis and a multidisciplinary approach are essential for successful management.

Basic science: definition and pathophysiology

The portal vein carries blood to the liver from the gastrointestinal tract and spleen, contributing two-thirds of the hepatic blood supply. Portal venous pressure is the product of blood flow and vascular resistance. Portal hypertension is defined by an increased hepatic venous pressure gradient between the portal and hepatic veins. A gradient of more than 12 mm Hg is necessary for the development of oesophageal varices. Portal hypertension leads to splenomegaly and the development of portosystemic collaterals at various sites, including the distal oesophagus, the anal canal, the falciform ligament and the abdominal wall. Large varices in the distal oesophagus are the usual cause of variceal bleeding.

Aetiology and clinical features

Portal hypertension typically presents with either haematemesis and/or melaena or splenomegaly or symptoms from underlying liver disease (jaundice, ascites, etc.). Portal hypertension in children may be due to:

- primary venous obstruction:
  - pre-hepatic, e.g. portal vein occlusion (PVO);
  - intra-hepatic, e.g. schistosomiasis;
  - post-hepatic, e.g. Budd–Chiari syndrome, venoocclusive disease;
- intrinsic liver disease, e.g. cirrhosis or fibrosis.

Chronic liver disease is the most common overall cause, but PVO is the most frequent cause of extra-hepatic portal hypertension.

In PVO, the liver is healthy but the portal vein is occluded and replaced by multiple venous collaterals (a cavernoma). Many cases are probably developmental malformations, but PVO can be acquired as a result of umbilical vein catheterization, umbilical sepsis, thrombophilic disorders, intraabdominal sepsis and trauma.

Intrinsic liver disease encompasses a wide variety of conditions, including biliary atresia, cystic fibrosis, autoimmune hepatitis, α-1-antitrypsin deficiency and congenital hepatic fibrosis.

Budd–Chiari syndrome is due to hepatic venous thrombosis, often secondary to an underlying myeloproliferative disorder or thrombophilic state. Clinical features include hepatosplenomegaly, intractable ascites and progressive cachexia.

Investigations

- *Haematology:* anaemia, leucopenia and/or thrombocytopenia may be due to hypersplenism. The prothrombin time is often prolonged in patients with intrinsic liver disease.
- *Biochemical liver function tests:* normal in PVO and often abnormal in chronic liver diseases. However, routine liver function tests can be normal in well-compensated cirrhosis.
- *Abdominal ultrasound scan:* large collateral veins and splenomegaly are evident. Abnormal hepatic echo texture may indicate chronic liver disease. Colour Doppler flow studies show the direction and velocity of flow in the portal and hepatic veins.
- *Gastrointestinal endoscopy:* oesophageal and gastric varices are seen. Large varices may show 'red signs' of recent or impending variceal haemorrhage.
- *Magnetic resonance imaging:* useful in evaluating focal liver lesions associated with portal hypertension and in Budd–Chiari syndrome. Magnetic resonance angiography or conventional angiography can confirm the diagnosis of PVO and determine the patency and calibre of veins throughout the portomesenteric system.
- *Percutaneous liver biopsy:* if there are no contraindications, then this is necessary to characterize chronic liver disease.

Management

In children with good liver function and bleeding varices, e.g. PVO, treatment is directed at the portal hypertension. In cirrhotic patients, the nature and severity of the underlying liver disease dictate management.

EMERGENCY MANAGEMENT OF VARICEAL BLEEDING

See Clinical scenario, p. 184.

PREVENTION OF RECURRENT BLEEDING

This can be achieved in various ways:

Endoscopic injection sclerotherapy or variceal ligation (banding)

These techniques provide effective treatment of oesophageal varices. Via a flexible gastrointestinal endoscope, varices are either injected with a sclerosant or occluded by the application of a rubber band. This induces variceal thrombosis. Major complications include oesophageal stricturing (which responds to dilation), recurrent oesophageal varices and bleeding from a treatment-induced ulcer. Banding offers more rapid eradication, with fewer treatment sessions and lower complication rates.

Surgery

Where anatomically feasible, portal vein bypass surgery should be performed for children with PVO and no underlying prothrombotic disorder. Other indications for surgery in portal hypertension are:

- uncontrolled bleeding from oesophageal varices (not responding to endoscopic treatment);
- bleeding from gastrointestinal varices that cannot be controlled endoscopically;
- massive splenomegaly causing severe hypersplenism or pain.

Possible surgical interventions include the following:

- Portosystemic shunt, e.g. mesocaval or spleno-renal shunt (Figure 20.4): this relieves portal hypertension by redirecting portal blood flow around the liver. Shunt thrombosis is a hazard and usually manifests as recurrent variceal bleeding. Encephalopathy is a potential complication in cirrhotics.
- Portal-vein bypass: the mesenterico-left portal (Rex) shunt connects the superior mesenteric vein with the intra-hepatic left portal vein located in the Rex recessus adjacent to the falciform ligament (Figure 20.4). The PVO is bypassed and portal hypertension resolves. This shunt is ideal for children with PVO, since it restores normal physiology, but it is not anatomically feasible in all cases.
- Non-shunt surgery: this is often disappointing in the long term, because of a high rate of rebleeding. Procedures have included splenectomy alone, suture ligation of varices, oesophagogastric transection and devascularization operations. Splenectomy may be necessary for massive splenomegaly causing severe hypersplenism or abdominal pain.
- Liver transplantation: the treatment of choice for most children with variceal bleeding complicating end-stage chronic liver disease.

Drugs

Propranolol reduces portal pressure and may help to prevent rebleeding.

Transjugular intrahepatic portosystemic stent shunt

With a transjugular intrahepatic portosystemic stent shunt (TIPS), an expandable metal stent is deployed between the hepatic and portal veins by an interventional radiologist (Figure 20.4). Stent occlusion is a major limiting factor in the long term. TIPS may be valuable in children with refractory variceal bleeding awaiting liver transplantation and selected patients with Budd–Chiari syndrome. PVO is a contraindication.

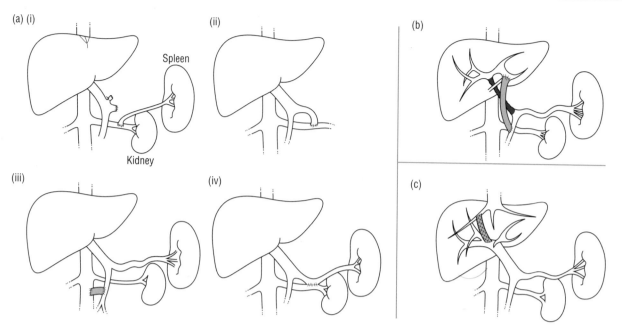

Figure 20.4 *Shunt procedures for portal hypertension. (a) Portosystemic shunts: (i) distal spleno-renal; (ii) proximal spleno-renal; (iii) mesocaval; and (iv) side-to-side spleno-renal. (b) Mesenterico-left portal (Rex) shunt. (c) Transjugular intrahepatic portosystemic stent shunt (TIPS).*

SURGICAL ANATOMY OF THE LIVER

The right and left liver lobes are separated by the attachment of the falciform ligament superiorly and the umbilical fissure and ligamentum venosum inferiorly. The internal anatomy of the whole organ can be subdivided on three levels:

- The right and left *hemi-livers* are divided by the midplane that lies between the medial margin of the gallbladder fossa and the inferior vena cava (Cantlie's line).
- Each hemi-liver is divided into two *sections*, based on the intra-hepatic anatomy of the hepatic artery and the bile duct. Thus, the right hemi-liver has anterior (segments 5 and 8) and posterior (segments 6 and 7) sections, and the left hemi-liver has medial (segment 4) and lateral (segments 2 and 3) sections (Figure 20.5).
- Segmental anatomy is based on Couinaud's eight *segments*, which relate to the intra-hepatic divisions of the portal vein. Each segment is also subserved by a hepatic artery and bile duct. The caudate lobe (segment 1) is defined by surface anatomy.

There are three main hepatic veins – right, middle and left. The left and middle hepatic veins usually unite to form a short common trunk before entering the inferior vena cava. Consequently, the left hepatic vein is potentially vulnerable during a right trisectionectomy and the middle hepatic vein during left hemi-hepatectomy. The middle hepatic vein occupies the midplane of the liver, and the right and left veins lie in the intersectional planes. During liver resection, the hepatic veins can be approached and ligated outside the liver or from within the parenchyma.

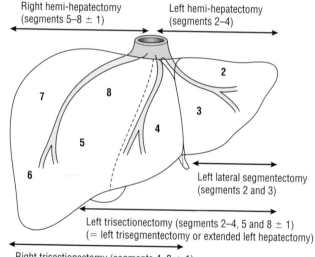

Figure 20.5 *Segmental anatomy of the liver and standard liver resections.*

The left branch of the portal vein and the left hepatic duct have a longer, more horizontal extra-hepatic course. Anatomical variations in the origin, course and number of the hepatic artery (or arteries) are common.

The diameter of the normal common bile duct is less than 6 mm in adolescents, less than 4 mm in children and less than 2 mm in infants. The cystic duct, common hepatic duct and undersurface of the right hemi-liver form the boundaries of Calot's triangle, an important landmark in cholecystectomy.

Variations in cystic duct anatomy are common and important. The right and left hepatic ducts divide within the liver into sectoral ducts, which have a variable anatomy. The common bile duct receives arterial blood from the right hepatic artery above and the retroduodenal and gastroduodenal arteries below; small arterial branches on the duct run in an axial direction and are located mainly at three and nine o'clock.

LIVER TRAUMA

After the spleen, the liver is the most commonly injured solid abdominal organ in children. Trauma is most often blunt but may be penetrating or iatrogenic. Road-traffic and recreational accidents are the most common causes of blunt trauma, but child abuse can also be a cause.

The structured approach to the child with major injuries advocated by the Advanced Paediatric Life Support Group programmes is essential. The focus of the *primary survey* is on airway and cervical spine, breathing, circulation and the control of bleeding, the assessment of conscious level, and a rapid overview of all injuries. The liver and spleen are more vulnerable in children because they are less well protected by the flexible ribcage. The abdomen must be inspected carefully for signs of patterned bruising, which indicates forceful compression against a rigid skeleton. This includes a seatbelt sign after rapid deceleration in a motor vehicle. In the shocked child with no obvious source of haemorrhage, intra-abdominal or intrathoracic bleeding should be considered.

The optimum radiological investigation of major abdominal trauma in the haemodynamically stable child is a double-contrast computed tomography (CT) scan; both intravenous and intragastric contrast are given, but the value of the latter is controversial. CT demonstrates parenchymal tears (Figure 20.6), disruption of major blood vessels and other intra-abdominal injuries, and allows an assessment of the volume of any free intraperitoneal blood. The need for emergency surgery relates more to the severity and persistence of intra-abdominal bleeding than to the extent of parenchymal injury observed on CT. Abdominal ultrasound scanning is quick and portable and can demonstrate free fluid and solid-organ injuries, but it is not as sensitive or specific as CT and it is more operator-dependent. Ultrasound scanning is more useful in the follow-up of blunt liver trauma. Biliary radioisotope scans can be helpful in the diagnosis and management of biliary trauma. Angiography is particularly valuable in the diagnosis and treatment (embolization) of haemobilia.

Most blunt liver injuries are associated with self-limiting haemorrhage. Isolated blunt liver trauma can be safely and effectively managed non-operatively in the majority of children, provided there is:

- haemodynamic stability after resuscitation with no more than 40–60 mL/kg of intravenous fluid;
- a good-quality CT scan;
- no evidence of hollow visceral injury;

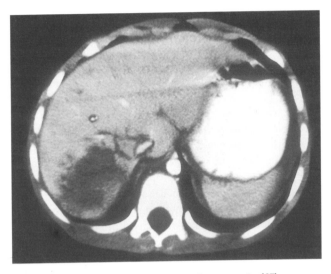

Figure 20.6 *Double-contrast computed tomography (CT) scan, showing barium contrast in the stomach and a large haematoma in the right hemi-liver following blunt abdominal trauma.*

- frequent, careful monitoring and immediate availability of appropriate surgical expertise.

Complications of non-operative management are uncommon but include haematoma rupture, infection and bile leaks. Bile leaks are typically managed by percutaneous drainage with or without ERC and temporary internal stenting of the bile duct. Uncomplicated cases of blunt liver trauma can be discharged home after five to seven days. Activity should be restricted for three to six weeks, and contact sports avoided until the haematoma has resolved, which may take up to three months after major trauma.

The relatively small proportion of children with evidence of continuing intra-abdominal bleeding (and those with major penetrating injuries) require urgent laparotomy. These cases have potentially fatal liver injuries and require a high degree of radiological and surgical expertise. Prompt arrest of major bleeding is critical to prevent prolonged hypotension, renal failure and the additional complications of coagulopathy, acidosis and hypothermia, all of which exacerbate haemorrhage. Rapid exposure of the abdominal cavity is achieved by a midline incision. Use of a cell saver is helpful. If a severe liver injury is confirmed, then the hepatic artery and portal vein are compressed in the free edge of the lesser omentum (Pringle manoeuvre), whilst parenchymal bleeding is controlled by peri-hepatic packing with large gauze rolls (Feliciano *et al.* 1981). This is followed by a rapid search for major injuries to other organs in the abdomen. Hepatic resection is required rarely now that the efficacy of intraoperative peri-hepatic packing has been proven.

PYOGENIC LIVER ABSCESS

Pyogenic liver abscess may occur at any age. Apparently healthy children and immunocompromised (e.g. chronic granulo-matous disease) children may be affected. There are several routes of infection: via the biliary tract (e.g. after Kasai porto-enterostomy or in association with stones or biliary obstruction), via the portal vein (e.g. complicating appendicitis), via the hepatic artery (e.g. from septicaemia coming from a distant source) or directly (e.g. from penetrating trauma). Abscesses may be single or multiple.

Staphylococcus aureus and *Escherichia coli* account for most cases of pyogenic liver abscess in children. Anaerobic organisms should be suspected if the abscess contains gas.

Pyogenic liver abscess usually presents with fever, anorexia, abdominal pain and general malaise. The liver may be enlarged and tender. Routine laboratory investigations often reveal anaemia and leucocytosis, with raised inflammatory markers. Disturbances of biochemical liver function and positive blood cultures are found in some patients. A plain chest radiograph may show an elevated right hemi-diaphragm or pleural effusion or, rarely, gas or a fluid level within the abscess. Ultrasonography is a sensitive method of detecting liver abscesses.

Treatment is guided by three principles:

1 Confirm the diagnosis and determine the anatomy of the abscess(es).
2 Treat with appropriate broad-spectrum intravenous antibiotics.
3 Add in percutaneous catheter drainage if there is no prompt clinical response.

Amoebic liver abscess is an extra-intestinal manifestation of amoebiasis and may occur in children. Multiple abscesses are common. Serologic tests are helpful but cannot differentiate between past and current infection. Diagnostic percutaneous aspiration of the abscess may be necessary, but characteristic 'anchovy sauce' is a variable finding. Treatment consists of metronidazole, with or without abscess drainage.

CLINICAL SCENARIO

A seven-year-old girl who underwent a Kasai porto-enterostomy for biliary atresia at ten weeks of age was admitted following a large haematemesis. Her pulse rate was 125 beats/minute, systolic blood pressure was 90 mm Hg and she had poor peripheral perfusion. Splenomegaly was noted. Her management was as follows:

- On admission, she had a secure airway and was given face-mask oxygen.
- Two peripheral intravenous cannulae (22 G) were inserted, and she was given a bolus of 20 mL/kg of 4.5% albumin and maintenance fluids with 5% dextrose.
- Full blood count, clotting, urea, creatinine, electrolytes, cross-match (3 units of packed cells), blood cultures and liver function tests were requested.

- Her fluid balance, cardiorespiratory status and blood glucose were monitored, and she was observed closely for signs of encephalopathy.

Haemoglobin (Hb) was 6.3 g/dL, prothrombin time 18 seconds (international normalized ratio (INR) 1.5), platelets 96×10^9/L and urea 8.3 mmol/L. Liver function tests showed an albumin of 32 g/L and bilirubin 23 μmol/L, with an abnormal liver enzyme profile. Her management was continued as follows:

- Transfusion of packed red cells *slowly*, aiming for Hb of about 10 g/dL.
- Intravenous vitamin K 5 mg given slowly and fresh frozen plasma held in reserve.
- She was started on an octreotide infusion (bolus dose 1 μg/kg intravenously, followed by infusion at 1–3 μg/kg/h (maximum 50 μg/h) via a dedicated line. Octreotide, an analogue of somatostatin, reduces splanchnic blood flow and portal pressure and is tolerated well.
- She was kept nil by mouth and given ranitidine 1 mg/kg intravenously three times daily and oral sucralfate.
- A 14F gauge paediatric Sengstaken-type tube was made available to be used if necessary.
- Urgent upper gastrointestinal endoscopy confirmed oesophageal varices as the source of bleeding. The varices were treated by banding.

Once there were no further signs of bleeding, octreotide was weaned gradually, she was allowed fluids and a soft diet, and she continued with further endoscopies to obliterate her oesophageal varices. Her liver function tests remained abnormal and it was anticipated that she would probably need a liver transplant in the future.

REFERENCES

Feliciano DV, Mattox KL, Jordan GL. Intra-abdominal packing for control of hepatic hemorrhage: a reappraisal. *Journal of Trauma* 1981; **21**: 285–90.

Miyano T, Yamataka A, Kato Y, *et al.* Hepaticoenterostomy after excision of choledochal cyst in children: a 30-year experience with 180 cases. *Journal of Pediatric Surgery* 1996; **31**: 1417–21.

FURTHER READING

Howard ER, Stringer MD, Colombani PM. *Surgery of the Liver, Bile-Ducts and Pancreas in Children*, 2nd edn. London: Arnold, 2002.

Spitz L, Coran AG. *Pediatric Surgery*, 5th edn. London: Chapman & Hall, 1994.

Stringer MD. Liver tumors. *Seminars in Pediatric Surgery* 2000; **9**: 196–208.

Abdominal wall defects

OLE HENRIK NIELSEN

Learning objectives

- To understand the types of abdominal wall defect.
- To understand the underlying embryopathogenesis.
- To be able to describe prenatal diagnosis and its implications.
- To be able to describe the postnatal presentation.
- To be able to describe the management, including the various surgical techniques.

INTRODUCTION

There are three main types of congenital abdominal wall defect:

- *Type 1:* hernia of the umbilical cord, or exomphalos minor.
- *Type 2:* exomphalos, or exomphalos major.
- *Type 3:* gastroschisis, or laparoschisis.

All present as protrusion of abdominal viscera in the umbilical area and represent a deficient closure of the abdominal wall in the midline. All elements of the abdominal wall are present, but they are displaced laterally at the site of the defect. In types 1 and 2, the protruding viscera are contained in the dilated root of the umbilical cord and thus covered by a membrane. In type 3, the defect is open. Exomphalos especially is often associated with other anomalies. The two other types occur mostly as isolated anomalies, although there may be a combination with the rare midline defects outside the umbilical area. Upper-midline defects comprise various degrees of sternal cleft, which may also include ectopia cordis. The most pronounced form is the pentalogy of Cantrell: umbilical defect (exomphalos or hernia of the cord), sternal cleft, anterior diaphragmatic defect, pericardial defect and cardiac defect (mostly ventricular septal defect). A lower-midline defect produces the bladder exstrophy complex, and combination with an umbilical defect means cloacal exstrophy, which includes exomphalos or hernia of the cord, and bladder exstrophy with a vesical cleft in the midline, through which protrudes an intestinal fistula. There is frequently also a sacral meningocele.

Because the viscera have been situated outside the abdomen during most of the pregnancy, the abdominal cavity has not grown to accommodate them. It has been said that the viscera have lost their right of domicile. This fact is of significance in the management, because it is the cause of some of the difficulties met when closure of the defects is attempted.

The overall incidence of these defects is around one in 3000 live births. There are many spontaneous intrauterine deaths with exomphalos, and after antenatal diagnosis there is an increasing number of terminations. These factors may modify the figures, which also tend to vary between different countries. In short, incidence figures are uncertain at best.

RELEVANT BASIC SCIENCE

The embryopathogenesis of abdominal wall defects is not documented fully, and there is some controversy about the details. There are, however, some established facts. The embryo has three sets of folds, the cephalic, lateral and caudal folds. Closure of the anterior abdominal wall is effected by fusion of these folds in the midline in the third week of gestation. Failure of fusion of the cephalic fold will result in an upper-midline defect – epigastric exomphalos. Failure of fusion of the caudal fold will result in a lower-midline defect – hypogastric exomphalos. Failure of fusion of the lateral fold will result in an umbilical defect – the types we are concerned with here. From gestational week five to ten, the midgut is situated temporarily in a peritoneal extension into the umbilical cord. This delays the total closure of the abdominal wall in the umbilical region, and in abdominal wall defects the return of the gut to the abdomen does not occur at all.

The experience gained by ultrasound scanning during pregnancy has provided additional knowledge about the sequential events. It has been noted that in exomphalos, the first organ to appear in the umbilical cord is the liver, rather than the gut, and it is reasonable to infer that this detail is of significance, since the liver is never displaced in normal development. In the other types, the liver is not in the cord, and this probably explains the difference in size of the various types of defect. The presence of the liver and the pattern of associated anomalies clearly point to a true congenital anomaly with a genetic background and place exomphalos in a totally different category from the other types of defect.

There are many features in common between hernia of the cord and gastroschisis, and the hypothesis that gastroschisis is really a hernia of the cord with intrauterine rupture of the membranes seems the most plausible explanation (Shaw 1975). Such a sequence has now been observed at serial antenatal ultrasound scanning.

DIAGNOSIS

There is no problem in identifying these conspicuous defects at birth. Diagnostic procedures are directed at other anomalies that might be present. Karyotyping should be performed, especially in covered defects, because chromosome anomalies, which are sometimes lethal, are frequent.

Antenatal diagnosis

abdominal wall defects are clearly visible on fetal ultrasound scanning. It is easy to see whether a membrane is covering the viscera, or whether a major part of the liver is outside the abdomen. Therefore, a precise diagnosis can almost always be made. This has made a change in the management: once the diagnosis is known before delivery, it is possible to make plans and avoid some of the dangers facing the fetus. If the diagnosis is made early enough (before the twentieth week of gestation), then termination of the pregnancy is possible.

Options after antenatal diagnosis

Options include:

- supplementary investigations;
- termination of the pregnancy;
- continuation of the pregnancy, with repeated ultrasound scanning;
- planning of the delivery in a tertiary centre;
- selecting the mode of delivery.

Further investigations at an early point are important, because the finding of an anomaly incompatible with life will make termination desirable. A careful search for other anomalies should be made, because a combination with other severe anomalies is of considerable prognostic significance. A chorion biopsy or amniotic fluid sampling should be done, with karyotyping, because a lethal chromosome anomaly (trisomy 13 or 18) may be identified.

The real advantage of antenatal diagnosis is the possibility of determining the mode and place of delivery (Nielsen et al. 1995). Spontaneous birth will often occur prematurely. Therefore, to avoid transport of a fragile baby, delivery should be planned in the centre where surgery will take place. The mode of delivery is often discussed, and caesarean section may be suggested by other members of the antenatal multidisciplinary team. There may be a clear obstetric indication for this, but there is no direct benefit from caesarean section for the treatment of abdominal wall defects (Nielsen et al. 1995). It is, however, the only certain way of timing the delivery precisely, if that should be desired. Vaginal delivery does not incur a greater risk of infection or of damage to the protruding viscera, even in gastroschisis.

All of these factors must be considered by the antenatal team. It is important that the parents are informed by the paediatric surgeon, because the surgeon is best placed to answer the inevitable questions that the parents will have. The decisions about the further management – pre- and postnatally – really belong to the parents, and the information they have must be as complete and precise as possible. This is not an easy task.

After 32 weeks of gestation, repeated ultrasound scanning at one- to two-week intervals is indicated, especially in gastroschisis, because the state of the protruding intestines can be estimated. If they are very dilated and the wall is thickened, then preterm delivery may be considered, because it may render reduction and closure easier, and possibly postnatal intestinal malfunction may be avoided. Another indication for the frequent scans during the last months of gestation is the high risk of sudden *in utero* death, especially in gastroschisis.

GENERAL PRINCIPLES OF MANAGEMENT

Total primary closure is optimal but not always possible. The surgical method should be selected carefully to suit each individual case.

The goal of treatment in all types of abdominal wall defect is reduction of the viscera and closure of all layers of the abdominal wall. When the peritoneum is open, this should be done without unnecessary delay, but the urgency is not such that it is necessary to operate between midnight and morning.

Primary closure is to be preferred, but this may not be possible because the defect is too large and the protruding viscera too voluminous. Intra-abdominal pressure can be measured and must not exceed 20 cmH$_2$O, otherwise the venous return will be compromised. The theoretically correct pressure to be measured is that of the inferior vena cava below the diaphragm, but an intragastric pressure is very good in practice. If primary closure cannot be achieved, then several options are available for delayed or staged closure.

HERNIA OF THE UMBILICAL CORD

- Incidence: one in 7000 live births.
- Small defect (<4 cm).
- Contains only midgut.
- Non-rotation and non-fixation are part of the anomaly.
- Associated anomalies are rare.
- Frequent persistent omphalo-enteric duct.
- May also be part of pentalogy of Cantrell and Beckwith–Wiedemann syndrome.
- Primary closure is always possible and easy.

Hernia of the umbilical cord appears as a relatively small protrusion in the umbilical area (Figure 21.1). The umbilical cord inserts into the left side of the defect. The inner lining of

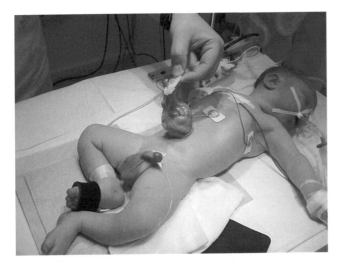

Figure 21.1   *Hernia of the cord, containing only midgut.*

the membrane is peritoneum, while the outer lining is amnion. Through the membrane, the intestines are seen.

Treatment

Operation is carried out in the first days of life. The membrane is excised, sparing the clamped umbilical cord. An omphalo-enteric duct is resected if present. The fascia is closed in the midline and the skin is sutured, if needed, after mobilization, but tension is rare. The umbilicus is preserved in the middle.

Discharge is usually possible on the day after surgery, but it is reasonable to perform ultrasonography as a screen for other anomalies, although they are rare.

Complications

Complications are rare. Sometimes, delivery staff, not realizing the nature of the anomaly, will clamp the sac instead of just the cord, which may result in injury to the intestine inside. Any injury will be looked for and repaired during surgery.

EXOMPHALOS

- Incidence: one in 7000 live births.
- Large defect.
- Contains much more than midgut, always including the liver and occasionally the stomach, spleen and large bowel.
- Non-rotation and non-fixation are part of the anomaly.
- The liver may be totally extra-abdominal, taking the vena cava with it. Instant reduction may result in total obstruction of the venous return, with intraoperative death, so primary closure is only rarely possible.
- Associated anomalies, which can be in any organ system, are very frequent (over 50 per cent).
- High proportion of chromosomal anomalies.

An exomphalos appears as a large membrane-covered bulge in the umbilical region. It is hemispherical, with a diameter of 5–12 cm. The umbilical cord usually inserts on the left side. The viscera are visible through the membrane. The liver occupies the majority of the space (Figure 21.2), with some intestines being seen in the lower part.

Treatment

An attempt at primary closure may be made if the volume and nature of the prolapsed viscera seem to allow it, but it is mostly unwise, because the distance between the borders of the rectus muscles is almost always too big. Closure with too high an intra-abdominal pressure will lead to deficient venous return, severe respiratory trouble and risk of intestinal ischaemia (abdominal compartment syndrome). As mentioned above, reduction of the liver may also be dangerous and possibly life-threatening. Slow, gradual reduction over several days is possible without danger, however. A nasogastric

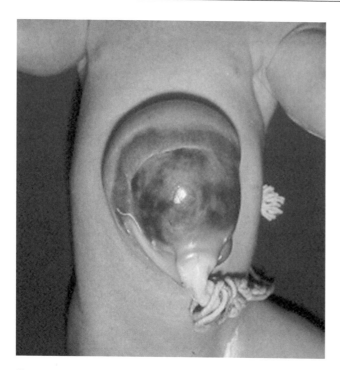

Figure 21.2 *Exomphalos major. A broad rim of skin is seen upon the amniotic sac. The liver is seen clearly through the sac.*

tube for drainage and monitoring of the abdominal pressure are important during this course. The main principle is still closure as early as possible, because of the danger of intraperitoneal infection by prolonged treatment.

Radical treatment of the abdominal wall defect is uncalled for if other lethal anomalies have been detected.

There are various options at hand for delayed closure:

- *Conservative treatment:* the sac is painted with disinfectant, and the development of an eschar is awaited. Gradually, the amniotic surface will be epithelialized, and at a later stage a secondary closure is attempted. This may take several stages and may continue for many years. Because of the long duration of this treatment, and because there is considerable morbidity and even mortality, it has largely been abandoned. It is the only option in really huge exomphalos.
- *Primary covering with skin:* this also has largely been abandoned. In this procedure, the skin is mobilized and closed over the viscera. The ventral hernia is closed later. The abdominal cavity will often still be too small, however, because the viscera have been placed under the skin, but on top of the rectus muscles.
- *Covering with prosthetic material:* suturing of prosthetic material to tissue lasts for only a short time (7–12 days), and it is important that the viscera are reduced and a full-layer closure achieved within that time. At the primary operation, the abdominal wall is stretched manually. If necessary, the intestines are emptied by irrigation to decrease their volume and facilitate

reduction. The method implies suturing of a 'chimney' containing the viscera to the fascia borders. Originally, silastic sheeting was used, being sutured into shape, but any tissue-neutral material may be used, such as blood bags, which are already shaped. The volume of the bag is then reduced gradually over the following period by strapping, clamping or suturing. The intra-abdominal pressure is monitored, starting in the operating room and continuing at the reduction sessions twice daily. Experience shows that the abdominal cavity will stretch surprisingly quickly. This method can be modified by suturing the prosthesis to the skin and retaining the intact amniotic sac, which will then be inverted gradually into the abdomen. However, the abdominal contents then cannot be inspected, and sometimes an anomaly may be missed.

- *Strapping the natural cover, i.e. the exomphalos sac:* this is possible sometimes and will make the prosthetic material unnecessary. If the sac seems reasonably sturdy, then this method should be the first choice. No anaesthesia is needed, but it is still important to monitor the abdominal pressure. The umbilical cord is lifted and cotton tape, about 1 cm wide, is strapped around the sac from above, thus reducing the viscera into the abdomen. The umbilical cord should be suspended without tension with tape from the roof of the incubator. The reduction procedure is repeated twice daily in the same manner as with the prosthetic bag. If the sac ruptures before full reduction is achieved, then it may be necessary to convert to a prosthetic bag (which, of course, requires anaesthesia).

Postoperative management

Since the management, irrespective of the method used, will always result in a period of increased abdominal pressure and respiratory problems, ventilatory assistance will be needed, at least for some days. It is usually necessary to start parenteral nutrition, but usually this is needed for only a short time.

There is some risk of infection, although rarely peritoneal, and antibiotic prophylaxis is indicated.

Prognosis

Prognosis is dependent largely on the associated anomalies. If no serious anomalies are present and no serious complications have occurred, then the child may have a perfectly normal life.

GASTROSCHISIS

- Incidence: one in 5000 live births.
- Small defect (<4 cm).
- Midgut protruding. Sometimes bits of other viscera may protrude (even including the testes).

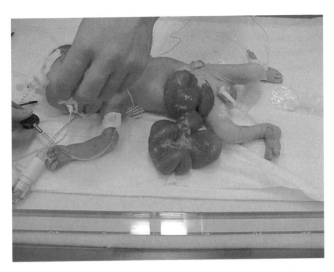

Figure 21.3   *Gastroschisis: the intestines are partly covered in fibrin and are thickened.*

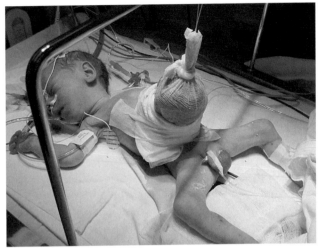

Figure 21.4   *Gastroschisis: staged closure with suspended bag, covered with towels.*

- Non-rotation and non-fixation are part of the anomaly.
- The intestines may be dilated, thickened and covered with a thick fibrin peel.
- Primary closure is mostly, but not always, possible.
- There is a risk of dehydration in the perioperative period.
- Associated anomalies outside the prolapsed viscera are rare. Intestinal atresia occurs in five to ten per cent (this is a complication rather than an anomaly).
- Closure should be undertaken as a semi-emergency ('immediately' after birth, but not necessarily between midnight and morning).

The midgut protrudes through a rather small defect, usually to the right of the umbilical cord (Figure 21.3) There is usually a small skin-covered bridge between the defect and the cord. The appearance of the intestines varies. They can be quite normal, or they can be dilated, thickened and covered with a thick fibrinous peel. At times, it is an inseparable mass. The intestinal changes are due to the narrow passage through the defect, with kinking of the intestine and compression of the mesentery and local intestinal ischaemia. The fibrinous cover is due to the contact with the amniotic fluid, especially in the final period, when increasing faecal matter is added. Occasionally, the intestinal ischaemia is so pronounced and so protracted that an atresia results.

Treatment

'Immediate' reduction and closure are indicated. In selected cases (i.e. when the intestines are not thickened and there is no peel), it may be possible to reduce the intestine without anaesthesia and cover the defect with the umbilical cord, secured with a suture (not compulsory). Obviously, this is possible only with gentle manipulation and only if the baby accepts it without crying. Alternatively, the bowel can be placed in a preformed silo while spontaneous reduction is awaited.

In other cases, the procedure is done under anaesthesia. If necessary, the bowel is emptied by irrigation. The abdominal wall is stretched digitally and the bowel reduced. If this cannot be done through the existing opening, then a midline incision upwards is indicated. If the viscera are fused together, then no attempt at separation should be made, even though an atresia might be present in the mass. A clearly visible atresia should be treated with primary anastomosis or temporary enterostomy, according to the circumstances. Abdominal testes should be brought down. The fascia is closed in the midline, and the skin is sutured. The umbilical cord is preserved.

The abdominal pressure is monitored. If reduction and closure cannot be achieved without undue pressure, then a bag should be constructed (Figure 21.4), as described for exomphalos, with continued reduction over the following days in the same way.

Postoperative management

Ventilatory assistance may be necessary, at least for some days. Parenteral nutrition is needed, on average, for three weeks but in favourable cases for seven to ten days and in rare cases for several months. This is due to impaired intestinal function, which seems to be rarer since the advent of antenatal scanning and preterm delivery. Oral feeding must be started, even in minimal doses, as soon as peristalsis begins, because this stimulation helps to restore normal function and prevent liver damage from cholestasis.

The intestinal malfunction may simulate obstruction by an atresia, and further investigation and second look should be done only if there are no signs of function at least three weeks after the primary operation.

Prognosis

There is some mortality from complications – mostly infections and other complications of prolonged parenteral nutrition – but survival should be over 90 per cent. If there is no permanent intestinal damage, then a totally normal life can be expected.

CLINICAL SCENARIOS

Case 1

A full-term boy is born, weighing 3500 g. He has an obvious hernia of the umbilical cord. The cord is clamped with care, away from the membrane. There are no other visible anomalies, and the baby is otherwise well, with fine Apgar scores. It is Saturday. The baby is allowed to suck. On the following Monday, the membrane is removed, the intestines are inspected and found to be normal, and all layers of the abdominal wall are closed. He is discharged the following day.

Case 2

At antenatal scanning at 26 weeks, a large exomphalos containing liver and intestinal loops is found. A ventricular septal defect is also diagnosed, and the baby is clearly small for dates. The parents are informed of the various possibilities, and they accept amniotic fluid sampling as advised. The karyotyping shows trisomy 18, and the parents are informed that their child will not be able to live beyond the neonatal period. They are also informed that termination of the pregnancy is no longer possible. Spontaneous intrauterine death occurs in 29 week, and a stillborn child is delivered. Psychological support is provided for the family.

Case 3

The antenatal scan at 16 weeks' gestation shows clear gastroschisis, with intestinal loops in the amniotic fluid. No other anomalies are detected. The parents are informed about the diagnosis and the good expected outcome, provided that no complications occur. They decide to continue the pregnancy. At 26 weeks' gestation, the scan is repeated every two weeks. At 32 weeks, dilation of some of the intestinal loops is noted; this is increased at 34 weeks. At 36 weeks, a marked thickening of the intestinal walls can be seen. The Doppler scan shows intestinal circulation, but to be on the safe side delivery is induced medically. An otherwise normal girl is born, with birth weight 2250 g. There are dilated and slightly thickened loops, but otherwise the intestines are normal, soft and pliable, and without peel. The baby is stable and without electrolyte derangement. At operation four hours after delivery, reduction and primary closure are achieved with no difficulty. Parenteral nutrition is instituted and ventilatory assistance is provided for two days. After two days, small amounts of breast milk are offered; the amounts are increased over the next week. Parenteral nutrition can be discontinued after ten days. The baby is moved to the surgical ward after eight days and discharged after 13 days. She is followed in the outpatient clinic for the next year, and is thriving and well.

REFERENCES

Nielsen OH, Kvist N, Brocks V. Abdominal wall defects in the era of prenatal diagnosis. *Pediatric Surgery International* 1995; **11**: 4–7.

Shaw A. The myth of gastroschisis. *Journal of Pediatric Surgery* 1975; **10**: 235–44.

FURTHER READING

Cooney DR. Defects of the abdominal wall. In: O'Neill JA, Rowe MI, Grosfeld JL, Fonkalsrud EW, Coran AG (eds). *Pediatric Surgery*, 5th edn. St Louis, MO: Mosby, 1998; pp. 1045–69.

22

Infantile hypertrophic pyloric stenosis

PAUL KH TAM AND KENNETH KY WONG

Learning objectives

- To understand the pathology and possible pathogenesis of infantile hypertrophic pyloric stenosis.
- To know the clinical features and imaging studies for diagnosis of infantile hypertrophic pyloric stenosis.
- To understand and to be able to correct the preoperative fluid and electrolyte abnormalities.
- To be familiar with the operative procedure of pyloric stenosis.

INTRODUCTION

Infantile hypertrophic pyloric stenosis is the most common surgical cause of non-bilious vomiting in infancy. The aetiology remains poorly understood. Once an invariably lethal condition, it is now associated with an almost negligible mortality rate. The main reason for this remarkable success was undoubtedly Ramstedt's introduction of pyloromyotomy as a simple, effective surgical cure. Results of treatment have been enhanced further by earlier diagnosis, improved preoperative management and safer neonatal anaesthesia. Laparoscopic pyloromyotomy has been introduced as an alternative treatment to open surgery. Nevertheless, morbidity has not been eliminated totally.

The incidence of pyloric stenosis is around two to three per 1000 live births in Caucasians, but it is lower (one per 1000) in Negroes and Asians. An increasing incidence was observed in the UK and the USA in the 1970s and 1980s, but more recently a decreasing incidence has been reported in Sweden. There is a male preponderance, with an average male/female ratio of four to one. Firstborns are more often affected and comprise 40–60 per cent of all cases.

Associated anomalies consisting mainly of urinary tract anomalies occur in one to 20 per cent. Association with Smith–Lemli–Opitz syndrome and various chromosomal disorders, including trisomy 18, trisomy 21 and Turner syndrome, is well documented. Association with asymptomatic joint hypermobility suggests a systemic abnormality of extracellular matrix. Familial occurrence is well described. With an affected mother, there is a 20 per cent risk for a son and a seven per cent risk for a daughter to develop pyloric stenosis. With an affected father, the respective risks are five and 2.5 per cent. The neuronal nitric oxide synthase (*NOS1*) gene has been described as a susceptible locus for pyloric stenosis.

Many hypotheses have been postulated for the pathogenesis of pyloric stenosis. A neurogenic origin is supported by findings of a reduction of non-adrenergic, non-cholinergic inhibitory nerves, especially those containing nitric oxide synthase and various neuropeptides, such as substance P and vasoactive intestinal peptide. The nerve-supporting cells, interstitial cells of Cajal (pacemaker cells) and nerve growth factor are all deficient in pyloric stenosis. There is also abnormal regulation of smooth muscle cells by growth factors such as transforming growth factor beta, insulin-like growth factor 1, epidermal growth factor and platelet-derived growth factor. However, it remains unclear whether these findings are primary or secondary.

The characteristic biochemical change is hypochloraemic alkalosis. This is mainly a result of excessive loss of gastric fluids rich in hydrogen and chloride (130–150 mmol/L), along with smaller sodium (60–100 mmol/L) and potassium (10–15 mmol/L) losses. In established pyloric stenosis, the patient is dehydrated, serum pH and bicarbonate levels are elevated, and the serum chloride and, to lesser extents, potassium and sodium levels are lowered.

Initially, alkaline urine is excreted to compensate for metabolic alkalosis. As dehydration worsens, maintenance of extracellular volume through sodium conservation becomes a more important priority. Increased sodium resorption by the renal tubules results in potassium loss, which is compensated by hydrogen excretion, resulting in paradoxical aciduria. Bicarbonate resorption, accompanying sodium resorption and hypokalaemia aggravate the alkalosis, setting up a vicious circle.

CLINICAL FEATURES AND DIAGNOSIS

The typical presentation is non-bilious vomiting, which usually begins at three to four weeks of age. The vomit is effortless, is not forcefully projectile at the start but soon becomes so, and is not preceded by discomfort. The child appears to be hungry all the time and feeds voraciously. There is an average delay of several days before the infant is admitted to hospital. Occasionally, there may be haematemesis due to oesophagitis. Rarely, vomiting starts as early as the first week of life and sometimes as late as several months. Late presentation is not uncommon in preterm infants, and often their vomiting is not projectile. Recognition of the condition may be delayed in patients with associated congenital anomalies or confounding medical conditions.

Constipation, passage of greenish 'hungry stool', 'starvation diarrhoea', failure to thrive, weight loss, lethargy, wasting and severe dehydration are clinical features related to starvation and persistent vomiting. These should be seen seldom nowadays. Jaundice is found in two to five per cent of patients as a result of unconjugated hyperbilirubinaemia secondary to hepatic glucuronyl transferase deficiency.

The infant has a worried look when he or she is about to vomit. Visible gastric contractions passing from left to right across the epigastrium are suggestive but not pathognomonic of pyloric stenosis. The definitive sign of pyloric stenosis is a palpable olive-shaped mass ('tumour') in the right upper quadrant. The infant's stomach should be emptied before the examination. The hand of the examiner should be placed in the epigastrium of the supine infant. Gentle deep palpation below the liver edge reveals the 'tumour', which can often be rolled under the fingers, like feeling a walnut through a blanket. A small feed with dextrose water (the 'test feed') facilitates the examination by

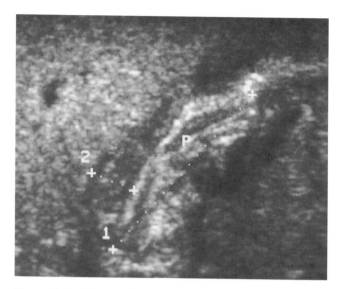

Figure 22.1 *Ultrasound image with a longitudinal view of the hypertrophic pylorus, showing an elongated pyloric canal (P) of length 21.6 mm (marked 1) and thickened pyloric muscle of thickness 4.6 mm (marked 2).*

relaxing the infant's abdominal muscles and stimulating the hypertrophied pylorus to contract and harden. For the inexperienced examiner, the caudate lobe of the liver and the upper pole of the kidney may occasionally be mistaken for a hypertrophied pylorus.

Imaging studies are required only in cases of uncertain clinical diagnosis. There is a worrying trend that increased reliance on imaging studies has resulted in declining clinical skills in the diagnosis of pyloric stenosis. Ultrasonography has now replaced barium-meal examination as the investigation of choice. The main advantages of ultrasonography are that it is non-ionizing and non-invasive and can be repeated safely in cases of evolving pyloric stenosis. However, the accuracy of ultrasonography is dependent on the expertise available. The diagnostic criteria of pyloric stenosis on ultrasound examination are: (i) pyloric muscle thickness greater than 4 mm, (ii) pyloric canal longer than 18 mm and (iii) non-passage of fluid into the duodenum despite vigorous gastric peristalsis (Figure 22.1).

Contrast studies for the diagnosis of pyloric stenosis have been in use since 1932. The typical findings are a distended stomach with delayed passage of contrast through an elongated, narrow pyloric canal – the 'string sign' (Figure 22.2). Other ancillary signs include the 'beak sign', representing the beginning of the elongated pyloric canal, the 'mucosal nipple sign', from the protrusion of the redundant pyloric mucosa into the antrum, the 'shoulder sign', produced by the impression of the hypertrophied pyloric muscle on the distal antrum, and the 'double-track sign', caused by barium encircling the thickened pyloric mucosa. One advantage of using contrast examination is to evaluate the possibilities of gastro-oesophageal reflux and malrotation as alternative causes of infantile vomiting.

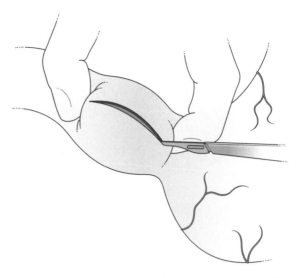

Figure 22.3 *The incision is made along the length of the pyloric tumour on the relatively avascular anterosuperior aspect.*

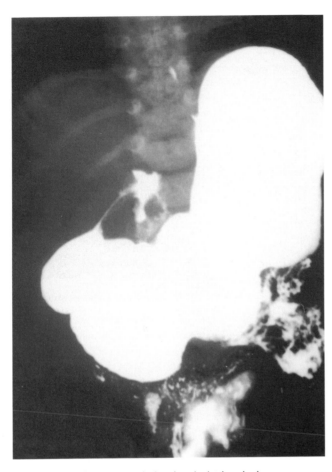

Figure 22.2 *Contrast meal, showing the 'string sign'.*

Upper-gastrointestinal endoscopy has been used for the diagnosis of pyloric stenosis. Conditions such as reflux oesophagitis also can be evaluated. However, since the procedure requires expertise and is invasive, its use remains limited.

TREATMENT

The standard treatment for pyloric stenosis is surgery. Proper preoperative preparation is the key to a successful surgical outcome. Oral feeding is discontinued and a nasogastric tube is passed to decompress the stomach and allow gastric losses to be measured. Dehydration and biochemical abnormalities should be corrected by intravenous fluid and electrolyte administration. The characteristic biochemical change is hypochloraemic alkalosis. The major electrolyte deficits are chloride and sodium. Potassium becomes depleted in advanced cases. These electrolytes should be replaced accordingly. A useful regimen is as follows:

1 *Mild dehydration/alkalosis:* 130 mL 0.45% saline/5% dextrose/kg/day plus replacement of gastric loss with an equal volume of normal saline with KCl 20 mmol/L. Add 40 mmol KCl to each litre of infused fluid. Check serum electrolytes and acid/base after 12–24 hours. Revert to

maintenance fluids when the HCO_3 is less than 25 mmol/L.

2 *Moderate dehydration/alkalosis:* 150 mL 0.45% saline/ 5% dextrose/kg/day plus replacement of gastric loss with an equal volume of normal saline with KCl 20 mmol/L. Add 40 mmol KCl to each litre of infused fluid. Check serum electrolytes and acid/base after 12–24 hours. Revert to usual maintenance fluids when HCO_3 is less than 25 mmol/L.

3 *Severe dehydration/biochemical changes:* similar to regimen 2, plus any other resuscitation measures as necessary.

Ramstedt's pyloromyotomy remains the procedure of choice. The standard approach is a transverse incision made in the right upper quadrant midway between the xiphisternum and the umbilicus, extending from the lateral border of the rectus towards the costal margin. After the external oblique aponeurosis is incised, the rectus may be split vertically or transversely. Alternatively, an umbilical incision may be used to give better cosmesis. The skin is incised above the umbilicus for 50–75 per cent of its circumference. The incision is then deepened on to the linea alba and can be extended superiorly or laterally for greater access.

On entering the peritoneal cavity, the firm pyloric 'olive' is identified readily by palpation and is delivered out of the wound using atraumatic tissue-holding forceps. Once delivered, the pylorus is held between the surgeon's left thumb and index finger (Figure 22.3).

An incision is made along the length of the pyloric mass on its relatively avascular anterosuperior aspect, down to the superficial part of the hypertrophied muscle. The risk of perforation is greatest at the site where the duodenal mucosal fold projects into the pylorus. The external landmark of the distal limit of the incision is the white line just proximal to the prepyloric vein, and the position is confirmed by invaginating

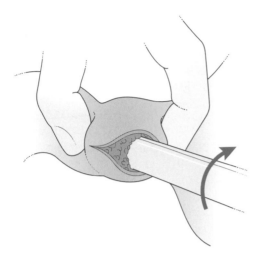

Figure 22.4 *The blunt end of a scalpel handle is inserted into the hypertrophied muscle along the length of the incision until it comes against the mucosa. It is then turned through 90 degrees, allowing the mucosa to bulge out, thus relieving the obstruction.*

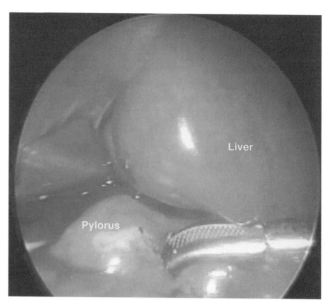

Figure 22.5 *Laparoscopic view, showing hypertrophied pyloric muscle being split with a spreader. See also colour Plate 3.*

the duodenal lumen against the gritty pyloric mass with the surgeon's left thumb. Proximally, the incision should extend well up on to the antrum. The blunt end of an empty scalpel handle is inserted into the hypertrophied muscle with its flat surface along the length of the incision until it comes against the mucosa. It is then turned through 90 degrees, splitting the muscle and allowing the mucosa to bulge out (Figure 22.4). Alternatively, a pair of artery forceps (with tips pointing upwards) or a pyloric spreader can be used for completion of the myotomy. Mucosal perforation is tested by injecting air into the stomach via the nasogastric tube. If present, it should be repaired with interrupted absorbable sutures with or without an omental patch. Minor oozing from venous engorgement at the myotomy site will usually stop when the pylorus is returned to the peritoneal cavity. The wound is closed with strong slow-absorbing sutures, and the skin is closed using an absorbable subcuticular suture.

Recently, the technique of laparoscopic pyloromyotomy has been advocated. In brief, a pneumoperitoneum of 8–10 mmHg is created and three 4-mm ports consisting of a telescope in the umbilicus and an instrumentation cannula in each upper quadrant are used. An atraumatic grasper is inserted into the right port to fix the duodenum. A retractable knife is inserted into the left port for the myotomy incision. The myotomy is completed as in the open procedure, using a special laparoscopic pyloric spreader (Figure 22.5). Some surgeons prefer to grasp the stomach from the patient's left and perform the pyloromyotomy from the patient's right. Completion of myotomy is indicated by bulging of the mucosa upon compression of the ends of the myotomy towards each other, or instillation of air via the nasogastric tube.

There are several postoperative feeding regimens after pyloromyotomy, which differ in the time of introduction of feeds and the speed with which full feeds are established. The reason for withholding feeds in the early postoperative period

is based on previous manometric findings that gastric peristalsis is absent in the initial four to six hours and is depressed for an additional 16–24 hours. Earlier feeding hence increases the incidence of vomiting. However, prolonged fasting in a hungry baby often results in more distress, and many authors have now advocated the use of *ad libitum* feeding. In studies comparing the use of *ad libitum* feeding and traditional methods, patients on *ad libitum* feeding experienced more postoperative emesis but tolerated full feedings sooner. Furthermore, no patient required additional therapy or readmission after discharge.

Alternatives to pyloromyotomy for the treatment of pyloric stenosis have also been described. These include pyloric traumamyoplasty, endoscopic balloon dilation and intravenous atropine treatment, but none is practised widely.

RESULTS AND OUTCOME

Results of surgical treatment of pyloric stenosis are highly satisfactory. Symptomatic relief is complete, and most patients are discharged within 24–48 hours postoperatively. Mortality is virtually zero, and most complications are minor.

Minor degrees of postoperative vomiting are not uncommon and need not deter feeding. Persistent and severe postoperative vomiting, however, should alert clinicians to underlying problems such as gastritis, reflux oesophagitis, mucosal perforation or incomplete myotomy. Wound infection remains the most common complication (one to ten per cent). The umbilicus is an important source of infection and should be sterilized meticulously. Wound dehiscence, incisional hernia and mucosal perforations are technical complications and typically occur more frequently when treatment is provided by general rather than paediatric surgeons. Myotomy bleeding, inadequate myotomy and negative laparotomy are complications encountered rarely.

There is a learning curve with laparoscopic pyloromyotomy, which means initially higher complication rates and longer operating times than with open pyloromyotomy. These disadvantages can be eliminated with increasing expertise of the laparoscopic procedure. In a recent review including a total of 266 patients, the average operating time was 25 minutes, the mucosal perforation rate was three per cent and the inadequate myotomy rate was 0.8 per cent. Advantages of the laparoscopic approach include superior cosmetic result, decreased wound infection and shortened hospital stay.

The sonographic appearance of the pylorus returns to normal within a few months of pyloromyotomy. There are conflicting data on long-term sequelae after pyloromyotomy, but even when abnormalities of pyloric motility can be demonstrated, patients appear well-compensated and few have clinical symptoms.

CLINICAL SCENARIO

A three-week-old male baby was admitted with a history of feeding problems due to recurrent vomiting for a week. The baby was a first-born child, with no significant antenatal history. He had had normal feeds and weight gain in the first two weeks of life, but by the third week he had developed non-bile-stained vomiting. His mother said that he was willing to feed, but 'projectile' vomiting was the invariable result. She took him to their general practitioner, who advised a change in the infant formula. There was no improvement, and the baby began to lose weight and had reduced urine output and bowel motions. He was then referred to a children's hospital.

Physical examination showed a crying baby with features of mild dehydration and visible gastric peristalsis. A junior doctor was unable to detect any abnormalities on abdominal palpation, but a senior doctor felt a palpable mass ('olive') in the epigastrium when a test feed was administered.

A clinical diagnosis of infantile hypertrophic pyloric stenosis was made. Blood tests revealed Na^+ 134 mmol/L, Cl^- 98 mmol/L, K^+ 3.3 mmol/L, HCO_3^- 30.6 mmol/L and pH 7.49. Ultrasound examination demonstrated marked thickening and elongation of the pylorus, thus confirming the diagnosis. The baby was resuscitated with intravenous fluids and replacement of the electrolyte losses. Biochemical normality was restored two days later, and Ramstedt's pyloromyotomy was carried out. Intraoperatively, a hypertrophied pylorus was found. Postoperatively, *ad libitum* feeding was resumed. The patient made an uneventful recovery and was discharged the following day.

FURTHER READING

Breaux CW, Jr, Hood JS, Georgeson KE. The significance of alkalosis and hypochloremia in hypertrophic pyloric stenosis. *Journal of Pediatric Surgery* 1989; **24**: 1250–52.

Downey EC, Jr. Laparoscopic pyloromyotomy. *Seminars in Pediatric Surgery* 1998; **17**: 220–24.

Carpenter RO, Schaffer RL, Maeso CE, *et al*. Postoperative ad lib feeding for hypertrophic pyloric stenosis. *Journal of Pediatric Surgery* 1999; **34**: 959–61.

Ohshiro K, Puri P. Pathogenesis of infantile hypertrophic pyloric stenosis: recent progress. *Pediatric Surgery International* 1998; **13**: 243–52.

Pranikoff T, Campbell BT, Travis J, Hirschl RB. Differences in outcome with subspecialty care: pyloromyotomy in North Carolina. *Journal of Pediatric Surgery* 2002; **37**: 352–6.

23

Intussusception

ELERI L CUSICK AND MARK N WOODWARD

Learning objectives

- To understand the pathogenesis of intussusception.
- To recognize and investigate a possible case of intussusception.
- To safely instigate non-operative and operative management of intussusception.
- To be aware of atypical presentations.

INTRODUCTION

Intussusception occurs when one segment of intestine (the intussusceptum) invaginates into the lumen of the adjacent more distal intestine (the intussuscipiens) (Figure 23.1). It is the most common cause of intestinal obstruction in infants and young children. Originally described in 1793 by John Hunter, intussusception remained a generally fatal condition until the late 1800s, when the first successful operative and hydrostatic reductions were described.

INCIDENCE

Intussusception occurs most commonly between the ages of two months and two years, with 50 per cent of cases occurring between three and ten months of age, and 65 per cent of cases occurring before age one year. There is a male/female preponderance of three to two. The reported incidence varies between 1.5 and four cases per 1000 live births.

PATHOGENESIS

Most cases do not have an identifiable cause, but seasonal clustering in spring and winter suggests a link with viral respiratory and enteric infections more common at these times. In addition, the incidence of intussusception was increased in the USA in association with the introduction of rotavirus vaccine in 1998, strongly supporting a causal relationship and resulting in withdrawal of the vaccine after one year (Peter and Myers 2002).

The lamina propria of the small intestine is a loose areolar network extending between intestinal glands and into the core of the villi, and containing scattered lymphocytes and isolated lymphatic nodules. These nodules are more numerous in the

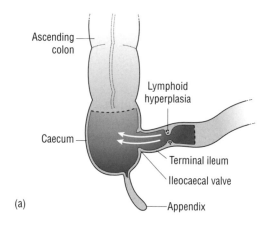

Ascending colon

Lymphoid hyperplasia

Caecum

Terminal ileum

Ileocaecal valve

Appendix

(a)

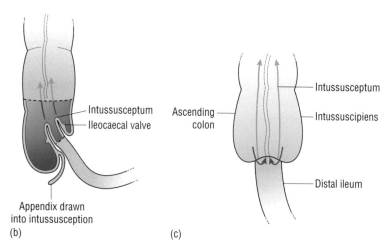

Intussusceptum
Ileocaecal valve

Appendix drawn into intussusception
(b)

Ascending colon

Intussusceptum

Intussuscipiens

Distal ileum

(c)

Figure 23.1 *In typical 'idiopathic' intussusception, lymphoid hyperplasia within the lamina propria of the terminal ileum (a) acts as a lead point. The resultant intussusceptum is peristalsed through the ileocaecal valve, drawing in the appendix (b), and progresses distally into the ascending colon (c).*

distal small intestine and may be sufficiently large as to occupy the whole mucosa. Visible masses of this lymphoid tissue may occur along the anti-mesenteric border of the ileum, up to 2 cm in length, and are known as Peyer's patches. Lymphoid hyperplasia within the intestine may result in enlarged Peyer's patches, which serve as the lead point for intussusception in 'idiopathic' cases (Figures 23.1 and 23.2).

The intussusceptum usually arises in the distal ileum and passes through the ileocaecal valve into the colon. As the intussusceptum progresses, distension of the distal encasing intestine and compression of the proximal internal intestine occurs. The accompanying mesentery will eventually be drawn into the distal bowel and also compressed, with resulting venous congestion and bowel wall oedema. Arterial obstruction will supervene if this is not relieved, with ensuing necrosis of the incarcerated proximal intestine.

A pathological lead point is a recognizable abnormality within the bowel that predisposes to intussusception and is present in two to eight per cent of cases. Small-bowel polyps (e.g. Peutz–Jeghers syndrome), submucosal haematomas, duplication cysts, Meckel's diverticula and small-bowel lymphoma are among the more common of these conditions. Intussusception may also be seen in Henoch–Schönlein purpura, as a result of submucosal haematoma, and in cystic

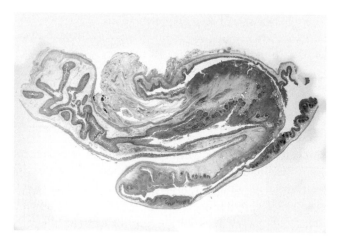

Figure 23.2 *Longitudinal section through terminal ileum following resection for irreducible intussusception, demonstrating ulcerated mucosa at the apex of the intussusceptum.*

fibrosis, secondary to inspissated stool. Pathological lead points occur more commonly outside the typical age range (over 20 per cent of children over two years of age have a pathological lead point) and should be actively sought in patients with recurrent intussusception.

CLINICAL PRESENTATION

The classic presentation is the sudden onset of symptoms in a previously well infant between five and nine months of age. Between 80 and 100 per cent of affected infants have colicky abdominal pain, usually with episodes of screaming and drawing up of the legs every 15–20 minutes and complete recovery in between. Vomiting is seen in 80 per cent; this may be an early reflex feature or bilious if complete obstruction has occurred. The passage of blood and mucus per rectum ('redcurrant jelly') may be seen in up to 60 per cent, whilst a smaller proportion (20 per cent) will simply have diarrhoea. The complete triad of vomiting, colicky pain and bloody stools is seen in approximately only one-third of patients. Occasionally, infants will present to the admitting paediatrician with severe lethargy and features suggestive of meningitis.

PHYSICAL EXAMINATION

If medical advice is sought early, then there may be little to find on clinical examination between bouts of pain, although careful abdominal examination in a quiet cooperative infant may reveal the presence of a right upper quadrant sausage-shaped mass in 60–80 per cent of cases. Rarely, the intussusceptum is visible on perineal inspection or palpable on digital rectal examination.

If there has been delay in seeking medical attention, then dehydration may have supervened, with a profoundly lethargic child with clinical signs indicative of dehydration or shock: tachycardia and prolonged capillary refill. Inspection of the nappy may reveal bloody stool, or this may be prompted by rectal examination. The presence of overt toxicity with fever and tachycardia reflects bacteraemia secondary to vascular compromise of the intussuscepted bowel.

INVESTIGATION

If the diagnosis is suspected, then the gold-standard radiological investigation is abdominal ultrasound, with a sensitivity of over 98 per cent and a specificity of 100 per cent in experienced hands (Shanbhogue *et al.* 1994). The characteristic finding is a 'target sign' on transverse section, consisting of two concentric rings of low echogenicity separated by a hyperechoic ring (Figure 23.3). The 'pseudo-kidney' sign is seen on longitudinal section and comprises superimposed hyper- and hypo-echoic layers representing the oedematous bowel walls of the intussusception (Figure 23.4). The amount of free fluid within the peritoneal cavity can be determined, and Doppler can be used to record blood flow within the intussusception.

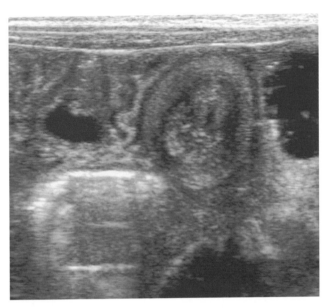

Figure 23.3 *Abdominal ultrasound, showing a central 'target-sign' appearance produced by the intussusceptum within the intussuscipiens.*

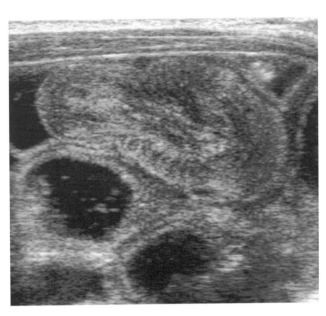

Figure 23.4 *Abdominal ultrasound, showing 'pseudo-kidney' appearance of intussusception in longitudinal section.*

Plain abdominal X-ray may show evidence of small-bowel obstruction (Figure 23.5) or rarely the classic appearance of the intussusceptum as an opacity within the gas-filled distal bowel (Figure 23.6). However, it should be remembered that the most common finding is a normal plain film. Rarely, where diagnostic doubt remains following ultrasonography, contrast enema may be diagnostic as well as therapeutic.

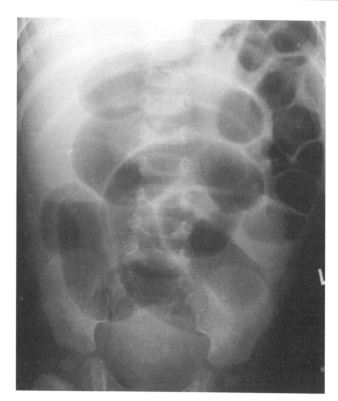

Figure 23.5   *Plain abdominal X-ray, showing multiple dilated small-bowel loops in an infant with small-bowel obstruction secondary to intussusception.*

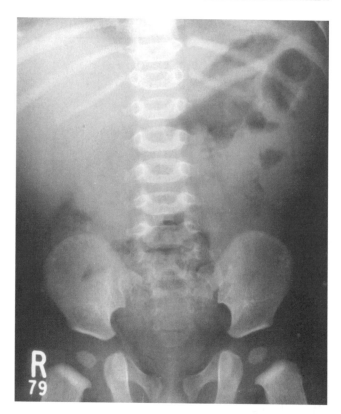

Figure 23.6   *Plain abdominal X-ray, showing the appearances of a right upper quadrant opacity, produced by the intussusceptum within the proximal transverse colon.*

NON-OPERATIVE MANAGEMENT

Intravenous access should be obtained and a nasogastric tube inserted if the infant is vomiting. A minimum fluid bolus of 20 ml/kg NaCl should be given before attempted reduction of the intussusception, and suitable intravenous antibiotics should be started, e.g. cefuroxime and metronidazole. Sedation for the procedure is rarely necessary.

Traditionally, barium was used in conjunction with fluoroscopy both to make the diagnosis of intussusception and for hydrostatic reduction; however, this has largely been superseded by the use of air, which is equally efficacious and causes minimal contamination if perforation occurs (Kirks 1995). More recently, saline reduction with or without ultrasound screening has been described; however, use of this is not currently widespread.

If 'air-enema' reduction is to be performed, then a member of the surgical team should be in the department with a cannula available to relieve the tension pneumoperitoneum that may occur following perforation and to help look after the child. Reduction is performed in accordance with guidelines produced by the British Society of Paediatric Radiology (www.bspr.org.uk/intuss.htm). The child is held immobile, a straight catheter is inserted into the rectum, and the buttocks are taped. The catheter is connected to a pressure-monitoring device with a cut-off at 120 mmHg. Initial attempts at reduction are made with pressures of 80–100 mmHg, usually with up to three attempts of three minutes' duration. The progress of the intussusceptum can be followed with intermittent fluoroscopic screening (Figure 23.7). A combined maximum of 15 minutes of attempted reduction is usually sufficient: over 90 per cent of successful reductions are performed with screening times of less than ten minutes.

Air-enema reduction is successful in 75–80 per cent of cases. This is confirmed radiologically with reflux of air back into the small intestine (Figure 23.8) (Palder *et al.* 1991). The child may take on a more normal colour and fall asleep. Failure of reduction is more likely to occur if symptoms have been present for more than 48 hours. Occasionally, the ileo-caecal valve may be oedematous, thus preventing air reflux; in this situation, a repeat ultrasound scan may be performed to confirm reduction. If reduction is unsuccessful but the patient is stable, then repeat reduction may be attempted two to four hours later. If reduction is successful, then the child is usually kept nil by mouth for 12 hours before fluids are restarted. Antibiotics may be discontinued at 24 hours if the child is afebrile, and discharge is usually possible at 48 hours.

Contraindications to non-operative management

Surgery is indicated if there are signs of peritonitis, if an ileo-ileal intussusception is suspected, e.g. in postoperative

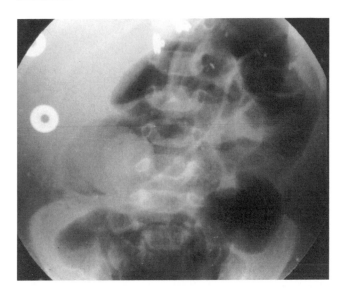

Figure 23.7 *Fluoroscopic appearances of the intussusceptum within the transverse colon during air-enema reduction.*

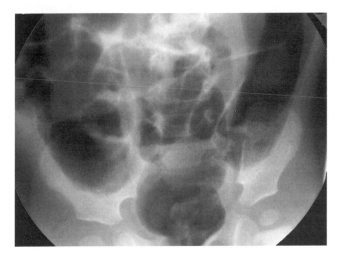

Figure 23.8 *Fluoroscopic appearances of multiple dilated small-bowel loops centrally, which arise following successful reduction of the intussusception.*

intussusception, and in a child with a condition such as Peutz–Jegher syndrome who develops intussusception.

OPERATIVE MANAGEMENT

Surgery is necessary if air-enema reduction fails and if a perforation is revealed during reduction.

A right-sided transverse muscle-cutting incision is made at the level of the umbilicus. The intussusceptum is palpated and reduced gently by pushing rather than pulling, attempting to avoid serosal injury (Figure 23.9). Following reduction, the bowel is inspected for viability and then palpated for lead points. The appendix is not removed routinely. It is usually

possible to start oral fluids 12–24 hours following operative reduction.

In 40–50 per cent of cases, reduction will be unsuccessful and/or the affected bowel may be necrotic; in this case, bowel resection is necessary (Figure 23.2) (Palder *et al.* 1991). This may take the form of a limited right hemi-colectomy with primary anastomosis, or simple resection and primary anastomosis of the reduced but non-viable section of small bowel that formed the apex of the intussusceptum. Fluids may be started when the postoperative ileus has resolved.

COMPLICATIONS AND OUTCOME

Perforation has been reported in approximately one per cent of air-enema reductions (Maoate and Beasley 1998). Massive abdominal distension secondary to pneumoperitoneum can cause rapid diaphragmatic splinting and respiratory compromise unless decompression is performed, but minimal peritoneal contamination is produced. Perforation is more likely in infants with a relatively long history (more than 48 hours).

Recurrence of intussusception is seen in five to seven per cent of cases. It occurs within 24 hours in 30 per cent, and within six months in 70 per cent, of affected cases. Recurrence may occur following either non-operative or operative reduction, but there are some data to suggest that recurrence is less likely following operative manual reduction. Children tend to present earlier with recurrent intussusception and are less unwell, often because their parents appreciate the significance of their symptoms more quickly. The success rate of air-enema reduction for recurrent episodes is comparable to that for initial episodes, even if previously this had failed and open manual reduction had been necessary.

Investigations for pathological lead points (including abdominal ultrasound and contrast studies) are usually performed if an infant under two years of age has more than two recurrences, and if a single recurrence occurs in a child over two years of age.

The mortality rate from intussusception has declined in recent years and currently is less than one per cent. Stringer *et al.* (1992) analysed the 33 deaths from intussusception in England and Wales that occurred between 1984 and 1989. They concluded that potentially avoidable factors contributing to death could be identified in almost two-thirds of cases. These factors included diagnostic delay (more than 24 hours), inadequate fluid resuscitation and antibiotic therapy, and delay in recognizing recurrent or residual intussusception following reduction.

POSTOPERATIVE INTUSSUSCEPTION

Postoperative intussusception is a rare form accounting for approximately five per cent of intussusceptions overall.

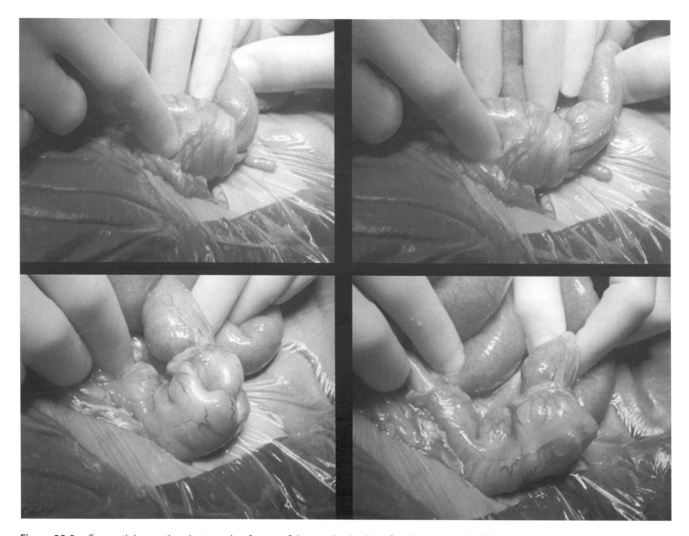

Figure 23.9 *Sequential operative photographs of successful manual reduction of an intussusception. The operating surgeon gently pushes on the apex of the intussusceptum, rather than applying proximal traction. See also Colour Plate 2.*

Postoperative intussusception may be seen following thoracic or abdominal surgery, particularly following retroperitoneal dissection, or if there has been a postoperative regimen of radio- and/or chemotherapy. The mechanism is unclear, but it is thought to occur as a consequence of proximal small-bowel peristalsis recovering when there is a persistent distal ileus.

The diagnosis requires a high index of suspicion, because usually the presentation is atypical, and it should be actively considered in any child who appears to have a prolonged ileus following surgery. Postoperative intussusception is usually ileo-ileal. Ultrasound scan is often diagnostic, although the diagnosis may be made at laparotomy for suspected adhesive small-bowel obstruction. Air- or contrast-enema reduction is usually unsuccessful, and the preferred treatment is operative reduction. Resection is rarely necessary, and there are no reports in the literature of recurrence after open simple manual reduction.

CLINICAL SCENARIOS

Case 1

A term infant presented at four months of age with a 14-hour history of vomiting, which initially had been clear but was subsequently bilious. He had been unsettled and had also passed a bloody stool. On admission, he was irritable but not dehydrated, with an abdominal mass palpable and frank blood in his nappy.

He was commenced on intravenous fluids, a nasogastric tube was passed and he was given intravenous antibiotics and morphine. Abdominal ultrasound scan confirmed the clinical diagnosis of intussusception. During air-enema, the apex of the intussusceptum was followed back until it was effaced in the caecum and the mass disappeared, but no air was observed to pass back into the small bowel. On review several hours letter, he was slightly unsettled and a sausage-shaped mass once again was palpable in the right upper quadrant. At repeat air-enema, the intussusceptum could not be moved back from its position in the transverse colon.

At laparotomy, firm sustained pressure of the encasing transverse colon was necessary to evacuate oedema from the intussusception before reduction by sequential squeezing distal to the intussusceptum permitted reduction of the ileocolic intussusception. He required 40 mL/kg of colloid intraoperatively (in addition to his preoperative saline bolus). He made an uneventful recovery, recommencing oral fluids on the third postoperative day and manifesting a pyrexial viral illness before discharge.

Case 2

A 15-month-old girl was admitted as an emergency with a previously undiagnosed incarcerated para-oesophageal hiatus hernia. She underwent a three-hour emergency procedure to mobilize the stomach and repair the defect. Postoperatively, she appeared to be recovering well, with decreasing nasogastric aspirates. She passed flatus after three days, at which stage she was commenced on oral fluids.

However, 36 hours later, she became unsettled, with abdominal distension, and her nasogastric aspirates became bilious and more copious. Abdominal ultrasound scan demonstrated a postoperative intussusception with marked proximal small-bowel distension. No attempt at air-enema reduction was made, and she underwent operative manual reduction of an ileo-ileal intussusception. Her postoperative recovery thereafter was uneventful. She recommenced oral fluids on the third postoperative day, and she was discharged home two days after this.

Case 3

A 16-week-old girl presented with a two-day history of cough and a 24-hour history of profuse vomiting, together with feed refusal but no diarrhoea. Despite this, a clinical diagnosis of gastroenteritis was made, and she was admitted under the paediatricians, having failed to tolerate oral fluids during a period of observation in the emergency department.

Her symptoms continued over the next three days, with some of the vomits being bilious. Following the development of abdominal distension and the recognition of blood-stained stools, together with lethargy and ongoing refusal of feeds, an abdominal X-ray was performed and a paediatric surgical opinion sought. The plain film demonstrated small-bowel obstruction, and a clinical diagnosis of intussusception was made. She subsequently underwent an emergency laparotomy, at which time a typical ileocolic intussusception was identified and reduced. She commenced oral feeds on the third postoperative day and was discharged home two days later.

REFERENCES

Kirks D. Air intussusception reduction: 'the winds of change'. *Pediatric Radiology* 1995; **25**: 89–91.

Maoate K, Beasley S. Perforation during gas reduction of intussusception. *Pediatric Surgery International* 1998; **14**: 168–70.

Palder S, Ein S, Stringer D, Alton D. Intussusception: barium or air? *Journal of Pediatric Surgery* 1991; **26**: 271–4.

Peter G, Myers M. Intussusception, rotavirus, and oral vaccines: summary of a workshop. *Pediatrics* 2002; **110**: 67.

Shanbhogue R, Hussain S, Meradji M, *et al.* Ultrasonography is accurate enough for the diagnosis of intussusception. *Journal of Pediatric Surgery* 1994; **29**: 324–7.

Stringer MD, Pledger G, Drake PP. Childhood deaths from intussusception in England and Wales, 1984–9. *British Medical Journal* 1992; **304**: 737–9.

FURTHER READING

DiFiore JW. Intussusception. *Seminars in Pediatric Surgery* 1999; **8**: 214–20.

Young DG. Intussusception. In: O'Neill JA, Rowe MI, Grosfeld JL, Fonkalsrud EW, Coran AG (eds). *Pediatric Surgery*, 5th edn, Vol. 2. St Louis, MO: Mosby, 1998; pp. 1185–98.

24

Gastro-oesophageal reflux in childhood

JUAN A TOVAR

Learning objectives

- To understand why gastro-oesophageal reflux is frequent in children.
- To understand why the clinical features of reflux are so variable in children.
- To be able to interpret the investigations for gastro-oesophageal reflux correctly.
- To understand the functional basis of anti-reflux treatment.

INTRODUCTION

Gastro-oesophageal reflux (GOR) is frequent in infancy and childhood. It often has a benign clinical course with a spontaneous tendency to disappear with the passage of time. However, it can also be a severe and even lethal condition requiring urgent treatment. In these cases, surgery is often required; this, and the frequent association of GOR with other surgical conditions and malformations, makes the close involvement of paediatric surgeons in the decision-making process highly desirable.

RELEVANT BASIC SCIENCE

The oesophagus is the only part of the digestive tract that is devoid of any digestive or absorptive functions and therefore serves only for the transit of the bolus of food from the pharynx to the stomach. In consequence, its mucosa, which is only minimally secretory, is not designed for prolonged contact with potentially harmful digestive juices. However, its muscle layers produce efficient peristaltic movements that propel the bolus of food into the stomach.

Swallowing triggers the onset of peristaltic waves that progress down the oesophagus. Simultaneously, there is relaxation of the upper and lower oesophageal sphincters, allowing the passage of the bolus into the stomach. Whenever there is a failure of the anti-reflux mechanism and gastric fluid enters a healthy oesophagus, non-deglutory peristaltic waves are triggered to achieve clearance. The vagal and sympathetic nerve fibres regulate these actions via the intrinsic neural network of the oesophagus.

The anatomical position of the oesophagus exposes it to a permanent threat: the stomach, located in the abdominal cavity and producing strong contractions, is permanently under positive intra-abdominal pressure, whereas the oesophagus, located mainly in the thorax, is subjected to strong negative pressure during inspiration. This creates a positive abdominothoracic pressure gradient that, at least during inspiration, should make the retrograde passage of gastric contents into the oesophagus (reflux) unavoidable. These conditions are somewhat reduced on standing, but they are aggravated by lying down – the predominant position throughout infancy and throughout life in most animals.

The risk of reflux created by the anatomy of the oesophagus is counteracted by a physiological anti-reflux barrier. This barrier is a complex mechanism involving two main and several minor components. The main components are the lower oesophageal sphincter and the diaphragmatic crural sling. They overlap anatomically and work synergistically to maintain the oesophagogastric junction permanently closed, except during swallowing, when the food bolus passes into the stomach. The sphincter consists of the circular or inner layer of the smooth lower oesophageal muscle, and its function consists of maintaining a permanent resting tone able to close the lumen at that level and relaxing only during swallowing. In contrast, the striated muscle fibres of the crural sling, which surround the terminal oesophagus, contract rhythmically during the respiratory cycle to permit ventilation and, at the same time, displace the gastro-oesophageal junction downwards, closing it tightly during each inspiratory movement when the intrathoracic negative pressure accentuates the abdominothoracic gradient. The synergy between the smooth muscle of the sphincter and the striated muscle of the sling is not unlike that of the internal and external anal sphincters that regulate continence and defecation.

The minor components of the gastro-oesophageal barrier are also important. The terminal portion of the intra-abdominal oesophagus is closed by permanently positive intra-abdominal pressure. If the angle of His is intact, then the presence of air and liquid in the gastric fundus compresses the terminal oesophagus, reinforcing the barrier effect; however, when the stomach is full, the angle of His tends to become more obtuse, which facilitates reflux.

In addition to the barrier and peristalsis, the oesophagus has some other defensive mechanisms. Saliva is alkaline and buffers any acid present in the lumen, together with the alkaline fluid secreted by the oesophageal submucous glands. The structure of the mucosa is the result of a permanent balance between desquamation of the outer cells and regeneration from the basal layers. Physical or chemical attack increases desquamation, but the mucosa is able to react only by increasing proliferation. The high content of epidermal growth factor (EGF) in the saliva suggests that stimulation of proliferation may be related to salivary secretion.

PATHOGENESIS OF REFLUX

The anti-reflux barrier may be distorted anatomically, as in a hiatus hernia, or functionally abolished, facilitating the appearance of GOR. However, in children and adults, the occurrence of long non-deglutatory sphincteric relaxations accounts for most episodes of GOR. The loss of permanent sphincter tone for long periods of time creates a common gastro-oesophageal cavity, which allows the abdominothoracic gradient to cause damage by permitting reflux. The cause of this relaxation is unknown, but it is probably related to failure of the neural or humoral regulation of the mechanism of closure.

In addition to these non-deglutory relaxations, there are some clinical conditions in which the barrier mechanisms are absent or modified, facilitating the appearance of GOR:

- *Brain damage:* patients with neurological disease of various origins are often lying down, have abnormal neural regulation with abnormal peristalsis, suffer from spasticity and constipation, which increase intra-abdominal pressure, and may have scoliosis, which further distorts the anatomy of the barrier. In consequence, they very often have GOR.
- *Congenital abnormalities:* children who were operated on as neonates with oesophageal atresia (OA), congenital diaphragmatic hernia (CDH) or an abdominal-wall defect (AWD) frequently have GOR. In OA, even with little or no tension, the anastomosis produces an oesophagus that is shorter than normal and has deficient intrinsic and extrinsic innervation. The intra-abdominal segment of the oesophagus is almost absent and there is no angle of His. The barrier fails and peristalsis is inefficient, creating the circumstances for significant GOR. In CDH, the hiatus is enlarged after closure of the hernial defect, and the increased negative thoracic pressure coupled with the increased positive abdominal pressure accentuate the normal gradient. In addition, the oesophagus is probably not very efficient in terms of peristalsis, since it is often dilated and atonic. These circumstances, together with the non-rotation of the bowel, facilitate the appearance of GOR. Neonatal closure of exomphalos and gastroschisis increase the intra-abdominal pressure, and their association with non-rotation or malrotation may facilitate GOR.
- *Distal obstruction:* pyloric stenosis, duodenal or jejunal stenosis and malrotation delay gastric emptying and facilitate GOR.

NATURAL HISTORY OF GASTRO-OESOPHAGEAL REFLUX IN CHILDHOOD

In contrast to adults, in whom GOR has no spontaneous tendency to improve, GOR often improves in children, particularly in infants, such that the expectation of improvement influences all subsequent diagnostic and therapeutic decisions.

It used to be thought that the gastro-oesophageal barrier was immature in the newborn and that progressive maturation alleviated the tendency to reflux. There is no serious manometric evidence to justify this explanation, however, since premature and term babies have adequate sphincteric pressures and peristalsis. However, other factors, such as recumbency, the relative size of the oesophagus and the stomach, and perhaps different pressure gradients between the abdomen and the thorax, make GOR more likely to occur in the newborn and young infant. This trend improves with time, and most patients lose their symptoms by the age of 12–18 months, at the same time as they stand upright. After two years of age, only a minority of patients remain symptomatic. These patients probably belong to a selected population in which the factors leading to GOR persist. This group is particularly important for paediatric surgeons because it contains most of the children requiring surgery. However, the disappearance of symptoms simply means that the babies stop vomiting and gain weight. Some of them may continue to reflux and become symptomatic much later on. GOR is extremely frequent in adults and many have a history of vomiting during infancy.

GOR in children with associated conditions (brain damage or previous operations for OA, CDH or AWD) does not tend to improve with time, and it would be a serious mistake to treat these children by following the guidelines developed for normal children with their generally favourable prognosis.

CLINICAL FEATURES

In children, GOR may present as the result of three different pathological pathways, which may coexist in the same patient.

Vomiting

Vomiting is the key symptom in neonates and young infants. It is frequent, rarely complete, often (but not always) postprandial and non-bilious. These children stop gaining weight and may become malnourished after some months. Regardless of the severity of the reflux, vomiting decreases in frequency and volume with time and usually resolves when the child starts walking. Even if GOR persists, children older than two years rarely vomit, or do so only when they have intercurrent disease or when they are in particular positions. Refluxing adults usually do not vomit, and children after the age of four or five years behave similarly.

Other consequences of the frequent presence of gastric contents in the oesophagus are bad breath (halitosis), which may provoke teasing at school, and deterioration of dental enamel (especially of the molars).

Oesophagitis

Repeated or prolonged exposure of the oesophagus to acid and/or alkaline reflux harms the mucosa, which desquamates and becomes infiltrated by neutrophils and eosinophils. Active regeneration from below thickens the basal layer, and the papillae come closer to the surface. If desquamation overtakes regeneration, then the papillary vessels are exposed and may bleed. In severe cases, the mucosa ulcerates and the inflammation reaches the deeper layers of the wall, leading to healing by fibrosis.

Any bleeding is usually microscopic and may be undetectable, except by occult blood testing of the stool. However, it may lead to iron-deficiency anaemia, which considerably decreases the potential for mucosal regeneration and hence aggravates the oesophagitis. In severe cases, the bleeding is macroscopic and may present as haematemesis or melaena.

The inflamed oesophagus becomes painful, and these patients show their discomfort in different ways: older children may express it as heartburn or retrosternal pain, but younger children may complain of 'abdominal pain', frequently periumbilically, or may cry bitterly without apparent explanation. During infancy, they may only be agitated during the night (writhing in bed) and are often 'irritable' or 'unfriendly'.

When the oesophageal wall inflammation involves the submucosa and the muscle layers, there is also dysphagia. This happens rarely in infancy and is not very frequent later on. Very occasionally, untreated refluxers, particularly those with brain damage, may have peptic strictures that make swallowing progressively more difficult or impossible and require urgent and aggressive treatment.

Occasionally, GOR is accompanied by peculiar neck postures or torticollis without a vertebral or muscular cause. This is Sandifer syndrome and needs to be recognized because it is often the only symptom of oesophagitis and dysphagia. (In some long-necked birds, deglutition is accompanied by strange head and neck movements; Sandifer syndrome can be viewed as a human version of the same difficult process of swallowing.)

Respiratory tract disease

This involves a very important group of symptoms that are known to be associated with reflux but that are often attributed to other causes, which delays the diagnosis. GOR may cause aspiration of gastric contents into the airway, leading to sudden death (Mendelson syndrome), asphyxia with missed sudden infant death (very rare), repeated pneumonia or atelectasis (more frequent) and recurrent bronchitis or respiratory tract infection (very frequent). Sometimes, the bronchitis is associated with bronchospasm, which makes it clinically similar to asthma. This creates confusion, in which it would be as inappropriate to pretend that GOR comes before the asthma as to maintain the opposite. GOR may cause bronchial constriction by local oesophagobronchial reflexes or by micro-aspiration. This in turn may contribute to sensitization of the respiratory epithelium to some alimentary allergens. On the other hand, atopic asthma, often treated with xanthines, which are known relaxants of the oesophageal sphincter, increases the gastro-oesophageal pressure gradient, thus facilitating reflux. The potential for confusion is obvious, and attribution of the symptoms to either of these conditions may be difficult. The correct diagnosis is important because, on the one hand, the treatment of the GOR will alleviate or cure the respiratory tract disease, whereas on the other hand, control of the GOR can be obtained only by treating the respiratory disease effectively.

Other symptoms should be carefully taken into account in order to make the correct diagnosis: family history, atopic symptoms, and increased immunoglobulin E (IgE) or positive skin tests may help to detect asthma as the origin of the GOR. Conversely, a history of vomiting during infancy or some pH probe features (see below) are more consistent with a primary GOR inducing secondary respiratory tract disease.

INVESTIGATIONS

GOR is, to some extent, a normal phenomenon, particularly after meals, and therefore the diagnosis becomes a quantitative problem. In other words, we all have some reflux, and its detection is not sufficient to make the diagnosis of a pathological condition. This is the reason for the apparently excessive number of tests used to detect GOR. The question is not to detect GOR but rather to measure how much, how many times and when it occurs. We shall describe briefly the investigations and give some basic guidelines for their use.

Radiology

Barium meal classically was the procedure used for diagnosis. However, although it may detect reflux, the need to reduce irradiation to a minimum makes quantification over time impossible. There are too many false-positives and it has poor specificity. It does, however, provide morphological information (hiatus hernia, oesophageal stenosis, absence of the angle of His, delayed emptying for liquids, malrotation) that can be crucial for decisions about treatment. Although it is the most widely available test, its use is limited to preoperative work-up and little more.

Scintigraphy

Using an isotope-tagged meal instead of barium allows detection of GOR episodes over a prolonged period of time with much less irradiation. It also allows an accurate assessment of gastric emptying for solids. However, the morphological information obtained is quite poor, and the equipment is so expensive that it cannot be used for the routine diagnosis of GOR.

Plain and colour Doppler-assisted ultrasonography

These procedures have the advantage of being harmless and may be used for some time in order to quantify the reflux. Widening of the junction and flow through it can be detected clearly by expert observers. Although these procedures probably are too operator-dependent, and the cost of the staff

required is considerable, it is likely that they will be used increasingly in the future.

Fibre-optic endoscopy and biopsy

Modern endoscopes greatly facilitate direct observation of irritation or inflammation of the mucosa and of the presence of exudates, stenosis and ulcers with limited discomfort. Biopsies can be taken through the operating channel of the instrument in order to assess histologically the presence of signs of oesophagitis (papillary lengthening, basal thickening, leucocyte infiltration, ulceration, Barrett's columnar dysplasia). However, oesophagitis is only one of the pathogenic pathways of GOR disease and, very occasionally, patients may die of reflux without oesophagitis. Nevertheless, the finding of oesophagitis is an important adjunct in the diagnosis of GOR.

Twenty-four-hour pH-probe

This is the best method for quantifying reflux. An antimony or glass electrode is located in the lower oesophagus and connected to a pH-meter with an additional electrode to close the circuit. The pH in the oesophageal lumen is measured every few seconds and recorded, together with other information, such as timing of meals, position of the patient, and so on, in a portable Holter-type device, which is the size of a personal cassette player. This information is later transferred to a computer and read with appropriate software in order to print and analyse the tracings. As the gastric enzymes do not work above a pH of 4, this is taken as the threshold of abnormal acid exposure. The number of dips below this level, the proportion of total time below pH 4, the number of episodes lasting for more than five minutes, and the duration of the longest episode are measured. Other variables, including the area under the curve and scores that put together all of these data, can be measured, but it has been our experience that the four classic parameters and a thorough analysis of the trace give the best information.

However, pH-probe measurement has some limitations that should be acknowledged. It measures only pH and not reflux; therefore, if the gastric content is not acid, then the oesophageal electrode will not read any episode of reflux. This is particularly bothersome in young children who receive five or six milk feeds every day. The gastric pH is buffered for at least two hours after each meal and, therefore, the oesophageal electrode will remain 'blind' to reflux for 12 out of the 24 hours, thus under-recording any GOR (Figure 24.1a).

The same artefact can occur if alkaline duodenogastric reflux occurs. In these cases, well known in adults but not very well studied in children, bile and pancreatic secretions activated by HCl and pepsin neutralize acid while creating a very harmful refluxate that cannot be detected by a pH-electrode located in the oesophagus (Figure 24.1b).

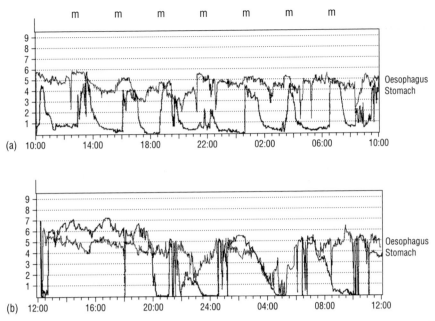

Figure 24.1 *Simultaneous gastric and oesophageal 24-hour pH-metering tracings, demonstrating the importance of interpreting the information obtained by the oesophageal electrode together with the information from the gastric electrode. (a) In this vomiting newborn baby, every milk feed (m) is followed by a two-hour period of gastric buffering, which hides the episodes of reflux for 50 per cent of the time. (b) This child had severe oesophagitis. There are several long falls of oesophageal pH below 4, particularly during the night, but the gastric electrode shows that there are long periods of gastric alkalinization, suggesting alkaline reflux and/or delayed gastric emptying. Oesophageal acid exposure is underscored by the oesophageal electrode in these conditions, which can be particularly harmful for the mucosa.*

We always use combined gastric and oesophageal pH electrodes in order to assess the pH of the stomach and the oesophagus simultaneously (Tovar *et al.* 1993).

Manometry

Direct measurements of the pressures within the lumen of the oesophagus make it possible to assess the function of the sphincter as well as peristalsis and thence to judge the status of the barrier and the ability of the oesophagus to clear the reflux.

Manometry requires expensive and complicated equipment consisting of multi-channel probes with lateral orifices perfused with pneumo-hydraulic pumps capable of creating constant high pressures within low-compliance systems. These in turn are connected to transducers that continuously deliver the information to recording devices.

Sphincteric manometry was performed by pulling the probe through the gastro-oesophageal junction or high-pressure zone. The gastric pressures were first recorded followed by a pressure 'plateau' corresponding to the sphincter and then by thoracic pressures. The introduction of perfused sphincteric sleeves has allowed stationary study of the sphincter revealing non-deglutatory relaxations as the cause of most episodes of GOR. This procedure is not used widely because measurement of the pressure is only really valuable when it is very reduced and the non-deglutory relaxations are difficult to record.

The assessment of peristalsis using stationary perfusion manometry is difficult in children: they move about, because the intra-oesophageal tubing is uncomfortable, which makes the measurements meaningless. However, it has been facilitated to some extent by the introduction of non-perfused solid-state probes. However, these are quite thick, making the procedure useful only in older children.

Manometry has contributed a great deal to the understanding of the phenomenon of GOR and the physiology of the oesophagus, but it cannot be considered a routine diagnostic method in children.

In each individual patient, the use of each different investigation must be governed by a knowledge of the natural history and the likely severity or particular nature of the GOR. When dealing with young infants who vomit, no investigation is indicated until a first therapeutic trial has failed. This approach excludes the vast majority of babies with reflux symptoms from relatively invasive and expensive tests. In those in whom the symptoms are of late-onset or persist beyond two or three years, a 24-hour pH-probe is indicated. Scintigraphy or ultrasonography can also be used as first-level tests. Oesophagoscopy is indicated only in children with symptoms suggesting the presence of oesophagitis (Vandenplas *et al.* 1993). Manometry or ambulatory manometry are justified only in children who are suspected of having motor disorders of the oesophagus. In respiratory patients, a 24-hour pH-probe is particularly useful, together with the recovery of lipid-laden macrophages from a tracheal aspirate.

TREATMENT

Medical

There is a general consensus about the need for a conservative approach to the treatment of GOR disease. Keeping in mind the generally favourable natural history, minimal measures should be instituted at first in most babies suspected of having GOR, before performing any investigations. In most cases, these measures will stop the symptoms. They consist of the maintenance of the upright supine or prone position around the clock and perhaps the introduction of a milk thickener if the baby is bottle-fed. Some authors advise reducing the volume of feeds while increasing their frequency, but this is not accepted uniformly. In older children, positional treatment consists of elevating the head of the bed in order to maintain the patient in a semi-upright position. At this age, a light early dinner is advisable, avoiding fatty meals and chocolate. Antacids such as alginates and other adsorbents such as sucralfate are still used, but histamine H_2 receptor blockers may be better.

If symptoms persist, then a prokinetic drug is indicated. Cisapride (0.8 mg/kg/day in three doses), a non-dopamine receptor blocker that improves oesophageal peristalsis, strengthens the sphincter and facilitates gastric emptying, was used with success for a long time until some untoward side effects on heart conduction were reported. It remains the best prokinetic drug and may still be indicated in certain cases, with all necessary precautions being taken. Domperidone (1 mg/kg/day), metoclopramide (0.5 mg/kg/day) and other prokinetics can be used instead, with some satisfactory results.

If evidence of oesophagitis appears or if the symptoms are controlled insufficiently, then inhibition of the secretion of gastric acid is indicated. H_2 receptor blockers, such as cimetidine (30 mg/kg/day) and ranitidine (10–15 mg/kg/day), are used but proton-pump inhibitors (e.g. omeprazole 10–40 mg/day) are more effective.

The success of treatment can be assessed only after several months. If the symptoms disappear, then treatment can be stopped after some time. If they recur, then the possibility of surgery should be discussed. If the symptoms do not disappear with treatment, then this can be called treatment failure and surgery should be considered (Vandenplas et al. 1993, 1997; Rudolph et al. 2001).

Surgical

Operation is considered only in patients in whom conservative medical treatment has failed. For the above-mentioned reasons, this is very rarely before the age of two years, in order to leave time for the usual tendency for improvement to occur.

Patients with respiratory symptoms and GOR should be treated surgically if there is a history of vomiting during infancy and repeated non-obstructive bronchial or parenchymal disease or if there are prolonged nocturnal episodes of reflux upon pH measurement. In these circumstances, a favourable outcome can be predicted in those cases where an initial energetic course of medical treatment has failed. In addition, after anti-reflux surgery, some atopic asthmatic patients are also improved in terms of reduced drug requirements and fewer asthmatic attacks.

There are some rare circumstances in which surgery should be considered early on, i.e. patients with symptomatic reflux in the context of previously treated malformations, such as OA, CDH and AWD. In these children, particular consideration should be given to surgical treatment, because a favourable natural history cannot be expected. After ruling out malrotation and delayed gastric emptying, early operation should be considered very seriously.

Children with brain damage and symptomatic reflux should also be considered for operation, because the causes of GOR will persist, irrespective of the duration or the nature of the medical treatment. A gastrostomy may be inserted at the same time.

A few babies with life-threatening apnoeic spells leading to near-miss sudden infant death may require early surgery. There are many other causes for these episodes and they should be ruled out before any operative decision is taken, but whenever GOR is documented in these children, and particularly if there are episodes of apnoea coinciding with GOR, then there should be no hesitation about the need for operation. Some of these children die of GOR and it is better to perform a relatively simple operation unnecessarily than to regret a preventable catastrophe.

Anti-reflux operations aim to reconstruct an effective anti-reflux barrier while maintaining the free passage of the food bolus through the gastro-oesophageal junction. In a Nissen fundoplication, the gastric fundus is used to construct a perioesophageal wrap that acts as a highly efficient pneumo-hydraulic valve (Figure 24.2). The wrap should be loose and not too long, in order to avoid gas-bloat and dysphagia. This is the most efficient anti-reflux operation and it should be considered the gold standard that other techniques should match. Anterior fundoplications were developed by Thal, Dor, Boix-Ochoa and Ashcraft, and posterior fundoplication has been introduced by Toupet. Other operations, such as anterior gastropexy, may be less effective.

All these procedures can be performed laparoscopically with approximately the same results as, and less discomfort than, their open counterparts. It is our impression that nowadays the majority of fundoplications should be performed laparoscopically, except when the local conditions may interfere with the procedure, such as some cases of GOR associated with OA or peptic stenosis. Children with delayed gastric emptying represent a particular problem. This may be suspected when the stomach is large in spite of the reflux or when prolonged postprandial gastric neutralization is detected upon simultaneous gastric and oesophageal pH-metry. Isotopic assessment of emptying time is then indicated. A pyloroplasty or antroplasty should be performed in

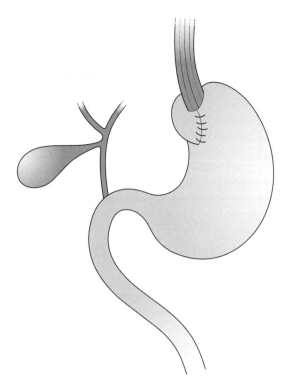

Figure 24.2 *Nissen fundoplication. The wrap is fashioned from the gastric fundus. It should be loose and relatively short, in order to avoid gas-bloat and dysphagia. This operation is done laparoscopically in most cases.*

these patients at the same time as fundoplication, to avoid undue pressure building up within the stomach, which cannot empty well and cannot vomit (Fonkalsrud and Ament 1996).

Peptic strictures initially should be dilated one or more times while continuing vigorous medical anti-reflux treatment. If resistant to dilation, then fundoplication should be performed. The acquired shortness of the oesophagus in these cases may make laparoscopic operation particularly difficult, and we prefer an open approach in such cases.

COMPLICATIONS OF FUNDOPLICATION

Anti-reflux operations are often dramatically effective, but up to ten per cent have side effects and complications that should be taken into consideration and explained fully to the child and the parents.

The use of the fundus for creating the wrap transiently reduces gastric volume, so it is impossible to eat large meals during the first postoperative weeks. Bread should be avoided initially, as it can stick in the oesophagus.

Long and/or tight wraps can cause entrapment of gas in the stomach (gas-bloat), which may be very uncomfortable and should be prevented by adhering strictly to a policy of a loose, short wrap. Gas-bloat is dangerous, as it may develop into acute gastric dilation, with reflex vagal slowing of the heart, which may progress to cardiac arrest. Gas-bloat requires urgent decompression, either by passing a nasogastric tube

or via the gastrostomy. This complication is rare if the wrap is performed around a very large intra-oesophageal tube.

Dumping syndrome is possible after fundoplication, particularly when a pyloroplasty or antroplasty is performed at the same time. This situation is very rare and generally transient, but it may be a considerable nuisance.

Wrap failure should not be a very frequent problem in children operated upon for GOR alone, but it is very frequent (up to 25 per cent of cases) in the long run in neurological patients and in patients operated on previously for OA, CDH or AWD, because all the mechanisms leading to GOR persist after the operation and the interposition of the wrap alone does not always suffice to maintain the situation in the long term.

CLINICAL SCENARIOS

Case 1

A two-month-old boy, born after an uneventful pregnancy and normal delivery and weighing 3400 g, was seen. He vomited frequently, particularly after feeds. Weight gain had stopped in the past week, and his mother reported nocturnal crying and distress. Physical examination was unremarkable. The initial advice was to maintain an upright position without any further tests, but he continued to vomit. With thickening of his feeds and a prokinetic drug, he improved clinically, and after six months he was asymptomatic.

Case 2

An eight-year-old girl who suffered severe brain damage during delivery was referred. She was severely retarded, had spastic quadriplegia and had to be treated for occasional seizures. She could not speak and she barely communicated. For the past year, she had been pale and miserable. She had lost weight and vomited frequently, often with small amounts of dark blood. For the past few days, she had refused her feeds. Her blood count showed severe microcytic anaemia, and endoscopy demonstrated severe oesophagitis of the distal third, with a stricture near the cardia. Biopsy showed ulceration and severe oesophagitis. After dilation of the oesophagus under anaesthesia, she was treated with omeprazole for some weeks and then underwent a laparoscopic Nissen fundoplication with gastrostomy. In the ensuing weeks, she became happier, ate better and received some additional feed through the gastrostomy, with considerable weight gain. Her family were very happy with the results of the operation and found the gastrostomy very useful.

Case 3

A six-month-old boy was operated on at birth for type C oesophageal atresia. He had an uneventful postoperative course and was discharged at the age of 20 days. He vomited frequently and had developed an anastomotic stricture requiring dilation under anaesthesia on four occasions during the previous five months. A 24-hour pH-probe performed with a double electrode showed that he had severe GOR, and therefore a Nissen operation was performed. He stopped vomiting and the stricture did not recur in the ensuing 12 months.

Case 4

A six-year-old girl was referred for assessment of her reflux by her paediatrician, who was treating her for asthmatic bronchitis. She had had frequent episodes of bronchoconstriction, with wheezing and severe discomfort, since the age of nine months. Skin tests were positive for house dust mite, insects and seafood. She had elevated IgE. A 24-hour pH-probe showed excessive lower-oesophageal acid exposure, with many short episodes of reflux during the day. No oesophagitis was found upon endoscopy. On the basis of the clinical history, the pH-probe result and the absence of oesophagitis, medical treatment of GOR was undertaken but did not improve the clinical picture.

Case 5

A nine-year-old boy who had had six episodes of pneumonia in the past five years was referred. No particular causative organism was found. He had a long history of vomiting during infancy and required positional and medical treatment, which were apparently successful. At present, he vomits only when he has a cold. He has halitosis and occasional retrosternal pain. A 24-hour pH-probe revealed severe GOR, with many episodes during the day and at least three during the night that lasted more than 30 minutes each. This suggests that he will be cured by fundoplication. After ruling out immune deficiencies and cystic fibrosis, positional advice and H$_2$ blockers greatly improved the symptoms. He was offered laparoscopic fundoplication, which was very successful.

REFERENCES

Fonkalsrud EW, Ament ME. Gastroesophageal reflux in childhood. *Current Problems in Surgery* 1996; **33**: 1–70.

Rudolph CD, Mazur LJ, Liptak GS, *et al*. Guidelines for evaluation and treatment of gastro-esophageal reflux in infants and children: recommendations of the North American Society for Pediatric Gastroenterology and Nutrition. *Journal of Pediatric Gastroenterology and Nutrition* 2001; **32** (Suppl 2): S1–31.

Tovar JA, Wang W Eizaguirre I. Simultaneous gastro-oesophageal pH monitoring and the diagnosis of alkaline reflux. *Journal of Pediatric Surgery* 1993; **28**: 1386–92.

Vandenplas Y, Ashkenazi A, Belli D, *et al*. A proposition for the diagnosis and treatment of gastro-oesophageal reflux disease in children: a report from a working group on gastro-oesophageal reflux disease. Working Group of the European Society of Paediatric Gastroenterology and Nutrition (ESPGAN). *European Journal of Pediatrics* 1993; **152**: 704–11.

Vandenplas Y, Belli D, Benhamou P, *et al*. A critical appraisal of current management practices for infant regurgitation: recommendations of a working party. *European Journal of Pediatrics* 1997; **156**: 343–57.

25

Inflammatory bowel disease

MARK BEATTIE AND D MERVYN GRIFFITHS

Learning objectives

- To understand the definitions, clinical features and strategies for the investigation of inflammatory bowel diseases.
- To be aware of who should be referred for investigation and of the differential diagnosis.
- To understand the clinical course and medical management, including, in particular, the importance of nutrition and the potential adverse effects of the diseases on growth and pubertal and emotional development.
- To understand the indications for surgery and to be aware of the operations available, including preoperative management and long-term outcome.

INTRODUCTION

Inflammatory bowel disease (IBD) usually implies Crohn's disease or ulcerative colitis. Rarer colitides include indeterminate colitis, food-allergic colitis and pseudomembranous colitis. Infective colitis is part of the differential diagnosis.

Ten to 15 per cent of patients with IBD present in childhood. The diagnosis should be considered in children who present with abdominal pain. Assessment includes panendoscopy and barium radiology. The clinical course is one of recurrent relapses. Particularly in adolescence, the diseases impact significantly on growth and development.

Medical management is complex, requiring multidisciplinary input and a major emphasis on nutrition. Surgery is frequently required in resistant Crohn's disease, but the relapse rate is high and usually continued medical therapy is required. Surgery can be curative for ulcerative colitis.

DEFINITIONS

Crohn's disease is a chronic inflammatory disease that can affect any part of the bowel, from the mouth to the anus. The most common sites are the terminal ileum, ileocolon and colon. The typical pathological features are transmural inflammation and granuloma formation, which may be patchy.

Ulcerative colitis is an inflammatory disease limited to the colonic and rectal mucosa. The characteristic histology is mucosal and submucosal inflammation, with goblet-cell depletion, cryptitis and crypt abscesses but no granulomas. The inflammatory change is usually diffuse rather than patchy.

Colitis means colonic inflammation. Characteristic features include abdominal pain, tenesmus, bloody diarrhoea and blood and mucus per rectum.

Ten to 15 per cent of colitis is indeterminate, which means that the histology is consistent with IBD but not characteristic of Crohn's disease or ulcerative colitis.

INCIDENCE AND AETIOLOGY

Up to 15 per cent of cases of IBD present under the age of 16 years. The incidence in childhood is 5.2 per 100 000 children, and 58 per cent of these have Crohn's disease. The mean age at diagnosis of Crohn's disease is 12 years. Ulcerative colitis presents at any age. In children under ten years of age, ulcerative colitis is the more likely diagnosis.

The aetiology of IBD is multifactorial. A family history is common, with an increased risk of IBD in first-degree relatives. Various candidate genes have been studied, and genetic susceptibility is clearly a factor. The trigger is unknown. It is thought that in a genetically susceptible individual, interaction between environmental factors and the host's intestinal microflora triggered by some event activates an immune response, the end result of which is chronic inflammation. Ongoing inflammation is thought to be an uncontrolled immune response to antigens from the normal bowel bacterial flora.

CLINICAL FEATURES

Crohn's disease

Children with Crohn's disease are almost always underweight at diagnosis (Figure 25.1a). As many as 50 per cent have significant growth failure, usually associated with delay in pubertal development. The common presenting symptoms are anorexia, abdominal pain, diarrhoea and blood per rectum. There may be other features, such as oral ulceration, perianal signs, rashes, uveitis and joint swelling.

The disease may be florid at presentation. The disease may, therefore, be insidious in onset and the symptoms episodic. The diagnosis therefore may be delayed, sometimes for many months or even years.

Abdominal pain is common in children. The presence of additional features as above and/or systemic upset should prompt further evaluation and/or investigations. Perianal skin tags, fistulae and resistant fissures make Crohn's disease likely. Perianal visualization is, therefore, an essential part of the assessment of a child with abdominal pain, particularly if the pain is chronic.

Nutritional status frequently is compromised at diagnosis. This is multifactorial:

- There is decreased food intake because of anorexia and abdominal pain following food, which reduces the desire to eat.

- There may be reduced absorption in the presence of bowel mucosal inflammation.
- There is an increase in energy requirements, chronic inflammation being associated with an increased metabolic rate.

EXTRA-INTESTINAL MANIFESTATIONS OF CROHN'S DISEASE

Extra-intestinal manifestations include:

- joint disease in ten per cent (ankylosing spondylitis rarely);
- rashes, e.g. erythema nodosum, erythema multiforme, pyoderma gangrenosum;
- liver disease (rare in childhood), e.g. sclerosing cholangitis, autoimmune liver disease;
- uveitis;
- osteoporosis.

COMPLICATIONS OF CROHN'S DISEASE

Complications include:

- growth failure, with delayed puberty;
- emotional disturbance, particularly the effect of chronic disease and pubertal delay, i.e. the patient may appear to be younger than he or she really is and may be treated accordingly, which has a major impact during adolescence;
- treatment toxicity, e.g. corticosteroids;
- long-term cancer risk.

Ulcerative colitis

Presentation may include:

- acute toxic colitis
- pan-colitis – mild, moderate or severe
- distal colitis.

The symptoms of colitis are diarrhoea, blood per rectum and abdominal pain. There may be significant pain before or during bowel movement, which is relieved by the passage of stool. Systemic disturbance can accompany more severe disease, e.g. tachycardia, fever, weight loss, anaemia, hypoalbuminaemia and leucocytosis. The presentation can be more indolent, with occult blood loss or non-specific abdominal pain. Constipation can be a feature, particularly in distal colitis.

Unusually, the disease can present with predominantly extra-intestinal manifestations, including liver disease (sclerosing cholangitis, autoimmune liver disease), arthropathy and erythema nodosum.

Complications of ulcerative colitis include toxic megacolon, growth failure, carcinoma and treatment toxicity.

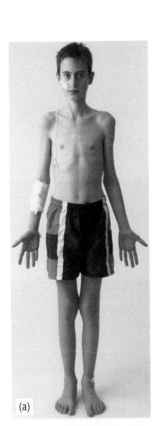

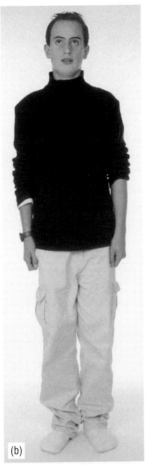

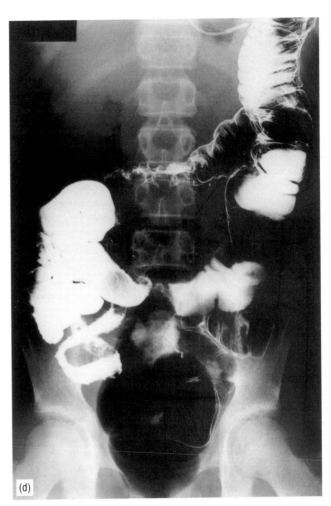

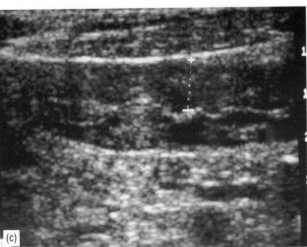

Figure 25.1   *(a) A 14-year-old boy, who presented unwell with anorexia, weight loss, severe epigastric and lower abdominal pain. Inflammatory markers were raised. Note the pallor, reduced subcutaneous fat and poor muscle mass. The nasogastric tube is for enteral nutrition. Investigation showed oesophageal, ileal and colonic Crohn's disease. He has done well, entering a sustained remission following initial treatment with corticosteroids, 5-acetylsalicylic (5-ASA) derivatives and nutritional support and achieving a final adult height above the ninety-seventh centile. (b) At age 15 years. (c) Typical radiological findings in Crohn's disease, seen in the same boy. Ultrasound scanning shows thickened bowel wall in the right iliac fossa at the terminal ileum (shown in transverse section). (d) Barium meal and follow-through with per oral pneumocolon shows narrowing at the terminal ileum with fissuring ulceration.*

DIFFERENTIAL DIAGNOSIS

The differential diagnosis of Crohn's disease includes abdominal tuberculosis, gut lymphoma and rare infections, including *Yersinia* enterocolitis. The differential diagnosis of colitis (Crohn's colitis or ulcerative colitis) is wider and includes infective and non-infective causes (Table 25.1).

INVESTIGATION

Abdominal pain is common in childhood, with more than ten per cent of children suffering recurrent symptoms at some stage. Most of this is functional, implying no serious underlying organic cause. Children with additional symptoms and physical signs, including anorexia, weight loss, diarrhoea, blood

Table 25.1 *Differential diagnosis of inflammatory bowel disease*

Infective colitis	Non-infective colitis
Salmonella	Ulcerative colitis
Shigella	Crohn's disease
Campylobacter pylori	Ischaemic colitis
Escherichia coli O157	Hirschsprung's enterocolitis
(and other *E. coli*)	
Clostridium difficile	Necrotizing enterocolitis
(pseudo-membranous colitis)	
Yersinia enterocolitica	Microscopic colitis
Tuberculosis	Food-allergic colitis
Cytomegalovirus	Behçet's disease
Entamoeba histolytica	

per rectum or more widespread systemic disturbance, require consideration of an underling organic cause, such as IBD.

Most children with active Crohn's disease will have raised inflammatory indices, e.g. C-reactive protein (CRP), erythrocyte sedimentation rate (ESR), neutrophilia, mild anaemia and thrombocytosis. Low serum albumin is common and reflects enteric loss. Iron deficiency and micronutrient deficiency (most commonly, zinc and selenium) can occur and should be screened for. Stores of fat-soluble vitamins, such as A, D and E, may be low. An abnormally low serum alkaline phosphatase is consistent with decreased bone turnover, reflecting impaired nutrition.

Inflammatory markers are less likely to be raised in ulcerative colitis, particularly if not florid. Iron deficiency, however, is common secondary to gastrointestinal blood loss. Investigations for other causes of bowel inflammation are important, e.g. stool culture (infection). Remember that enteric infection can trigger a non-infective colitis.

Endoscopy is indicated in all cases in order to get a tissue diagnosis and assess the disease extent. Endoscopy should include upper-gastrointestinal endoscopy and ileocolonoscopy in most cases. Most children in the UK have endoscopy under general anaesthetic, although some centres will investigate children using controlled sedation. Adequate bowel preparation is essential, as a good mucosal view will be obtained only if the bowel is clear. Ileocolonoscopy and upper-gastrointestinal endoscopy with biopsy (in conjunction with barium radiology) provide information about disease severity and extent as well as a tissue diagnosis in most cases. The disease extent will influence the choice of treatment and follow-up. Limited distal examination, e.g. sigmoidoscopy, may miss more proximal disease. It is essential to take biopsies, as there may be no endoscopic abnormality but significant histological change.

The preparation and technique of endoscopy is covered well in Cotton and Williams (1996). The reader is referred also to the Internet, where endoscopic atlases are readily accessible, showing typical features of the different inflammatory disorders. Typical changes of Crohn's disease are shown in

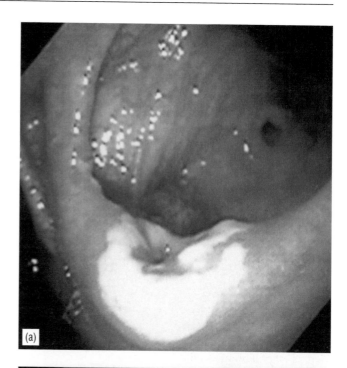

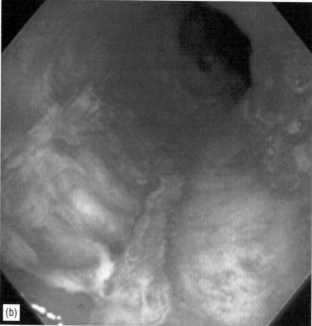

Figure 25.2 *(a) Ulceration of the ileocaecal valve seen at colonoscopy in a child with ileocaecal Crohn's disease. Note the appendix orifice. (b) Transverse ulceration and cobble-stoning of the transverse colon, seen at endoscopy in a child with Crohn's colitis. See also Colour Plate 3.*

Figure 25.2. It is crucial to have good access to expert histology for biopsy interpretation. The differences between ulcerative colitis and Crohn's disease are listed in Table 25.2.

Small-bowel disease is best assessed by either barium meal and follow-through or small-bowel enema. Ultrasound will assess bowel-wall thickening and is specific but less sensitive (Figure 25.1b).

Table 25.2 *Differences between Crohn's disease and ulcerative colitis*

Crohn's disease	Ulcerative colitis
Pan-enteric	Colon only
Skip lesions	Diffuse
Transmural	Mucosal
Granulomas	Crypt abscesses
Perianal disease	

White-cell scanning can be used to assess colitis but is not a particularly sensitive investigation for small-bowel disease. Although it may in selected cases help with the ongoing assessment of colitis, it is not a diagnostic test.

Magnetic resonance imaging (MRI) is useful in the assessment of complex perianal disease with multiple fistulae.

Histology is indeterminate in a significant number of children with colitis (indeterminate colitis). In these cases, serological markers may help in the assessment (perinuclear anti-neutrophilic cytoplasmic antibody (pANCA) positive in 70 per cent of ulcerative colitis; perinuclear anti-*Saccharomyces cerevisiae* antibody (pASCA) positive in over 50 per cent of Crohn's disease).

CLINICAL COURSE

IBD runs a chronic relapsing and remitting course. A single episode of active disease followed by a sustained clinical remission is rare. The chronic nature of the inflammatory process leads to ongoing growth failure, usually with delayed onset of puberty (particularly Crohn's disease). Many children will miss periods of schooling, and their illness may disrupt their social and psychological wellbeing. They often look younger than their peers and, therefore, get treated as if they are younger. Children who are chronically ill and who lag behind physically, educationally and socially may struggle during their adolescent years and into adulthood.

MEDICAL MANAGEMENT

A multidisciplinary approach is important. Key professionals include a paediatric gastroenterologist, general paediatrician, paediatric surgeon, radiologist, histologist, paediatric dietician, nurse specialist and psychologist. Close liaison with educational services, and with other local services if seen in a specialist centre, is essential.

Crohn's disease

The aim is to induce remission and to normalize growth and development, while minimizing treatment impact and complications.

The initial treatment will be determined by the clinical state of the child and the disease extent. In most children, enteral nutrition is appropriate as first-line treatment. This may be in addition to corticosteroids or as sole therapy. Additional therapies, however, are often required because of the frequently relapsing nature of childhood Crohn's disease. Surgical input may be required in up to 50 per cent of cases.

Basic anthropometry, including height and weight and pubertal assessment, is an essential part of the initial clinical and follow-up assessment.

ENTERAL NUTRITION

The use of a formula feed exclusively to substitute for normal diet for a period (four to eight weeks) will induce disease remission in 70–80 per cent of children if patients are selected appropriately and compliance is good. Large volumes are required, with individualized volume and feed concentrations, to achieve weight gain and to prevent hunger. The volume of feed is increased over five to seven days, depending on tolerance. Often, children require 120 per cent or more of their predicted calorie requirements. Most children tolerate their feed orally, divided evenly through the day. The formula can be flavoured to improve compliance. Nasogastric feeding is an option and is most useful in children who cannot tolerate a volume large enough to meet their calorific needs by mouth.

The formulation used most frequently in the UK is Modulen IBD®. This is a polymeric feed designed specifically for use in IBD. EO28®, an elemental feed, is an effective but less palatable alternative. There have been no published controlled trails comparing types of feed. Both induce improvement in symptoms. Often, an improvement in wellbeing is felt in a matter of days. Weight gain is often established in the first week when the feed is tolerated well. Inflammatory markers almost universally improve within two weeks of treatment in children who are going to do well.

Motivation (patient, family, healthcare professionals) is key, and ongoing support is needed to maintain compliance. Reintroduction of food after a period of enteral nutrition is staged and begins with low-residue foods, new food groups being added every few days over a period of four to eight weeks. Enteral nutrition is weaned slowly during this period.

CORTICOSTEROIDS

The use of corticosteroids is considered in children with severe disease or isolated colitis and in those who do not respond to enteral nutrition alone. Corticosteroids are an effective treatment for Crohn's disease, with a similar efficacy to enteral nutrition, although they can impact on growth, at least in the short term. Steroids are usually given as prednisolone 1–2 mg/kg (maximum dose 40–60 mg) by mouth, although occasionally intravenous steroids are required. High-dose prednisolone is continued until remission is achieved, and then the dose is weaned by reducing the daily dose by 5 mg each week. The side effects of steroid therapy are listed in Box 25.1.

Box 25.1 Side effects of steroid therapy

Immunosuppression, with increased susceptibility to
  infection
Inappropriate weight gain and fluid retention
Acne and striae
Osteopenia/osteoporosis
Hypertension
Glucose intolerance
Depressed mood
Growth suppression

MAINTAINING REMISSION

Between 50 and 90 per cent of people diagnosed with Crohn's disease will relapse within the first 12 months. Maintaining remission is, therefore, a major challenge.

5-Acetylsalicylic acid (5-ASA) derivatives are used to help maintain remission. Sulfasalazine in syrup form is most appropriate for younger children. Mesalazine, given as either controlled- or delayed-release preparations, is used for older children. Controlled-release preparations (e.g. Pentasa®) work better proximally, and delayed-release preparations (e.g. Asacol®) work better distally.

Some children are continued on their enteral feed formula at a lower volume as a dietary supplement, whereas others may use different products, according to their individual needs. Continued emphasis on good nutrition is essential. Symptoms induced by the intake of food can result in reduced intake. Malabsorption may be a factor, and, as with any chronic disease, basal metabolic rate will be increased. Most children require higher than normal requirements when well, and use of high-calorie-density supplements is often required.

Children with long-term nutritional needs may benefit from gastrostomy placement for supplementary feeding.

FURTHER MANAGEMENT

Relapse is most often defined clinically and is usually associated with rising inflammatory markers. Enteral nutrition and steroids remain therapeutic options. In the case of steroid-dependent (require steroids to remain well) and steroid-resistant (remain unwell despite the use of steroids) children, other treatments need to be considered, such as azathioprine and other immunosuppressants.

Azathioprine and 6-mercaptopurine are highly effective steroid-sparing agents. They are effective in 60–80 per cent of patients, inducing a sustained remission and growth spurt in many cases. Azathioprine is used most commonly in the UK and may be introduced early in therapy for severe disease. More than 50 per cent of children with Crohn's disease are likely to need azathioprine. The usual indication is to give azathioprine after two to three relapses, particularly if the relapses have been over a short period. Some centres advocate introduction at diagnosis in particularly difficult cases. Short-term

hypersensitivity is seen in ten per cent. The side effects of azathioprine include bone-marrow suppression, pancreatitis and hepatitis; thus, close monitoring of blood count and liver function is essential. There is a theoretical long-term cancer risk. More powerful immunosuppressive agents may be required in resistant or severe disease. These include ciclosporin, thalidomide, methotrexate, tacrolimus and infliximab (anti-tumour necrosis factor monoclonal antibody). There is less experience with the use of these therapies in childhood Crohn's disease, and they are reserved for use under the supervision of specialist centres. See Bremner and Beattie (2002) and Escher *et al.* (2003) for more detailed accounts of these other treatment options.

OESOPHAGITIS

Crohn's disease can affect all parts of the bowel, and inflammatory infiltration of the oesophageal mucosa may or may not be symptomatic. Most children with oesophageal involvement present with disease elsewhere in the bowel. Treatment of symptomatic oesophagitis or gastritis with a proton-pump inhibitor is helpful, particularly if corticosteroids are also being given.

ORAL AND PERIANAL DISEASE

Oral manifestations of Crohn's disease may occur as recurrent aphthous ulceration, orofacial granulomatosis or a manifestation of pan-enteric disease. Oral disease in isolation is managed with systemic antibiotics, such as metronidazole and ciprofloxacin, and systemic steroids. However, oral disease may also respond to enteral nutrition. Topical tacrolimus and oral thalidomide have been used.

Perianal Crohn's disease represents a particularly difficult challenge. Active perianal disease is often associated with active Crohn's disease in other locations. Treatment of the active disease will often result in improvement of perianal disease and/or closure of fistulae. Specific therapeutic strategies have used include 5-ASA derivatives, local and systemic corticosteroids and other immunosuppressants, including azathioprine, and antibiotics, particularly metronidazole. Tacrolimus may be administered topically, although systemic treatment can be used if conventional treatments fail. Tumour necrosis factor monoclonal antibody has been used in resistant cases with reasonable efficacy.

Ulcerative colitis

ACUTE TOXIC COLITIS

Acute toxic colitis implies that the child has colitic symptoms in addition to systemic upset, with pyrexia, tachycardia and abdominal tenderness/distension. Toxic megacolon (colonic dilation on plain abdominal X-ray) is a life-threatening complication of this. It is important to get multiple stool cultures to exclude infection and to request *Clostridum difficile* toxin testing specifically.

Crohn's disease can occasionally present as acute toxic colitis.

The practical management of toxic colitis is detailed as follows:

- Fluid resuscitation with saline bolus, if required, for reduced peripheral perfusion.
- Blood transfusion if haemoglobin (Hb) less than 8 g/dL.
- Intravenous fluids: initially 0.45% saline/dextrose with 20 mmol KCl/500 ml, modified depending on fluid balance and electrolyte results.
- Intravenous hydrocortisone 10 mg/kg in four divided doses – maximum 50 mg four times daily (higher doses are occasionally used).
- Broad-spectrum intravenous antibiotics if pyrexial.
- Plain abdominal X-ray: if toxic megacolon (colonic dilation), repeat every 12–24 hours or if patient deteriorates clinically.
- Abdominal ultrasound to look at bowel-wall thickening.
- Surgical review (at presentation): up to 50 per cent of patients with toxic megacolon will require colectomy, although most with an acute toxic colitis (not megacolon) will settle.
- Once the child is stable, fluids and a light diet can be allowed (milk-free initially).

PAN-COLITIS: MILD, MODERATE, SEVERE – NOT TOXIC

This is the more usual presentation in childhood. Children with colitis need upper-gastrointestinal endoscopy and barium radiology to exclude small-bowel disease. Acute gastritis is seen occasionally in children with ulcerative colitis.

Prednisolone and mesalazine should be started. Sulfasalazine syrup can be given to younger children. Methylprednisolone is used occasionally, although mild cases may respond to 5-ASA derivatives alone. Exclusive enteral nutrition has no role. Milk exclusion is helpful occasionally. Dietetic input is helpful, as most children with colitis will be energy-deficit and have high calorie needs.

The main indications for azathioprine in ulcerative colitis, as in Crohn's disease, are steroid-sensitive, frequently relapsing disease, steroid-dependent disease and steroid-resistant disease. The aim is to improve clinical wellbeing and reduce steroid requirements. It usually takes two to three months to take effect, and frequent blood monitoring is required. Ciclosporin and methotrexate are used occasionally. The medical management of ulcerative colitis is discussed in Bremner and Beattie (2004) and Escher et al. (2003).

DISTAL COLITIS

This usually requires systemic treatment. Local preparations are not tolerated well in children. Prednisolone or hydrocortisone enemas can be used. 5-ASA derivatives can also be given locally.

Table 25.3 *Inflammatory bowel disease: indications for surgical intervention*

Diagnostic
Upper-/lower-gastrointestinal endoscopy
Biopsy of mouth or perianal lesions
Biopsy of chance findings at laparotomy, e.g. for suspected appendicitis
Therapeutic
Emergency
Acute toxic colitis
Abscess/fistula/perianal disease
Elective/semi-elective
Disease resistant to medical therapy
Disease resistant to medical therapy plus growth failure/delayed puberty
Obstruction (partial or complete) due to stricture
Complications from/intolerance of medical therapy
Long-standing chronically active pan colitis in which there is an increased cancer risk
Malignancy
Resistant perianal disease

SURGICAL MANAGEMENT

Historically, up to 50 per cent of children with Crohn's disease and 25 per cent of children with ulcerative colitis required surgery within five years of diagnosis, although these figures may overestimate the rates now, with increased use of newer immunosuppressants. IBD starting in childhood seems to be more likely to require surgery than IBD developing later.

Diagnostic operations include upper- and lower-gastrointestinal endoscopy, together or separately, biopsy of the mouth or perianal lesions, and biopsy of chance findings at laparotomy, e.g. suspected appendicitis (Table 25.3).

Therapeutic operations can be either emergency or elective. Emergency operations are for either toxic megacolon or perianal abscess. Elective operations are much more problematic and are never purely a surgical decision. Careful planning is essential, including multidisciplinary assessment and, most importantly, involvement of the patient and their family. For example, maximal growth will be achieved if surgery is performed before puberty.

Indications for surgery

EMERGENCY OPERATION

Toxic megacolon, with a colonic diameter of more than 6 cm accompanied by a rapid clinical deterioration, may progress to perforation and an increased mortality. Subtotal colectomy and ileostomy may be life-saving.

Perianal Crohn's disease may present as an abscess, which requires simple incision and drainage.

ELECTIVE OPERATION

Surgery is indicated for disease resistant to medical management, often accompanied by poor growth, delayed puberty and recurrent abdominal pain (Figure 25.3). Subacute obstruction due to strictures, intolerance or complications of medical therapy, fistulation and resistant perianal disease are less common indications in children. Long-term indications, such as the malignancy risk of pan-colitis, are rare in children.

Preoperative management

Nutrition must be optimized and immunosuppression reduced as much as possible before surgery to reduce the risks of postoperative complications from sepsis, poor wound healing and thrombosis.

Most older children on steroids should have subcutaneous heparin (e.g. enoxaparin 20 mg daily), although there is no evidence for its efficacy.

Before an ileostomy is performed, both the child and the family need to be prepared thoroughly. The child may be more accepting of the stoma than the family. They need to be seen by a paediatric stoma nurse and hopefully to meet another child of the same age and gender with a stoma. The optimal site should be marked with an indelible pen and then protected with an Opsite dressing, which is removed just before skin preparation in theatre. There is a lower complication rate for stomas formed through the rectus sheath.

Operations for inflammatory bowel disease

In both ulcerative colitis and Crohn's disease, the surgeon has to remember that a temporary or permanent ileostomy is likely at some point, so the right lower quadrant must be kept unscarred. Although paediatric surgeons like to use transverse incisions, these are contraindicated in IBD surgery, except in children in whom everything can be done through a supraumbilical transverse incision (e.g. a right hemicolectomy in a nine-year-old). The optimum incision will be a personal choice, but the author uses a left paramedian skin incision, leading obliquely down to a midline linea alba incision. This puts the scar and any mucous fistula as far as possible from any stoma, and the midline linea alba incision is easier to open and subsequently close.

CROHN'S DISEASE

The operations for Crohn's disease vary in type and results, depending on the site and extent of disease.

Pure ileal disease

Isolated segments causing subacute obstruction may be resected with primary anastomosis. If possible, a 2-cm margin should be left beyond any macroscopic disease. Multiple resections may result in short bowel syndrome. Anastomotic sites should be marked with Ligaclips to aid any subsequent radiological investigations. Stricturoplasty should be performed for

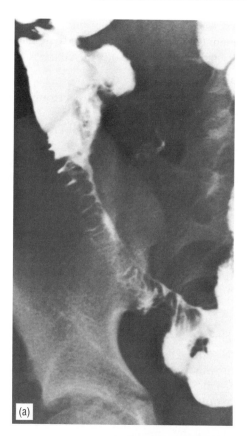

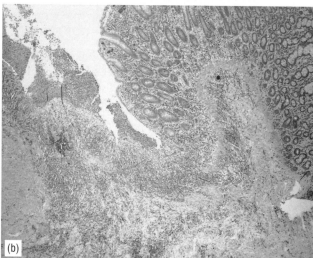

Figure 25.3 *Barium radiology in a 13-year-old boy with terminal ileal Crohn's disease, diagnosed at age 11 years, who, despite enteral nutrition, corticosteroids and azathioprine, had persistent abdominal pain with food, resulting in the need for long-term enteral nutrition. Note the significant persistent terminal ileal abnormality (a). He has done well, with symptom relief and a growth spurt, following limited ileocaecal resection. Histology of the terminal ileum and valve showed mostly fibrotic change with deep-fissuring ulceration (b) and significant stricturing of the bowel lumen. See also Colour Plate 4.*

fibrotic strictures, particularly if there is no surrounding inflammation. Following small-bowel resection, the length of the remaining small bowel should be measured.

Ileocaecal disease

Limited or extended right hemicolectomy to include colonic disease with primary anastomosis is usually safe. The anastomoses should be marked with Ligaclips and the small bowel measured. Although terminal ileal disease may appear to spare the ileocaecal valve, this is very rare, and limited right hemicolectomy avoids subsequent stenosis and disease at the anastomosis or valve.

Colitis

Toxic colitis in Crohn's disease is very rare but, like pan-colitis, requires a subtotal colectomy, ileostomy and mucous fistula. However, Crohn's colitis can occur in an isolated segment, and debate rages as to the role of segmental colectomy. Historically, subtotal colectomy had the benefit of a single operation but was associated with increased morbidity. Segmental colectomy produced a better quality of life, but, especially in children, often multiple reoperations were required until a subtotal colectomy and ileostomy was performed. Since the advent of adjuvant immunosuppression, segmental resection may be performed.

If the sigmoid and rectum are inflamed only mildly, then subtotal colectomy, ileostomy and a mucous fistula to the bottom of the abdominal incision allow decompression and the local installation of steroids. If the sigmoid and rectum are very inflamed, then the rectum can be divided and oversewn (Hartmann procedure), with no increased risk of pelvic sepsis.

Results of surgery in Crohn's disease

No operation for Crohn's disease is curative. However, wellbeing, development of puberty, catch-up growth and psychological improvement through adolescence can all be achieved. Up to 50 per cent of children require reoperation within five years; the recurrence rate is highest for colonic and pan-enteric disease, and the best outcome follows hemicolectomy for ileocaecal disease. After surgery, most children should continue on immunosuppressants, which will reduce disease recurrence. The recurrence is often at a new site. In children, reoperation is more often for new disease resistant to medical management than for specific complications, e.g. stricture.

Figure 25.4 shows the resected specimen in severe colonic Crohn's disease refractory to medical management.

ULCERATIVE COLITIS

Following suitable counselling, the operations for ulcerative colitis vary only in their staging and the method of potential reconstruction. Surgery will be required in 15 per cent of children within five years of diagnosis and 25 per cent within ten years.

Subtotal colectomy and temporary ileostomy

This can be performed as an emergency or electively, leaving a rectal stump as short as is practical. The ileostomy can be constructed safely in ileum that exhibits 'backwash ileitis'.

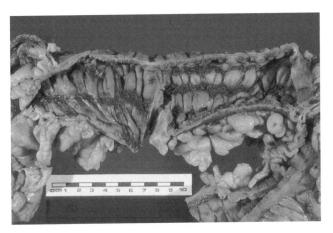

Figure 25.4 *Resection specimen, showing colonic Crohn's disease. Note the deep-fissuring ulceration, cobble-stoning and bowel-wall thickening, with extensive fat deposition on the serosal surface. See also Colour Plate 5.*

Reconstruction

This is often timed after puberty to coincide with the holidays after school examinations (aged 16+). As the child is eventually going to have to be transferred to a sympathetic adult colorectal surgeon for long-term care, it is the author's view that this should occur before surgical reconstruction.

A J-pouch performed by stapling the terminal 20 cm of ileum back on itself, and then anastomosing the apex to the rectal stump, is unlikely to affect continence, although residual mucosal disease may be troublesome. A Soave-type pull-through was also recommended, as it removed all the diseased mucosa and avoided pouchitis.

Twenty per cent of patients prefer a permanent ileostomy combined with excision of the rectal stump, especially if there have been multiple complications following reconstruction. These patients already have previous experience of ileostomy and are able to make rational choices.

Results of surgery for ulcerative colitis

Colectomy is curative from the point of view of the colitis, and catch-up growth occurs in 45 per cent, especially if prepubertal, with no further deterioration in the remainder. Following reconstruction, bowel frequency will be 10–12 times per day initially, reducing to three to four times per day by one year following surgery. However, there may be major long-term morbidity from faecal incontinence, defecation at night, adhesion obstruction and problems with the rectal stump. Pouchitis affects at least 33 per cent of all pouches, although antibiotics may be helpful if given intermittently.

CANCER SURVEILLANCE

Patients with active colitis for more than ten years are at increased risk of colonic cancer, and regular colonoscopic surveillance, with colectomy if there is dysplasia, is recommended.

OTHER COLITIDES

Food–allergic colitis

- Secondary to food allergens, most commonly milk.
- Presents with rectal bleeding usually in otherwise healthy infants.
- Responds to milk exclusion using a substitute (hydrolysed) milk.
- Usually self-limiting.

Pseudomembranous colitis

- Secondary to *C. difficile*, a Gram-positive anaerobe.
- Risk factor is disruption of the normal intestinal flora by antibiotics.
- Clinical features of *C. difficile* colonization vary from asymptomatic carriage to life-threatening pseudomembranous colitis.
- Pathogenesis is through toxin production.
- Treatment is with vancomycin (oral) or metronidazole (intravenous or oral). Probiotics may have a role. Surgery is required occasionally.
- Relapse rate is 15–20 per cent.

CLINICAL SCENARIOS

Case 1

A 15-year-old boy presents with a six-month history of abdominal discomfort with loose stools. He has lost weight and has had a reduced height velocity (< 4 cm/year) over the past 12 months. He has not yet entered puberty. He has missed more than 50 per cent of school. He looks pale and unwell. Basic investigations show a mild normochromic anaemia, thrombocytosis, raised CRP and low serum albumin. Crohn's disease is suspected. Further investigations, including upper-gastrointestinal endoscopy, ileocolonoscopy and barium radiology, confirm ileocaecal Crohn's disease.

Management priorities include getting him well, establishing weight gain, promoting growth and the onset of puberty, and getting him back into school.

He is treated with enteral nutrition given as sole therapy for eight weeks, which induces a clinical remission. He is then well for more than six months, with good weight gain. Unfortunately, he relapses and requires a further course of enteral nutrition. Steroids are avoided because of the potential toxicity, and azathioprine is introduced as steroid-sparing therapy. He then has a more sustained remission, with improved linear growth and the onset of puberty. The final adult height is normal.

Medical therapy will suffice in most cases of ileocaecal Crohn's disease, particularly with the early introduction of azathioprine as steroid-sparing medication. Newer agents, such as infliximab, can be used. If the disease proves resistant to medical management, particularly if there are persistent symptoms or structuring disease and/or persistent growth failure, then ileocaecal resection is appropriate, which will effect a remission, although recurrent disease is common.

Case 2

An eight-year-old girl presents with abdominal discomfort associated with frequent loose stools containing blood and mucus. Investigations show mild anaemia with thrombocytosis but no other abnormalities. Stool cultures are negative. Colonoscopy shows a pan-colitis, with no normal mucosa. Histology is consistent with ulcerative colitis. She does well initially with corticosteroids and 5-ASA derivatives. Her disease, however, relapses three times in the first year. Despite further steroids and a trial of milk exclusion, she becomes steroid-dependent, with poor growth and mood disturbance. She is started on azathioprine. This induces a more sustained remission. However, four years later, she is less well, with steroid-dependent disease and significant toxicity. Repeat colonoscopy shows a featureless 'hosepipe' colon. After appropriate preoperative counselling, she undergoes a subtotal colectomy with ileostomy and mucous fistula formation and does well with a symptom-free adolescence. She will be a good candidate for future reconstructive surgery after she has completed her school examinations.

ACKNOWLEDGEMENTS

Dr R Bremner, Dr J Fairhurst and Dr I Moore for help with the figures. The child in Figure 25.1a for his consent to publish his pictures.

REFERENCES

Bremner ARF, Beattie RM. Therapy of Crohn's disease in childhood. *Expert Opinion on Pharmacotherapy* 2002; **3**: 809–25.

Bremner ARF, Beattie RM. Therapy of ulcerative Colitis in childhood. *Expert Opinion on Pharmacotherapy* 2004; **5**: 37–53.

Cotton P, Williams C. *Practical Gastrointestinal Endoscopy*, 4th edn. Oxford: Blackwell Science, 1996.

Escher JC, Taminiau JA, Nieuwenhuis EE, *et al.* Treatment of inflammatory bowel disease in childhood: best available evidence. *Inflammatory Bowel Diseases* 2003; **9**: 34–58.

FURTHER READING

Incidence and aetiology, including genetics

Podolsky DK. Inflammatory bowel disease. *New England Journal of Medicine* 2002; **347**: 417–28.

Sawczenko A, Sandhu BK, Logan RF, et al. Prospective survey of childhood inflammatory bowel disease in the British Isles. *Lancet* 2001; **357**: 1093–4.

Endoscopy

Numerous atlases of endoscopy are available on the Internet by keying 'atlas of endoscopy' into one of the search engines.

Medical management of inflammatory bowel disease in childhood

Carter MJ, Lobo AJ, Travis SP, et al. On behalf of the British Society of Gastroenterology. Guidelines for the management of inflammatory bowel disease in adults. *Gut* 2004; **53**(Suppl V): v1–16.

Hyams JS, Markowitz J, Wyllie R. Use of infliximab in the treatment of Crohn's disease in children and adolescents. *Journal of Pediatrics* 2000; **137**: 192–6.

Pearson DC, May GR, Fick G, Sutherland LR. Azathioprine for maintaining remission of Crohn's disease. *Cochrane Database of Systematic Reviews* 2000; (2): CD000067.

Surgical management of inflammatory bowel disease in childhood

Besnard M, Jaby O, Mougenot JF, et al. Postoperative outcome of Crohn's disease in 30 children. *Gut* 1998; **43**: 634–8.

Mclain BI, Davidson PM, Stokes KB, Beasley SW. Growth after gut resection for Crohn's disease. *Archives of Disease in Childhood* 1990; **65**: 760–62.

Shand WS. Surgical therapy of chronic inflammatory bowel disease in childhood. *Baillière's Clinical Gastroenterology* 1994; **8**: 149–80.

Gastrointestinal duplication

DAVID M BURGE

Learning objectives

- To understand the types of intestinal duplication.
- To understand the complications of duplication cysts and the ways in which they can present.
- To be able to describe the imaging characteristics of duplications.
- To be able to describe the surgical techniques that might be required to excise a duplication.

INTRODUCTION

Congenital duplication of the gastrointestinal tract can take many forms, can occur in any part of the enteric system from mouth to anus, and can present in very many different ways. Although the term 'duplication cyst' is used commonly, 10–20 per cent are tubular structures (Pinter *et al.* 1992) that can communicate at either or both ends with the gut lumen. The spectrum of the condition includes small cysts within the wall of bowel or within other organs such as the pancreas, large tense cysts on the mesenteric border of the bowel causing luminal obstruction by stretching, and long tubular duplication or triplication of entire sections of the gastrointestinal tract. Symptoms produced by duplications vary according to their position, size, type and histology. Features common to all duplications are attachment to the gastrointestinal tract, a well-developed smooth-muscle coat and an epithelial lining of gastrointestinal origin. Multiple duplications can occur in the same patient, and other congenital anomalies may be present.

RELEVANT BASIC SCIENCE

Awareness of the embryology of duplication cysts will alert the surgeon to looking for associated phenomena, e.g. hemivertebrae, enteric cysts within the spine. Knowledge of the pathology will help in the understanding of the mechanisms of clinical presentation.

Given that duplication anomalies are a heterogeneous group, it is unlikely that they have a common embryological cause. Some enteric duplications are densely adherent to the spinal column, are associated with hemi-vertebrae, have a cystic intraspinal component, or open as an enteric fistula on the skin of the back. A concept that explains these less common, but clinically important, variants is that of the split notochord (Faris and Crowe 1975). The notochord is a structure that develops in the midline of the embryo during the third week. It is destined to remain in part as the nucleus pulposus of the intravertebral discs, but in early embryonic life it plays a vital role in organizing symmetry of the embryo and in the development of the spine. Its presence separates developing endoderm (destined to be intestine) from ectoderm (destined to be skin).

If a longitudinal split develops in the notochord, then endoderm and ectoderm can connect. This connection may result in a complete fistula from bowel to skin that passes through the spinal cord and column. Variations include intraspinal cysts that can enlarge and cause spinal compression with neurological signs.

The histology of enteric duplications usually reflects that of the neighbouring gastrointestinal tract. Thus, gastric epithelium predominates in foregut lesions, while cysts further down the gastrointestinal tract will contain small- and/or large-bowel mucosa. However, different types of lining can be found in cysts at any site, and even pancreatic tissue and neural tissue can be present. The presence of these types of mucosa explains mechanisms of presentation, e.g. haemorrhage from gastric acid irritation and pain from pancreatitis. The lesions are invested in a full intestinal muscle wall that may merge with the wall of neighbouring bowel. This wall is easily visible on ultrasound scanning, and this facilitates diagnosis.

GENERAL FEATURES AND INVESTIGATIONS

Clinical features arising from duplications vary with their site and are dealt with below. About 30 per cent present in the neonatal period (Holcomb *et al.* 1989), and most have presented by the age of ten years. The diagnosis can be made on prenatal ultrasound. Preoperative diagnosis of the exact nature of thoracic or abdominal cystic lesions is not always possible. The presence of a vertebral anomaly on plain X-ray is indirect evidence that the associated lesion may be a foregut duplication cyst (Figure 26.1). The ultrasound appearance of abdominal duplications may clearly show the inner mucosal layer and outer-muscle wall coats (Figure 26.2). Cross-sectional imaging using computed tomography (CT) or magnetic resonance imaging (MRI) may give valuable information and is essential if an intraspinal component is suspected. Gastrointestinal contrast studies may yield useful information, particularly about the extent of hindgut tubular duplications (Figure 26.3). The presence of ectopic gastric mucosa, which is found in 35 per cent of duplications, may be demonstrated by ^{99m}Tc-pertechnetate radionuclear scanning (Figure 26.4).

ANATOMICAL TYPES

Thoracic duplications

Approximately 20 per cent of duplications arise from the oesophagus (Holcomb *et al.* 1989). Presentation is usually in the neonatal period, with respiratory distress from birth or within the first few days of life as the lesion continues to fill with secretions produced by its lining mucosa and

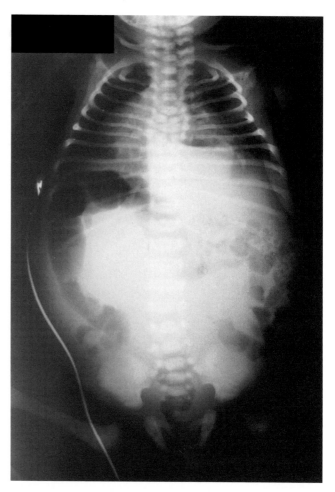

Figure 26.1 *X-ray showing multiple thoracic vertebral anomalies with an intrathoracic duplication.*

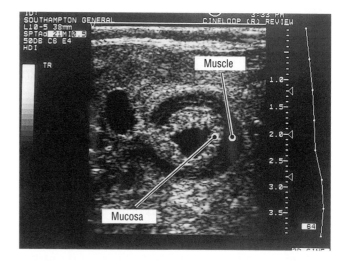

Figure 26.2 *Ultrasound of duplication cyst, whose wall contains both mucosal and muscular layers.*

compresses the lung hilum (Figure 26.5). A high proportion of these lesions contain gastric mucosa, which can cause ulceration into the oesophagus or trachea, producing gastrointestinal bleeding or haemoptysis.

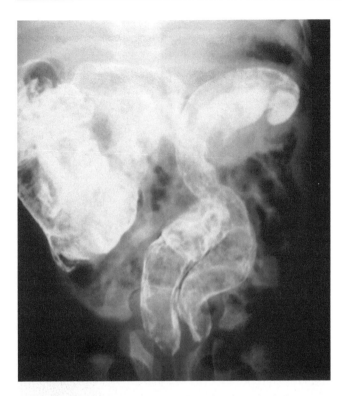

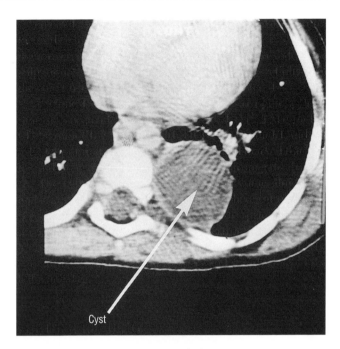

Figure 26.5 *Computed tomography (CT) scan of the chest, showing stretching of the left main bronchus over a thoracic duplication.*

Figure 26.3 *Contrast enema revealing a long rectal tubular duplication.*

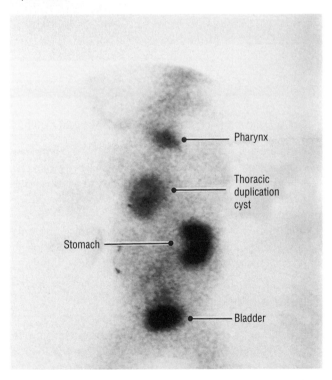

Figure 26.4 *Technetium scan demonstrating ectopic gastric mucosa within a thoracic duplication.*

Thoracic lesions may extend across the diaphragm and, in some cases, the bulk of the duplication is intra-abdominal. For this reason, careful abdominal imaging should be undertaken. Once the lesion has been confirmed as cystic, the main differential diagnosis is bronchogenic cyst or cystic teratoma. It is in this group of duplications that the presence of vertebral anomalies and abnormal uptake on ^{99m}Tc-pertechnetate radionuclear scanning may help in preoperative diagnosis.

Treatment is by thoracotomy and excision. Particular care must be taken if the cyst is within the wall of the oesophagus or densely adherent to the trachea or lung hilum. Large lesions may involve extensive dissection. Thoracoabdominal lesions can be removed by staged surgery, approaching the end causing the presenting symptoms in the first instance.

Gastroduodenal duplications

Gastric duplications usually arise from the greater curve of the stomach (Figure 26.6). A large lesion may present as an abdominal mass, as an acute abdomen or with gastrointestinal bleeding. Smaller lesions may present with pancreatitis (see below).

Pyloric and duodenal duplications usually present by causing obstruction to the intestinal lumen or pancreatitis. These lesions usually are quite small. Those sited in the duodenum are located on its posteromedial border. This can make them hard to find at surgery, especially if peptic irritation or pancreatitis has occurred.

Acute pancreatitis, sometimes recurrent or associated with pseudo-cyst formation, has been reported as a presenting feature of duplications. Such lesions may contain ectopic pancreatic tissue and an accessory duct connection with the main pancreatic duct system.

The most helpful investigations in this group of duplications are ^{99m}Tc-pertechnetate radionuclear scanning and cross-sectional imaging. Endoscopic retrograde cholangio-pancreatography (ERCP) may demonstrate abnormal

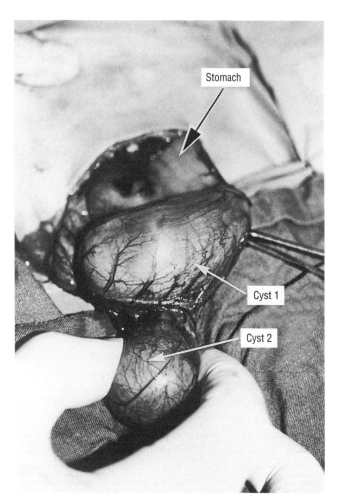

Figure 26.6 *Two cystic duplications on the greater curve of the stomach.*

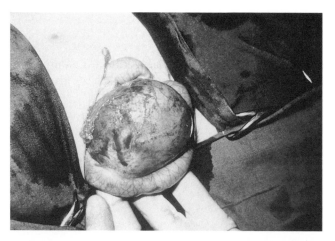

Figure 26.7 *Ileal cystic duplication on the mesenteric border. On this occasion, despite its size, the cyst is not compressing the ileum.*

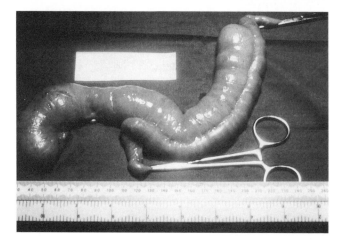

Figure 26.8 *Colonic tubular duplication.*

pancreatic duct anatomy, in some cases with pancreatitis. Surgical excision is the treatment of choice. With some gastric duplications, this can be accomplished without breaching the mucosa of the stomach.

Intra-abdominal cystic duplications

Most abdominal cystic duplications are small bowel in origin (Holcomb *et al.* 1989).They arise from the mesenteric border, and the muscle coats merge with those of the adjoining bowel, with which they share a blood supply (Figure 26.7). The most common presentation in neonates is with a large abdominal mass, but they may be detected on prenatal ultrasound. They may also present acutely in older children with abdominal pain simulating appendicitis, as intussusception with the duplication as the lead point, as intestinal obstruction due to stretching of the adjacent bowel or volvulus, or with perforation.

Lesions in this site are less likely to be associated with vertebral anomalies and the presence of ectopic gastric mucosa. They will be identified as a cystic mass on ultrasound scanning.

The differential diagnosis includes mesenteric (lymphangiomatous) cyst, choledochal cyst and, in females, ovarian cyst. A skilled ultrasonologist will often be able to give a precise diagnosis. It is advisable to obtain a chest X-ray in such cases, as thoracic duplications may coexist.

Treatment is by surgical excision. This usually requires the removal of the adjacent small bowel, although occasionally this can be preserved without damage to its blood supply.

Tubular duplication

This is the most common type of duplication affecting the colon (Figure 26.8), although small-bowel tubular duplications occur. Presentation depends to some extent on the anatomy and on the type of lining epithelium. A tubular duplication that communicates with the intestinal lumen proximally but not distally may present as an abdominal mass due to ballooning of the distal blind end with intestinal contents. Abdominal pain or gastrointestinal bleeding is the likely mode of presentation when ectopic gastric mucosa is present. Colonic tubular duplications may open in the perineum with anal duplication or may be associated with other obvious external abnormalities.

In many cases, the exact nature and extent of tubular duplications will not be appreciated until laparotomy. If the diagnosis is suggested by external signs, then contrast enema studies may aid the planning of surgery.

The surgical treatment of tubular duplications may be very difficult. If a long segment of small bowel is involved, then simple excision of the duplication and adjacent bowel may risk short bowel syndrome. In such cases, it is possible to incise the muscle coat, strip out the mucosal lining and close the points of communication with the bowel lumen. Long colonic duplications often require temporary colostomy with subsequent detailed radiological investigation of the anatomy before final corrective surgery.

Rectal duplication

This rare variety of duplication is worth special description as its methods of presentation may mimic other conditions. It may present as a retro-rectal mass causing constipation and thus be confused with sacrococcygeal teratoma or anterior meningocoele or as a cause of rectal bleeding, or it may be mistaken for simple fistula-in-ano. Excision is best achieved via a posterior sagittal approach.

OUTCOME

The majority of children with gastrointestinal tract duplications will survive without long-term morbidity (Holcomb *et al.* 1989). At most risk are children with intraspinal involvement and children with long small-bowel tubular duplications. Complete excision of the entire lesion, or at least its mucosal lining, is essential to prevent recurrent cyst formation or complications arising from ectopic gastric mucosa. Malignant tumours, including carcinoid, adenocarcinoma and squamous cell carcinoma, have been reported in a number of duplications.

CLINICAL SCENARIOS

Case 1

Antenatal scan at 20 weeks' gestation showed an abdominal cyst measuring 3 cm in diameter. Subsequent scans showed the cyst persisting. The infant was thought to be a girl. At this stage, the differential diagnosis included ovarian cyst, mesenteric (lymphatic) cyst and choledochal or hepatic cyst. Postnatally, the baby was asymptomatic, but ultrasound scanning showed a cyst 7 cm in diameter with a clearly visible muscle coat. Technetium scanning showed no abnormal uptake.

Chest X-ray was normal. The parents were advised that the cyst should be excised because of the potential for volvulus, gastrointestinal bleeding or pain from peptic irritation within the cyst. The cyst was excised along with a few centimetres of adjacent small bowel as an elective procedure when the infant was three months old.

Case 2

A six-month-old infant presented with dark red rectal bleeding for 12 hours. On admission, the abdomen was slightly tender but no masses were palpable. The child was tachycardic (140 beats/min) but normotensive. Haemoglobin level on admission was 79 g/L. The differential diagnosis included intussusception, Meckel's diverticulum, duplication, intestinal haemangioma, peptic ulceration and colitis. After fluid and blood resuscitation, ultrasound scanning was performed but was normal. Technetium scanning showed abnormal uptake in the central abdomen. Laparotomy was performed, suspecting a Meckel's diverticulum, but a tubular duplication cyst of the right colon was found and right hemicolectomy was performed.

Case 3

A three-year-old boy had a chest X-ray performed when he had a chest infection. This showed a right-sided mediastinal mass and a hemi-vertebra at T4. On CT scanning, the mass was cystic and sited in the posterior mediastinum. Technetium scanning showed abnormal uptake in the right chest but also in the abdomen. Elective surgery was performed a few weeks later, requiring a combined thoracoabdominal approach to excise a duplication extending across the diaphragm and behind the peritoneum.

REFERENCES

Faris JC, Crowe JE. The split notocord syndrome. *Journal of Pediatric Surgery* 1975; **10**: 467.

Holcomb GW, Gheissari A, O'Neill JA, *et al.* Surgical management of alimentary tract duplications. *Annals of Surgery* 1989; **209**: 167–74.

Pinter AB, Schubert W, Szemledy F, *et al.* Alimentary tract duplications in infants and children. *European Journal of Pediatric Surgery* 1992; **2**: 8–12.

FURTHER READING

Nayar PM, Freeman NV. Gastrointestinal duplications. In: Freeman NV, Burge DM, Griffiths DM, Malone PS (eds). *Surgery of the Newborn.* Edinburgh: Churchill Livingstone, 1994; pp. 255–66.

Abdominal pain

RAJENDRA SURANA

Learning objectives

- To be able to diagnose the causes of abdominal pain.
- To understand the management of acute appendicitis.
- To understand the complications of appendicectomy.
- To understand the principles of managing recurrent abdominal pain.

INTRODUCTION

Acute and recurrent abdominal pain in childhood are separate and distinct problems. *Acute* abdominal pain may be defined as abdominal pain of short duration (up to a week). *Recurrent* abdominal pain (RAP) is abdominal pain of any duration with more than two attacks over a three-month period.

The precise incidence of acute or recurrent abdominal pain is difficult to establish. Acute abdominal pain is a commonly encountered problem in childhood and constitutes about five per cent of total paediatric admissions and up to 20 per cent of surgical admissions. The management of acute abdominal pain in children is easy on the one hand and difficult on the other. It is easy because of the narrow spectrum of differential diagnoses and difficult because of communication difficulties and atypical presentations.

RAP is common and is estimated to affect up to 15 per cent of children.

RELEVANT BASIC SCIENCE

The differential diagnosis of acute abdominal pain is shown in Table 27.1.

Table 27.1 *Diagnosis of admissions with acute abdominal pain*

Diagnosis	Proportion of total admissions with acute abdominal pain (%)
Acute non-specific abdominal pain	55–65
Appendicitis	25–40
Urinary infection	1–2
Others	2–7

Aetiopathogenesis

The precise aetiopathogenesis of acute non-specific abdominal pain (ANSAP) or acute appendicitis is unknown. Various theories from viral infection to bowel dysmotility are proposed as the aetiological factors for ANSAP. The factor that is considered responsible for appendicitis is luminal obstruction, either by a faecolith or by inflammatory swelling.

Pathology of appendicitis

ACUTE APPENDICITIS

The typical acutely inflamed appendix is congested and oedematous, with submucosal or transmural neutrophil infiltration.

GANGRENOUS APPENDICITIS

In more advanced stages, ischaemia causes grey-green or blackish areas of gangrene in the wall of the appendix. The lumen may contain pus. The peritoneal fluid is increased and is usually purulent. Histologically, there is a loss of normal tissue architecture.

PERFORATED APPENDICITIS

Perforations can be macroscopic or microscopic and are usually on the antimesenteric border. The peritonitis may be localized because of its anatomical position, such as in the paracolic gutter or pelvis. In other children, the peritonitis may be generalized. Rarely, infective thrombi may travel up the portal system, causing portal pyaemia and liver abscess.

APPENDIX MASS

This includes an inflammatory mass and an abscess. An inflammatory mass is formed by the localization process and usually consists of the appendix surrounded by small bowel and omentum.

An analysis of the pathological findings of patients with appendicitis is shown in Table 27.2.

Table 27.2 *Analysis of appendicitis patients*

Diagnosis	Preschool children (%)	Other children (%)
Acute appendicitis	22	67
Perforated appendicitis	56	14
Appendix mass	19	8
Histological normal appendix	3	11
Total	100	100

CLINICAL PRESENTATION

The classic triad in appendicitis is abdominal pain, vomiting and fever. The abdominal pain of acute appendicitis begins around the umbilicus and moves to the right iliac fossa. The initial (referred) pain is colicky, but the right iliac fossa pain is constant and due to localized peritonitis. The pain with appendicitis is exacerbated by abdominal movement. Younger children may not actively complain of abdominal pain but instead may show increasing irritability and disinclination to move about.

Nausea and, initially, non-bilious vomiting are typical. The temperature may be normal but is usually elevated in children with perforated appendicitis, usually in the range of 38–38.5 °C. A temperature over 39 °C suggests perforation with generalized peritonitis or a non-surgical condition, e.g. viral illness or urinary tract infection (UTI).

Constipation is not a common feature. Diarrhoea, if present, is of significance. Twenty per cent of preschool children complain of diarrhoea at presentation (Surana, Quinn and Puri 1995). Viral gastroenteritis may mimic appendicitis.

A history of recent illness, such as upper respiratory tract infection, cough and dysuria, and use of analgesics/antibiotics should be sought, as it may alter the clinical findings. Previous attacks are uncommon in children with appendicitis.

Examination should begin by assessing the general condition of the child, pyrexia, dehydration and progressive tachycardia. Ear, nose and throat (ENT) examination may suggest mesenteric adenitis as the cause of the abdominal pain. Respiratory signs may be obvious on inspection and auscultation, which point to pneumonia as the diagnosis.

Abdominal examination should be gentle and thorough and should always begin with inspection, including hernial orifices and genitalia. Palpation should begin as far away as possible from the area of maximum pain. Localized tenderness and guarding in the right iliac fossa in a relaxed child or generalized guarding are diagnostic of appendicitis. Percussion and auscultation are usually not useful. Appendicitis is unlikely if the child can jump up and down.

Rectal examination is usually unnecessary, especially if a definitive diagnosis has been made. However, if the history suggests it and the child is ill, then it may be possible to diagnose pelvic appendicitis only by gentle rectal examination.

INVESTIGATIONS

In the majority of patients, careful physical examination is all that is necessary to arrive at a diagnosis. Laboratory and radiological investigations are neither sensitive nor specific. Establishment of evidence-based clinical pathways with ongoing monitoring, continued education and identification of key pathway team members responsible for the pathway system might result in decreased hospital costs, reduced hospital stays and fewer unnecessary tests (Warner *et al.* 2002).

White cell count

Leucocytosis with neutrophilia has been considered to be of significance in appendicitis. However, the decision to operate should not be based on white cell count alone, as leucocytosis has been noted in patients who do not have appendicitis and a normal white cell count can occur in patients with perforation and peritonitis.

Other blood tests

A routine serum amylase is unnecessary in children with abdominal pain and should be done only if pancreatitis is a real possibility. Urea and electrolyte tests may be required in sick, dehydrated children. Elevated C-reactive protein has been reported to have a specificity of up to 75 per cent in appendicitis.

Urine microscopy and culture

Two per cent of girls admitted with acute abdominal pain have a bacteriologically proven urinary infection, and this should always be considered in children with known urological abnormalities. Abnormalities on microscopy are commonly found in patients with appendicitis.

Radiology

Plain radiographs rarely help to establish the diagnosis of acute abdominal pain but may be more useful in children aged under three years, when a faecolith may be seen. Urinary calculi are found occasionally. The non-specific features of appendicitis include scoliosis, blurring of the right psoas margin and an abnormal gas pattern in the right lower quadrant.

Ultrasonography

There has been increasing use of ultrasound in children with acute abdominal pain. It is a quick, non-invasive and well-tolerated investigation. The diagnostic features are a turgid appendix, decreased echogenicity of the surrounding fat and the presence of a poorly defined hypo-echoic round or oval structure adjacent to the caecum and separated from other bowel loops. Criteria for perforated appendicitis are clear asymmetry in the wall thickness, with indistinctness of the wall layer or the presence of an air–fluid collection around the appendix. False-negative results may be obtained in as many as 16 per cent of patients, even in experienced hands, and may contribute to a delay in diagnosis and treatment.

Computed tomography (CT) and magnetic resonance imaging (MRI) are usually unnecessary in the management of patients with acute abdominal pain.

MANAGEMENT OF ACUTE ABDOMINAL PAIN

At this point, the diagnosis and the institution of appropriate management may be possible. However, in any case, patients should be divided into three categories:

- No significant abnormality: the patient can be discharged with clear instructions to return if their condition has not settled or is worsening.
- Acute appendicitis requiring appendicectomy.
- Diagnosis uncertain, with surgery not required at that point. These patients are admitted for active observation and/or further investigations.

Active observation

The objective of active observation is to achieve an accurate diagnosis and avoid unnecessary surgery. The assumption is that appendicitis is an evolving process and definitive diagnosis may not be possible at the time of initial presentation. Therefore, in patients with an uncertain diagnosis, a conscious decision is taken to keep the patient under surveillance until the pain has either gone (or almost gone) or intervention is required. Children are allowed clear fluids as the operation can then be performed without undue delay. Active observation differs from other types of observation in that the doctor commits himself/herself to visiting the patient within a specific predetermined interval without waiting to be called because of any change in the patient's condition. This interval is determined by the clinical condition of the patient and the likelihood of surgery being required.

Active observation entails admission to hospital and serial monitoring of temperature and pulse at one-, two- or four-hourly intervals, depending on the patient's condition. At every visit, parental and nursing reports should be obtained and the temperature and pulse chart scrutinized carefully before examining the child. In a hospital setting, and with the increasing use of shift systems, more than one doctor may well see the patient, so careful documentation of each visit is necessary.

A definite diagnosis may not be possible at the second visit, so a third visit is planned, and so on. An effort is made to establish a diagnosis at each visit. A clear explanation should be given to the parents each time the child is seen. As time goes by and diagnosis of appendicitis becomes unlikely, diet may be introduced. During this period, an alternative diagnosis becomes evident in some children; in others, pain resolves, thus avoiding unnecessary surgery. The objections to this policy come from the fear that any delay in surgery will lead to an increased incidence of perforation and postoperative morbidity. Although in a small number of patients this practice may allow appendicitis to progress significantly, our data have shown that there is no real increase in the number of perforations in patients who undergo appendicectomy after active observation, and certainly the morbidity was no worse in these patients. The advent of better antimicrobial agents and intravenous therapy has certainly minimized the effect of the delay (Surana, O'Donnell and Puri 1995).

Appendicectomy

The treatment of appendicitis is appendicectomy. However, surgery may need to be postponed, as very sick children need adequate resuscitation before surgery, and this may take several hours. Appendicectomy is necessary in the middle of the night only rarely (Surana *et al.* 1993). If an operating theatre is made available during the daytime, then one-third of nocturnal operations will be avoided and junior staff will not have to operate on a 'doubtful abdomen'. However, any unnecessary delay in operating should be avoided.

Preparation

Prophylactic or therapeutic antimicrobial agents against Gram-negative bacilli and anaerobes are commenced.

EXAMINATION UNDER ANAESTHESIA

Before proceeding to surgery, the abdomen should be examined properly under anaesthesia to ascertain whether there is a mass. If an appendix mass is identified, then there are two approaches to further management: to defer the surgery and treat the appendix mass conservatively with intravenous fluids and antibiotics, or to proceed with the operation (see p. 237).

POSTOPERATIVE CARE

Antibiotics are continued prophylactically postoperatively for three doses in uncomplicated appendicitis and are continued for five to seven days in children with perforated appendicitis, depending on clinical progress.

Regular oral analgesics are prescribed for at least the first 48 hours or more, and then as required. Nasogastric tubes are required rarely in children. Patients with acute appendicitis are usually ready to start oral fluids 12–24 hours after the operation, while those with severe peritonitis may require intravenous fluids for longer. Intravenous fluid requirements are assessed regularly and discontinued as soon as possible.

Postoperative course and follow-up

Most patients with uncomplicated appendicitis are ready to be discharged home within 48 hours. They may be seen in the community by the paediatric community nurse, or they may be followed up after a week or so to check on the histology and to ensure that they have no postoperative infective complications, such as a wound infection or an intra-abdominal abscess, which presents with pyrexia, vomiting, diarrhoea and abdominal distension.

Table 27.3 *Postoperative complications (n = 870)*

Complication	n	%
Wound infection	16	1.8
Scrotal inflammation	1	0.1
Intra-abdominal abscess	14	1.6
Adhesive obstruction	6	0.7
Total	37	4.2

Postoperative complications

With the advent of better antimicrobial agents, especially against anaerobes, the incidence of postoperative complications has decreased (Table 27.3).

WOUND INFECTION

Wound infection occurred in 1.8 per cent of the patients in our series and included patients who developed wound infection after discharge. All these patients were managed with antibiotics, opening the edge of the wound, or incision and drainage. Complications such as necrotizing fasciitis are rare. Need for debridement and resuturing is unusual.

SCROTAL INFLAMMATION

In young patients, when the processus vaginalis is patent, any infection may track down into the scrotum.

INTRA-ABDOMINAL ABSCESS

Postoperative intra-abdominal abscess occurred in 1.6 per cent in our series. Common sites are in the pelvis and right paracolic gutter; more rarely, they occur in the subphrenic space. With aggressive use of antibiotics, most intra-abdominal abscesses will resolve and are best monitored by clinical course and serial ultrasound scans. Abscesses that fail to respond need drainage. Well-localized abscesses are best drained percutaneously under ultrasound control.

Pelvic abscesses should be allowed to drain rectally. Only rarely will open drainage be required.

FEMALE INFERTILITY

There is still some controversy about the role of intra-abdominal sepsis, especially pelvic sepsis, in the causation of infertility. Careful follow-up of women at risk have shown that prepubertal sepsis will not necessarily result in diminished fertility (Puri *et al.* 1989).

MORTALITY

Deaths due to childhood appendicitis are rare. Such deaths are usually due to inadequate preoperative resuscitation of the patient or overdependence on antibiotics in patients who should have had earlier post-appendicectomy drainage of an abscess.

Management of appendix mass

The management of appendix mass is controversial. Conventional thinking is to treat preoperatively diagnosed appendix masses with intravenous fluids, antibiotics and delayed-interval appendicectomy. However, the dilemma occurs when the diagnosis is made under general anaesthesia. Some advocate continuation of conservative management. Continuation of conservative management results in about ten per cent of patients requiring early intervention, but there are complications from delayed-interval appendicectomy in only a minority of patients. Others, however, advocate proceeding with a difficult appendicectomy under the same anaesthetic.

DIFFERENTIAL DIAGNOSIS OF OTHER CAUSES OF ACUTE ABDOMINAL PAIN

Urinary tract infection

UTI (see also Chapter 52) is an uncommon cause of acute abdominal pain in childhood, especially if it is not accompanied by urinary symptoms such as dysuria, frequency or haematuria. Constitutional symptoms such as fever, vomiting and anorexia are not unusual. If the child has a previous history of proven UTI or has a congenital urinary tract anomaly, then the possibility of UTI should be considered. A clinical diagnosis of UTI in other patients in the absence of urinary symptoms is unwise. A pelvic appendicitis may mimic UTI.

Mesenteric adenitis

Clinically, children with mesenteric adenitis present with abdominal pain and pyrexia (39 °C or higher). Vomiting is not common and appetite may be normal. There is often an associated upper-respiratory infection, with enlargement of neck lymph nodes. The tenderness is usually medial to McBurney's point and guarding is usually not present. The pain and tenderness may shift medially if the child is rolled to the left side. The condition usually settles within 24–48 hours, and the abdominal pain disappears.

Constipation

Although frequently considered as a differential diagnosis of acute abdominal pain, constipation of two to three days' duration is unlikely to be a frequent cause of acute abdominal pain. The diagnosis is more likely if a suppository relieves the pain. Enemas should be used with caution and only when appendicitis has been ruled out.

Meckel's diverticulitis

Although uncommon, children with Meckel's diverticulitis may present with acute abdominal pain indistinguishable from acute appendicitis. Up to one-third of patients may have perforation and peritonitis. Patients with Meckel's diverticulitis usually present with periumbilical pain; the tenderness is usually medial but may be anywhere in the lower abdomen. The treatment is laparotomy with resection of the diverticulum. It must also be looked for in patients undergoing appendicectomy where the appendix appears normal. Less than one per cent of operations for acute abdominal pain in children are for complications of Meckel's diverticulum.

Pancreatitis

Although pancreatitis is uncommon, and routine amylase investigation in acute abdominal pain is unnecessary, it should be suspected in children with predisposing causes such as choledochal cyst and patients presenting with severe upper abdominal pain radiating to the back, with tenderness and guarding in the upper abdomen. Occasionally, body-wall ecchymoses, such as Cullen's sign at the umbilicus or Grey Turner's sign in the flanks, will be evident. The diagnosis of pancreatitis is made by a serum amylase activity four times the upper limit of normal or lipase activity twice the upper limit of normal. Serum lipase has high specificity as it remains increased for a longer period than amylase and there are no other sources of lipase. Plain X-ray findings are unreliable and include a sentinel loop, local or generalized ileus, a colon cutoff, a renal halo sign and, rarely, retroperitoneal gas. These are non-specific but may help to exclude other pathology, such as a perforated viscus. Ultrasound may be unhelpful in confirming the diagnosis, but a swollen pancreas, free fluid, gallstones, dilated bile ducts or a choledochal cyst may be identified. A CT scan is more helpful and is recommended in severe cases three to ten days after admission.

C-reactive protein measurement over 210 mg/L in the first four days or over 120 mg/L at the end of the first week suggests severe disease. Three or more positive Ranson or Glasgow scoring criteria on initial admission, or over 48 hours, indicate severe disease.

MANAGEMENT OF PANCREATITIS

Mild acute pancreatitis

These children are treated with intravenous fluids and basic monitoring of temperature, pulse, blood pressure and urine output. There is no role for routine antibiotics, unless specific infections, such as chest infection, occur. Although aprotonin, glucagons and somatostatin have been used, none has any proven value and therefore they are not recommended.

Severe acute pancreatitis

This is uncommon but associated with a high mortality. The initial management involves full resuscitation and a multi-disciplinary approach. These patients should be managed in an intensive care unit. Peripheral venous and central lines, a urinary catheter and a nasogastric tube are required. The following should be measured hourly: pulse, blood pressure, central venous pressure, respiratory rate, oxygen saturation, urine output, temperature and fluid balance. There is some evidence to support the use of prophylactic antibiotics. Confirmed infections will necessitate treatment in their own right. All patients with mild or severe pancreatitis will require ongoing assessment to monitor recovery or possible development of life-threatening complications. Ongoing assessment consists of clinical, biochemical, radiological and bacteriological assessment. Necrotizing pancreatitis requires an experienced endoscopist and pancreatobiliary surgeon (British Society of Gastroenterology 1998).

Gastroenteritis

Copious diarrhoea and vomiting, with hyperactive bowel sounds and without any localizing signs, suggest gastroenteritis, usually caused by viruses such as rotavirus and astrovirus. Remember that diarrhoea may be a presenting feature of acute appendicitis.

Ovarian pathology

Abdominal pain secondary to ovarian pathology usually occurs in peripubertal girls. The pain is in a lower quadrant or midline and may be associated with nausea and vomiting. The ovarian cysts *per se* rarely cause abdominal pain, but haemorrhage into the cyst or torsion of the cyst or normal adnexa can present with acute abdominal pain. Occasionally, ovulation-induced haemorrhage causes localized peritonitis; this is termed 'mittelschmerz'. Ultrasound is helpful in diagnosing ovarian pathology. The treatment for patients with torsion is early laparotomy to salvage the ovary and remove the cyst. Oophorectomy is rarely necessary and should be avoided if at all possible. Contralateral oophoropexy has been recommended, as excessive mobility and hormonal activity may cause similar problems on the other side of the body.

Primary peritonitis

Primary peritonitis is a rare cause of acute abdominal pain in children. It is more common in girls than boys. The diagnosis is often made at a laparotomy for suspected appendicitis when no pathology is identified. The causative agent is usually either *Pneumococcus* or *Streptococcus*. It is usually associated with other associated medical condition, such as nephrotic syndrome. The precise causation is unknown but is hypothesized to be either haematogenous or retrograde passage through the female genital tract or through transmural migration of the microbes through the gastrointestinal tract.

Henoch–Schönlein purpura

This is a systemic vasculitis of unknown origin with a pathognomonic rash that is initially urticarial but becomes haemorrhagic (purpuric), involving the ankles, buttocks and perineal areas. Two-thirds of patients present with abdominal pain. Associated features include nausea, vomiting, bloody stools, nephritis and, occasionally, scrotal inflammation. The symptoms are due to haemorrhage into the bowel wall or complications such as intussusception, obstruction and perforation. Ultrasound is a valuable tool for distinguishing complications requiring surgery from intestinal intramural haemorrhage. Intussusception in these patients can be monitored with ultrasound, with resolution in many patients.

Irreducible inguinal hernia and torsion of testes

Children with these problems may present with lower abdominal pain, but exposure of the abdomen to the mid-thigh and careful examination will point to the obvious cause.

Non-abdominal causes

Right-sided basal pneumonia may present as right upper quadrant pain, and acute subhepatic appendicitis may cause a sympathetic pleural effusion. The diagnosis is usually based on the abdominal and chest findings. Chest X-ray will demonstrate the consolidation. However, appendicitis can occur in the presence of pneumonia.

RECURRENT ABDOMINAL PAIN

Incidence

It is difficult to measure the incidence of RAP, but it is estimated that 15 per cent of school children experience RAP at some point, with almost 20 per cent of these having severe bouts, significantly affecting their activity.

Causes

The causes of RAP are usually grouped into functional, psychogenic and organic.

FUNCTIONAL CAUSES

Irritable bowel syndrome
The criteria for the diagnosis of irritable bowel syndrome (IBS) are that the child should be old enough to provide an accurate history of the pain, the abdominal discomfort and pain have been present for at least 12 weeks, not necessarily consecutively over the previous 12 months, the abdominal discomfort is relieved with defecation and associated with a change in stooling form or frequency, and any structural or metabolic abnormalities that might explain the symptoms are absent.

Abdominal migraine

Abdominal migraine is defined as three or more paroxysmal episodes of intense, acute midline abdominal pain lasting from two hours to several days, with intervening symptom-free intervals lasting weeks to months, in the preceding 12 months and with no evidence of metabolic, gastrointestinal, central nervous system, structural or biochemical diseases, and with two of the following features: headache during episodes, photophobia during episodes, family history of migraine, headache confined to one side only, and aura. However, it is important to exclude any organic cause of the pain (Hyman *et al.* 2000). The functional gastrointestinal disorders may be due to alterations in motility and visceral hypersensitivity.

PSYCHOGENIC CAUSES

Parental depression and major life events, such as parental separation, financial difficulties or serious illness in the household, can trigger RAP. The personality of the child may predispose him or her to RAP. Children who are 'strivers' (ambitious, perfectionist, overachieving) are sometimes trying to live up to the expectations of ambitious parents. Management of the child's anxiety depends on building up his or her confidence through reassurance, hard work and experience.

There may be problems at school, especially if the child has an unsympathetic teacher. The child's educational abilities may need to be assessed formally. Bullying and lack of self-esteem are common problems.

ORGANIC CAUSES

Constipation

Constipation is one of the most commonly cited gastrointestinal causes of abdominal, especially left iliac fossa, pain. The prominent symptom is infrequent passage of hard stools. Overuse of laxatives can cause colicky abdominal pain, so a detailed laxative history should be taken.

Inflammatory bowel disease

In Crohn's disease, any pain is usually in the right lower quadrant and may begin as a diffuse, vague abdominal discomfort. In the majority of patients, abdominal pain is minimal or overshadowed by failure to thrive and other bowel symptoms. Clinical anaemia and a right lower quadrant mass should raise suspicions of Crohn's disease.

Peptic ulcer disease

Peptic ulcer disease is uncommon in children. There is an increased familial incidence. Patients are usually of school age, and boys are affected more commonly than the girls. Patients may also present with vomiting, haematemesis, melaena and anaemia. Physical examination is usually not helpful, apart from occasional epigastric tenderness. Endoscopy will demonstrate that duodenal ulcers are more common than gastric ulcers. Endoscopy is preferred over contrast studies. Management is with histamine H_2 receptor antagonists such as ranitidine or proton-pump inhibitors such as omeprazole, giving appropriate treatment for *Helicobacter pylori* infection, if required. Surgery is indicated rarely. Zollinger–Ellison syndrome is rare; therefore, serum gastrin levels are not required routinely.

Gynaecological pathology

Endometriosis, pelvic inflammatory disease, dysmenorrhoea and intermittent ovarian torsion can cause RAP.

Neoplasia

The most serious but fortunately very rare cause of RAP is neoplasia. This is often the major, but unspoken, parental worry. Lymphoma, neuroblastoma and Wilms tumour may cause abdominal pain but should have associated features, such as unexplained weight loss, anorexia, other constitutional symptoms or a mass.

CLINICAL SCENARIOS

Case 1

A nine-year-old boy presented with abdominal pain of six hours' duration, which started centrally and was now in the right side of the abdomen. He felt nauseated and had two non-bilious vomits. There were no other symptoms and no other positive history. General examination revealed a distressed child with minimal dehydration, pulse rate 112 beats/min and temperature 37.8 °C. Chest and other examination was normal. Abdominal examination showed tenderness and guarding in the right iliac fossa. Full blood count showed leucocytosis with neutrophilia. The clinical diagnosis was acute appendicitis. Intravenous fluids were started, along with prophylactic antibiotics. After informed consent, appendicectomy was performed. At operation, an acute suppurative appendix was removed with peritoneal lavage. Postoperatively, feeds were established by 24 hours and the child was discharged. The risk of adhesive obstruction was explained.

Case 2

A three-year-old girl was brought in by her parents. She had been irritable, unwell and unhappy to touch her tummy for four days. She was seen by her general practitioner, thought to have an upper respiratory infection and given paracetamol. However, the pain did not settle and she was referred for paediatric assessment unit at a local hospital. The paediatric senior house office thought it was a viral illness and discharged her. She was later brought back to the accident and emergency department, as she was unwell and lethargic. The surgical registrar was called, who thought her abdomen was rigid. She was resuscitated and a laparotomy was performed. At operation, there was free pus in the abdomen, with a perforated appendix. A thorough peritoneal lavage was performed and the wound was closed. Intravenous triple antibiotics (penicillin, gentamicin, metronidazole) were continued. Her abdomen remained distended for 48 hours and then her bowels gradually got going. However, on day five, she started having a spiking temperature and diarrhoea. Her white cell count was elevated and ultrasound confirmed the clinical suspicion of a pelvic collection. Her peritoneal swab had grown Gram-negative bacilli with anaerobes. She was continued on the appropriate antibiotics, with gradual improvement in her white cell count. Ultrasound confirmed the resolution of the pelvic collection. She was discharged home after ten days.

Case 3

A four-year-old boy presented with a four- to five-day history of being unwell, with irritability and abdominal pain and with no improvement with painkillers. On examination, he looked well, but abdominal examination revealed a fixed 10-cm mass in the right iliac fossa, which was marked with a felt-tip pen. A diagnosis of appendix mass was made, which was confirmed on ultrasound. He was commenced on triple antibiotics, his condition improved, and the mass became smaller clinically. Ultrasound was repeated after one week, and the mass had resolved. His parents were counselled and he was readmitted for interval appendicectomy after four weeks. At operation, a fibrotic appendix was removed and he was discharged 36 hours later.

Case 4

A 13-year-old girl was admitted with vague lower abdominal pain for 12 hours. There was no associated vomiting, diarrhoea or constipation. Examination showed some tenderness in the right lower quadrant. White cell count and midstream urine were normal. She was admitted for active observation. There was no change in her vital signs despite persistent minimal right lower quadrant tenderness. Ultrasound was normal. She remained well, the pain resolved after 36 hours of admission, and she was discharged home with a presumptive diagnosis of ANSAP.

REFERENCES

British Society of Gastroenterology. United Kingdom guidelines for the management of acute pancreatitis. *Gut* 1998; **42** (Suppl 2): S1–13.

Hyman PE, Rasquin-weber A, Fleisher DR, *et al.* Childhood functional gastrointestinal disorders. In: Drossman DA (ed.). *The Functional Disorders*, 2nd edn. Lawrence, KS: Allen Press, 2000; pp. 533–75.

Puri P, McGuiness EPJ, Guiney EJ. Fertility following perforated appendicitis in girls. *Journal of Pediatric Surgery* 1989; **24**: 547–9.

Surana R, Quinn FMJ, Puri P. Is it necessary to perform appendicectomy in the middle of the night in children? *British Medical Journal* 1993; **306**: 1168.

Surana R, O'Donnell B, Puri P. Appendicitis diagnosed following active observation does not increase morbidity in children. *Pediatric Surgery International* 1995; **10**: 76–8.

Surana R, Quinn F, Puri P. Appendicitis in preschool children. *Pediatric Surgery International* 1995; **10**: 68–70.

Warner BW, Rich KA, Atherton H, Andersen CL, Kotagal UR. The sustained impact of an evidence-based clinical pathway for acute appendicitis. *Seminars in Pediatric Surgery* 2002; **11**: 29–35.

FURTHER READING

Cope Z, Silen W. *Cope's Early Diagnosis Of Acute Abdomen*. Oxford: Oxford University Press, 2000.

O' Donnell B. 1990 *Abdominal Pain in Children*. Oxford: Blackwell Scientific.

28

Acquired conditions of the anorectum and perineum

SPENCER W BEASLEY

Learning objectives

- To describe the significance of the various presentations of rectal bleeding in infants and children.
- To identify when rectal prolapse is secondary to identifiable organic disease.

INTRODUCTION

Several unrelated conditions may affect the anorectal and perineal areas in children (Box 28.1). Most are minor, but sometimes they are manifestations of more extensive disease, such as the perianal disease seen in Crohn's disease. Others, such as necrotizing enterocolitis, volvulus and intussusception, are potentially life-threatening and require a high index of suspicion if the correct diagnosis is to be made early and appropriate treatment instituted.

Anal fissure is by far the most common condition. It may present at any age with pain on defecation and a small amount of bright red blood on the surface of the stool or immediately after defecation. The fissure is found in the midline and normally heals within days. It may be a reflection of a tendency to constipation, and treatment of the underlying constipation will reduce the likelihood of its recurrence.

A variety of other conditions also produce apparent rectal bleeding in children. They are best considered in relation to the way in which they present, as this will give some clues as to their likely cause (Table 28.1). The two important surgical causes of rectal bleeding in the neonate are necrotizing enterocolitis and malrotation in which volvulus of the midgut has supervened.

Anal fissures, although more common in older children, may occur in the neonatal period. If the infant has swallowed maternal blood, either during delivery or from a cracked nipple, then blood may be evident in the stools. Haemorrhagic disease of the newborn also may produce blood in the stools and is prevented by routine administration of vitamin K.

Box 28.1 Acquired conditions of the anorectum and perineum in children

Anal fissure
Rectal polyp
Rectal prolapse
Perianal abscess and fistula
Inflammatory bowel disease
Straddle injuries
Labial adhesions

Table 28.1   *Presentation of rectal bleeding in children*

Clinical setting	Typical causes
Neonatal	Necrotizing enterocolitis Volvulus with ischaemia Haemorrhagic disease of the newborn (vitamin K deficiency) Anal fissure Swallowed maternal blood
Small amount of bright blood in a well child	Anal fissure (by far the most common) Rectal polyps Unrecognized rectal prolapse Haemorrhoids (idiopathic)
Ill child with acute abdominal condition	Intussusception Gastroenteritis Henoch–Schönlein purpura
Major haemorrhage from gastrointestinal tract	Oesophageal varices Peptic ulcer Meckel's diverticulum Tubular duplications
Chronic illness with diarrhoea	Crohn's disease Ulcerative colitis Non-specific colitis

MILK ALLERGY

Cows' milk protein is the most common cause of protein intolerance in children. It may produce a variety of features, including specks of bright blood in the stools, occult blood loss, acute colitis, diarrhoea, vomiting and coeliac-like syndrome. It may also result in eczema, urticaria and wheeze. The infant's symptoms will resolve on withdrawal of cows' milk and relapse on introduction. Goats' milk and soy formulae have similar antigenic properties to cows' milk.

SMALL AMOUNT OF BLOOD IN A WELL CHILD

This is a common presentation. The cause of the bleeding can often be determined by the history alone.

Anal fissure

An anal fissure occurs when passage of hard stool splits the mucosa of the anus, usually in the midline posteriorly or anteriorly. The child suffers pain on defecation, and a small amount of bright red blood may be seen on the surface of the stool or immediately following it. The fissure heals rapidly, but if it has been recurrent, it may produce a small mount of oedematous skin, just external to the fissure, as a 'sentinel pile'. The diagnosis can be confirmed by gently parting the anus laterally to expose the anal mucosa anteriorly and posteriorly. Healing of

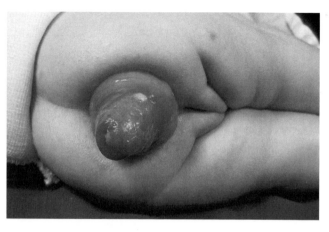

Figure 28.1   *Rectal prolapse.*

the fissure is facilitated by treating the underlying constipation. Liquid paraffin oil and lactulose are effective in softening the stools and acting as lubricants. Sometimes, an anal fissure can develop after an episode of severe diarrhoea. The key to treatment is to ensure that the child does not develop a pattern of inappropriate 'holding on' and reluctance to defaecate for fear of pain, leading to chronic rectal distension and faecal loading.

Rectal polyp

A juvenile polyp is a benign hamartomatous lesion that is usually located in the rectum and should be suspected when there is intermittent rectal bleeding in the absence of constipation or pain on defecation, and where there is no fissure evident on clinical examination. The diagnosis is made on digital examination of the rectum or proctoscopy, at which time the polyp can be removed. A rectal polyp may prolapse, in which case it must be distinguished from rectal prolapse. If the polyp has prolapsed, then its base can be ligated without anaesthesia. Otherwise, the polyp can be located through a proctoscope, withdrawn to demonstrate its stalk, and sutured. Recurrence is unusual and malignancy is extremely rare.

Rectal prolapse

Prolapse of the rectum (Figure 28.1) is diagnosed from the history, as it is almost always observed by the parents after the child has been straining at stool. The rectum may prolapse with each attempt at defecation. When the prolapsed rectum becomes congested or traumatized, it may ulcerate and bleed. Prolapse is common in toddlers. Although it may occur frequently for several months, it almost always resolves spontaneously without any residual sequelae. In a minority of children with rectal prolapse, there is an underlying organic cause (Table 28.2). Predisposing factors in idiopathic rectal prolapse are believed to be excessive straining during defecation in a child with constipation, and precipitate or explosive defecation. The prolapse appears at the anus painlessly and usually reduces spontaneously, although manual replacement

Table 28.2 *Causes of rectal prolapse*

Cause	Comment
Idiopathic	By far the most common type
Neurological (paralysis of anal sphincters)	Myelomeningocele (spina bifida), sacral agenesis, and after spinal trauma
Ectopia vesicae (bladder exstrophy)	Or cloacal exstrophy
Following anorectoplasty for congenital anorectal malformation, e.g. imperforate anus	Redundant rectal mucosa may prolapse after anorectoplasty and resemble rectal prolapse
Nutritional	Marasmic undernourished hypotonic infants
Cystic fibrosis	Prolapse also seen in children with malabsorption and chronic diarrhoea

is sometimes required. The use of a stool softener (e.g. paraffin oil) sometimes is helpful in reducing the force of straining. The differential diagnosis includes prolapse of the rectal polyp and intussusception. Haemorrhoids are rare in children.

GROUP A STREPTOCOCCAL PERIANAL ERYTHEMA

Perianal erythema (also called perianal dermatitis) may occur in neonates with frequent loose bowel actions or in association with streptococcal infection. The erythema in streptococcal infection often looks quite florid but resolves with a course of penicillin.

ILL CHILD WITH ACUTE ABDOMINAL CONDITION

In this clinical setting, the symptom of rectal bleeding is additional to other more obvious features suggesting significant pathology. Intussusception presents with symptoms of vomiting, colicky abdominal pain, pallor and lethargy, usually in children between the ages of three months and two years. In only about half of the patients is there evidence of blood in the stools – the characteristic 'redcurrant jelly' stool.

Patients with severe gastroenteritis may have vomiting and colicky abdominal pain, and blood may be mixed with the loose stools. In children under two years of age, the initial diagnosis may be difficult to distinguish from intussusception.

The arthralgia and a rash over the extremities typical of Henoch–Schönlein purpura may not appear until well after the commencement of abdominal symptoms, making early diagnosis of the underlying condition difficult. Submucosal haemorrhages in the bowel wall may cause abdominal pain, the passage of blood rectally and, occasionally, intussusception.

MAJOR HAEMORRHAGE PER RECTUM

In these patients, the haemorrhage may be severe enough to cause anaemia or require transfusion. Causes range from oesophageal varices and peptic ulcer to a bleeding Meckel's diverticulum and tubular duplications of the bowel.

If a Meckel's diverticulum contains ectopic gastric mucosa, the acid it produces may ulcerate the mucosa of the adjacent ileum. Bleeding may be profuse and present as brick-red stools. Sometimes the child complains of vague abdominal pain. The bleeding usually stops spontaneously without the need for emergency surgery. The definitive investigation is surgery (usually laparoscopy), but in many instances a technetium scan may demonstrate a hotspot in the region of the ectopic gastric mucosa.

PERIANAL ABSCESS

Perianal abscess (Figure 28.2) is a common condition in infants, particularly in the first year of life, and arises from infection in one of the anal glands that open into the crypts of the anal valves. Although there is an internal opening at the level of the anal valves, the abscess itself almost always points superficially through the skin 1–2 cm from the anal verge. Drainage of the abscess alone is often inadequate, as recurrence is likely. Appropriate treatment involves opening the entire fistulous tract from the internal opening in the anal canal to the abscess cavity: this is performed under general anaesthesia.

Some children may develop a superficial subcutaneous infection in the buttock or near the anus, which may produce a subcutaneous abscess. This tends to occur secondary to nappy rash or poor hygiene, or as a result of infection with skin organisms. Antibiotics and simple drainage (if there is an abscess) are curative.

INFLAMMATORY BOWEL DISEASE

Since the 1970s, there has been a dramatic increase in the incidence of Crohn's disease in children. The incidence of ulcerative colitis has remained unchanged. Crohn's disease can involve any part of the gastrointestinal tract and is characterized by a transmural inflammatory process. Perianal disease is common. Perianal abscesses and fissures tend to be chronic and indolent and, unlike the usual type of anal fissure, are often placed laterally. They may give surprisingly little discomfort.

The great variability of presentation in Crohn's disease may lead to considerable delay between the onset of symptoms and diagnosis. A diagnosis of Crohn's disease should be considered in any child who has an unusual perianal abscess or fissure away from the midline. There may be a history of recurrent abdominal pain and weight loss. In the adolescent,

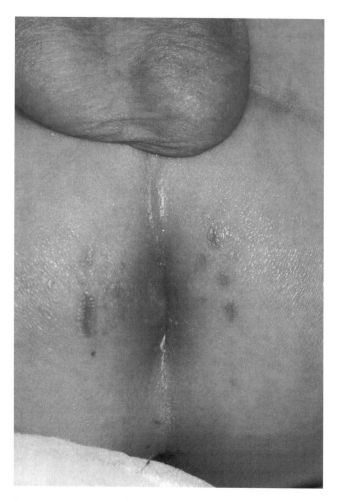

Figure 28.2 *Perianal abscess.*

the first manifestations of disease may be growth failure with delayed onset of puberty.

FEMALE GENITALIA

Labial adhesions

This is a common acquired condition of girls in which there is midline adherence of the labia minora, which usually commences posteriorly and may extend as far anteriorly as the clitoris. Labial adhesions (or fused labia) should not be confused with congenital absence of the vagina, as such an error in diagnosis may cause parents much unnecessary anxiety. Labial adhesions have never been reported at birth. Whether symptomatic labial adhesions should be treated remains controversial. In young toddlers, they can be separated without anaesthesia by sweeping them apart with the blunt end of a thermometer or by exerting gentle lateral traction on the labia minora. Occasionally, particularly in older children, they may be more densely adherent and require separation under general anaesthesia. There is a tendency for refusion following separation, so parents should be encouraged to apply petroleum jelly to the raw area on the medial side of the labia minor for about two weeks until complete re-epithelialization has occurred. Topical application of oestrogen cream also has been used to separate labial adhesions.

Imperforate hymen

This condition is very much less common than labial adhesions and often presents at birth. The vagina secretes mucus, which accumulates beneath the imperforate hymen to form a mucocolpos. Sometimes an imperforate hymen is not noticed until puberty, when an adolescent presents with primary amenorrhoea and haematocolpos or with cyclical attacks of abdominal pain. Removal of the hymen is curative.

CLINICAL SCENARIO

A three-year-old boy presented with a four-month history of pain on passing stools. He appeared to be inappropriately 'holding on' when he clearly had the urge to defecate. On several occasions, his mother noticed a small amount of fresh blood on the surface of the stools. On examination, he had an acute posterior anal fissure, with an oedematous swelling immediately external to it. Examination of his abdomen was unremarkable, apart from faeces palpable in his sigmoid colon. He was prescribed paraffin oil for three months, after which he had pain-free defaecation and return of normal bowel habit.

Abdominal trauma

JENNY WALKER

Learning objectives

- To appreciate the importance of trauma as a cause of morbidity and mortality in childhood.
- To understand the management of abdominal trauma, both blunt and penetrating.
- To be able to perform resuscitation, as per the Advanced Paediatric Life Support and Advanced Trauma Life Support systems.
- To know the significant points of abdominal trauma and the varieties of injury and their management.
- To understand the principles of safety and organ preservation by non-operative management and close observation.
- To recognize abdominal trauma in non-accidental injury victims.
- To understand the prevention of accidents and the consequent decrease in trauma to children as an important target for governments.

INTRODUCTION

Trauma kills over 350 children every year in the UK. It is the most common cause of death in children aged over one year and well into adult life in the UK. The major killer is from head injury, but isolated abdominal trauma and abdominal injuries as part of multiply injured children have significant serious outcomes. Trauma is much more common in boys than girls, in part due to their natural daring, inquisitiveness and desire for speed. Blunt trauma is much more common than penetrating trauma in children.

Abdominal trauma follows accidents on the road, in the home and at play. On the road, children are most commonly injured as pedestrians or in pushchairs, by being knocked off a bicycle, by falling on to the handlebars of a bicycle, and as passengers in cars. In the home, they are injured accidentally by falls, e.g. down stairs or on to solid objects and non-accidentally by blows directly to the abdomen or lower back. At play, they are injured by falling from trees, by falling off equipment in playgrounds and by being kicked by horses.

Abdominal trauma can easily injure the intra-abdominal organs in children. The abdominal wall is thin and less muscular than in adults, providing less protection. Compared with adults, the diaphragm is more horizontal and the liver and spleen are more anterior and less protected by the ribs, which are very elastic and easily compressible, crushing the solid organ underneath.

Direct blows produce injury directly to a solid organ, bowel or mesentery, especially if there is a rigid surface, e.g. the lumbar spine and/or the ground, behind the child. Deceleration injuries produce shearing forces between the fixed and the relatively mobile parts of the gastrointestinal tract, in particular to the bowel and to the mesentery at the duodenojejunal flexure, the ileocaecal junction and the sigmoid colon.

RELEVANT BASIC SCIENCE

Accurate knowledge of the anatomy of the peritoneal cavity and its relationships with the organs and their blood supplies is essential in the prediction of injuries and the ability to manage them surgically if required. The physiology of the systems and the consequent effects of damage or rupture of that system are also important to enable appropriate management during the recovery phase.

PRESENTATION

The child is brought to hospital either because of symptoms or because of concern due to the mechanism of injury. If the child has symptoms or signs, then it is not difficult to ensure that they are managed correctly. However, serious organ injuries, e.g. ruptured liver, spleen, kidney or bowel, may not present immediately if the degree of injury is lesser and there is no associated hypovolaemia, severe pain or peritonism; symptoms or signs may not present for many hours after the event. Any child with a significant history must be assessed carefully and repeatedly and kept in for observation, if appropriate.

RESUSCITATION

The child should be managed by the Advanced Paediatric Life Support (APLS)/Advanced Trauma Life Support (ATLS) system, with airway management and cervical spine control; high-flow oxygen administration, breathing assessment and support, as required; repeated circulatory assessment of pulse rate, capillary refill time and blood pressure measurement; insertion of two relatively large-bore cannulae (intraosseous, if needed); and the sending of blood samples for full blood count (FBC), clotting, group and cross-match (the type – O-negative/group-specific/full cross-match – and volume of blood required depending on the circulatory state of the child), urea and electrolytes, amylase and liver function tests, if indicated. Fluid resuscitation depends on the circulatory status but is 20 mL/kg of crystalloid, colloid or blood, as indicated, and repeated as necessary. Further monitoring of the circulatory parameters, blood tests, capillary gases, calcium and blood sugar depends on the patient's injuries and condition.

PRIMARY/SECONDARY SURVEY

Some indication of a significant abdominal injury may be demonstrated in the primary survey, when hypovolaemia is not found to have an intra-thoracic cause. However, it may not present until later, when the child is stable and the secondary or even tertiary survey is undertaken in a multiply injured child. The surgeon involved with the patient must have a high index of suspicion at all times, until an intra-abdominal injury has definitely been excluded.

MECHANISMS OF INJURY

The history of the injury is very important, in particular the area of the body that struck the solid object, be it a bumper or handlebar, the ground, a rock or a fist. The injury may be the result of a direct blow to the organ, compression of that organ against the solid ground or the lumbar spine, or shearing forces at a fixed site.

EXAMINATION

Abdominal examination must be gentle and repeated frequently. The pain of intraperitoneal blood or leaking bowel content or pancreatic juices may not initially be significant to the child, especially if the accident has given him or her another painful injury, such as a bony fracture, which distracts the child from complaining about the abdomen. If the child has a head injury, then the level of consciousness may be decreased, again interfering with the assessment of abdominal pain and tenderness.

If the patient is severely injured and is intubated and ventilated, then abdominal signs must be assessed closely and repeatedly, as some injuries can be missed for several days, e.g. ruptured bowel. The presence of bruising on the abdominal wall may be visible, either immediately if the injury is severe or later (after a day or two), and this should raise the alarm about possible intra-abdominal injury.

Abdominal assessment is hampered by a distended stomach or bladder. Trauma and stress both cause acute gastric dilation in children, and a gastric tube should be passed to empty the stomach. Whether the tube is passed via the nose or the mouth will depend on any associated head and facial injuries. If the gastric contents are blood-stained, then concern about injury to the stomach or, more likely, the duodenum should be raised. Emptying the bladder may be spontaneous, but urethral or suprapubic drainage and hourly monitoring may be required. The passage of a urethral catheter in a boy is not without its dangers, and the decision to do so should be made by the paediatric surgeon in charge.

Early rectal examination is not indicated in children with trauma, as it rarely contributes to the knowledge of the patient's injuries and will not affect immediate management. It may be performed later as part of the secondary survey by a consultant surgeon if it is felt that it will change the management. Vaginal examination in girls under the age of 16 years is an assault and must not be performed without a general anaesthetic and reasonable suspicion of injury.

INVESTIGATIONS

Ongoing regular cardiorespiratory monitoring should continue, with appropriate resuscitation as required. If the child is unstable and the circulation cannot be maintained without continued blood transfusion, then the child may require an urgent laparotomy and the consultant surgeon will be involved. If the child is not in a centre with paediatric surgeons, then the general surgical consultant will decide whether the child requires a laparotomy in that centre to save life by stopping ongoing haemorrhage or whether the child can be stabilized enough for transfer to a paediatric centre.

If the child is stable, then investigation of a suspected abdominal injury can be undertaken.

The gold standard is a double-contrast (intravenous and intragastric contrast) computed tomography (CT) scan, which will show whether solid organs, e.g. liver and spleen, are damaged, their perfusion, renal function (the site and function of both kidneys), the presence of free fluid and, possibly, bowel rupture. Unfortunately, CT scans must be performed in the X-ray department, where assessment, monitoring and resuscitation are less easy. The patient must be accompanied to the CT scanner by appropriate medical and nursing staff with access to appropriate equipment.

If a child has had a significant head injury, then they will undoubtedly be undergoing a head CT scan, and consideration must be given to whether an abdominal CT scan should be performed at the same visit to the scanner. Paediatric surgeons should encourage their district general hospital colleagues to perform abdominal CT scans whenever appropriate.

Abdominal ultrasound is easier, and the necessary equipment can be brought to the patient in the accident and emergency department if necessary. However, serious injuries to solid organs, retroperitoneal haematomas, bleeding and bowel rupture can be missed on ultrasound. A normal ultrasound does not exclude even life-threatening intra-abdominal injury.

Plain abdominal X-ray may show free air if there is a bowel perforation. However, apart from confirming the position and adequacy of the gastric tube, there is little else to recommend this investigation.

Diagnostic peritoneal lavage is never indicated in injured children nowadays, as positive results do not necessarily change the management, and it produces peritoneal irritation for about 48 hours, which hinders repeated abdominal assessment.

MANAGEMENT OF SPECIFIC INJURIES PRODUCING HYPOVOLAEMIA

The majority of children with intraperitoneal bleeding can be managed by judicial fluid resuscitation with crystalloid, blood and clotting factors as required, with close monitoring and waiting for the ruptured liver, spleen or kidney to stop bleeding. Even enormous lacerations across the liver parenchyma and largely mashed spleens can stop bleeding with non-operative observation. Laparotomy always disturbs the clot and releases the relative tamponade and leads to partial hepatectomy, splenectomy or nephrectomy. Complete bed-rest with adequate analgesia, antibiotics, fluid and nutritional support will allow over 95 per cent of patients to recover with their organs intact. This approach has also been adopted in the adult sector over the past ten years, with increasing numbers of trauma patients keeping their solid organs. The child with intraperitoneal bleeding must be managed in a paediatric surgical centre, where surgical intervention and intensive care are available if and when required.

Mesenteric bleeding can lead to immense uncontrollable hypovolaemia, necessitating emergency laparotomy. Mesenteric bleeding can also stop; however, if any bowel has become devascularized and, hence, becomes ischaemic, then it may necrose or perforate, or heal with later stricture formation. Therefore, these injuries may require laparotomy, either sooner or later.

The retroperitoneum can also be the source of massive haemorrhage, leading to instability and requiring urgent laparotomy. The bleeding may be coming from short veins injured by shearing forces, e.g. hepatic or pancreatic veins. These are very difficult to identify at laparotomy, and bleeding may be impossible to control successfully. The expectant tamponade approach is to be hoped for.

MANAGEMENT OF SPECIFIC INJURIES PRODUCING PERITONITIS

Duodenum

The duodenum is the most common piece of bowel to be injured after a direct blow to the abdomen, as the duodenum is a fixed and retroperitoneal structure crushed against the lumbar spine and may rupture after, for instance, being punched in the epigastrium, falling on to the handlebars of a bicycle, or being kicked by a horse. The duodenal wall may not always rupture but may be severely bruised. The haematoma can cause functional obstruction for some weeks. A diagnostic laparoscopy may help identify the source of the peritonitis. The child may need a feeding jejunostomy while the duodenal repair heals if there is severe adjacent bruising.

Pancreas

Pancreatic injuries can occur from the same mechanisms as for the duodenum. A raised serum amylase is expected, and management as for acute pancreatitis is necessary. A CT scan and magnetic resonance cholangiopancreatography (MRCP) can identify the site of pancreatic rupture, which may help guide whether urgent partial pancreatectomy is necessary. If early surgery is not indicated, then the early passage of a nasojejunal feeding tube will enable early enteral feeding, with consequent early recovery as well as avoidance of total parenteral nutrition. A pancreatic pseudo-cyst develops in about 20 per cent of cases of pancreatic injury. This pseudo-cyst will resolve spontaneously in over half of patients, but the other half (about five to ten per cent overall) may require ultrasound-guided drainage, or laparotomy and surgical drainage.

Small or large bowel

Bowel rupture can be by direct injury, or by mesenteric injury leading to bowel ischaemia and subsequent rupture. Laparotomy may be as an emergency for control of blood loss, or later on for primary repair, resection and primary anastomosis, or temporary defunctioning stoma formation.

OTHER INJURIES

Renal tract

Kidneys can rupture and produce hypovolaemia, requiring urgent laparotomy and nephrectomy to stop the bleeding. However, the majority will settle with bed-rest and antibiotic cover. Even a kidney split into two parts can heal and function well. The retroperitoneal haematoma may produce an ileus, requiring intravenous nutrition. Regular ultrasound scans must be performed to ensure that the urine is draining into the collecting system and down to the bladder. Urinomas and collections need to be drained if they do not resolve after a couple of weeks of ultrasound-monitored observation, as this suggests a continued leak and is a site of potential infection. The drainage may be performed percutaneously by a radiologist, or by endoscopic stenting; only rarely is surgical intervention required, as this often leads to more loss of renal function. Ureteric and bladder injuries often heal with adequate urine drainage.

Penetrating injury

Penetrating injury is very rare in the UK. It demands the usual initial assessment and resuscitation and, depending on the depth of penetration, a laparotomy. Surprisingly, it is possible to have a stab wound that penetrates the peritoneal cavity without solid-organ or vascular injury. If the patient is stable, then it may be decided to monitor the patient closely and to perform laparotomy only in cases where clinical signs require it. If there is any doubt, then an exploratory operation is essential, with appropriate management of the injuries as located.

Chance fracture

Chance fracture refers to the injury pattern seen after a hyperflexion injury. The injury occurs due to acute vehicle deceleration while the passenger is either unrestrained or restrained only in by a lap seatbelt. The patient has a crush fracture of the lumbar spine, with or without serious spinal-cord injury, and with or without gastrointestinal injuries, e.g. to the duodenum or pancreas. Management is directed at all aspects of the injury. The possibility of neurogenic shock due to spinal-cord transection must be taken into account during resuscitation.

NON-ACCIDENTAL INJURY

Non-accidental injuries with solid-organ or bowel rupture in children are, fortunately, very rare. They may, however, have a delayed or more chronic presentation, with symptoms of intestinal obstruction, if the blow has caused bruising and haematoma and consequent obstruction of, for instance, the duodenum. As in all cases of childhood injury, a careful history must be obtained, and any concern about non-accidental injury must be brought to the attention of the on-call paediatric medical team and social services, if necessary. As well as managing the abdominal injury, the child must be placed in safe care.

ACCIDENT PREVENTION

There are many areas in which accidents can be prevented, and considerable energy is put into this in the UK, both nationally and locally, with schemes to make children wear bright clothing when cycling, to encourage cycling proficiency and to make road safety an important part of a child's education. Safety at home is also targeted, and recently renewed energy has been invested into surveillance of non-accidental injury.

CLINICAL SCENARIOS

Case 1

A healthy six-year-old boy fell 3 m out of a tree and landed on a pyramid-shaped stone in his epigastrium. He stood up and walked with his friend for a few steps and then fell down, pale and quiet. He was brought to the accident and emergency department by 999 ambulance. He was talking sensibly but very pale, with a thready pulse of over 200 beats/minute and a capillary refill time of over six seconds. Two large-bore cannulae were inserted, blood was sent for appropriate tests, and a bolus of 400 mL of 0.9% NaCL solution was given (20 mL/kg), having estimated his weight to be 20 kg according to the formula (age + 4) × 2. No injury was found in his chest. He was complaining of abdominal pain and had a tense and tender abdomen with a small graze in the epigastrium. On reassessment, there was no improvement in his cardiovascular parameters, with tachycardia and prolonged capillary refill time, and he remained hypotensive. He had a further saline bolus and then required a unit of O-negative blood. His cardiovascular measurements began to improve whilst waiting for the group-specific and then fully cross-matched blood. He required another two units of blood, given more slowly, before his cardiovascular measurements remained stable, and a repeat haemoglobin after that third unit of blood was 9 g. He had received 1200 mL of blood, which is three-quarters of his blood volume, as well as half his blood volume of saline. A nasogastric tube was inserted and his stomach aspirated of air and fluid. When he was stable, he had a CT scan with intravenous contrast, which showed a complete laceration of the liver down to the porta, with free intraperitoneal blood. He was managed with bed-rest, intravenous analgesia and cefuroxime, close monitoring of his cardiovascular parameters, and judicious fluid/blood replacement to maintain normal pulse, capillary refill time, blood pressure and adequate urine output. His ileus recovered after a few days, his analgesic requirements settled, and he began to tolerate fluids and diet. He was gradually mobilized after 12 days, and he was discharged home after 16 days in hospital. His ultrasound of liver looks completely normal after six weeks, and he is back to full activity, although he is not climbing trees again … yet.

Appropriate resuscitation and careful monitoring and non-operative management can be successful even with severe solid-organ damage. The patient must be managed in a paediatric surgical centre where emergency surgery can be performed if required.

Case 2

A three-year-old healthy boy ran out of the garden into the path of a car passing at 30 mph. He was thrown into the air and landed on the grass verge and was unconscious at the scene. He arrived at the accident and emergency department by 999 ambulance. He was unconscious but breathing spontaneously with 100 per cent saturation on facemask oxygen. His cardiovascular parameters were normal. Cannulae were inserted, blood was sent for testing, and the patient was electively intubated and ventilated, as his Glasgow Coma Scale (GCS) score was only 8. An urgent CT scan of his head and abdomen showed a contusion of the brain but no solid-organ damage and no free fluid. He was managed on the paediatric intensive care unit, still ventilated for his head injury management. Three days later, he was found to have abdominal distension, with an ileus, and bruising was now visible over his right iliac fossa. Ultrasound of his abdomen showed free fluid. Abdominal X-ray showed obstruction. At laparotomy, he was found to have an isolated ileal perforation, with local peritonitis, which required surgical repair. Following this, he made a steady and full recovery.

The mechanism of injury must always be remembered with continuing suspicion of intra-abdominal injury until it has been excluded. Patients who are paralysed and ventilated for management of their head injury may not show abdominal signs early on.

Case 3

An 18-month-old boy was admitted urgently to hospital with a history of collapse while in the care of his mother's partner. He had a tender and distended abdomen. He was cardiovascularly stable but with obvious peritonitis. Imaging did not show the cause of the problem. After appropriate resuscitation, he had a laparotomy, which showed a completely disrupted duodenum from the jejunum at the duodenojejunal flexure, with severe bruising and damage to the adjacent bowel. Surgical repair was successful. No true history of the presumed injury was ever obtained. He has recovered fully from the surgery and is now back in the care of his mother and her new partner, with close supervision from social services.

FURTHER READING

Advanced Life Support Group. *Advanced Paediatric Life Support: The Practical Approach*, 4th edn. Oxford: Blackwell Science, 2005.

American College of Surgeons Committee on Trauma. *Advanced Trauma Life Support for Doctors*, 7th edn. Chicago, IL: American College of Surgeons, 1997.

Part 3

Thoracic surgery

30

Congenital diaphragmatic hernia

NICOLA P SMITH AND PAUL D LOSTY

Learning objectives

- To gain appropriate knowledge for antenatal counselling of parents when a fetus is diagnosed with congenital diaphragmatic hernia.
- To understand the rationale and evidence base behind currently available treatment strategies for congenital diaphragmatic hernia.
- To be aware of the long-term outcomes for survivors with congenital diaphragmatic hernia.
- To appreciate the contribution of basic science and experimental models in aiding future developments in congenital diaphragmatic hernia care.

INCIDENCE AND OUTCOMES

Congenital diaphragmatic hernia (CDH) has an incidence of approximately one in 3000 births, with a new case every 24–36 hours in the UK. Despite advances in antenatal diagnosis and neonatal care, the mortality for CDH remains around 40–60 per cent. Recent studies claiming markedly improved survival figures should be interpreted with caution, as many include only liveborn infants or infants undergoing delayed surgery. The hidden mortality in CDH persists: recent reports from Liverpool (Beresford and Shaw 2000) and Newcastle (Stege *et al.* 2003) note persistently high mortality (~60 per cent) when all antenatal cases of CDH were included. For isolated CDH, the major determinant of mortality is the degree of associated pulmonary hypoplasia. Associated anomalies such as cardiac defects are not uncommon, their presence indicating a dismal prognosis, with mortality rising to 93 per cent in some series.

HISTORY

Bochdalek first described the posterolateral congenital diaphragmatic defect that bears his name in 1848. This was preceded by reports of diaphragmatic defects, both congenital and traumatic, dating back as far as 1575. The first (unsuccessful) repair of a diaphragmatic defect was carried out in 1888, but it was not until the 1940s that a series of successful repairs were reported by Ladd and Gross (1940). Initial impressive success rates began to decline as surgery was attempted on newborns with poor respiratory function, who previously would have succumbed before surgery. Edith Potter, a pathologist, in 1953 first made the association between congenital diaphragmatic defects and pulmonary hypoplasia, with Areechon and Reid in 1971 later documenting in detail the morphometric changes in the human hypoplastic lung. Thus, the link was explained between a simple anatomical diaphragmatic defect and lethal pulmonary hypoplasia, the major determinant of survival.

ANTENATAL DIAGNOSIS AND PROGNOSTIC FACTORS

CDH is diagnosed on antenatal ultrasound scan in approximately 50 per cent cases. The diagnosis should prompt a detailed scan for associated anomalies. Although in the majority of cases CDH is an isolated defect, genetic associations include trisomies 13 and 18 and syndromes including Fryn (MIM229850), Coffin–Siris (MIM135900) and Denys–Drash (MIM194070). The presence of associated anomalies has been shown to have a detrimental impact on outcome: up to 93 per cent of cases perish antenatally. Technological improvements in antenatal diagnosis have stimulated considerable interest in determining reliable prognostic indicators for isolated CDH. Many prognostic indices have been suggested, including gestational age at diagnosis, the site and size of the defect, polyhydramnios, and the presence of the liver in the thoracic cavity ('liver-up' cases). Determining the extent of pulmonary hypoplasia in the antenatal period has been an area of extensive research. Measurements such as the lung-to-head ratio (LHR) and the lung-to-thoracic ratio (LTR) have been suggested as ultrasound predictors of the degree of lung hypoplasia. The LHR calculates the ratio between the circumference of the skull (to normalize for fetal size) and the diameter of the lung contralateral to the diaphragmatic defect. An increasing number of reports have defined limits for this variable to correlate with outcome. An LHR below one is almost universally fatal, and a value greater than 1.4 is likely to imply a favourable outcome. Although promising as a useful tool to assess the adequacy of lung development in the fetus, all studies to date have been retrospective. A large prospective trial is warranted to confirm the validity of this measure as a prognostic marker. Fetal magnetic resonance imaging (MRI) lung volumetry also has been reported, but at present its use remains largely experimental.

At birth, a range of prognostic indicators have been proposed, including ventilatory indices, five-minute Apgar scores and birth weight, some of which are now largely historical. Of interest, a recent large multicentre retrospective review from Scandinavia (Skari *et al.* 2000) assessing prognostic indicators for liveborn infants with CDH found that prenatal diagnosis, one-minute Apgar score and right-sided CDH were independent predictors of mortality.

DELIVERY PLAN

If the diagnosis of CDH is established antenatally, then this provides an ideal opportunity to formulate a plan for delivery. Antenatal counselling with a paediatric surgeon, obstetrician and neonatologist permits adequate discussion regarding the timing and mode of delivery and likely postnatal management. The infant should be delivered at a centre with easy access to paediatric surgical services to avoid lengthy postnatal transfers. Delivery by caesarean section is usually reserved for obstetrical indications.

POSTNATAL MANAGEMENT

Up to 50 per cent of cases of CDH may not have been detected antenatally. These newborns often present with respiratory distress within the first few minutes of life. A scaphoid abdomen and mediastinal shift away from the side of the lesion support the diagnosis. Radiographs typically reveal an absent diaphragmatic outline together with loops of bowel herniated into the chest (Figure 30.1). If necessary, the position of the tip of a nasogastric tube within the thorax, along with an upper-gastrointestinal contrast study or postnatal ultrasound scan (in experienced hands), will help to differentiate CDH from lesions such as cystadenomatoid malformations.

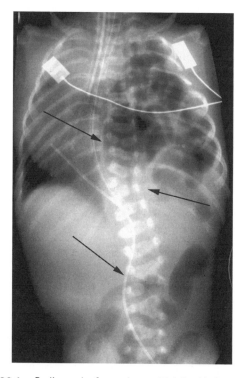

Figure 30.1 *Radiograph of a newborn with left-sided congenital diaphragmatic hernia (CDH). Multiple loops of bowel are herniated into the left thoracic cavity, with the mediastinum displaced to the right. Note the associated vertebral anomalies (arrows), part of the global embryopathy of CDH.*

At birth, or following diagnosis, the newborn should be intubated and a large-bore nasogastric tube passed. Both interventions are designed to prevent any dilation of the intrathoracic bowel, which would cause further respiratory embarrassment. Early postnatal management is aimed at providing adequate tissue oxygenation, whilst avoiding high ventilatory pressures, which cause damage to the neonatal lung through barotrauma. Traditionally, this is achieved through routine use of sedation, with or without paralysis, to prevent the infant 'fighting' the ventilator. Peak inspiratory pressure and positive end-expiratory pressures are adjusted to maximize oxygenation and prevent the development of acidosis. Minimal handling and maintenance of normal pH are applied to avoid aggravating pulmonary hypertension, which inevitably accompanies pulmonary hypoplasia. Failure of conventional ventilation to provide adequate oxygenation may necessitate the use of adjuncts to ventilation. These include high-frequency oscillatory ventilation (HFOV), inhaled nitric oxide (iNO) and extracorporeal membrane oxygenation (ECMO).

VENTILATORY ADJUNCTS

High-frequency ventilation

HFOV was designed to increase oxygenation whilst minimizing barotrauma to the neonatal lung. The principle is to increase the ventilator rate to 100–150 breaths/minute, with gas exchange occurring through bulk diffusion rather than mass flow. Mean airway pressure is maintained at a high level (typically 18–20 cmH$_2$O) to encourage alveolar recruitment; fluctuations around this mean pressure are minimized. Despite the outcome of an early multicentre randomized trial in North America suggesting no benefits in preterm neonates with respiratory failure, several anecdotal reports continue to report improvements in CDH. A recent Italian study reported on the outcome of 44 infants treated over a ten-year period showing an increase in survival from 67 to 94 per cent by employing HFOV in the preoperative management of CDH. Surgical repair has also been undertaken whilst maintaining the infant on high-frequency ventilation.

Nitric oxide

NO is a selective pulmonary vasodilator used in the treatment of persistent pulmonary hypertension of the newborn. Initial trials in infants with persistent pulmonary hypertension of the newborn were very encouraging, some demonstrating a universal increase in systemic arterial oxygen saturation (SaO$_2$). Studies in infants with CDH have shown a more variable response, with many infants manifesting no benefit. A recent meta-analysis and Cochrane Review (Finer and Barrington 2001) showed an improvement in perinatal outcome only in infants with persistent pulmonary hypertension who do *not* have CDH. Despite a lack of evidence for beneficial effects, favourable anecdotal reports support the continued use of iNO in CDH-related pulmonary hypertension.

Permissive hypercapnia

Wung et al. (1995) reported a novel ventilatory technique in CDH infants with improved survival and decreased incidence of chronic respiratory distress. The basic principle is to avoid the use of high airway pressures, thus minimizing the effect of barotrauma on neonatal lungs. This strategy, termed 'permissive hypercapnia' or 'gentilation', allows the infant to ventilate spontaneously, strictly limits the peak inspiratory pressure (ideally below 25 cmH$_2$O), and minimizes the fraction of inspired oxygen (FiO$_2$) to produce preductal saturations above 90 per cent, whilst allowing the partial pressure of carbon dioxide (pCO$_2$) to rise, e.g. to 60–65 mmHg. If this mode of ventilation fails (pCO$_2$ continues to rise or worsening metabolic acidosis develops), then the infant is switched to high-frequency ventilation with a similar positive inspiratory pressure (PIP). The use of higher PIP is stringently avoided. The New York group that originally described the method reported their ten-year experience with 120 CDH infants treated in this manner. Survival to discharge for live CDH babies recruited to the study was 84 per cent, with 13 per cent requiring ECMO support when respiratory function deteriorated. This is a very promising technique that is now gaining wider acceptance in North America.

Extracorporeal membrane oxygenation

Persistent severe refractory hypoxia promoted the use of ECMO in CDH. ECMO, introduced in the late 1970s, involves placing the infant on cardiopulmonary support to allow a period of 'lung rest' and reduction in pulmonary vascular resistance, whilst providing the baby with oxygenated blood via an artificial circuit. ECMO is an accepted treatment modality for management of respiratory failure in newborns. In the UK, its use is restricted to designated paediatric ECMO centres. Evidence to support the use of ECMO in CDH is conflicting. Early favourable reports were flawed by the use of historical controls. A North American study (Azarow et al. 1997; Wilson et al. 1997) addressed the relative outcomes from two centres, one offering ECMO (Boston) and the other offering conventional respiratory care (Toronto). This report failed to show any consistent improvement in outcome with the use of ECMO. The results of a multicentre trial in the UK, whilst demonstrating benefits in newborns with respiratory failure, failed to support the use of ECMO in CDH. This study has been criticized for having excessively stringent entry criteria necessitating near-unsalvageable respiratory failure before inclusion of infants with CDH. Elbourne et al. (2002) showed a significant survival advantage for all infants with respiratory failure. However, the benefits were least significant in CDH. Despite a lack of clear evidence for its use, ECMO continues to be employed as an important rescue strategy in CDH.

SURGERY

The timing of surgery for CDH has been debated for several years. Traditionally, CDH repair was performed as an emergency. This was based on the theory that immediate reduction of the hernia and repair of the defect would relieve pulmonary compression and, thus, improve respiratory mechanics and gas exchange. However, during the 1980s, surgeons and intensivists noted that early surgery was associated with deterioration in ventilatory parameters and a worsening of pulmonary hypertension. This observation led to preoperative stabilization aimed at maximizing respiratory function. Moyer *et al.* (2002), examining early versus delayed surgery for CDH, found no clear benefit for the latter. The majority of institutions, however, continue to employ a period of preoperative stabilization.

The most popular operative approach for CDH is transabdominal repair. This allows gentle reduction of viscera into the abdominal cavity, followed by clear visualization of the defect. Correction of the 'unrotated' midgut by division of Ladd's bands with or without appendicectomy should be discouraged.

A subcostal muscle-cutting incision is made on the side of the defect. A careful inspection is carried out to identify any hernial sac, present in approximately 20 per cent cases. If present, the sac should be excised.

Most cases of diaphragmatic hernia defects can be corrected by primary repair, involving direct closure of the margins of the defect. The posterior rim is often sparse; dissecting free an adequate rim of native tissue to include in the primary repair may prove challenging. The defect should be repaired with interrupted non-absorbable sutures (e.g. Ethibond™) (Figure 30.2). Where insufficient natural tissue exists, prosthetic material, e.g. Gore-Tex (W. L. Gore & Associates, Flagstaff, AZ, USA), may be utilized to complete closure. Other innovative techniques include the creation of a muscle flap from either the latissimus dorsi or the rectus abdominus to close the diaphragmatic defect. Similarly, if primary abdominal closure is difficult or complicated by unacceptably high ventilatory pressures, then a prosthetic patch may be incorporated into the abdominal wall. Patients on ECMO present a technical challenge. The use of anticoagulation to maintain the ECMO circuit precludes aggressive dissection of native diaphragmatic tissue. In such cases, prosthetic patch closure is common.

Laparoscopic repairs of diaphragmatic defects have been described, most frequently in adults. Case reports of children and neonates have been restricted to stable infants with good respiratory function. Caution should be exercised in the deployment of this technique in high-risk CDH babies.

LONG-TERM OUTCOMES

Long-term outcome data in patients following CDH repair are restricted largely to historical studies of cases undergoing

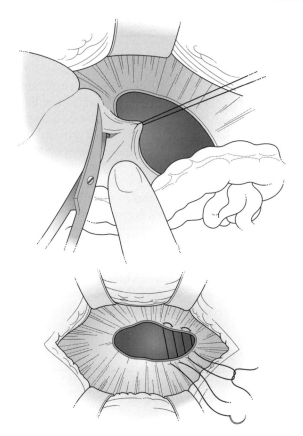

Figure 30.2 *Surgical technique for congenital diaphragmatic hernia (CDH) repair. The posterior rim of the diaphragm is mobilized before interrupted non-absorbable sutures are placed to close the defect.*

surgery in the 1940s and 1950s. More recent reports involving the era of advances in intensive care clearly identify a population of children with ongoing respiratory and gastrointestinal morbidity. Aside from neurological sequelae resulting from chronic neonatal hypoxia, a high proportion of patients have chronic respiratory insufficiency secondary to pulmonary hypoplasia and the consequences of iatrogenic lung injury. Gastro-oesophageal reflux and its attendant complications are perhaps related to diaphragmatic malfunction and may entail anti-reflux surgery. Deformity of the spine and/or chest wall following CDH repair similarly may require surgical treatment. In particular, results of a long-term follow-up study following CDH patch repair in San Francisco indicates the need for close scrutiny, since nearly 50 per cent will suffer from patch failure and recurrent herniation.

It is equally important to assess the long-term outcome for infants treated with ECMO. The UK collaborative ECMO trial published four-year follow-up data for infants recruited to the study, including CDH and other causes of severe respiratory distress. Strikingly, although the authors reported a 60 per cent incidence of neuromuscular disability, they found no significant differences between those treated conventionally and those who received ECMO. Further evidence will continue to evolve as ECMO survivors reach adolescence.

EXPERIMENTAL THERAPIES

Fetal surgery

The traditionalists' 'compression theory' of lung hypoplasia promoted the idea that intrauterine repair of a diaphragmatic defect may reduce pressure on the developing lung, permitting lung growth and alleviating postnatal respiratory failure. Early experimental fetal surgery in lambs with a surgically created diaphragmatic hernia was a prelude to the evolution of human fetal surgery programmes. However, attempts at fetal repair in humans were disappointing and open surgical techniques have been abandoned.

The seminal observation that fetuses with laryngeal atresia (preventing the normal efflux of intraluminal lung liquid) developed pulmonary hyperplasia led to the novel concept that occluding the trachea in utero would increase lung growth in CDH. Trials using the lamb model of surgically created diaphragmatic hernia followed by open tracheal occlusion produced significant increases in lung volume. However, hysterotomy resulted in a high incidence of premature labour and fetal loss. Studies evaluating this experimental therapy (the 'PLUG': Lug the lung Until it Grows) in humans were limited to fetuses deemed to have a poor prognosis. Harrison's group in San Francisco currently use a combination of 'liver-up' and low lung-to-head ratio to select fetuses for antenatal surgery. Early reports on PLUG mirrored the animal data, with increases in lung growth at term, but revealed high rates of fetal morbidity. This prompted the development of a less invasive method to access the fetal trachea, fetal endoscopy ('FETENDO') surgery. Endoscopic instruments are utilized to enter the uterine cavity and access directly the fetal trachea, allowing insertion of an occluding balloon. A study from the University of California, San Francisco (UCSF) evaluating 40 infants treated with FETENDO surgery produced some encouraging pilot data, which led to a National Institutes of Health (NIH) randomized trial. The trial has shown, strikingly, no survival benefits over standard conventional postnatal care for the high-risk CDH fetus (Harrison et al. 2003). Moreover, UCSF pathology studies in CDH non-survivors undergoing tracheal occlusion when grouped by post-conceptual age showed no statistically significant differences with respect to lung-to-body weight ratio, radial alveolar count, mean alveolar length or relative arteriolar media thickness compared with conventionally treated CDH infants. Fetal surgery for CDH requires reappraisal.

Antenatal steroids

Administration of antenatal steroids to mothers with threatened premature labour is widespread. Glucocorticoids have been shown to enhance maturation of premature lungs and reduce the incidence and severity of respiratory distress syndrome. Antenatal glucocorticoids improve both pulmonary compliance and maturation of hypoplastic lungs from both the nitrofen and lamb CDH models (see below). Small case series suggest similar benefits in humans. At the time of writing, a multicentre trial is attempting to evaluate this therapy.

Liquid ventilation

The concept of liquid ventilation was first investigated during the 1950s for astronauts and divers. Theoretical advantages are that liquid will diffuse evenly through the lung and decrease surface tension at the alveolar surface. Initial attempts with electrolyte solutions were unsuccessful; however, the discovery of perfluorocarbons regenerated liquid ventilation as a potential therapy. Perfluorocarbons are high-density inert biological polymers that have an oxygen-carrying capacity in excess of blood and are eliminated by vaporization, so limiting toxicity. Experimental studies of their use in animal models of respiratory distress had very encouraging results, with increases in oxygen saturation and pulmonary compliance. American phase II and III clinical trials have been initiated to evaluate the use of partial liquid ventilation (PLV) in adults and children with respiratory distress. One study has reported growth-promoting effects of constant pressure lung inflation with perfluorocarbons whilst oxygenating the CDH patient with ECMO. This therapy may offer promise for improving survival in infants with CDH.

BASIC SCIENCE AND LUNG DEVELOPMENT

Experimental models of CDH and pulmonary hypoplasia have permitted study of the pathophysiology of this birth defect. As the aetiology of CDH remains largely unknown, models cannot mimic precisely the human condition. However, the use of experimental models has provided important advances in understanding and developing novel therapies.

Lamb model

The lamb model of diaphragmatic hernia involves the surgical creation of a diaphragmatic defect in previously normal animals during the mid-trimester of development (pseudoglandular phase of lung development). At term, they animals exhibit a diaphragmatic hernia, intrathoracic herniation of viscera along with pulmonary hypoplasia and lethal pulmonary hypertension. This model has been used extensively to aid development of techniques for human fetal surgery. The main advantages of the model are in permitting physiological studies, particularly the influence of interventions on respiratory mechanics and gas exchange. However, the creation of a diaphragmatic defect in previously normal lambs implies that no information regarding the embryogenesis of CDH can be obtained.

Nitrofen rodent model

In the early 1980s, it was discovered that administration of the herbicide nitrofen to pregnant rodents resulted in the development of CDH and pulmonary hypoplasia in a proportion of newborns. The resultant phenotype bears close similarity to the human condition, with mainly left-sided CDH and pulmonary hypoplasia associated with a similar range and frequency of cardiac, limb and skeletal defects. Administration of nitrofen early in gestation allows detailed investigation of embryogenesis. The main limitation of the model is the difficulty in performing complex physiological studies.

Transgenic models

Several genetic knockout models include a diaphragmatic defect in their phenotype. However, the spectrum of associated anomalies differs widely from that seen in humans. For example, deletion of both copies of the gene encoding for the murine retinoic acid receptor results in a high incidence of cranial, vertebral, limb, cardiac, foregut and pulmonary malformations, but a low incidence of CDH. Thus, information from these animal studies needs to be translated to the human situation with caution. Homozygous deletion of the WT1 gene in rodents leads to diaphragmatic, renal and limb defects. Scientists in Scandinavia, however, failed to find evidence of WT1 mutations in human infants with CDH and their families. It seems that although mutations of the WT1 gene can lead to CDH in rodents, its role in the genesis of the human phenotype remains unclear.

Pulmonary hypoplasia: theories and advances

Traditional surgical teaching suggests that pulmonary hypoplasia in CDH results from compression of the developing lung by herniated abdominal viscera. Use of teratogenic models and development of organotypic lung culture systems has enabled investigation of the earliest stages of pulmonary organogenesis. These studies have identified abnormalities in pulmonary development that correlate with and precede the development of a diaphragmatic defect. Thus, there may be an intrinsic lung defect, i.e. pulmonary hypoplasia may not be due simply to compression. These experimental observations were supported and extended by the development of the 'dual-hit' hypothesis, suggesting that the lungs were subject to a primary intrinsic defect before being further impaired by secondary visceral herniation. The knowledge that 30–50 per cent of infants with CDH have an associated anomaly supports the concept of a 'global embryopathy'.

Vitamin A

Vitamin A is important in lung development. In 1953, Wilson and colleagues noted a high incidence of CDH in the pups of vitamin A-deficient rats. Interestingly, it has been noted that human infants with CDH have significantly reduced levels of retinol and retinol-binding protein compared with age-matched controls. A strain of transgenic mice in which both copies of the retinoic acid receptor (vitamin A binding receptor) gene have been deleted display CDH together with left lung agenesis and significant right lung hypoplasia. Experimental studies into the possible restorative role of vitamin A in hypoplastic CDH lungs have had interesting results. Thebaud and colleagues (1999) have shown that prenatal treatment with vitamin A in the nitrofen model of CDH reduces the incidence of CDH at term, as well as demonstrating improvements in lung growth and maturation in perinates. The pivotal role of vitamin A has been addressed further by the retinoid hypothesis proposed by Greer and colleagues (2003).

Growth factors

Mammalian lung development requires the complex interplay of growth factors and cell signalling pathways. Evidence for the roles of specific components of these pathways has been elucidated from studies in mice and the fruit fly, *Drosophila melanogaster*. *Branchless* and *breathless* are *Drosophila* mutants lacking fibroblast growth factor (FGF) and its receptor (FGFR), respectively. Similar knockouts involving members of the FGF signalling pathway have been developed in mice. All such knockouts show abrogated airway branching. This knowledge led to the study of the effects of adding exogenous growth factor to normal and hypoplastic lungs in organ culture (Figure 30.3). Experiments have revealed a role for many mammalian FGFs in branching morphogenesis in both normal and hypoplastic lungs (including FGF-10, FGF-9, FGF-7, FGF-1 and FGF-2). It has been postulated that disturbance of the FGF pathway may comprise at least part of a signalling defect in pulmonary hypoplasia.

MECHANICAL FACTORS IN LUNG DEVELOPMENT

The importance of mechanical factors in the maintenance of normal lung development increasingly is being recognized. At a cellular level, stretch promotes growth and differentiation of both respiratory epithelial and smooth muscle cells. In whole lung, the role of both fetal breathing movements and lung liquid are being characterized. Fetal breathing movements are observed from mid-trimester; their abolition in experimental models through phrenic nerve or cervical section leads to pulmonary hypoplasia. Another mechanical factor that appears to be coupled to lung growth *in vitro* is the spontaneous phasic contractions of developing airways (termed 'airway peristalsis'). Airway peristalsis is abnormal in experimental lung hypoplasia; however, the precise link between

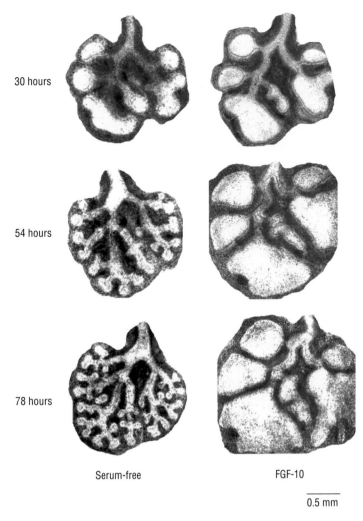

30 hours

54 hours

78 hours

Serum-free

FGF-10

0.5 mm

Figure 30.3 *Experimental lung primordia in organotypic culture. Photomicrographs taken following 30, 54 and 78 hours in vitro. The left column shows lungs cultured in standard serum-free media. Those on the right have been cultured with the addition of 50 ng/mL fibroblast growth factor 10 (FGF-10) to the medium. FGF-10 has significantly increased the lung lumen area at all three time points.*

this activity and *in vivo* lung growth remains unknown. Harnessing these mechanical stimuli to enhance the antenatal growth of hypoplastic lungs may represent a future advance in CDH care.

DIAPHRAGMATIC EVENTRATION

Eventration of the diaphragm may be congenital or an acquired anomaly. Eventration may result from phrenic nerve injury (secondary to birth trauma or following thoracic surgery) with diaphragmatic paralysis. The embryological origins of the congenital form remain unclear. Typically, the diaphragm exhibits an area of thinned or absent muscular development. At worst, the diaphragm may resemble the membranous sac seen in CDH. Congenital eventration is often associated with pulmonary hypoplasia, which is the major determinant of mortality of this condition.

Eventration may be diagnosed on a routine chest X-ray or may present with variable respiratory symptoms, which may include pneumonia, severe respiratory distress or ventilator dependency following traumatic delivery. Diagnosis is confirmed by an abnormally raised hemi-diaphragm on chest X-ray, the smooth diaphragmatic outline differentiating the condition from CDH (Figure 30.4). If doubt remains, then dynamic imaging by ultrasound scanning or fluoroscopy may show paradoxical diaphragmatic movement and can confirm the diagnosis. Milder acquired cases may not warrant surgery. A degree of functional recovery is expected, particularly following incomplete nerve section. Some infants and children therefore may be managed expectantly with positive pressure ventilation. Surgical intervention is reserved for those with prolonged ventilator dependency.

We recommend a transabdominal surgical approach. This permits clear visualization of the diaphragm, bilateral repair through a single incision where needed, and surgical correction of the coexistent visceral malrotation where present.

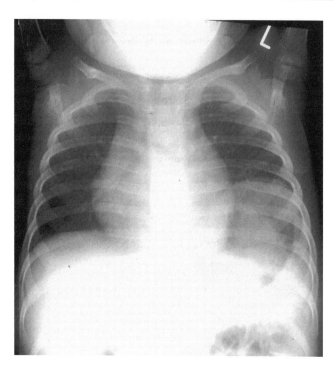

Figure 30.4 *Radiograph of a newborn with left diaphragmatic eventration. The left diaphragmatic outline is raised. The smooth upper border differentiates this from a congenital diaphragmatic hernia.*

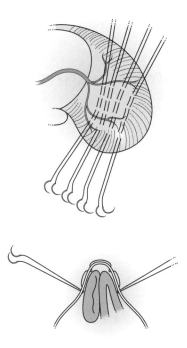

Figure 30.5 *Surgical technique for repair of a left-sided diaphragmatic eventration. Interrupted non-absorbable sutures are placed in the diaphragm, taking care to avoid the expected course of the intradiaphragmatic phrenic nerve. The sutures are then tightened to plicate the loose muscle. From* Operative Paediatric Surgery, *5th edn, Spitz L and Coran A (eds) (1995), London: Chapman & Hall, with permission.*

Some authors advocate a thoracic approach on the right, as this avoids the need to mobilize the liver. The most commonly employed technique is to plicate the 'floppy' diaphragm using non-absorbable sutures (Figure 30.5) in the hope of functional recovery. Where there is an area of membranous amuscular diaphragm this may be resected and the free edges repaired with non-absorbable sutures. Plication is more frequently employed since this minimizes the risk of damage to the intramuscular branches of the phrenic nerve which may be difficult to visualize. Outcomes following surgery depend largely on the associated degree of pulmonary hypoplasia. Most infants and children however, appear to be successfully weaned from the ventilator, and have few long-term respiratory symptoms. The majority of follow-up studies suggest that plication remains intact – with minimal attenuation of the diaphragmatic muscle.

CLINICAL SCENARIO

A 24-year-old female has a fetus with a CDH indicated on an ultrasound at 18 weeks' gestation. No other structural abnormalities were identified. Amniocentesis following the scan revealed no chromosomal abnormalities.

Q: What information regarding prognosis should the parents be given in light of the scan findings?
A: In an isolated case of CDH, the prognosis at this early stage is for approximately 40–50 per cent survival. There are currently no reliable prognostic indicators to give a more accurate outlook.

Q: The parents contact you a week later, having searched the internet for CDH. They enquire about the possibility of fetal intervention. What can you tell them?
A: Although fetal intervention is the subject of trials in the USA, it is not offered routinely in either Europe or America. The evidence for fetal surgery suggests that it offers no benefit over conventional postnatal management. New procedures, including the FETENDO procedure for tracheal ligation, are currently under investigation for 'liver-up' cases. As yet, there is no clear evidence that a benefit exists (Harrison *et al.* 2003).

Q: The mother was induced at 38 weeks' gestation, and the baby was delivered vaginally. What should the immediate management be following delivery?
A: The infant should be intubated and ventilated and a large-bore nasogastric tube should be passed. This serves the dual purpose of providing oxygenation for the infant whilst preventing gastric dilation, leading to further respiratory embarrassment. Vascular access – both venous and arterial – will be needed in the early neonatal period. A right radial arterial line is extremely helpful for monitoring preductal oxygen saturations. The infant will require a full clinical examination to assess her

physiological state and to check for any associated anomalies. Vitamin K should be given according to the unit's protocol.

Q: What investigations should be carried out in the early neonatal period?
A: The diagnosis may be confirmed on a plain chest/abdominal radiograph. If there continues to be doubt, then an upper-gastrointestinal contrast study or abdominal/thoracic ultrasound scan may be helpful. The infant will need arterial blood gases to help assess the degree of respiratory support needed. Baseline blood tests, including a coagulation screen and blood cross-match, should be carried out. The infant will require an echocardiogram in the first hours of life – and definitely before surgery – to check for any associated cardiac defects.

The baby was transferred to the neonatal intensive care unit, sedated and ventilated.

Q: What information should the parents now be given regarding timing of surgery?
A: There is no case for emergency surgery. The operation is carried out routinely when the baby is physiologically stable. Moyer *et al.* (2002) demonstrated no adverse effects from delaying surgery. This remains the protocol employed in most units in the UK.

At five days of age, the infant continues to be ventilated by conventional ventilation, with a PIP of 20 cmH$_2$O, positive end expiratory pressure (PEEP) of 5 cmH$_2$O and FiO$_2$ of 35 per cent. Arterial blood gases are satisfactory. The baby is taken to theatre, undergoes a primary diaphragmatic hernia repair, and is then returned to the neonatal intensive care unit.

REFERENCES

Azarow K, Messineo A, Pearl R, *et al.* Congenital diaphragmatic hernia: a tale of two cities – the Toronto experience. *Journal of Pediatric Surgery* 1997; **32**: 395–400.

Beresford MW, Shaw NJ. Outcome of congenital diaphragmatic hernia. *Pediatric Pulmonology* 2000; **30**: 249–56.

Elbourne D, Field D, Mugford M. Extracorporeal membrane oxygenation for severe respiratory failure in newborn infants. *Cochrane Database Systematic Review* 2002; (1): CD001340.

Finer NN, Barrington KJ. Nitric oxide for respiratory failure in infants born at or near term. *Cochrane Database Systematic Review* 2001; (4): CD000399.

Greer JJ, Babiuk RP, Thebaud B. Etiology of congenital diaphragmatic hernia: the retinoid hypothesis. *Pediatric Research* 2003; **53**: 726–30.

Harrison MR, Keller RL, Hawgood SB, *et al.* A randomized trial of fetal endoscopic tracheal occlusion for severe fetal congenital diaphragmatic hernia. *New England Journal of Medicine* 2003; **349**: 1916–24.

Ladd WE, Gross RE. Congenital diaphragmatic hernia. *New England Journal of Medicine* 1940; **223**: 917–23.

Moyer V, Moya F, Tibboel R, *et al.* Late versus early surgical correction for congenital diaphragmatic hernia in newborn infants. *Cochrane Database Systematic Review* 2002; (3): CD001695.

Skari H, Bjornland K, Haugen G, Egeland T, Emblem R. Congenital diaphragmatic hernia: a meta-analysis of mortality factors. *Journal of Pediatric Surgery* 2000; **35**: 1187–97.

Stege G, Fenton A, Jaffray B. Nihilism in the 1990s: the true mortality of congenital diaphragmatic hernia. *Pediatrics* 2003; **112**: 532–5.

Thebaud B, Tibboel D, Rambaud C, *et al.* Vitamin A decreases the incidence and severity of nitrofen induced congenital diaphragmatic hernia in rats. *American Journal of Physiology* 1999; **277**: L423–9.

Wilson J, Roth CB, Waekany J. An analysis of the syndromes of malformation induced by maternal vitamin A deficiency: effects of restoration of vitamin A at various times during gestation. *American Journal of Anatomy* 1953; **92**: 189–217.

Wilson JM, Lund DP, Lillehei CW, Vacanti JP. Congenital diaphragmatic hernia: a tale of two cities – the Boston experience. *Journal of Pediatric Surgery* 1997; **32**: 401–5.

Wung JT, James LS, Kilchevsky E, James E. Management of infants with severe respiratory failure and persistence of the fetal circulation without hyperventilation. *Pediatrics* 1985; **76**: 488–94.

FURTHER READING

Bohn D. Congenital diaphragmatic hernia. *American Journal of Respiratory Critical Care Medicine* 2002; **166**: 911–15.

Boloker J, Bateman DA, Wung JT, Stolar CJ. Congenital diaphragmatic hernia in 120 infants treated consecutively with permissive hypercapnea/spontaneous respiration/elective repair. *Journal of Pediatric Surgery* 2002; **37**: 357–66.

Henderson-Smart DJ, Bhuta T, Cools F, Offringa M. Elective high frequency oscillatory ventilation versus conventional ventilation for acute pulmonary dysfunction in preterm infants. *Cochrane Database of Systematic Reviews* 2001 (3): CD000104.

Hirschl RB, Philip WF, Glick L, *et al.* A prospective, randomized pilot trial of perfluorocarbon-induced lung growth in newborns with congenital diaphragmatic hernia. *Journal of Pediatric Surgery* 2003; **38**: 283–9.

Smith NP, Jesudason EC, Losty PD. Congenital diaphragmatic hernia. *Paediatric Respiratory Review* 2002; **3**: 339–48.

31

Structural anomalies of the airway and lungs

DAVID M BURGE AND SRINIVASAN R BABU

Learning objectives

- To understand the different causes of airway obstruction and the types of stridor that may occur, depending on the level of obstruction.
- To know how to manage the different types of airway obstruction, especially in patients presenting acutely.
- To understand the different types of congenital lung lesion and arguments for and against treatment in asymptomatic cases.

INTRODUCTION

Most of the conditions described in this chapter present with respiratory difficulty. The precise manifestation of this depends on the anatomical level of the lesion (Table 31.1). Conditions affecting the nasal airway and pharynx tend to produce obstructive apnoea; those of the larynx, inspiratory stridor; and those of the trachea, biphasic stridor. Lung lesions present with respiratory distress without obstructive features. All grades of severity of these features may be encountered. Although many of these conditions may produce mild symptoms that may be self-limiting, in their severe forms they can cause death or cerebral damage from hypoxia.

Table 31.1 *Structural anomalies of the airways and lungs*

Upper airway	Larynx	Trachea and bronchi	Lungs	Pleura
Choanal atresia/stenosis	Laryngomalacia	Tracheal agenesis, stenosis	Agenesis	Chylothorax
Transient nasal obstruction	Vocal cord palsy	Vascular ring	CLE	
Craniofacial anomalies	Subglottic stenosis	Tracheomalacia	CCAM	
Pierre Robin syndrome	Haemangioma	Bronchomalacia	Pulmonary sequestration	
Extrinsic tumours	Laryngeal cleft		Bronchogenic cyst	
Intrinsic tumours	Miscellaneous, e.g. web, cysts			
Macroglossia				

CCAM, congenital cystic adenomatoid malformation; CLE, congenital lobar emphysema.

UPPER AIRWAY

Choanal atresia/stenosis

Choanal atresia is a congenital obstruction of the posterior nares at the level of the posterior border of the nasal septum. Although it has an incidence of about one in 10 000, the perceived incidence in the neonatal period is less than this because unilateral cases, which are more common, may not produce clinical features at birth. In ten per cent of cases the obstruction is only membranous, but in the remainder the obstruction is bony. In some cases, choanal atresia is the presenting feature of the CHARGE association: coloboma of the retina and/or iris, heart abnormalities, atresia choanae, retardation (which may be physical and mental), genital anomalies and ear anomalies (Pagon *et al.* 1981). It is important that any baby with choanal atresia is screened carefully for these other features, because the associated developmental implications may be considerable.

CLINICAL FEATURES

Babies within the first few weeks of life are obligatory nose-breathers. This explains the marked respiratory difficulty that choanal atresia can produce, considering that all the baby has to do to overcome the obstruction is to open its mouth to breath. Some babies will do this readily and present with breathing difficulty only with feeding, when the mouth is otherwise occupied. Other infants present with cyanosis at rest and become pink only when they open their mouths to cry. Unilateral atresia may become apparent in the neonate if the other nostril is blocked by oedema or secretions. In most cases, it presents in later childhood with unilateral nasal discharge.

INVESTIGATION

The diagnosis usually is suggested by failure to pass a suction catheter beyond the posterior nares. A simple test of nasal patency is to listen with a stethoscope at the external nares. Confirmation of the diagnosis is best achieved by someone who has seen the condition before probing the nose gently with a small metal sound. Contrast can be instilled into the nostril with a baby probe to obtain radiological confirmation (Figure 31.1), but this is not usually required. Computed tomography (CT) or magnetic resonance imaging (MRI) should be performed in every case to clarify the bony anatomy. This not only identifies the type of atresia (bony or membranous) but also shows the bone thickness. More importantly, it will demonstrate the anatomy of the postnasal space, which may be considerably narrowed in many cases. This information is essential before attempting surgical correction to prevent damage to adjacent structures.

TREATMENT

If the atresia is membranous, then simple perforation and dilation under general anaesthesia may suffice. Bony atresia can be treated by a transnasal or transpalatal approach. The latter

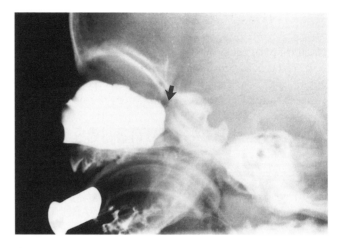

Figure 31.1   *Lateral skull radiograph of an infant with bilateral choanal atresia who has had contrast instilled into the nostrils. Whilst this investigation indicates clearly the level of the atresia, at the posterior nares (arrow), it is not usually required in the assessment of children with this condition.*

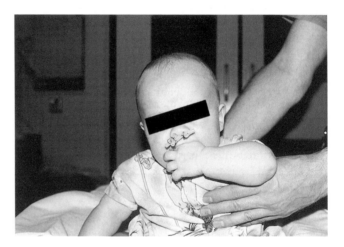

Figure 31.2   *Postoperative nasal stenting after surgery for choanal atresia.*

provides better visualization of the area to be resected but can cause palatal damage. Most surgeons still practise the transnasal approach. The atretic area should be visualized endoscopically from in front (zero-degree telescope) and behind (120-degrees telescope). The bony wall should be perforated and resected using a drill or forceps. Once a reasonable passage has been created, it should be stented to reduce the risk of stenosis. This is best achieved using thick-walled silastic tubing passed down one nostril and up the other with a fenestration sited posteriorly (Figure 31.2). A cross-bar of the same tubing is then placed across the two external limbs and sutured in place. This prevents inward movement of the stent. The stent is usually needed for up to 12 weeks, and repeated dilations under anaesthetic may be needed in the first months. With the advent of powered instrumentation and routine postoperative revision endoscopy, prolonged stenting may be avoided.

Transient nasal obstruction

Nasal mucosal oedema is a common cause of nasal obstruction in the newborn. It can be distinguished from choanal atresia by the passage of a nasopharyngeal tube. It is a transient condition. Nasal decongestants may be helpful.

Craniofacial anomalies

Conditions in which there is abnormal maxillary development may be associated with posterior nares or nasopharyngeal obstruction. These include Treacher Collins, Crouzon and Apert syndromes.

Pierre Robin syndrome

This condition is characterized by micrognathia, posterior displacement of the tongue (glossoptosis) and cleft palate. Babies with all three features clearly fall into the syndrome, but those with some but not all features are often included. This has resulted in a wide variation in the reported incidence of the syndrome, from one in 10 000 to one in 2000. The degree of micrognathia can be very severe (Figure 31.3) and can persist into childhood, requiring mandibular surgery. It can be postulated that micrognathia is the primary defect and that posterior tongue displacement is secondary and in itself causes palate maldevelopment.

CLINICAL FEATURES AND MANAGEMENT

Airway obstruction is caused by the tongue obstructing the hypopharyx (Benjamin and Walker 1991). This can be profound and cause severe hypoxia. The cause of obstruction usually can be deduced because of the obvious micrognathia and, where present, the cleft palate. Confirmation that glossoptosis is the cause usually can be obtained by positioning the baby prone. This allows the tongue to fall forwards and relieves obstruction. This may be all the treatment that is needed; however, in some cases this is not adequate. Passage of a nasopharyngeal tube – a standard suitable diameter endotracheal tube passed through one nostril to a position behind the tongue and above the larynx – may produce an adequate airway, both through the tube and alongside it. If this fails, then intubation of the trachea may be needed, but this is notoriously difficult in these cases because the position of the tongue makes visualization of the larynx very difficult. In rare cases, tracheostomy may be required.

Spontaneous improvement in airway obstruction occurs gradually as the child gets older. Surgery is needed for palatal repair and sometimes for mandibular lengthening later in childhood. The likely difficulty in intubation for these procedures should be brought to the attention of the anaesthetist.

Head and neck tumours

Extrinsic tumours anywhere in the neck can cause respiratory obstruction. The most common tumours are cystic hygroma,

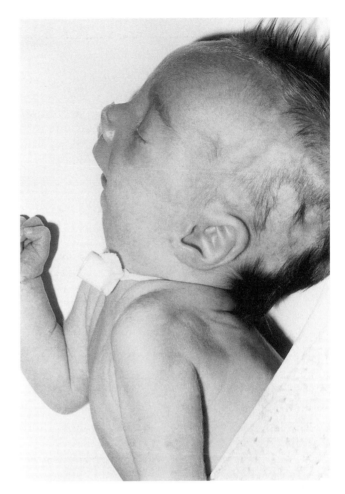

Figure 31.3 *Infant with Pierre Robin syndrome with severe micrognathia requiring tracheostomy.*

cervical teratoma (Figure 31.4) and haemangioma. In these conditions, relief of obstruction can be very difficult or even impossible. Anatomical distortion may impede both tracheal intubation and tracheostomy. In such cases, the careful siting of a nasopharyngeal tube may be life-saving.

Intrinsic smaller space-occupying lesions may cause obstruction, depending on the position. These include nasopharyngeal lesions (dermoid, encephalocele, rhabdomyosarcoma) and oro/hypopharyngeal lesions (lingual thyroid, vallecular cysts, haemangioma, etc.). Cross-sectional imaging and careful endoscopy are required to establish the diagnosis.

Macroglossia

This may be secondary to a generalized disorder (hypothyroidism, Beckwith–Weidemann syndrome) or localized pathology (haemangioma, lymphangioma), or it may be an isolated abnormality. It is important to consider Beckwith–Weidemann syndrome, because this may be associated with neonatal hypoglycaemia and subsequent neurological impairment, which may be prevented if the diagnosis is made early. Surgical

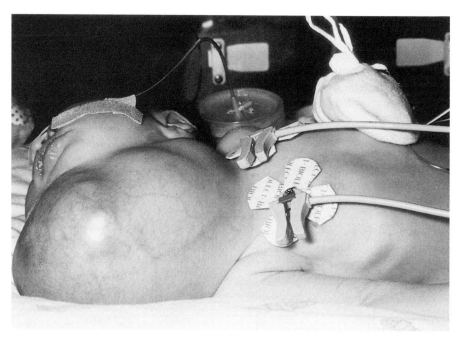

Figure 31.4   *Infant with massive cervical teratoma.*

reduction of the tongue may be possible, although haemangiomatous lesions are difficult to treat.

LARYNX

Laryngomalacia

CLINICAL FEATURES

This is the most common cause of laryngeal stridor in infants. The inspiratory stridor may not be present at birth but develops over the first few days or weeks of life. It is due to inherent floppiness of the aryepiglottic folds, the cuneiform cartilages and, to some extent, the epiglottis itself, all of which are sucked into the larynx on inspiration and expelled on expiration. Classically, the condition does not distress the infant, despite the quite dramatic stridor that it may produce. Although the stridor may vary in severity with crying, the cry itself is normal.

INVESTIGATION

In the past, this condition often has been diagnosed without endoscopy based on the clinical features and the knowledge that it is the most common cause of these features in babies. However, there is now a greater tendency to perform endoscopy to ensure precise diagnosis. This approach is to be encouraged, as some conditions producing laryngeal stridor can be progressive and may cause complete obstruction and death, e.g. laryngeal cysts, subglottic haemangioma. Worsening stridor in an infant is an absolute indication for endoscopy.

Endoscopy may be performed under sedation using a fine flexible bronchoscope, but in some centres rigid endoscopy

with general anaesthesia is used. It is essential that the larynx is inspected with the child breathing spontaneously in order for the diagnosis to be made.

MANAGEMENT

In most cases, the stridor decreases over the first one to two years of life, although it may worsen again temporarily with respiratory infection. In rare cases, hospital admission may be required during infections, but most cases require no treatment. Very severe forms may require tracheostomy.

Vocal cord palsy

Cord palsy in the neonate is usually unilateral and self-limiting. A common cause is birth trauma. As a result, there may be other features of a traumatic delivery, such as Erb's palsy or phrenic nerve palsy. Unilateral palsy may be so mild as to go unnoticed but when clinically apparent, it presents with a weak cry, a tendency to aspirate secretions and choking with feeds. Bilateral palsy causes severe stridor and cyanosis. Although recovery may occur in the first six months, tracheostomy is usually required until then. Diagnosis of unilateral cord palsy is particularly difficult and requires considerable experience of infant endoscopy.

Subglottic stenosis

This may be congenital or acquired. With improved neonatal intensive care techniques and endotracheal tube materials, acquired stenosis is now much less common than it was. In fact, it is quite surprising how rarely it occurs nowadays, given that many small infants with chronic lung disease still undergo prolonged intubation. The narrowest point in the airway is at the level of the cricoid ring. It is at this site that acquired stenosis secondary to prolonged intubation may occur. Stenosis is suggested clinically when attempts to extubate an infant after prolonged ventilation fail and are accompanied by evidence of obstruction (stridor, sternal and subcostal recession, etc.).

In many cases, extubation failure is due to a combination of subglottic oedema or stenosis and chronic lung disease. The relative importance of these may be hard to define, but endoscopy is valuable in determining optimal management. If oedema alone is present, then a course of steroids – which may also improve coexisting chronic lung disease – may enable subsequent extubation. Minor granulations require no treatment. Thin web stenoses can be resected by laser. More severe fibrous scarring often is circumferential, and tracheostomy with subsequent laryngoplasty with bone grafting may be needed. More recently, surgical incision of the cricoid over the indwelling endotracheal tube without the need for tracheostomy has been described.

Congenital subglottic stenosis is rare. It usually presents with stridor, but this may not be apparent at birth, presenting later during respiratory infection. The added airway narrowing produced by such infection may compromise the airway sufficiently as to make intubation necessary. As a result, further oedema occurs, making extubation difficult. Most children with congenital stenosis require no treatment and improve with age. Severe cases require tracheostomy and laryngoplasty.

Haemangioma

Subglottic haemangiomas present with stridor in infancy. Like other haemangiomas, the lesion may be absent or very small at birth but may enlarge over the first few months, only to regress in the first two to five years. Thus, stridor may not be present at birth, but once present it may become increasingly severe. As this process may be quite rapid, any infant with worsening stridor requires urgent endoscopy. Diagnosis is usually possible without resort to biopsy. Cutaneous haemangiomas are present in the head and neck region in 50 per cent of cases. Another association is with sternal clefting. Tracheostomy usually is required, followed by expectant treatment awaiting resolution or medical (steroids, radiotherapy) or surgical (laser resection, cryosurgery) treatment.

Laryngeal cleft

Congenital clefting of the larynx with or without trachea may occur alone or in combination with other anomalies, such as oesophageal atresia, congenital heart disease, cleft lip and palate and genitourinary anomalies. It probably arises from incomplete separation of the foregut into trachea and oesophagus. It has been classified into four types (Benjamin and Inglis 1989):

- *Type I:* interarytenoid cleft.
- *Type II:* partial cricoid cleft.
- *Type III:* total cricoid cleft.

- *Type IV:* clefting extending into the trachea; severe forms extend to the carina.

Presentation varies with the extent of clefting but includes feed aspiration, recurrent pneumonia, stridor and weak cry. Complete stage IV clefts may result in total tracheal collapse, requiring intubation from birth.

The diagnosis of minor clefts is difficult and they are often missed. Laryngoscopy must include careful inspection of the posterior commissure. Surgical treatment of minor clefts is usually straightforward, but gastro-oesophageal reflux must be looked for and treated if present. Children with longer clefts require tracheostomy and major reconstruction. The prognosis for this group is poor, and few children with complete tracheal clefting have survived.

Miscellaneous anomalies

Various types of webs and cysts can cause laryngeal obstruction (see Benjamin *et al.* 1994).

TRACHEA AND BRONCHI

Tracheal agenesis and stenosis

Tracheal agenesis is extremely rare. It comprises failure of development of the trachea, although the extent of this failure and the subsequent anatomy varies. Seven different anatomical types have been described. In the most common (56 per cent) variety, the trachea ends blindly at or just below the vocal cords and arises again from the lower oesophagus. Presentation is with immediate cyanosis and impossible endotracheal intubation. In 80 per cent of patients, improvement occurs with positive-pressure ventilation via the oesophagus. No long-term survivors with this condition have been reported, although various techniques have been employed that have kept the baby alive in the short term. With this in mind, accurate diagnosis must be obtained by endoscopy, and the parents must be counselled regarding the fact that oesophageal ventilation may need to be discontinued and the baby allowed to die. New techniques such as lung transplantation and tracheal transplantation may arise for this condition, and any baby in whom this diagnosis is made or suspected should be discussed with a specialist paediatric ear, nose and throat (ENT) or thoracic surgical department.

Congenital tracheal stenosis is characterized by loss of the pars membranosa of the trachea, such that the tracheal rings, which are normally horseshoe-shaped, are complete circles. This abnormality may extend to the bronchial cartilages. Although the whole of the trachea may be involved, the stenosis more commonly is confined to a section of the trachea. Presentation is with respiratory distress. This can usually be relieved by positive-pressure ventilation, even if the endotracheal tube will not pass through the affected area. The diagnosis is confirmed by bronchoscopy, although bronchography may be required to determine the extent of tracheal/bronchial involvement. Because of the reported association with pulmonary artery slings, echocardiography should be performed. Treatment of short stenoses is by surgical resection of the stenotic segment and primary anastomosis. Up to 66 per cent of the length of trachea can be resected in this way. Tracheal longitudinal incision and cartilage grafting are required for longer segments but are hazardous.

Vascular ring

Abnormalities of development of the major vessels near the trachea can result in compression of the trachea by a double aortic arch, pulmonary artery sling or other vessels. In double aortic arch, one branch passes in front of the trachea and one behind. One branch is usually larger than the other. All affected infants present with stridor, but this may not become apparent until the child is a few years of age. Aortic arch abnormalities may also cause dysphagia. Pulmonary artery slings, however, are notorious for producing life-threatening obstruction, which may in part be due to associated tracheal stenosis (see above). In most cases, the left pulmonary arises from its partner on the right and passes between the trachea and oesophagus. Investigation for these anomalies should include a contrast swallow and bronchoscopy. If these suggest a vascular anomaly, then echocardiography and arteriography may be required. Double aortic arch is treated by division of the smaller branch. Pulmonary artery sling surgery is more complex and may involve resection of tracheal stenosis if this coexists.

It is debated whether the innominate artery can cause symptomatic tracheal compression. Although in the normal adult this vessel runs to the right of the trachea, it was noticed in some infants with stridor that it ran across the trachea from left to right and was thought to be compressing the trachea in these cases. Subsequent reports have shown that this course of the innominate artery is found in many normal children. The condition certainly overlaps with tracheomalacia.

Tracheomalacia

This is a common cause of tracheal (biphasic) stridor. In paediatric surgical practice, it is most commonly encountered in association with oesophageal atresia (OA) and tracheo-oesophageal fistula (TOF) (Chapter 15, p. 123). In its common mild form, it is responsible for the so-called 'TOF cough'. However, tracheomalacia can occur in isolation or as a result of external tracheal compression by cysts or tumours or from long-term intubation. The primary abnormality is defective development of the tracheal cartilage rings that support the trachea during respiration. Instead of being horseshoe-shaped, the rings are opened out posteriorly as well as often collapsing inwards anteriorly.

Clinical presentation in OA is with the TOF cough, which in more severe cases is combined with stridor and 'dying spells'. In these life-threatening events, the trachea collapses completely but usually reopens as the child relaxes when consciousness is lost. The diagnosis can usually be made easily on bronchoscopy under conditions that allow spontaneous respiration. In the absence of OA as an underlying explanation, a search for another causative lesion, e.g. a mediastinal cyst or a vascular ring, should be made. Although the condition is usually self-limiting, such that stridor may be gone at a few months of age and TOF cough at a few years of age, severe cases will require aortopexy (Filler et al. 1992). This procedure approximates the aorta to the sternum, which has the effect of pulling the anterior wall of the trachea forwards, increasing the tracheal lumen. It is most suited for the treatment of short-segment tracheomalacia. If the whole trachea is involved, then tracheostomy may be required. Such severe cases may eventually improve spontaneously, allowing removal of the tracheostomy after a few years, but in other cases, tracheal reconstruction (pericardial patch, slide tracheoplasty) may be required. Different techniques described for tracheomalacia of different segments include anterior cricoid suspension for high tracheomalacia, pulmonary artery trunk-pexy (PA-pexy) for distal bronchomalacia, and balloon-expandable metallic stents for longer-segment tracheobronchomalacia in patients in whom conventional therapy has failed.

The same process of weakness of cartilage support may also involve the bronchi (bronchomalacia). This may be an isolated defect or may be found in conjunction with tracheomalacia. If unilateral, it may present as recurrent pneumonia, but if bilateral and combined with tracheomalacia, it can cause serious respiratory obstruction. This may be treatable, but in some cases it is fatal.

LUNGS

Agenesis

This rare anomaly is a result of primary arrest of lung-bud development. In about 50 per cent of cases, other anomalies coexist, such as cardiac lesions, vertebral and skeletal anomalies, oesophageal atresia and gastrointestinal anomalies. Mortality is high in the neonatal period and usually due to the associated anomalies. In surviving infants, the diagnosis is usually made on routine chest X-ray. Although lobar agenesis can occur, pulmonary agenesis is more common. The condition requires no treatment, but the dramatic radiological features of mediastinal displacement in a child who has presumably had sufficient symptoms in the first place to merit X-ray usually result in further investigations being considered, the most useful being a ventilation/perfusion (V/Q) scan, bronchoscopy and bronchography.

Congenital lobar emphysema

DEFINITION

Congenital lobar emphysema (CLE) is defined as overexpansion of the alveolar spaces of a lung segment or lobe. It is thought to result from cartilaginous deficiency in the tracheobronchial tree, which produces a check-valve type of obstruction and air trapping within a lobe. Compression of the adjacent lung may compromise ventilation, depending on the volume occupied by the emphysematous lobe.

This condition has various aetiologies, as indicated by histopathological analysis:

- Intrinsic bronchial obstruction resulting from bronchomalacia or abnormal bronchial cartilage support is seen in 35–50 per cent of patients.
- Congenital or post-infective alveolar septal fibrosis.
- Pulmonary alveolar hyperplasia or polyalveolar lobe, found in one-third of CLE patients. A polyalveolar lobe is characterized by a normal number of bronchi, but the acini contain three to five times the normal number of alveoli of normal size and a decreased number of arterial branches per unit volume of the emphysematous lobe.
- Extrinsic bronchial compression resulting in CLE can occur in association with an enlarged heart due to congenital cardiac anomalies (ventricular septal defect, patent ductus arteriosus, tetralogy of Fallot, dilated atria) or aneurysmal dilation of the major vessels in 15 per cent of infants. Bronchogenic cysts are known to cause regional CLE from external bronchial obstruction.
- Pulmonary hypoplasia due to diminished number of bronchial branches and abnormal small arteries.
- Lobar emphysema also can be an acquired disorder, particularly in preterm neonates and small-for-date infants who have been on long-term ventilation, in whom bronchial obstruction may occur due to redundant bronchial mucosa, inspissated mucus plugging the bronchus, and torsion of the bronchus.

PATHOPHYSIOLOGY

In complete bronchial obstruction, regional hyperinflation is due to a check-valve mechanism in the collateral ventilation through the alveolar pores of Kohn, the broncho-alveolar channels of Lambert or the interbronchiolar channels. In partial obstruction of the bronchus, air is allowed through in inspiration, but during expiration the bronchus is occluded completely, resulting in overinflation and overexpansion of the lung and breakdown of alveolar septae.

In polyalveolar lobes, the number of bronchial branches is normal but there is an abnormal increase in the number of alveoli in each acinus, with a decrease in the number of arteries per unit volume of emphysematous lung. Infants with polyalveolar lobe present early. The condition is indistinguishable from other forms of CLE.

The distribution of lung involvement is shown diagrammatically in Figure 31.5.

CLINICAL FEATURES

CLE presents dramatically within hours of birth with rapidly progressive respiratory distress in 50 per cent of affected

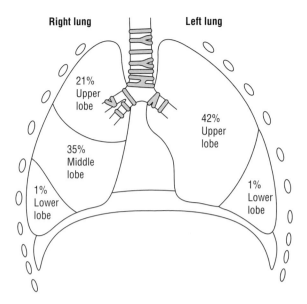

Figure 31.5 *Distribution of lobar involvement by congenital lobar emphysema (CLE). In cases where CLE is bilateral, the right middle and left upper lobes are affected most commonly.*

neonates. In other cases, presentation is delayed for days or even months, but symptoms usually become apparent in the first six months of life. Males are affected three times more often than females. The earlier the onset of symptoms, the more probable the progression to life-threatening progressive pulmonary insufficiency from compression of normal adjacent lung. Tachypnoea, dyspnoea and cyanosis form the complex of symptoms; hyper-resonance and diminished breath sounds over the affected area are the detectable physical signs.

CLE has been detected on antenatal ultrasonography, the features being either echogenic or a cystic lung lesion detected early in gestation . Although these lesions may regress or resolve antenatally, some patients become rapidly symptomatic postnatally due to air trapping and should have ready access to postnatal surgical intervention.

DIFFERENTIAL DIAGNOSIS

The differential diagnoses includes giant congenital cystic adenomatoid malformation, tension pneumothorax, atelectasis of one lung or lobe with compensatory emphysema in the other as a result of inspissated mucous plugging or torsion of the bronchus, and pneumatocoele.

INVESTIGATIONS

The diagnosis is usually suspected on review of a chest X-ray performed because of respiratory symptoms (Figure 31.6). Radiological features include:

- hyperlucent overexpanded lung;
- herniation of the emphysematous segment into the opposite side anterior to the heart and great vessels;
- wide separation of bronchovascular structures;
- shift of the mediastinum;

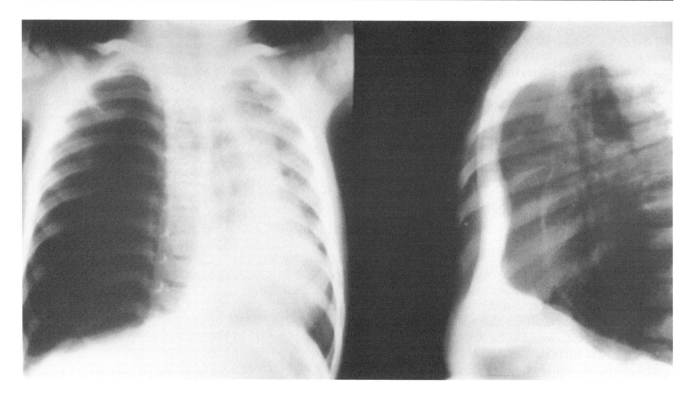

Figure 31.6 *Chest X-ray of a newborn infant with congenital lobar emphysema.*

- compression and atelectasis of the adjacent lung structures, depending on the magnitude of overexpansion;
- depression of the ipsilateral diaphragm.

In most cases, no other form of investigation is needed and, indeed, may delay urgently required surgery. In cases where the onset of symptoms has been gradual, CT scanning can be useful to demonstrate a causative lesion such as a bronchogenic cyst. V/Q scanning is useful in long-term follow-up and assessment of the unaffected segments of the lung and of the affected segment when conservative treatment has been adopted. Echocardiography may be used to define cardiac abnormalities, as 15 per cent of these patients have major cardiac anomalies.

TREATMENT

Surgical lobectomy is the treatment of choice. Urgent surgical intervention is indicated when there is a life-threatening progressive pulmonary insufficiency from compression of adjacent lung structures. There is no role for bronchoplastic procedures. In occasional cases, rapid deterioration occurs under anaesthesia due to positive-pressure ventilation of the obstructed lobe with increased air trapping. For this reason, spontaneous respiration should be adopted until the chest is opened. At thoracotomy, usually the emphysematous lobe is impossible to compress. This can make access to the hilum of the lung difficult, although in some cases the affected lobe can be delivered through the wound, improving access. Once the hilum is identified, resection usually is straightforward.

Infants over two months of age presenting with mild to moderate respiratory symptoms and normal bronchoscopic findings have been successfully treated conservatively. However, these children require close follow-up, and the family should be warned about acute deterioration. Selective bronchial intubation can be used in acquired forms to isolate the affected lung and, thereby, hasten resolution.

RESULTS

Lobectomy is usually tolerated well provided that the remaining lobes are normal. Long-term follow-up has shown no symptomatic functional impairment, although respiratory flow rates are diminished to about 80 per cent of normal. Long-term evaluation of surgically and conservatively managed children has shown that the pulmonary function has remained equivalent in both groups and an asymptomatic hyperlucent overdistended lobe may not impair the normal development of the remaining lung.

Congenital cystic lung abnormalities

The nomenclature and pathological classification of congenital cystic lung abnormalities is confusing. A number of publications suggest new classifications (Bush 2001; Langston 2003). The two main conditions encountered by paediatric surgeons are congenital cystic adenomatoid malformation (CCAM) and pulmonary sequestration. For the purposes of this chapter, these two traditional terms will be used and the conditions discussed separately. However, the pathological features of these two conditions may coexist (Conran and Stocker 1999). To some extent, the details of pathological definition are not relevant to the surgeon. If a decision is made to operate on the basis of either symptoms or the risk of potential complications (see below), then the main problems facing the surgeon are how much lung to remove and what gross anatomical variations may be encountered.

The main anatomical variations relate to the presence of anomalous systemic blood supply. This is particularly well reported in pulmonary sequestrations and is described below, but given the overlap between CCAM and sequestration, the surgeon should be aware of the possibility of anomalous supply in any cystic lesions, should attempt to identify it on preoperative imaging, and should approach surgical dissection with caution.

CONGENITAL CYSTIC ADENOMATOID MALFORMATION

This abnormality was first described in 1949. Although uncommon, it is being encountered more frequently as a result of prenatal ultrasound screening. The incidence is often quoted at one in 25 000, but in the authors' experience, about one in 10 000 pregnancies are associated with a diagnosis of CCAM/sequestration.

Definition
CCAM is a multicystic mass of pulmonary tissue in which there is a proliferation of bronchial structures at the expense of alveoli. In rare cases, skeletal muscle may be present in the cyst walls.

Pathology and embryology
Histopathologically, there is an abnormal proliferation of mesenchymal elements and failure of maturation of bronchiolar structures. Proliferation of polypoid glandular tissue occurs at the expense of alveolar development. CCAMs communicate with the tracheobronchial tree. Air trapping occurs secondary to lack of cartilaginous bronchi. The absence of bronchial cartilage and the high incidence of associated anomalies suggest that the prenatal insult has occurred before 31 days of gestation; the mixture of epithelial and mesenchymal structures suggests that the insult occurs after the two lung buds appear at 26–28 days.

Classification
This is based upon the clinical and histopathological characteristics that Stocker initially delineated into three types but has now revised to five subgroups:

- *Type 0:* solid small lungs (previously known as acinar dysplasia). Composed of bronchial-type airways, abundant mesenchyme and smooth muscle. Incompatible with life.
- *Type 1:* single or multiple cysts over 2 cm in diameter that are lined by pseudo-stratified columnar epithelium. Relatively normal alveoli may be present between the cysts.
- *Type 2:* multiple small cysts up to 2 cm in diameter that are lined by ciliated cuboidal or columnar epithelium.

Respiratory bronchioles and distended alveoli may be present between the cysts. There is a high frequency (26 per cent) of other congenital anomalies.
- *Type 3:* large, bulky non-cystic lesion. Bronchiole-like structures are lined by ciliated cuboidal epithelium and separated by masses of alveolar size structures lined by non-ciliated cuboidal epithelium.
- *Type 4:* large cysts (up to 10 cm) lined by flattened epithelium.

Overlap among these types is known to occur.

Clinical features
CCAM usually presents to the paediatric surgeon in one of three ways: on prenatal ultrasound, as respiratory distress in the newborn or infant, or as recurrent chest infections in later childhood. However 25–35 per cent of affected infants will never present to a surgeon, as they are affected so severely that they are stillborn or die rapidly after birth with severe pulmonary insufficiency. This should be borne in mind when considering the management of prenatally diagnosed CCAM (see below).

POSTNATAL SYMPTOMATIC CONGENITAL CYSTIC ADENOMATOID MALFORMATION

Neonatal presentation is usually with gradually progressive respiratory distress as the lesion enlarges postnatally due to air trapping. The rapidity of development of symptoms depends not only on the size of the lesion but also on the degree of pulmonary hypoplasia in the rest of the ipsilateral and contralateral lung induced by *in utero* compression – exactly analogous to the situation occurring in congenital diaphragmatic hernia. Hyper-resonance of the affected hemi-thorax is found with displacement of the cardiac apex.

In the great majority of patients, a single lobe is involved. Any lobe can be affected. Rarely, two or more lobes are involved. For this reason, careful cross-sectional imaging of the chest should be performed if time allows. The affected lobes are not always grossly abnormal macroscopically, and it is possible to resect one lobe only to find that further resection is needed a week or two later.

Associated anomalies have been reported with CCAM and include diaphragmatic hernia, jejunal atresia, prune belly syndrome and hydrocephalus.

Radiological investigations
The diagnosis of CCAM usually can be made on chest X-ray (Figure 31.7). However, the radiological features are variable and include marked hyperlucency of the hemi-thorax with mediastinal and diaphragmatic displacement mimicking tension pneumothorax or congenital lobar emphysema (usually type 1 lesions), multiple smaller cysts full of air and fluid mimicking diaphragmatic hernia (type 1 or 2 lesions), and solid space-occupying mass (type 3 lesions) (Figure 31.8). It is essential to perform an abdominal X-ray to demonstrate a normal abdominal gas pattern and exclude congenital diaphragmatic hernia. If the baby is deteriorating clinically due to

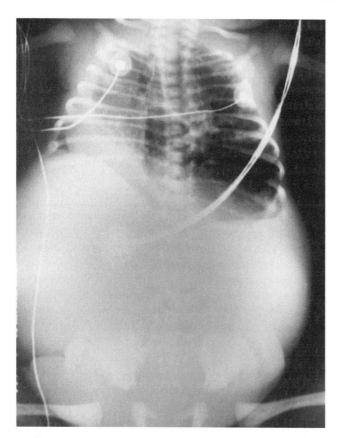

Figure 31.7 *Chest X-ray of a newborn infant with a large left lower lobe type 1 congenital cystic adenomatoid malformation (CCAM) causing mediastinal and diaphragmatic displacement. The lesion had been detected prenatally. The remaining lung was severely hypoplastic and the baby died, despite surgical resection of the CCAM.*

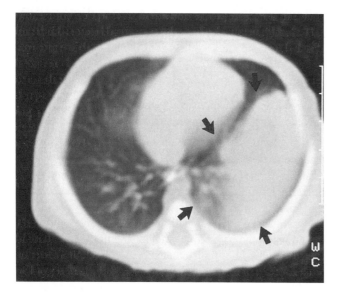

Figure 31.8 *Computed tomography (CT) scan of the chest of a newborn infant with a type 3 congenital cystic adenomatoid malformation (arrows).*

increasing air trapping, then this may be the only imaging that time allows before urgent surgery. There is no place for elective delay in surgery as in diaphragmatic hernia.

If the baby's condition allows, then further imaging in the form of CT scanning is useful to determine whether more than one lobe is affected. Since there is overlap between CCAM and pulmonary sequestration, an attempt should be made to determine whether there is an anomalous systemic arterial supply from, for example, the abdominal aorta. This is particularly important if the lesion appears to be affecting the lower lobe. Such vessels may be detected by Doppler ultrasound but are usually seen better on CT san with intravenous contrast. Although MRI will also identify anomalous vessels, any procedure other than corrective surgery that might involve general anaesthesia should be avoided, because positive-pressure ventilation will usually increase the cyst size and worsen the baby's condition.

Management of symptomatic congenital cystic adenomatoid malformation

The treatment of symptomatic CCAM is excision of the affected lobe(s). Fortunately, most infants with symptomatic CCAM will have fairly mild respiratory symptoms. When preoperative stabilization is required, it is essential to try to avoid positive-pressure ventilation, as this will risk further air trapping and can result in rapid deterioration. Clearly, this also affects anaesthetic management and, if possible, the infant should be allowed to breath spontaneously until the chest is opened. Mobilization of the affected lobe should include careful examination to exclude an anomalous vascular supply. Whilst most CCAMs are supplied by the pulmonary circulation, some, particularly those arising from the lower lobe, are supplied systemically. If a lower-lobe CCAM is found, then the inferior pulmonary ligament should be inspected carefully before division. It is possible to unwittingly divide or avulse what is often a very large systemic artery as it comes through the diaphragm. This vessel will then retract out of site, usually followed by death of the baby from haemorrhage. Lobectomy is otherwise usually straightforward. Local segmental resection is not usually required but can be employed to preserve lung tissue in bilateral cases.

In most cases, recovery from surgery is uneventful. However, persistent fetal circulation akin to that found in congenital diaphragmatic hernia may occur, requiring aggressive treatment, including extracorporeal membrane oxygenation (ECMO). Long-term outcome is normal in most cases.

Prenatal diagnosis

Detection of CCAM by prenatal ultrasound is now commonplace and has altered our knowledge of the natural history of the condition. Such knowledge is essential for prenatal counselling. It is now clear that CCAM will follow one of three courses. First, the lesion may become so large *in utero* as to distort the heart and great vessels and produce cardiac failure, which is manifest as hydrops. This will result frequently in death *in utero*. Second, the fetus may survive and be symptomatic at birth, as described above. Third, and perhaps most commonly, the infant will be born asymptomatic. Regression of CCAMs can occur *in utero*, and there are many reports of them diminishing in size or vanishing completely.

Lesions producing hydrops are usually solid, Stocker type 3 lesions. Whilst these can rarely resolve, the only treatment affecting outcome after development of hydrops is fetal surgery. Large cystic lesions rarely cause hydrops, although they are amenable to *in utero* shunting. The role of fetal surgery in CCAM is controversial. Adzick *et al.* (1993) have reported successful *in utero* resection of types 2 and 3 CCAMs, with reversal of fetal hydrops and good long-term outcome. However, selecting those fetuses that may benefit from intervention is difficult, as even large lesions can regress spontaneously before delivery.

Controversy exists about the postnatal management of asymptomatic infants with CCAM. Given that regression of these lesions can occur *in utero*, then perhaps further regression can occur postnatally, such that the lesion will never cause a problem. However, it is well reported that recurrent and severe infections can occur in CCAM in later life. Perhaps even more worrying is the reported development of malignancy in CCAM (see below).

MANAGEMENT OF ASYMPTOMATIC CONGENITAL CYSTIC ADENOMATOID MALFORMATION

Asymptomatic infants with CCAM should have a chest X-ray done within hours of birth. This will often show the affected area of lung to be radio-opaque due to delayed clearance of lung fluid (Figure 31.9a). This area will clear after 24–48 hours; subsequent X-rays may show air-filled cysts or may appear normal (Figure 31.9b). However, on close scrutiny, subtle changes are often visible and CT scanning frequently will show the lesion to be much more dramatic than expected (Figure 31.10). Whatever the decision made in the newborn period, the lung should not be declared normal until CT or MRI has been performed.

RISKS ASSOCIATED WITH ASYMPTOMATIC CONGENITAL CYSTIC ADENOMATOID MALFORMATION

One of the most difficult dilemmas in advising parents about the management of asymptomatic congenital lung cysts is our inadequate knowledge about potential complications. It is known that these lesions are at risk of both infection and malignant change. Infection may present with pneumonia or empyema during childhood or in adult life, but the incidence of this complication is not known. To await infective complications in an otherwise asymptomatic child would seem acceptable practice. Far more difficult is the uncertainty surrounding the risk of malignant change. Various malignancies, including pulmonary blastoma, bronchioalveolar carcinoma (BAC) and rhabdomyosarcoma, have been reported, both in childhood and in adult life. Evidence (MacSweeney *et al.* 2003) suggests that the histological features of type 4 CCAM are probably indistinguishable from grade 1 pleuropulmonary blastoma. Some early reports of sarcomas arising in CCAMs are now

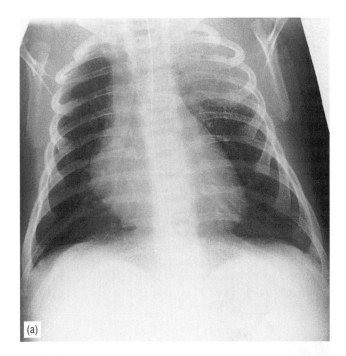

(a)

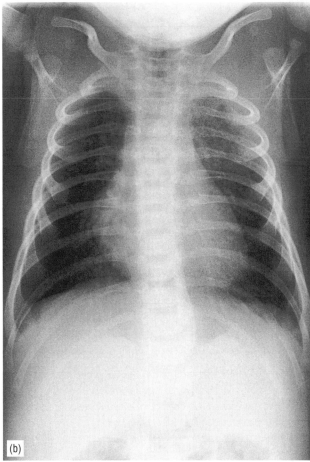

(b)

Figure 31.9 *(a) Chest X-ray taken on day one of life in an infant with prenatally diagnosed left upper lobe type 1 congenital cystic adenomatoid malformation (CCAM), showing opacity due to delayed clearance of lung fluid. (b) Chest X-ray in the same infant on day two of life.*

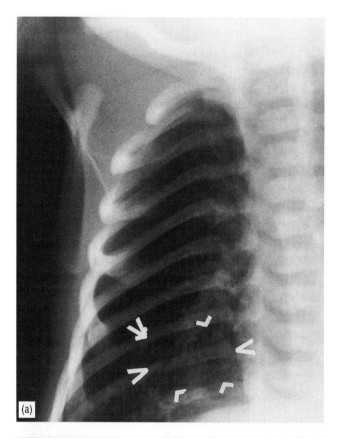

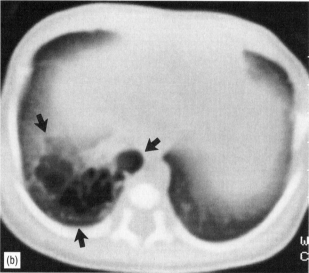

Figure 31.10 *(a) Chest X-ray of an infant diagnosed as having right lower lobe congenital cystic adenomatoid malformation (CCAM) on prenatal ultrasound. Although outlined with arrows, the lesion is virtually undetectable. (b) Computed tomography (CT) scan of the same infant, showing clear cystic changes in the right lower lobe.*

series have suggested that the incidence is less than one per cent. Unfortunately, the authors do not comment on the mode of presentation or indications for surgery in these patients, but it may be assumed that microscopic BAC was an incidental finding. The five patients ranged from six months to 36 years of age. None developed recurrence of BAC; indeed, only one patient in the literature has been reported to have died from metastatic disease. The degree of risk resulting from an asymptomatic CCAM of any type remains unclear. However, once the concept of possible malignancy has been discussed with the parents, many request resection.

PULMONARY SEQUESTRATION

Definition and clinical features

CCAM and pulmonary sequestration are known to be associated, and in some cases there is an overlap of the two pathologies within the same patient (Conran and Stocker 1999). They may well represent a spectrum of cystic lung lesions. Pulmonary sequestration is defined as a congenitally abnormal area of non-functioning lung tissue that does not communicate with the tracheobronchial tree and that receives its blood supply from anomalous systemic vessels, directly from the infradiaphragmatic aorta in 77 per cent. Two main types occur: intralobar, in which the sequestrated lobe is contained within the normal lung, and extralobar, in which the sequestration has its own visceral pleura and is separate from the normal pulmonary lobe. Up to 50 per cent of sequestrations may be atypical or associated with another anomaly. To facilitate management, sequestrations should be described according to their connection to tracheobronchial tree, visceral pleura, arterial supply, venous drainage, foregut communication, histology, multiplicity and associated anomalies.

Intralobar pulmonary sequestration (IPS) occurs predominantly in the posterior lateral basal segment of the left lower lobe. Arterial blood supply is by solitary or multiple moderate-sized vessels arising from the abdominal aorta (75 per cent) or by arteries arising from the thoracic aorta or other abdominal vessels (25 per cent). Venous drainage is usually into the pulmonary vein, although drainage into the hemiazygos and azygos veins occurs in one-third of the cases. IPS usually presents in older children as recurrent pneumonia; however, it has been detected on prenatal ultrasonography.

Extralobar pulmonary sequestration (EPS) has been diagnosed by antenatal ultrasound scans at 19–20 weeks' gestational age. It is characteristically seen as a hyperechogenic mass in the posterior basal part of the left hemi-thorax. More often, EPS is detected as an incidental finding during the management of infants with thoracic or cardiac anomalies. In 60 per cent of EPS patients, there is associated left-sided diaphragmatic hernia; there is a high incidence of other associated congenital anomalies (John *et al.* 1989), such as CCAM, congenital cardiac anomalies, pericardial defects, pectus excavatum, bronchogenic cysts and vertebral anomalies. EPS also may occur below the diaphragm (Figure 31.11) and can present as an echogenic suprarenal mass on the antenatal scan.

thought to be low-grade pulmonary blastoma, an entity not recognized at the time of these reports (Langston 2003). Rather worryingly, in MacSweeny and colleagues' series, five of 16 type 1 CCAMs had microscopic foci of BAC. Other

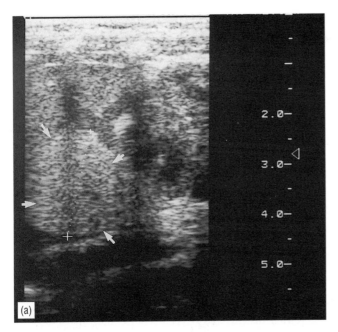 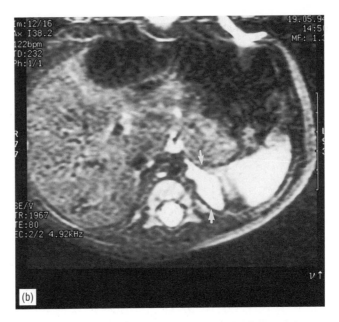

Figure 31.11 *(a) Prenatal ultrasound of fetus with a left-sided suprarenal extralobar pulmonary sequestration EPS (arrows). (b) Postnatal magnetic resonance scan in the same infant, showing the lesion still present but proportionally smaller. The lesion was asymptomatic but was excised at nine months of age after the onset of respiratory symptoms (not due to the lesion) and increased parental anxiety. (Reproduced with permission.)*

Investigation

Plain radiology alone is not sufficient to make the diagnosis, and some form of imaging to demonstrate the systemic arterial supply is required not only for diagnosis but also to facilitate surgery. Doppler ultrasonography scan is often able to do this. Although angiography previously was popular, MRI has now supplanted it.

Treatment

The treatment of pulmonary sequestration is resection. This usually involves lobectomy for IPS, although EPS usually can be resected in isolation. Care must be taken in identifying the anomalous vessels and in securing control of these blood vessels to avoid torrential haemorrhage and operative mortality. Preoperative embolization of the anomalous arterial supply with the help of interventional radiology may be a useful adjunct. If conservative management is adopted following prenatal diagnosis, then long-term follow-up is indicated because of the risks of infection and possible malignancy, given the overlap with CCAM. There is also the possibility of haemodynamic complications of the significant vascular shunting that occurs in some patients.

Bronchogenic cyst

These congenital cysts are derived form the primitive foregut and probably represent abnormal bronchial budding. They are rare, but they can present in adult life or are found incidentally at post-mortem. They can occur in the mediastinum, where they represent about five per cent of mediastinal masses in children, in the lung parenchyma, in the neck or attached to the chest wall. They vary in diameter from 2 to 10 cm. They contain viscid, milky mucus. Occasionally, they communicate with the airway.

Presentation is in one of four ways: as an incidental finding of a smooth mediastinal mass on chest X-ray (Figure 31.12); as a cause of respiratory distress in infancy due to pressure on the airway; as a cause of recurrent or persistent pneumonia, when the cyst communicates with the bronchial tree; and on prenatal ultrasound scan.

Investigations should include plain radiology of the chest and cross-sectional imaging (CT or MRI) to define the exact location of the lesion and to help with the differential diagnosis, particularly from solid lesions such as lymphoma and other tumours.

Treatment is by excision. This is usually very easy, but it may be more difficult if the lesion is within the oesophageal or tracheal wall or the lung parenchyma. There is a temptation to manage asymptomatic lesions conservatively, and this might be justifiable. However, with the knowledge that these lesions may become symptomatic if they enlarge and cause bronchial compression, and that sarcomatous change has been reported in such cysts, most authors still recommend excision.

One pitfall for the surgeon is that a bronchogenic cyst may cause bronchial compression and air trapping in the neonate, producing a clinical presentation and radiological features identical to those of congenital lobar emphysema. For this reason, careful inspection of the lung hilum at thoracotomy is essential before lobectomy for CLE.

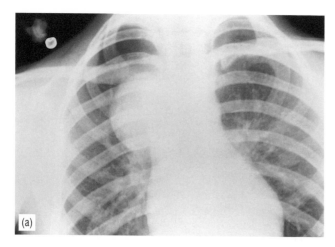
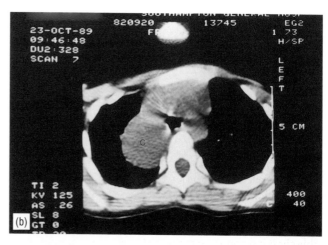

Figure 31.12 *(a) Chest X-ray, showing a right-sided bronchogenic cyst. (b) Computed tomography (CT) scan of the same child as in (a), showing the cyst (C).*

PLEURA: CHYLOTHORAX

Chylothorax can occur secondarily to thoracic surgery or central venous thrombosis, but it may also occur as a primary congenital phenomenon, possibly due to abnormal thoracic duct development. It is one of the causes of fetal pleural effusion and may produce sufficient fetal compromise to merit prenatal drainage.

Postnatal presentation is with respiratory distress with clinical and radiological features of pleural effusion. Diagnosis can be made on sampling the pleural fluid, but this will have the typical milky colour of chyle only if the infant is receiving milk feeds. The diagnostic feature of the fluid is its high leucocyte content, of which 80–90 per cent are lymphocytes.

Treatment involves tube drainage for about three weeks, during which time the volume of chyle being produced should be minimized by the use of enteral feeds containing medium-chain triglycerides or by the use of parenteral nutrition. If the chyle leak persists after three weeks, then surgical ligation of the thoracic duct leak (if it can be located), pleurodesis or pleural-fluid shunting should be undertaken. Persistence with conservative management carries a high mortality.

CLINICAL SCENARIOS

Case 1

A 3150-g male neonate, delivered normally at full term, was found to have excess salivation and respiratory distress. A chest X-ray with nasogastric tube confirmed the diagnosis of OA and distal tracheo-oesophageal fistula. There were no associated cardiac or other abnormalities. A bronchoscopy revealed moderate tracheomalacia and no proximal fistula. Primary repair was performed through a right thoracotomy. Oral feeds were commenced on day five, but the child continued to have

respiratory distress and oxygen requirement. A chest X-ray excluded aspiration pneumonia, and the child was treated with anti-reflux medication for gastro-oesophageal reflux. A repeat laryngobronchoscopy on day ten confirmed severe tracheomalacia. Repeated attempts to wean from oxygen failed and episodes of respiratory obstruction occurred with increasing frequency. An aortopexy was performed at three weeks of age. Following this, there was a rapid improvement in the respiratory distress and oxygen requirement, and he was discharged ten days later. At three months' follow-up, there was good weight gain and no further problems.

Case 2

A full-term 2800-g neonate was found at 24 hours' baby check to have respiratory distress, cyanosis and oxygen requirement during breast feeds, although the symptoms improved during crying. A chest X-ray and cardiac echo were normal, but attempts at passing a nasogastric tube failed because of resistance at the back of the nose. An oropharyngeal airway improved the symptoms and the baby was fed via an orogastric tube. A CT scan performed on day seven revealed membranous atresia with suspicion of bony elements, occluding both posterior nares. On day 12, under general anaesthesia, via a transnasal approach, the atresia was drilled and posterior nares were dilated. Bilateral stents were inserted. Following this, there was a marked improvement in respiratory distress. The baby was able to breastfeed and was discharged two weeks after surgery. Repeat endoscopy six weeks after surgery showed well-healed nasal passages, and the stents were removed.

Case 3

A 28-year old female, gravida 1, during antenatal scans at 22 weeks was found to have a female fetus with features of

CCAM of the right lung. The follow-up scans showed no increase in size, and at 37 weeks a 3050-g neonate was delivered by spontaneous vaginal delivery. There was no respiratory distress at birth and a chest X-ray was normal. A repeat chest X-ray was also normal on day three. The baby fed well and was discharged home. At one month of age, a CT scan with intravenous contrast showed an abnormal right lower lobe, with multiple cysts of varying size. The remaining lung tissue was normal and there was no evidence of a systemic blood supply. The child remained asymptomatic and the parents were counselled about the long-term complications of recurrent infection, malignancy and the need for a careful follow-up. At one year, there was no change in size of the CCAM on repeat CT scan. However, there was a single episode of a possible chest infection and the parents opted for a surgical excision. At 18 months of age, via a right thoracotomy, a right lower lobectomy was performed. The child recovered well and was discharged from follow-up at the age of 24 months.

REFERENCES

Adzick NS, Harrison MR. Management of the fetus with a cystic adenomatoid malformation. *World Journal of Surgery* 1993; **17**: 342–9.

Benjamin B. Airway obstruction. In: Freeman NV, Burge DM, Griffiths DM, Malone PS (eds). *Surgery of the Newborn*. Edinburgh: Churchill Livingstone, 1994; pp. 409–24.

Benjamin B, Inglis A. Minor congenital laryngeal clefts: diagnosis and classification. *Annals of Otology, Rhinology, and Laryngology* 1989; **98**: 417–20.

Benjamin B, Walker P. Management of airway obstruction in the Pierre Robin sequence. *International Journal of Pediatric Otorhinology* 1991; **22**: 29–37.

Bush A. Congenital lung disease: a plea for clear thinking and clear nomenclature. *Pediatric Pulmonology* 2001; **32**: 328–37.

Conran RM, Stocker JT. Extralobar sequestration with frequently associated congenital cystic adenomatoid malformation, type 2: report of 50 cases. *Pediatric and Developmental Pathology* 1999; **2**: 454–63.

Filler RM, Messineo A, Vinograd I. Severe tracheomalacia associated with esophageal atresia: results of surgical treatment. *Journal of Pediatric Surgery* 1992; **27**: 1136–41.

John PR, Beasley SW, Mayne V. Pulmonary sequestration and related congenital disorders: a clinical-radiological review of 41 cases. *Pediatric Radiology* 1989; **20**: 4–9.

Langston C. New concepts in the pathology of congenital lung malformations. *Seminars in Pediatric Surgery* 2003; **12**: 17–37.

MacSweeney F, Papagiannopoulos K, Goldstraw P, *et al.* An assessment of the expanded classification of congenital cystic adenomatoid malformations and their relationship to malignant transformation. *American Journal of Surgical Pathology* 2003; **27**: 1139–46.

Pagon RA, Graham JM, Zonana J, Yong S-L. Coloboma, congenital heart disease and choanal atresia with multiple anomalies: CHARGE association. *Journal of Pediatrics* 1981; **99**: 223–7.

Samuel M, Burge DM. Extra-lobar intra-abdominal pulmonary sequestration. *European Journal of Pediatric Surgery* 1996; **6**: 107.

FURTHER READING

Prescott CAJ. Nasal obstruction in infancy. *Archives of Disease in Childhood* 1995; **72**: 287–9.

Stocker JT, Madewell JE, Drake RM. Congenital cystic adenomatoid malformation of the lung. *Human Pathology* 1977; **8**: 155–77.

Wiatrak BJ. Congenital anomalies of the larynx and trachea. *Otolaryngologic Clinics of North America* 2000; **33**: 91–110.

Chest-wall deformities

DAVID CRABBE

Learning objectives

- To recognize the different types of chest-wall deformity.
- To understand the principles of surgical correction of pectus deformities.

INTRODUCTION

A variety of deformities of the chest wall appear during childhood. Pectus deformities are the most common. Whilst these do not have serious physiological consequences, they frequently cause a great deal of anxiety.

Cultural changes have significantly altered the perception and tolerance of pectus deformities, and increasing numbers of children are now seeking surgery. Many children have minor deformities and require only reassurance. However, children with significant pectus deformities should not be denied treatment, because good or excellent results can be expected in the majority of cases.

Major congenital chest-wall deformities are rare. They can be difficult, if not impossible, to repair and may be associated with major respiratory or cardiac disease.

INCIDENCE AND CLASSIFICATION

Chest-wall deformities are classified in Box 32.1. Pectus deformities affect about one per cent of the population. Boys are affected more frequently than girls, by a factor of four to one. Pectus excavatum is the most common deformity and is characterized by an inward depression of the sternum. Pectus carinatum is less common and is characterized by a forward angulation of the sternum. Both carinatum and excavatum deformities can be symmetrical or asymmetrical, with varying degrees of torsion of the sternum, which throws the costal cartilages into prominence on one side.

Sternal clefts may be partial or total. They are obvious at birth because the heart and great vessels lie beating visibly immediately under the skin. The heart is structurally normal. In the neonatal period, it is usually possible to bring together the two halves of the sternum without causing significant

---

Box 32.1 Classification of chest-wall deformities

Pectus excavatum
Pectus carinatum
Sternal clefts, upper, lower
Jeune's dystrophy
Spondylothoracic dystrophy
Cantrell's pentalogy

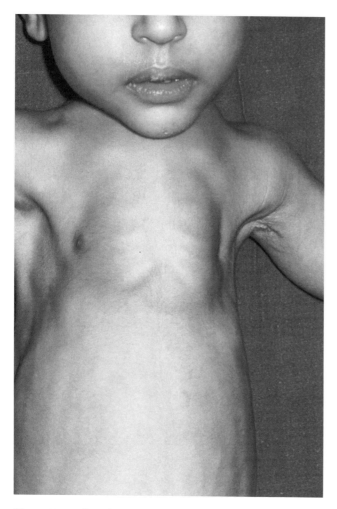

Figure 32.1 *Jeune's asphyxiating thoracic dystrophy.*
Courtesy of the Wellcome Foundation, with permission.

cardiac compression. In older children, this is not possible and the defect has to be repaired with a prosthetic patch.

Cantrell's pentalogy is characterized by a lower sternal defect, a ventral defect in the diaphragm, an apical pericardial defect, exomphalos major and a cardiac defect, usually a ventricular septal defect or Fallot's tetralogy. The heart lies covered by the amnion of the exomphalos. The nature of the cardiac defect is the major determinant of survival.

Jeune's disease is an autosomal recessive condition characterized by a narrow rigid chest, which is typically bell-shaped as a result of short horizontal ribs (Figure 32.1). Some degree of pulmonary hypoplasia is inevitable, but the degree of respiratory insufficiency is variable, and this determines outcome. Surgical attempts to increase the volume of the thorax generally are not successful.

Spondylothoracic dysplasia, the Jarcho–Levin syndrome, is a rare autosomal recessive disorder. The condition is associated with multiple rib and vertebral anomalies. The ribs are described as 'crab-like'. The thorax is small and misshapen. Death from respiratory failure usually occurs in early infancy.

BASIC SCIENCE

The cause of pectus deformities is unknown. Most are isolated abnormalities. The primary abnormality appears to lie in dystrophic growth of the costal cartilages, and the sternal angulation is a secondary phenomenon. Subtle abnormalities in collagen morphology have been demonstrated in the costal cartilages of children with pectus deformities, but it is not clear whether these are of causal significance. A family history of chest-wall deformity is seen in about one-third of cases, although a genetic link has not been established.

Pectus excavatum is seen in children with connective tissue disorders, including Marfan syndrome, Ehlers–Danlos syndrome, osteogenesis imperfecta and homocystinuria. Pectus excavatum occurs with an increased frequency in children with congenital heart diseases and Down syndrome. Pectus deformities are common in children following repair of congenital diaphragmatic hernias, especially if the original defect was large and repaired with a prosthetic patch. Approximately five per cent children with a pectus deformity will have a concomitant scoliosis.

PECTUS EXCAVATUM

Presentation

The deformity of a pectus excavatum is obvious but of variable severity (Figure 32.2). In about 80 per cent of cases, a minor deformity first appears in early infancy. The deformity becomes more obvious during the pubertal growth spurt.

Sternal recession is commonly seen in young infants with laryngomalacia. Inspiratory stridor causes a paradoxical movement of the sternum. This deformity improves as the laryngomalacia settles and the skeleton becomes more rigid. Progression to a fixed pectus excavatum in this group of children is rare. In other children with pectus deformities, there is no evidence that the deformity improves with time.

Symptoms reported by children with pectus excavatum are variable and, to some extent, age-related. Young children are asymptomatic. Older children and adolescents may complain of vague chest and back pains, particularly on exertion. Fatigue and reduced exercise tolerance are common, but these symptoms are probably more related to habitual inactivity than directly to the pectus deformity. Children with pectus deformities become progressively more self-conscious during adolescence.

Function

The physiological consequences of pectus excavatum have been the subject of extensive study. Mild restrictive defects in pulmonary function are common but by no means universal in children with pectus deformities. Rotation and displacement of the heart into the left thorax is common in severe deformities.

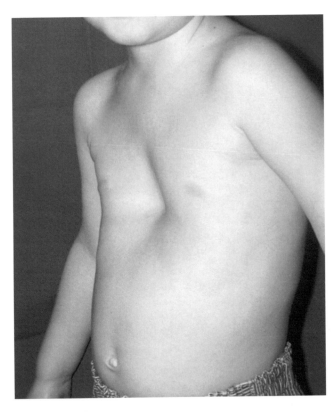

Figure 32.2 *Pectus excavatum.*

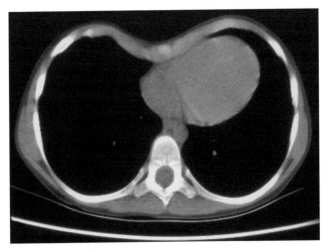

Figure 32.3 *Pectus excavatum: computed tomography (CT) scan, showing the sternal depression.*

Some studies have shown that cardiac output increases by a rise in heart rate because of a limited capacity to increase stroke volume. Mitral valve prolapse can be documented in about 20 per cent children with pectus excavatum, and it is thought that anterior compression of the heart deforms the mitral annulus. Mitral valve prolapse resolves in about 50 per cent of children after repair of the pectus deformity.

Considerable effort has been expended attempting to demonstrate consistent improvement respiratory and cardiac function following repair of the deformity. No consensus exists and there is, to date, no reliable evidence that correction of the deformity has any measurable physiological benefit. Despite this, there is a widespread perception by parents that the child's stamina increases after successful repair of a pectus deformity, and there is no doubt that self-esteem can improve dramatically.

Clinical assessment and investigations

The clinical signs of pectus excavatum are obvious. These children slouch to hide the deformity. The severity of the defect is variable. The presence of any rotational deformity of the sternum (i.e. asymmetry) should be noted. Height and weight should be recorded, and marfanoid features suggesting of connective tissue disease should be documented.

A plain radiograph of the chest, lung function tests and clinical photographs should be obtained. Cardiac ultrasound is indicated if there is concern about mitral valve prolapse or Marfan syndrome, but it is not necessary as a matter of routine. A non-contrast computed tomography (CT) scan of the thorax is the only way to record accurately the three-dimensional anatomy of the deformity (Figure 32.3). The severity of the pectus deformity can be assessed by the pectus index. This measurement is calculated from the transverse diameter of the chest divided by the anterior–posterior diameter of the chest measured from the underside of the deepest point of the sternum to the anterior aspect of the vertebral column. A pectus index greater than 2.5 is significant, and an index greater than 3.2 generally is regarded as a severe deformity.

Management

CONSERVATIVE

Physiotherapy has little role to play in the management of pectus deformities, other than in encouraging good posture. Exercise programmes and external bracing are of no proven value.

OPERATIVE

Numerous surgical procedures have been described to correct pectus deformities. Many entailed substantial destruction of the thoracic skeleton and most have not stood the test of time. Disguising the deformity with a subcutaneous silicone implant has been reported, although, of course, this does not correct the underlying skeletal deformity.

In 1949, Ravitch described a technique for correction of pectus excavatum, which remains the most commonly performed procedure today. Ravitch's operation involves resection of the deformed costal cartilages and a transverse sternal osteotomy to correct the sternal depression. The anterior chest wall is exposed through a vertical midline sternal or preferably a submammary incision. The pectoralis major muscles are reflected from the chest wall to expose the ribs. Deformed costal cartilages are removed by subperichondral resection.

Some regeneration of cartilage does occur. It is frequently necessary to resect four or five costal cartilages on each side.

Although excellent results can be achieved with the Ravitch procedure, there are a number of potential complications. Blood loss can be significant. Unless the sternum is supported with a metal strut after cartilage resection, the chest is flail in the early postoperative period, with attendant pulmonary problems. Within a few weeks, sufficient fibrosis ensues to anchor the sternum in place, and this problem is self-limiting. Recurrence of the deformity may occur if inadequate cartilage resection is performed. However, extensive cartilage resection at a young age may result in a permanent disturbance of chest-wall growth, probably caused by damage to the growth plates at the costochondral junctions. The late result is an asphyxiating osteodystrophy, with a small scarred anterior chest wall and a restrictive lung defect.

In 1997, Nuss reported a minimally invasive technique for the correction of pectus excavatum. The Nuss procedure involves implanting a curved metal bar through the chest, which exerts continuous pressure on the underside of the sternum. Immediate correction of the deformity is achieved. The soft malleable nature of the paediatric chest is ideally suited to this technique, although it can be applied to adults. The bar remains in place for two to four years, during which time remodelling of the thoracic skeleton occurs, such that removal of the bar does not result in recurrence of the deformity.

The length of the bar is determined by measurement of the anterior chest wall from mid-axillary line to mid-axillary line. The bar is curved to fit the shape of the chest. Two lateral chest-wall incisions are made to accommodate the ends of the bar. Through these incisions, a track is developed carefully through the right pleural cavity, behind the sternum and through the left pleural cavity. The curved bar is then pulled into place and flipped over, so that the ends come to lie on the lateral chest wall. The bar is then sutured firmly to the chest wall (Figure 32.4).

The Nuss technique has become very popular. However, with the initial surge of enthusiasm for this technique, a number of problems emerged. The procedure is painful, and thoracic epidural analgesia is highly desirable, if not mandatory.

Secure fixation of the lateral ends of the bar is vital to prevent displacement. This complication is most likely to occur in the early postoperative period. This risk is reduced considerably if a lateral stabilizing plate is used. The pectus bar transgresses both pleural cavities and small postoperative pneumothoraces are very common but rarely significant. Pericarditis and bar infection have been reported. The original operative description involved blind passage of a clamp through the thorax. As a result of a single report of non-fatal cardiac laceration, the technique was modified, and progress of the bar through the chest is now monitored either by thoracoscopy or by the surgeon's finger inserted through a small subxiphisternal incision. Older children and adults not infrequently continue to experience significant pain for several weeks postoperatively. It is usually possible for children to return to school after a few weeks, although abstention from sporting activities for two to three months is advisable.

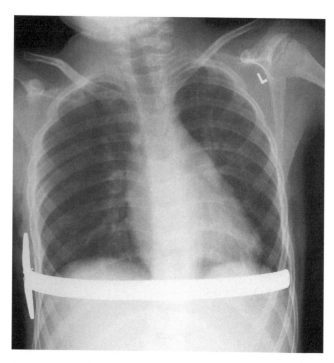

Figure 32.4 *Chest radiograph, showing the pectus bar in place, with a lateral stabilizer on the right side.*

Correction of pectus excavatum is simplified considerably by circumventing the need for cartilage resection and sternal osteotomy. More importantly, the risks of chest-wall growth disturbance are avoided and consequently the procedure can be performed safely in younger children. The ideal age for performing the Nuss procedure is 7–12 years. The procedure can be used to correct pectus deformities in teenagers and adults, although the thorax becomes progressively less malleable with advancing age. Frequently, it is necessary to implant two bars to distribute the increased load necessary to remodel the deformity in large adolescents and adults.

PECTUS CARINATUM

Pectus carinatum is less common than pectus excavatum. Like excavatum deformities, carinatum deformities affect boys more frequently than girls, by a factor of about three to one. A family history of chest-wall deformity is found in about 25 per cent. Carinatum deformities are characterized by an anterior angulation of the sternum (Figure 32.5). There is considerably more variation in the nature of the carinatum deformity than with pectus excavatum. Torsion as well as angulation of the sternum is seen in about ten per cent cases, and this is associated with protrusion of the costal cartilages on one side of the chest and recession on the other side. It is not uncommon for carinatum deformities to be noticed first in early adolescence, with progression during the pubertal growth spurt. Despite the anecdotal association of pectus carinatum with asthma, no consistent abnormalities of cardiovascular or respiratory function have been identified in these children.

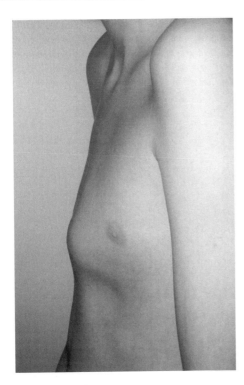

Figure 32.5 *Pectus carinatum.*

Table 32.1 *Results and complications of surgery for pectus excavatum*

	Nuss (n = 273)	Ravitch (n = 251)
Results	(n = 76 removed)	
Excellent	54 (71%)	97% very good or excellent
Good	16 (21%)	
Failed	6 (7.8%)	
Complications		
Wound seroma	0	12
Pleural effusion	0	13
Pneumonia	3 (0.9%)	12
Pneumothorax	52% (2.7% required treatment)	6
Pericardial effusion/ pericarditis	8 (2.4%)	3
Recurrence needing further surgery	6	5 (3 revision)
Protruding cartilage remnants	0	21 (5 revision)
Hypertrophic scar	0	35
Mortality	0	0
Wound infection	7 (2.1%)	Not stated
Bar displacement	29/329 (8.8%)	NA

NA, data not applicable.

The Ravitch procedure is effective for correction of carinatum deformities. The general principle is the same as for correction of an excavatum deformity, except that the sternal osteotomy is wedged open with a fragment of resected costal cartilage to angle the sternum backwards into a neutral position. The osteotomy becomes more complex if there is a rotational element to correct, and a certain degree of ingenuity is often required to restore a normal contour to the chest. The optimum age for correction of carinatum deformities is probably early adolescence.

OUTCOMES

Results and complications of the Nuss and Ravitch procedures are compared in Table 32.1 using data from two series. The results are impressive, but it should be borne in mind that both series are reported by experienced surgeons in the field. The Nuss procedure is not suitable for correction of carinatum deformities, which must be repaired by the Ravitch technique.

Pectus deformities in children with Marfan syndrome represent a technical challenge. These children tend to have marked pectus deformities often associated with a scoliosis. Correction of the pectus *per se* is straightforward, but the risk of recurrence is high, regardless of which technique is used, because of the underlying connecting tissue disorder. In these children, surgery is best postponed until late adolescence. If the Nuss technique is used, the bar(s) should remain in place for three to four years.

CLINICAL SCENARIO

A nine-year-old boy presents with an obvious excavatum. He was born with an unremarkable chest shape, but over the past three years he has acquired a 'dipping-in chest bone'. His mother thinks that his left arm is shorter than the right and is becoming impatient with his frequent complaints that the chest is painful and tender. She insists on surgery within the year. Although he clearly has pectus on examination, there is also an asymmetry in the anterior aspect of the chest that you cannot account for.

Pectus is not usually congenital, but it often appears within the first few years of life. The short arm and curious thoracic asymmetry may be a clue to an incomplete Poland syndrome, so look again and check whether there is unilateral absence of the pectoralis minor. Thirty per cent of patients with pectus have associated discomfort. However, the vast majority suffer significant pain following Nuss repair, for a period measured in months, which must be considered carefully when deciding whether to operate.

Technically, a minimally invasive repair of the excavatum is clearly feasible, but many surgeons would wish to wait until the child has sufficient mental capacity to play an active role in the decision-making. This is particularly important when treating a pathology whose manifestation is primarily cosmetic.

Just who wants this surgery: mother or child?

No patient can insist on a specific treatment, but you have a duty to ensure that an appropriate referral is made to another specialist if you decline to operate.

FURTHER READING

Fonkalsrud EW, Dunn JCY, Atkinson JB. Repair of pectus excavatum deformities: 20 years of experience with 375 patients. *Annals of Surgery* 2000; **231**: 443–8.

Haller JA, Kramer SS, Lietman S. Use of CT scans in selection of patients for pectus excavatum surgery: a preliminary report. *Journal of Pediatric Surgery* 1987; **22**: 904.

Nuss D, Croitoru DP, Kelly RE, *et al*. Review and discussion of the complications of minimally invasive pectus excavatum repair. *European Journal of Pediatric Surgery* 2002; **12**: 230–34.

Ravitch MM. *Congenital Deformities of the Chest Wall and their Operative Correction*. Philadelphia, PA: WB Saunders, 1977.

Empyema

DAKSHESH H PARIKH

Learning objectives

- To understand the pathogenesis of empyema.
- To understand the rationale behind the investigations.
- To be able to discuss different management options of empyema.

INTRODUCTION

Empyema thoracis is an accumulation of infective exudates (pus) within the pleural cavity. The name is derived from the Greek *empyein*, meaning pus-producing. Antibiotics and improved nutrition have helped to reduce the incidence of empyema. However, recently, the incidence of empyema has been increasing in the western world for unknown reasons. Early recognition and management are known to significantly reduce morbidity and mortality of this age-old disease in children. The role of drainage in the management of empyema was recognized by Hippocrates and Vesalius. The French surgeon Paré described evacuation of infected blood from the pleural cavity in the sixteenth century. Kuster suggested decortication in 1889. The management, planning and selection of the most appropriate treatment require a good understanding of the empyema disease process.

RELEVANT BASIC SCIENCE

Empyema is usually a sequel of bacterial pneumonia in children, which in turn is often preceded by viral chest infections. Empyema may occur (although rarely in children) secondary to infection in traumatic haemothorax, penetrating injury, post-thoracotomy, intrathoracic rupture of the oesophagus, and infection in the sympathetic effusion following pancreatitis or subphrenic abscess.

Lung parenchymal infection causes intense inflammation, associated with increased permeability of capillary walls and transudation of fluid. The transudate crosses the visceral pleura, forming a para-pneumonic effusion. This may remain uncomplicated and resolve spontaneously; however, if bacteria translocate into the effusion, then the subsequent suppuration leads to the exudative phase of an empyema. Progression of the disease depends on the virulence of the organisms, opposed by the host's natural resistance and the use of appropriate antibiotics. The consistency of pus in empyema may vary with the type of bacterial infection and the body's immune response.

Depending on the extent of the lobar consolidation and the rapidity with which pus accumulates within the pleural space, respiratory compromise can ensue. A large untreated empyema in some cases may spontaneously drain to the surface, usually through the perforating vessels in the second intercostal space anteriorly. This is called empyema necessitans; if situated on the left side, the swelling transmits the pulsations of the heart and great vessels, and it is then called a pulsating empyema. The pus in the empyema can rupture into the airway or spread to surrounding organs, such as the heart and pericardium. In septic children, the infection has been known to spread to the brain and bone. Occasionally, during the acute phase of staphylococcal pneumonia and rarely with streptococcal and *Haemophilus influenzae* pneumonia, necrosis and liquefaction of the lung parenchyma produces a pneumatocele. Most pneumatoceles and lung abscesses gradually decrease in size with effective antibiotic management; however, some may rupture, resulting in either a pyopneumothorax or a tension pneumothorax.

As the inflammation advances, the coagulation cascade is activated and the fibrinolytic response is suppressed, thus favouring fibrin deposition. Invading fibroblasts deposit fibrin strands within the pleural cavity, causing loculation. The proliferated fibroblasts intermingle with cells and bacteria, forming a pyogenic membrane. This deposited fibrin forms septa within empyema-forming loculations and a purulent covering over the lung. Antibiotics have low penetrance into the empyema loculations and are of little use without drainage of pus and debridement.

The fibroblasts deposit layers of fibrous tissue on both the visceral and the parietal pleura within the empyema cavity. This produces a fibrous rind around the collapsed lung and prevents it from expanding, causing respiratory compromise. This is the organization phase of empyema. Septic foci within the organized empyema contribute to the child's chronic ill health, failure to thrive and breathlessness with poor respiratory reserve. In the organization phase, the fibrous rind causes permanent loss of function in the affected lung.

The causative organisms in children are usually Gram-positive, i.e. *Staphylococcus aureus, Streptococcus pneumoniae, Streptococcus pyogenes, H. influenzae* and, rarely, *Klebsiella pneumoniae, Bacteroides* and anaerobic organisms. Atypical infection, such as with *Mycoplasma*, incites a variable reaction, while tuberculous and fungal infections lead to chronic empyema.

DIAGNOSIS

Clinically, the diagnosis of empyema can be suspected by attention to the history and physical signs. Childhood empyema usually presents early because of the acute respiratory distress caused by the pneumonic consolidation and mediastinal shift. The signs and symptoms of empyema vary somewhat according to the location of the infection and its severity. Patients usually exhibit clinical features of pneumonia, including fever, cough, fatigue, breathlessness and chest pain. They may prefer to lie on the side of the body affected by the empyema. Family members may notice halitosis. Some children with high spiking fever may become dehydrated, while others may cough up blood or greenish-brown sputum. Abdominal pain, distension and occasionally ileus associated with sepsis may intensify the respiratory compromise. In subacute cases, where the child has been treated partially or the organism is of lesser virulence, the presentation may be delayed.

The white blood cell count and inflammatory markers rise in bacterial infections. Blood, sputum and/or nasopharyngeal

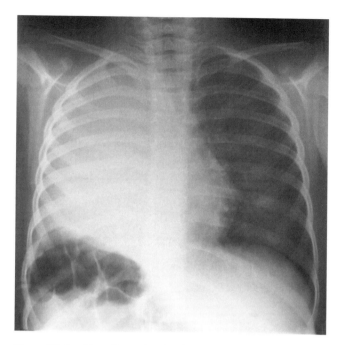

Figure 33.1 *Chest X-ray, showing fluid meniscus and right lower lobe consolidation.*

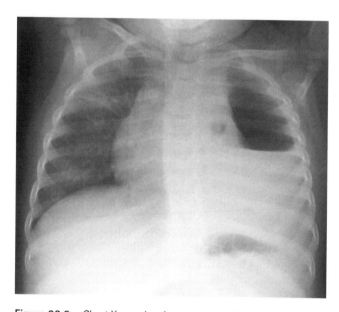

Figure 33.2 *Chest X-ray, showing pyopneumothorax with spontaneous infective bronchopleural fistula.*

aspirate should be sent for cultures. Done early, these investigations are extremely useful in identifying the pathogen and the selection of antibiotics according to the microbial sensitivities. A plain chest X-ray during the exudative phase shows a fluid meniscus with an associated mediastinal shift and pneumonic consolidation (Figure 33.1). It may also demonstrate a lung abscess or pneumatoceles and a pyopneumothorax (Figure 33.2). As the exudates solidify, the plain X-ray cannot differentiate empyema from tumours. Some tumours, such as pulmonary blastoma, can be mistaken for empyema, as the clinical presentation and some of the radiological features

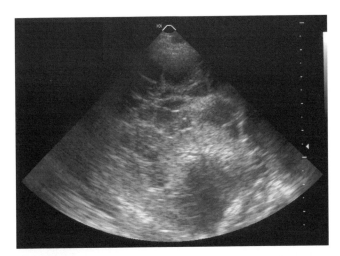

Figure 33.3 *Chest ultrasonography, illustrating exudative phase with fibrinous septa and loculation.*

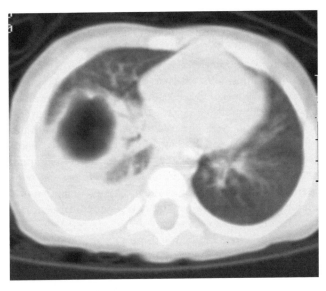

Figure 33.4 *Computed tomography (CT) scan with contrast, showing underlying consolidation, pneumatocele and empyema.*

are similar (Manivel *et al.* 1988). Therefore, the plain chest radiograph in the fibropurulent and organization phases of empyema is suggestive but not diagnostic of empyema.

Ultrasonography is a valuable tool in the diagnosis of empyema as well as in locating the fluid for thoracocentesis (McLoud and Flower 1991). Ultrasound is portable and, therefore, available for immediate evaluation of critically ill patients needing rapid bedside examination. Ultrasound can also help to diagnose loculations and gives some idea of density of the fluid (Figure 33.3). As the intercostal spaces narrow, the value of ultrasound becomes limited (McLoud and Flower 1991). Ultrasound examinations have been graded by some radiologists as either low-grade (anechoic fluid, no evidence of fibrinous organization) or high-grade (evidence of fibrinous organization, i.e. fronds, septations, loculations or thickening of visceral pleural surface). The key limiting factors of sonographic evaluation of the chest are based on the physical limitations of the ultrasound beam. Occasionally, homogeneous solid lesions may appear to be fluid-filled on sonography. While ultrasonography has limitations for identifying the pathology in the underlying lung and mediastinum, computed tomography (CT) scanning with intravenous contrast is extremely valuable and complements ultrasonography (McLoud and Flower 1991; Donnelly and Klosterman 1998). CT scanning with intravenous contrast distinguishes the rare lung tumours presenting as empyema in childhood as well as identifying mediastinal pathology, thickened pleural rind, consolidated lung and associated lung pathology (Donnelly and Klosterman 1998) (Figure 33.4). The identification of underlying lung pathology is a poor prognostic indicator. Complex empyema is the term coined to represent empyema with significant lung pathology, such as lung abscesses and infective bronchopleural fistula, and also bilateral empyema, atypical infection and secondary empyema.

Diagnostic thoracocentesis is mandatory before any definitive management is undertaken. A diagnostic tap might fail in the presence of a thick peel or viscid pus. Clinical and radiological data should be thoroughly evaluated and assessed before undertaking definitive management. Pleural fluid should be sent urgently for microscopy, Gram staining, culture and biochemistry for pH, glucose level and lactic dehydrogenase (LDH). The turbid and purulent appearance of the aspirated pleural fluid and biochemical analysis showing sugar below 2.2 mmol/L, pH below 7.2, LDH over 1000 IU/dL, protein over 25 g/L and specific gravity over 1.018 are diagnostic of empyema. Thin sterile fluid with a pH greater than 7.2 and a glucose level above 2.2 mmol/L represent parapneumonic effusion.

The issue of diagnostic thoracocentesis is controversial. Some surgeons would elect to proceed with definitive management on the basis of clinical features and imaging. In this case, the empyema fluid can be sent for laboratory analysis at the time of the operative procedure.

MANAGEMENT

Early recognition and aggressive antibiotic treatment for suspected pathogens of lobar pneumonia reduce the incidence of empyema. The cardinal principles of empyema management are administration of appropriate antibiotics in combination with adequate drainage, so as to achieve full expansion of the lung. Significant parapneumonic effusions may require either repeated thoracocentesis or intercostal tube drainage. The timely chest tube inserted in an appropriate place is preferable to the discomfort and inefficiency of repeated thoracocentesis. The very small empyema with minimal symptoms may respond to conservative management with antibiotics and active observation. The medical management should be optimized before referral for surgery. While many patients respond to chest tube drainage and antibiotics, some authors advocate the addition of fibrinolytic therapy (Thomson *et al.*

2002). In most children with effective initial management, radiological and clinical resolution takes place and white cell count returns to normal. In these children, no further surgical therapy is indicated.

However, it is difficult to predict with any accuracy the pathological phase of the empyema with any of the investigations currently available. It is safe to assume that the empyema is in the fibropurulent phase when the aspirated pus is thick. Effective drainage in this phase is imperative to reduce morbidity and progression of the disease to the organization phase. Individual surgical experience in childhood empyema may dictate the application of the most appropriate surgical option. However, it is imperative to recognize treatment failure to avoid disease progression.

Closed intercostal tube insertion with administration of antibiotics may be effective in some cases when loculation is negligible. An interventional radiologist may be able to insert a pigtail catheter under ultrasound guidance and achieve effective drainage. A low-grade suction applied to a catheter, combined with administration of a fibrinolytic agent such as urokinase into the pleural space, helps to dissolve fibrinous material, breaks down loculations and achieves the effective drainage of empyema (Thomson *et al.* 2002). Pigtail catheter drainage is less invasive than any other surgical method. The use of this technique has avoided open drainage in many children. However, it is important to realize that this therapy has its limitations, and its failure should be recognized early in order to avoid disease progression.

With the advent of video-assisted techniques, many surgeons are challenging the traditional approaches to empyema management in children. Video-assisted techniques offer distinct advantages in the accurate staging of the disease process and in the effectiveness of management of the fibrinous pleural disease when separating the loculi under vision (Angelillo-Mackinlay *et al.* 1996). This technique is less invasive than thoracotomy and in experienced hands is as effective in achieving the therapeutic goal. Thoracoscopy, however, requires expertise and a well-trained operating team familiar with the equipment. In the presence of a thick pyogenic membrane covering both the visceral and the parietal pleura, there is a likelihood of damaging the inflamed lung while removing the peel. Indeed, the current trend in the management of suspected infected pleural space disease is towards primary thoracoscopic pleural evacuation and subsequent chest tube drainage. Many paediatric surgeons not proficient with thoracoscopy continue to drain the empyema as effectively using a mini-thoracotomy.

Open drainage by mini-thoracotomy breaks down the fibrinous septae and achieves the objective of full expansion of the lung more readily than any other mode of drainage (Chan *et al.* 1997). Muscle-sparing thoracotomy can be employed effectively instead and is less painful. Thoracotomy and drainage of the fibrinous coagulum and pyogenic material after breaking of loculations of the fibropurulent empyema has been described wrongly in the literature as 'early decortication' (see below). Video-assisted thoracoscopy or thoracotomy should

be used as the therapeutic option for the late fibropurulent phase and in failed cases of the chest tube drainage or urokinase therapy (Chan *et al.* 1997).

Inadequate drainage in the fibropurulent phase, or prolonged use of antibiotics without drainage, allows the empyema disease process to continue, leading to organization and formation of a thick fibrous peel restricting lung expansion. Therefore, early effective drainage in the exudative and fibropurulent phases avoids empyema organization and morbidity. Surgical management of the organization phase of empyema carries significant morbidity. It requires excision of the fibrous peel covering the collapsed lung in order to achieve its expansion, known as 'decortication'.

Formal decortication requires sharp dissection and excision of both the peel covering the visceral pleura, together with the parietal peel, through a standard posterolateral thoracotomy. The aim of the procedure is to find the plane between the visceral pleura and the inner visceral membrane that constitutes the inner surface of the peel. Once this plane has been identified, it is usually possible to dissect the membrane away from the pleura. However, the excision of the visceral rind may result in significant bleeding and air leak in areas where separation is impossible and the visceral pleura is breached inadvertently.

The excision of the parietal peel may also cause bleeding and damage to nerves, because the parietal pleura should be excised *en bloc* with the peel. No attempt should be made to continue the parietal dissection over the mediastinum, for fear of damaging underlying structures.

Postoperative morbidity and occasional mortality have been described with formal decortication, although recognition of the fibrous stage and early excision minimizes these complications. Treated adequately, the prognosis for the near-normal lung function in most cases is excellent. However, if the fibrous peel of the organized chronic empyema is not managed appropriately, then associated chronic sepsis and restrictive lung disease lead to failure to thrive, anaemia and chronic ill health. Fibrosis also causes rib crowding and in the growing child results in scoliosis.

Complex empyema

EMPYEMA WITH LUNG ABSCESS

The empyema should be managed according to its stage of development. The abscess within the lung should be left alone and treated with appropriate antibiotics, as these can treat most lung abscesses effectively without the need for surgical drainage. The morbidity involved in excision of the lung abscess in the presence of infection is significant.

SPONTANEOUS BRONCHOPLEURAL FISTULA AND RESULTANT PYOPNEUMOTHORAX

A large bronchopleural fistula is usually obvious because of the copious volumes of pus in the sputum. In this situation, there is a real danger of infected effusion fluid entering the bronchial tree via the fistula, filling the airway and spreading to the contralateral healthy lung. This danger is greatest when the child is anaesthetized in a supine position, possibly with the affected side raised to facilitate placement of the intercostal tube. This hazardous situation may be avoided by inserting the tube into a sitting patient, but the final management must depend upon an expert thoracic surgical opinion, obtained before any procedure is attempted.

Thoracotomy for the effective drainage of the pus, separating all the adhesions with partial excision of the parietal pleura surrounding the fistula, is advisable. Primary muscle thoracoplasty brings blood supply to the necrotic area and helps in healing. A number of other grafts, such as pericardium, intercostal muscles, greater omentum and jejunum, have been described. An aggressive one-stage approach to the infective bronchopleural fistula results in expansion of the lung, with healing of the fistula, thus reducing the morbidity and mortality associated with pyopneumothorax (Figure 33.5). Previously, a staged approach was described for the management of the spontaneous bronchopleural fistula. Repeated thoracotomy and chronic infection lead to fibrosis and, therefore, increase the morbidity, reduce the chances of the bronchopleural fistula healing and may result in restrictive lung disease.

BILATERAL EMPYEMA

This is encountered in some infants and occasionally in immunocompromised children. The management should be similar to that for the pathological stage in which the empyema presents (Figure 33.6). Bilateral chest drains and/or bilateral operations are significantly more painful and therefore increase the time to re-expand the collapsed lungs and increase hospital stay.

Postoperative care and follow-up

The successful postoperative outcome of achieving full expansion of the collapsed lung depends upon the maintenance of the chest tube drainage until necessary, good physiotherapy and administration of the correct or best-guess intravenous antibiotics in effective doses. Good nutritional care is essential in the postoperative period to accommodate the high-energy needs of the child with infection. A prophylactic oral antibiotic for a further period of four weeks is advisable to avoid the risk of recurrent chest infection during the recovery phase. The antibody status for pneumococcal and *H. influenzae* influenza should be assessed approximately six weeks from discharge and appropriate vaccinations given to those patients lacking in immunity. The long-term clinical prognosis for adequately treated empyema is excellent. Complex empyema carries significantly higher morbidity and longer hospital stay compared with simple empyema.

CLINICAL SCENARIO

A two-year-old girl presents from a local hospital with an 18-day history of systemic illness, dyspnoea and weight loss. The working diagnosis is empyema, and the local paediatricians have prepared the parents for decortication. Throughout her history, broad-spectrum antibiotics have been given, both orally and intravenously.

On arrival at your centre, she is pyrexial and tachypnoeic but not distressed. The pathology is on the left side, with bronchial breathing in the upper zones, and stony dullness in the lower zone. The trachea is found slightly to the right of the midline.

Her imaging consists of a series of chest X-rays, which show a progressive loss of volume in the left hemi-thorax over her weeks of admission, with increasing mediastinal shift to the right. In the most recent film, there is radiolucency in the left upper zone, reported by the district general hospital radiologist as 're-expansion of the left upper lobe'.

No attempt has been made to sample the fluid within the pleural space.

This child is clearly ill. If the clinical diagnosis is confirmed, then she will need some form of intervention. Given the time scale, and her continued pyrexia and systemic state, it is unlikely that this is merely a pneumonia that has failed to resolve. However, it is clear that the pneumonia persists (bronchial breathing, lack of volume in hemi-thorax), together with fluid in the pleural space (stony dull), which is under pressure (mediastinal shift). The outstanding issues are (i) whether the persistent effusion is an otherwise uncomplicated parapneumonic effusion, or whether there is empyema formation, and (ii) could the radiolucency in the upper zone represent a bronchopleural fistula?

The latter needs to be considered carefully if intercostal drainage is being proposed.

An ultrasound scan should be performed to ascertain parietal and visceral pleural thickness, and to determine whether there are substantial rafts of protein or loculation within the pleural space. It is this potential protein load that will support the diagnosis of empyema. This information should be gathered before drainage is attempted, because the ultrasonography is facilitated by the presence of the effusion. Assuming a fluid collection is seen around the lung, then the time scale of this illness and the mediastinal shift would mandate its drainage. Whether urokinase should be instilled depends upon the degree of empyema formation, demonstrated by ultrasound scanning. Even at this stage in the illness, urokinase can be expected to resolve the visceral pleural thickening, but the underlying pneumonia will then need to be treated aggressively to inflate the consolidated lung.

Decortication is now a rare event in children with empyema. Adult thoracic surgeons recommend waiting several months before decortication, if at all possible, to minimize the potential trauma to the underlying lung.

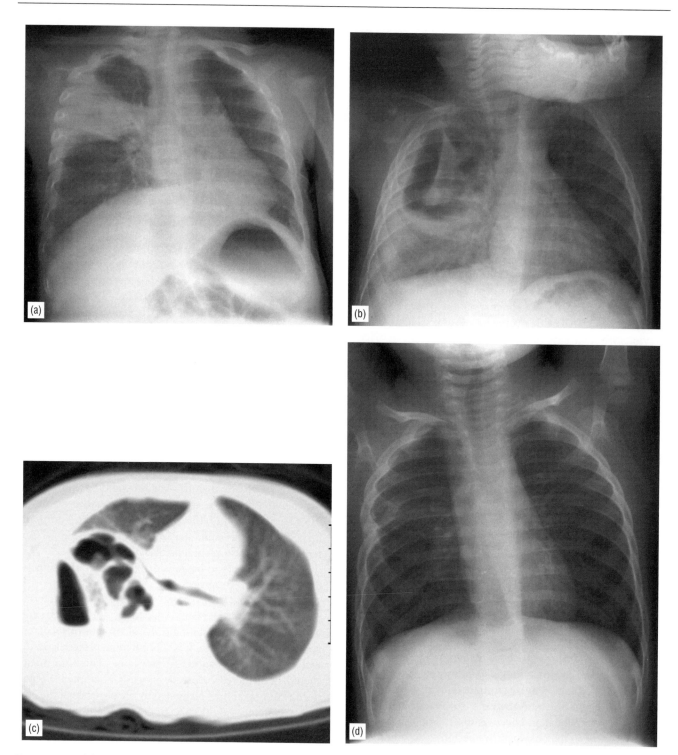

Figure 33.5 *(a) Chest X-ray in a six-month-old child, showing pneumonic right upper lobe, (b) Progression of disease, with pneumatocele formation. (c) In spite of intravenous antibiotics for Gram-positive cover, the disease progressed to develop spontaneous infective bronchopleural fistula, as shown on a computed tomography (CT) scan: lung abscess and fluid level in the pleural cavity. (d) Postoperative result after a one-stage approach of partial decortication, insertion of a digitation of the serratus anterior muscle flap on the fistula and chest drain. (From Hallows MR, Parikh DH,* Journal of Paediatric Surgery *2004;* ***39****: 1122–4.)*

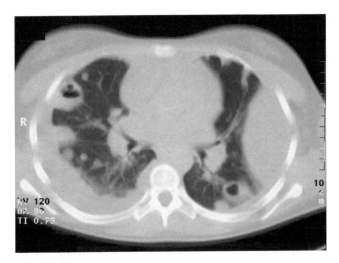

Figure 33.6 *Computed tomography (CT) scan, showing bilateral empyema and multiple lung abscesses.*

REFERENCES

Angelillo-Mackinlay T, Lyons GA, Chimondeguy DJ, *et al*. VATS debridement versus thoracotomy in the treatment of loculated post pneumonia empyema. *Annals of Thoracic Surgery* 1996; **61**: 1626–30.

Chan W, Keyser-Gauwin E, Davis GM, Nguyen LT, Laberge J-M. Empyema thoracis in children: a 26-year review of the Montreal Children's Hospital Experience. *Journal of Pediatric Surgery* 1997; **32**: 870–72.

Donnelly LF, Klosterman LA. The yield of CT of children who have complicated pneumonia and non-contributory chest radiography. *American Journal of Roentgenology* 1998; **170**: 1627–31.

Manivel CJ, Priest JR, Watterson J, *et al*. Pleuropulmonary blastoma. *Cancer* 1988; **62**: 1516–26.

McLoud TC, Flower CDR. Imaging the pleura: sonography, CT, and MR Imaging. *American Journal of Roentgenology* 1991; **156**: 1145–53.

Thomson Ah, Hull J, Kumar MR, Wallis C, Balfour Lynn IM. Randomised trial of intrapleural urokinase in the treatment of childhood empyema. *Thorax* 2002; **57**: 343–7.

Thoracic trauma

VIVIEN McNAMARA AND EVELYN H DYKES

Learning objectives

- To understand the common mechanisms of thoracic injury in children.
- To understand the anatomical and physiological characteristics of the paediatric thorax.
- To know the presenting features of the common types of thoracic injury.
- To be able to describe the main investigations and treatments that may be required.

INTRODUCTION

Thoracic trauma is commonly associated with injuries affecting other systems, including major head and abdominal injuries. This is related directly to the smaller target of the paediatric victim, with injuries commonly crossing anatomical boundaries. Mortality is increased significantly in children with multiple injuries. Blunt trauma, such as that sustained in motor vehicle accidents or falls, may deliver tremendous forces on to the chest of a child. These include not only direct blunt trauma to the chest wall but also associated compression and acceleration/deceleration forces, all of which have the potential to cause major intrathoracic damage.

Children may have very significant intrathoracic injuries with little external evidence of trauma. They may display few physical signs and symptoms on presentation and yet have sustained potentially life-threatening injuries, such as pneumothorax, haemothorax, pulmonary laceration/contusion or ruptured diaphragm. Prompt treatment of these injuries is usually curative, with little long-term morbidity. Rare thoracic injuries seen in children include an open pneumothorax and a flail chest. Cardiac injuries are more common with penetrating trauma, but myocardial and great vessel injury can occur as a result of severe blunt trauma. The clinician should always consider the possibility that a chest injury sustained in a child may be the result of a non-accidental mechanism, including injuries sustained over a period of time.

ANATOMY AND PHYSIOLOGY

There are significant differences in the anatomy and physiology of the paediatric thorax compared with that of an adult, and these influence the response to trauma. This is particularly evident in relation to the child's airway, chest wall and cardiorespiratory physiology. These differences also impact upon the presentation of specific chest injuries and must be recognized by health professionals caring for the injured child. The major

Table 34.1 *Relevant anatomical and physiological features in children compared with adults*

Difference seen in children	Consequence
Small stature	Energy dissipated over small target, leading to multisystem injuries
Infants (<6 months) obligate nasal breathers, blocked with blood or secretions	Airway obstruction
Large tongue, small oral cavity	Airway obstruction, difficult intubation
Narrow airway	Airway obstruction
Anterior/superior glottis	Emergency nasal intubation difficult
Short trachea	Endobronchial intubation
Mobile mediastinum	Readily displaced by pneumo/haemothorax
Pliable chest wall	Fractured ribs less common
Large head (risk of cervical spine injury)	Additional care required during intubation
Fractured ribs	Indicate significant intrathoracic injury
Diaphragmatic breathing in babies and infants	Increased respiratory distress with abdominal distension
Higher metabolic demands	Rapid cardiorespiratory deterioration
Increased oxygen consumption	Greater risk of hypoxia
Low functional residual capacity	Greater risk of hypoxia
Smaller absolute total blood volume	Rapid haemodynamic compromise
Weaker musculature	Rapid ventilatory deterioration
Greater surface area/volume ratio	Poor thermoregulation

Table 34.2 *Summary of clinical features suggestive of intrathoracic injury*

Clinical sign identified	Underlying potential injury or problem
Cyanosis, dyspnoea	Inadequate oxygenation
Noisy breathing	Airway obstruction with vomit, blood, teeth, etc.
Hyper-resonant chest on percussion or absent breath sounds	Ipsilateral pneumothorax
Dull percussion note, absent breath sounds	Ipsilateral haemothorax
Tracheal deviation*	Tension pneumothorax, massive pneumothorax
Hoarseness, stridor, difficulty with phonation	Direct laryngeal or tracheal injury
Cutaneous emphysema	Tracheal or bronchial laceration, oesophageal perforation
Bowel sounds heard in left chest	Left diaphragmatic rupture
ECG changes, with ectopic beats, arrhythmias (often atrial), ST segment changes or heart block	Cardiac contusion, myocardial ischaemia
Jugular venous engorgement*, hypotension, pulsus paradoxsus >10 mmHg*	Cardiac tamponade
Heart failure (basal crepitations), new or loud systolic murmur, hypotension despite volume resuscitation	Valvular injury, acute ventricular septal defect
Unequal limb pulses, radiofemoral delay*, unequal limb SaO$_2$	Acute aortic injury

*Difficult to identify in younger children.
ECG, electrocardiogram; SaO$_2$, systemic arterial oxygen saturation.

anatomical and physiological features specific to children and relevant to thoracic trauma are summarized in Table 34.1.

INITIAL MANAGEMENT

The initial assessment and resuscitation must occur simultaneously. The airway, breathing and circulation are examined rapidly during the primary survey and problems are corrected as they are identified. Airway management, appropriate fluid resuscitation, supplemental oxygen, adequate analgesia and decompression of the stomach will do much to support the child with thoracic injury. Intercostal chest drainage for pneumothorax or haemothorax is the most common invasive intervention required for a thoracic injury. Additional measures of endotracheal intubation and ventilatory support are required less commonly. Chest radiographs are the most

common form of imaging in the child with thoracic trauma. Further information and detail can be afforded with computed tomography (CT) scans. These are especially sensitive at identifying small, often anterior, pneumothoraces or pulmonary contusions and lacerations. Occasionally, additional investigations may be indicated, including echocardiography (both transthoracic and transoesophageal), bronchoscopy, angiography, oesophagoscopy and upper-gastrointestinal contrast studies. Certain clinical signs are suggestive of specific intrathoracic injuries and should be actively sought and managed (Table 34.2).

Having stabilized the child and treated life-threatening injuries, most thoracic injuries are identified on plain chest radiographs. It must be recognized that initial chest X-ray may be normal. Progressive clinical deterioration despite an apparently normal investigation should alert the clinician to reassess all investigations, looking for subtle signs that may have been missed. When a mechanism of injury would suggest potential significant intrathoracic pathology, repeated or alternative imaging should be considered.

Box 34.1 Indications for thoracotomy

Penetrating wounds of the heart or great vessels
Massive or continuous intrathoracic bleeding
Open pneumothorax with a major chest-wall defect
Aortogram indicating injury to the aorta or major
  branches
Massive or continuing air leak indicating a major
  airway injury
Cardiac tamponade
Oesophageal perforation
Diaphragm rupture

Following initial assessment, resuscitation and stabilization, all children with thoracic injuries should be admitted to an appropriate paediatric surgical or intensive care facility. Most injuries can be managed conservatively or require intercostal chest-drain insertion, although a small number will require operative intervention. Indications for emergency thoracotomy are massive bleeding, massive air leak and cardiac tamponade (Box 34.1). Emergency-room thoracotomy is a more contentious issue with less convincing evidence and provokes much debate.

CHEST–WALL INJURY

The chest wall of a child is elastic and very compliant. Blunt trauma or crushing injuries of the chest rarely fracture ribs. Deaths from major intrathoracic injuries continue to occur, even without bony injury. External signs of injury, including bruising and clothing imprints, can be absent. Knowledge of the mechanism of injury is vital, and with a high index of suspicion of likely complications, a directed clinical assessment will reduce the chances of missed or late diagnoses.

Bruising and abrasions and/or clothing and tyre imprints may be evident on visual inspection. These are signs of significant trauma and should be actively looked for, both anteriorly and posteriorly, on the child's chest. The child usually appears to have local chest-wall pain, with shallow rapid breathing. This may not be obvious in the face of other more significant or painful injuries, or in a frightened and uncooperative child. Local tenderness, crepitus and soft-tissue swelling may be obvious on palpation. The increased work of breathing seen with more significant chest-wall injuries causes the child to tire quickly, with increasing hypoxia, cyanosis and, ultimately, respiratory failure. Bradycardia is a late and ominous sign of hypoxia, rapidly progressing to cardiac arrest unless corrected promptly.

Initially, supplemental oxygen and analgesia are required. Uncomplicated rib fractures will require chest physiotherapy to prevent pulmonary atelectasis, collapse and the retention of secretions. Associated soft-tissue damage of the chest wall is treated according to standard general surgical principles.

Sternal fractures are uncommon in the paediatric population, but if present, or if there is bruising over the anterior chest wall, then one should consider the possibility of underlying cardiac injury. This occurs most commonly secondary to rapid deceleration, in which the mediastinum hits the back of the sternum and may result in cardiac contusion.

PULMONARY CONTUSION

Pulmonary contusions are the most common form of intrathoracic injury seen in children. They are usually associated with blunt thoracic trauma, either as a consequence of motor-vehicle accidents or from a fall from a great height. Since the acceleration/deceleration forces imparted on to the pliable chest wall rarely fracture ribs, at the time of presentation the intrapulmonary injury may not be clinically apparent, and other injuries (both thoracic and extra-thoracic) may appear more significant or dramatic. Knowledge of the mechanism of injury should arouse clinical suspicion; appropriate review and investigation over the following hours and days are necessary.

Over time, the child will demonstrate increasing tachypnoea, dyspnoea, increased work of breathing and haemoptysis. Oxygen requirement will increase and may progress rapidly to severe hypoxia, cyanosis and respiratory failure. On auscultation, areas of poor air entry may be detected, often at the lung bases. Within the lung, there are areas of ventilation–perfusion (V/Q) mismatch, which adds to the degree of venous admixture and increasing hypoxia. This is compounded by pulmonary oedema and haemorrhage. Initial chest X-ray may appear normal, but radiological signs may progress rapidly, with fluffy infiltrates, areas of collapse and, occasionally, pleural collections (Figure 34.1a).

Treatment is of a supportive nature. Adequate pain control is vital to allow the child to cough effectively. With regular directed physiotherapy, using additional aids such as an incentive spirometer, areas of atelectasis are re-expanded and bloody secretions are cleared promptly before significant pulmonary collapse and subsequent infection complicate the post-injury phase. Supplemental oxygen is commonly required, as may be ventilatory support with either continuous positive airways pressure (CPAP) or intubation and intermittent positive-pressure ventilation (IPPV). Fluid restriction is usually adopted, but the routine use of diuretics, steroids and antibiotics has not yet been established.

More focal intrapulmonary bleeding gives rise to a pulmonary haematoma. This should be evident on plain chest X-ray, but it will also be demonstrated by a CT scan (Figure 34.1b). As with pulmonary contusions, usually pulmonary haematomas resolve with a non-operative approach but occasionally they may be complicated by pleural collection, infection with or without abscess formation and the late appearance of a pneumatocoele. Most resolve within months and do not require surgery.

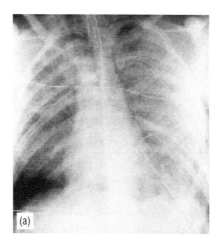
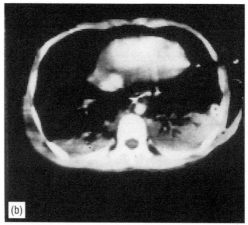

Figure 34.1 *Chest X-ray (a) and computed tomography (CT) scan (b) 12 hours following severe blunt chest trauma, showing significant pulmonary contusion and haemorrhage. Initial chest X-ray was normal. Note posterior drainage of blood due to prolonged supine position.*

PNEUMOTHORAX

A pneumothorax is one of the more common complications of thoracic trauma seen in the paediatric population. It may result from either penetrating or blunt trauma to the thoracic cage.

Many children are asymptomatic, but others display increasing degrees of tachypnoea, dyspnoea, distress and hypoxia. Visible signs of chest-wall damage may be evident, but often there is little to see on inspection. Careful palpation will demonstrate local tenderness, suggesting possible rib fractures, and may identify crepitus, indicating cutaneous emphysema, with air escaping from the lung parenchymal surface. The percussion note on the side of the pneumothorax may be hyper-resonant, and breath sounds may be diminished. Auscultation may be normal and is certainly difficult within a busy and noisy accident and emergency department.

When identified radiologically, and if the child remains asymptomatic, a small pneumothorax can be observed. With signs of respiratory compromise, if the child is being transferred to another hospital or in a child in whom an anaesthetic is subsequently planned, an intercostal drain should be inserted. In the latter situation, IPPV can rapidly convert a small simple pneumothorax into a tension pneumothorax, with dire consequences.

Insertion of an intercostal chest drain is advised for most cases of pneumothorax following chest trauma. The tube should be inserted using the open technique without the trocar. The ideal site of entry is within the triangle of safety (Figure 34.2). Tube position and resolution of the pneumothorax should be confirmed radiologically.

TENSION PNEUMOTHORAX

A tension pneumothorax usually results from blunt thoracic trauma. By virtue of a one-way valve system, air accumulates

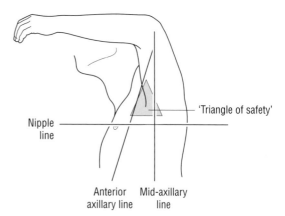

Figure 34.2 *'Triangle of safety' for insertion of chest drain to relieve pneumo/haemothorax.*

within the pleural cavity under increasing tension but cannot escape. Each inspiratory breath adds to the accumulated air, and the expanding pneumothorax displaces mediastinal structures further towards the contralateral side, compounding respiratory embarrassment. Tachycardia and tachypnoea develop, and the child becomes increasingly distressed. On examination, the ipsilateral chest is hyper-resonant to percussion, with diminished breath sounds, and the trachea should be deviated away from the side of the tension pneumothorax. Cyanosis is a late feature. With increasing mediastinal displacement impairing drainage of the vena cavae, the venous return to the right side of the heart becomes obstructed. Engorgement of the neck veins may be apparent in the older child. As cardiac filling is compromised, cardiac output is diminished. This may be rapid and potentially fatal unless the tension pneumothorax is relieved promptly.

As an immediate measure, needle thoracocentesis is performed in the second intercostal rib space using a needle or intravenous cannula and can help to decompress the tension pneumothorax before the insertion of an intercostal chest drain. The diagnosis of tension pneumothorax is a clinical one, and treatment must not be delayed to allow a confirmatory chest X-ray. Radiological assessment after drain insertion will confirm the position of the intercostal drain, demonstrate that the lung has re-inflated and identify other thoracic injuries requiring treatment.

A tension pneumothorax should always be considered in any child with a history of chest trauma, especially if ventilated, when there is a sudden clinical deterioration. Cardiac tamponade may resemble a tension pneumothorax, but the mediastinum should remain central and both lung fields should percuss normally.

HAEMOTHORAX

Following both blunt and penetrating thoracic trauma, a pneumothorax is frequently associated with a haemothorax. The blood may be derived from the systemic circulation (intercostal and internal mammary vessels) or from the lung parenchyma. Systemic loss may require operative intervention to control the bleeding. In contrast, blood loss from the lung parenchyma itself will usually stop spontaneously, since the pulmonary circulation is a low-pressure system. Both require the insertion of an intercostal drain, ensuring drainage of the haemothorax and full lung expansion. The fully inflated lung acts to obliterate the pleural cavity and tamponade the blood loss. The presence of blood within the pleural cavity may cause local defibrination and thus prolong bleeding from the lung surface. Despite the absence of continued active bleeding, the surgical evacuation of a clotted haemothorax may be required to secure haemostasis.

An expanding haemothorax, with or without pneumothorax, can cause respiratory embarrassment, displacement of the mediastinum and impaired venous return to the heart. The cardiorespiratory compromise is compounded by the effects of hypovolaemia resulting from the blood lost within the pleural cavity.

In a child, a significant proportion of the circulating blood volume may be lost from the intravascular compartment into the pleural cavity within minutes of a major vascular injury. Recognition and rapid fluid resuscitation are required. Indications for operative intervention include immediate drainage of more than 20 per cent of the child's estimated blood volume, drainage greater than 1–2 mL/kg/h, continued haemodynamic instability despite adequate volume resuscitation, and failure to evacuate blood and clots with inadequate lung expansion.

DIAPHRAGMATIC RUPTURE

Diaphragmatic injuries require considerable external compressive forces and are usually associated with multiple injuries, including major head injuries, intra-abdominal solid-organ damage and thoracic fractures. Such injuries usually result

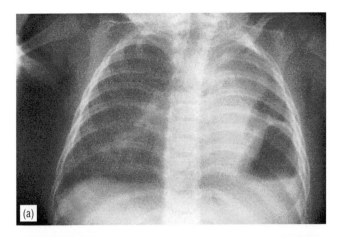

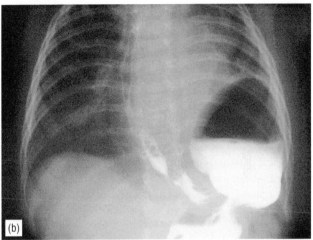

Figure 34.3 *Chest X-ray (a) and contrast study (b) of a child presenting six months after blunt abdominal trauma treated conservatively. The stomach is in the chest, confirming diaphragmatic rupture. Chest X-ray and computed tomography (CT) scan at the time of admission did not show this abnormality, but the child was intubated and ventilated for the initial investigation. (Courtesy of Dr D MacIver.)*

from abdominal crush insults, falls from a great height and motor-vehicle accidents. These injuries are rare in children.

In blunt trauma, left-sided injuries predominate (90 per cent), with relative protection of the right hemi-diaphragm afforded by the liver. Only half of these injuries are associated with rib fractures. In the face of multiple trauma, this injury may easily be missed and present late (Figure 34.3). Bruising over the chest and abdominal wall on the side of the injury is often evident on inspection. At initial assessment, the child may be asymptomatic or may display a varying degree of cardiorespiratory compromise, depending on the volume of herniated abdominal contents, the degree of lung compression and the associated mediastinal shift. In addition to chest and abdominal pain, shoulder-tip pain may be apparent in the conscious child. Bowel sounds may be heard within the left chest and are diagnostic, although they may be difficult to identify in a noisy accident and emergency department.

With right-sided rupture, damage to the liver and the inferior vena cava can result in life-threatening blood loss. Injuries to the diaphragm may be radial or circumferential and usually involve the central tendon. In cases of blunt trauma, they are usually radial.

Between 30 and 50 per cent of cases may have normal chest radiographs on initial examination, especially in ventilated patients, where the stomach and intra-abdominal contents are prevented from herniating into the chest because of the positive intrapleural pressures. With normal breathing, negative intrapleural pressure will encourage herniation of the stomach and bowel into the chest, which can be demonstrated on a chest X-ray. The abnormal position of a nasogastric tube coiled within the left chest is diagnostic of a left diaphragmatic rupture.

Diagnosis may be difficult, with other injuries often appearing more significant. CT scanning plays a useful role in the diagnosis, and sometimes an upper-gastrointestinal contrast study is indicated, although rarely within the acute setting.

Initial treatment includes securing the airway, supplemental oxygen, intravenous fluid resuscitation, analgesia and insertion of a nasogastric tube. Acute gastric distension with further respiratory compromise is a real risk, especially in paediatric patients. Definitive management is surgical, via an abdominal approach. This allows for primary repair of the diaphragmatic rupture and also a thorough assessment and correction of any associated intra-abdominal visceral injury.

TRACHEOBRONCHIAL INJURY

Tracheobronchial injuries are uncommon in children. They may result from blunt or penetrating trauma. Most acceleration/deceleration tears occur within 2.5 cm of the carina and appear as a circumferential laceration, which may disrupt the continuity of the airway. Signs and symptoms suggestive of direct airway damage include cough, haemoptysis, massive cutaneous emphysema and stridor. Features suggesting airway compromise include tachypnoea, dyspnoea and cyanosis.

Failure of the lung to re-expand and a continued massive air leak after chest drain insertion are suggestive of major tracheobronchial injury. Radiologically, the 'dropped lung' sign, in which the lung shadow is seen low in the pleural cavity, adjacent to the cardiac silhouette, is highly suggestive of a major bronchial disruption.

Small lacerations may heal without surgery, especially those affecting the membranous trachea or bronchial tears affecting up to one-third of the circumference of a bronchus. Large tears require specialist operative intervention.

Late presentations are seen. During the healing phase, stricture formation may result with features that suggest atelectasis secondary to distal bronchial narrowing. Recurrent episodes of pneumonia and even established bronchiectasis are recognized late-presenting problems.

OESOPHAGEAL INJURY

Most oesophageal injuries in children result from the ingestion of caustic liquids or from penetrating trauma, usually from instrumentation. Forceful vomiting can cause oesophageal tears, with the mechanism of injury dependent upon a rapid rise in intraoesophageal pressure, as gas is expelled from the stomach. The presence of cutaneous emphysema may suggest oesophageal perforation. The child is pyrexial and tachycardic and may complain of chest pain. Early detection allows for appropriate and prompt management, including intravenous fluids and broad-spectrum antibiotics. Surgical repair is best undertaken soon after injury. Late diagnosis may require supportive treatment with diversion and staged repair.

GENERAL FEATURES OF CARDIAC AND GREAT VESSEL INJURIES

Most paediatric cardiac and major vascular injuries are managed by cardiothoracic surgeons. However, the paediatric surgeon may be faced with the emergency management of such injuries before the arrival of specialist assistance. Blunt trauma sufficient to cause major cardiac or vessel injury is usually multisystem and rapidly fatal, but the rise in the incidence of penetrating trauma in adolescents, especially in urban areas, may make such injuries more common in paediatric practice.

Initial examination of the child may be unremarkable, even with a significant cardiovascular injury. Bruising over the precordium may be evident, in addition to upper-body cyanosis and unexplained hypotension. Cardiac dysrhythmias are seen, most commonly ventricular ectopics or atrial fibrillation. However, both continuous electrocardiogram (ECG) monitoring and a 12-lead ECG may be normal. Early chest radiographs may also be normal, even with a significant mediastinal or great vessel injury.

Repeat radiographs may help to identify cardiovascular injuries. Echocardiography, in experienced hands, is excellent at identifying even small pericardial fluid collections and associated structural cardiac injuries and cardiac dysfunction. This non-invasive imaging modality can be repeated as required. Further information regarding major vessel injuries is obtained from contrast-enhanced CT scans and even angiography. The three most common major cardiovascular consequences of injury are cardiac tamponade, major vessel disruption and cardiac contusion.

CLINICAL SCENARIOS

Case 1

A 15-year-old boy was injured severely in a high-speed motor accident in which he was the front-seat passenger. He was wearing a seatbelt but still sustained multiple injuries, including head trauma and a fractured femur. Initial chest X-ray showed multiple fractured ribs and bilateral pneumo/haemothoraces. Bilateral chest drains were inserted with good effect, and the re-expanded lung fields appeared normal. With positive-pressure ventilation, his respiratory status appeared stable. Within six hours, he deteriorated. Repeat chest X-ray showed fluffy infiltrates indicative of pulmonary contusion. These worsened rapidly, requiring increasing ventilatory pressures and fraction of inspired oxygen (FiO_2). At 36 hours following injury, he became impossible to ventilate and died. Post-mortem showed severe extensive intrapulmonary haemorrhage in addition to his cerebral contusion and skeletal fractures.

Case 2

A 12-year-old boy was stabbed in the back of the lower left chest. On admission, his vital signs were stable but chest X-ray showed a small left pneumothorax. Some crepitus was felt in the area surrounding the entry wound, which was 2 cm in length. He was treated conservatively, but over the ensuing 12 hours his oxygen requirement increased and breathing became more laboured. Ultrasound of the left chest showed a small pulmonary effusion. A chest drain was inserted and drained large amounts of serosanguinous fluid. He developed a rising tachycardia and required increasing fluid resuscitation. Surgical exploration was undertaken 30 hours after injury and revealed a laceration through the left lower lobe of lung, a 4-cm tear in the left hemi-diaphragm, a small splenic laceration with a subcapsular haematoma and perforation of the gastric fundus. Postoperatively, he made a good recovery.

FURTHER READING

Allshouse MJ, Eichelberger MR. Patterns of thoracic injury. In: Eichelberger MR (ed.). *Pediatric Trauma: Prevention, Acute Care, Rehabilitation*. St Louis, MO: Mosby, 1993; pp. 437–48.

Holmes JF, Sokolove PE, Brant WE, Kupperman N. A clinical decision rule for identifying children with thoracic injuries after blunt torso trauma. *Annals of Emergency Medicine* 2002; **39**: 492–9.

Peclet MH, Newman KD, Eichelberger MR, *et al.* Thoracic trauma in children: an indicator of increased mortality. *Journal of Pediatric Surgery* 1990; **25**: 961–6.

Reynolds M. Pulmonary, esophageal and diaphragmatic injuries. In: Buntain WL (ed.). *Management of Pediatric Trauma*. Philadelphia, PA: WB Saunders, 1995; pp. 238–47.

Roberts SR, Holder T, Ashcraft KW. Cardiac and major thoracic vascular injuries. In: Buntain WL (ed.). *Management of Pediatric Trauma*. Philadelphia, PA: WB Saunders, 1995; pp. 248–64.

Roux P, Fisher RM. Chest injuries in children: an analysis of 100 cases of blunt chest trauma from motor vehicle accidents. *Journal of Pediatric Surgery* 1992; **27**: 551–5.

Wesson DE. Thoracic injuries. In: O'Neill JA, Rowe MI, Grosfeld JL, Fonkalsrud EW, Coran AG (eds). *Pediatric Surgery*, 5th edn. St Louis, MO: Mosby, 1998; pp. 245–60.

Part 4

General surgery of infancy and childhood

Herniae and hydroceles

A EWEN MacKINNON

Learning objectives

- To recognize the risk of incarceration of inguinal herniae, particularly in the first year of life.
- To recognize the particular points relevant to neonates.
- To recognize the high chance of resolution of infantile hydroceles.
- To recognize the need to identify femoral herniae.
- To recognize the high chance that umbilical herniae resolve, even after the age of five years.

INTRODUCTION

This group of pathological conditions represents the most common indications for surgery in children. Even so, particularly with inguinal herniae in infancy, the technical aspects can be among the most demanding in paediatric surgery. Conversely, surgery is often recommended for umbilical herniae in spite of the fact that resolution may well occur throughout childhood.

INGUINAL HERNIAE

Evidence of a surgical approach to the management of inguinal herniae dates back nearly 2000 years. Skinner and Grosfeld (1993) outline the historical development of hernia surgery, with herniotomy, i.e. simple division of the hernia sac alone, being described at the beginning of the twentieth century.

Basic science

The gonad begins to develop during the fifth week of intrauterine life. Elongation of the body stalk results in a relative caudal migration, but the first phase of the testicular descent is under the influence of Müllerian inhibiting hormone. At the lower pole of the gonad, a strand of mesenchymal cells develops into a band-like structure, which becomes the gubernaculum in the male and the round ligament in the female. The former reaches outside the superficial inguinal ring by 30 weeks' gestation and then migrates to the lower pole of the scrotum under the influence of testosterone, while the round ligament never enters the labium. At about the eighth week of development, a peritoneal prolongation appears, passing through the layers of developing abdominal-wall muscle along the course of the developing gubernaculum or round ligament. The testis then migrates down the peritoneal canal or processus vaginalis, which is still patent at birth in about 90 per cent of children. Failure of this processus to close leads to the potential of an inguinal hernia or

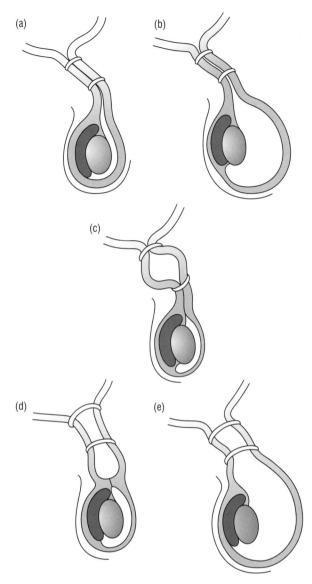

Figure 35.1   *Outcome of processus vaginalis: (a) normal obliteration; (b) communicating hydrocele; (c) hydrocele of cord; (d) inguinal hernia: bubonocele; and (e) inguinal hernia: complete.*

bubonoceles (Figure 35.1d), are said to account for 95 per cent of inguinal herniae.

Once the abdominal muscles have developed, the processus vaginalis emerges through the deep inguinal ring lying antero-lateral to the cord structures in the male or round ligament in the female. It then passes along the inguinal canal lying anterior to these structures and emerges through the superficial ring to pass into the scrotum in boys and may reach the labium major in girls. The inguinal canal measures less than 2 cm in the first year of life and more than doubles by age four years, the deep ring always being medial to the midpoint of the inguinal ligament. This has implications on the choice of surgical technique and the placing of the skin incision.

The medial boundary of the deep inguinal ring comprises the deep inferior epigastric vessels. The surface marking of the deep ring therefore is a point just above and medial to the point where the femoral artery passes under the inguinal ligament, just medial to the midpoint of the inguinal ligament. This is the key to placing the incision during surgery. The sac wall is lined by the mesothelial prolongation of the peritoneum, covered by a thin layer of connective tissue and some smooth muscle cells. Adherent to the sac is the vas in boys and the round ligament in girls. Other vestigial structures are present in 1.5 per cent of excised sacs (Popek 1990); these include adrenocortical rests and embryonal tubular structures, which can be confused microscopically with the vas. A sliding element may be present in a number of cases, particularly in a girl where the ovary on a mesovarium and accompanying Fallopian tube is found. Bowel wall or bladder wall may also present as part of the sac. Inguinal herniae are commonly present in patients with bladder extrophy and may also be associated with specific syndromes, including Ehlers–Danlos syndrome, Hurler–Hunter syndrome and complete androgen insensitivity syndrome (CAIS). The latter is important in girls, as the initial presentation may be with an inguinal hernia. This has led to some authors recommending karyotyping in all such cases.

Direct inguinal herniae are extremely rare in children, although it has been suggested that there may be a direct element in one per cent of indirect herniae. However, it is possible that this is an iatrogenic finding.

Clinical features

The most common presentation is of an intermittent swelling in the groin at the point of the deep inguinal ring, possibly extending to the scrotum or labium. If, on examination, this is not present, then it may be demonstrated by raising the intra-abdominal pressure if the child cries or is made to laugh or cough. If there is still no visible evidence, supportive signs include thickening of the cord structures or, if there is a very wide sac, rolling the cord between finger and pubic tubercle may give a feeling of rubbing together two layers of silk.

Confusion over the diagnosis is uncommon. However, in male infants, it can be difficult to differentiate herniae from

hydrocele. The mechanism of closure is still uncertain, but there is evidence that calcitonin gene-related peptide plays a role possibly through hepatocyte growth factor (Cook *et al.* 2000). Certain differences in the muscle fibres found on excised hernia sacs may have some relevance to this closure mechanism or may be a secondary feature.

Figure 35.1 illustrates the possible variations that arise when the processus vaginalis fails to close in part or in whole. Theoretically, if a wide canal persists, then a hernia may develop; if a narrow canal persists, then a hydrocele may develop. However, a wide processus may be associated with no clinical abnormality, a hydrocele, or both hernia and hydrocele, particularly if the neck is partly obturated by omentum or a Richter's type of hernia. Incomplete hernia sacs, or hydroceles. It may not be easy to decide whether one can 'get above' the swelling, the classic distinguishing feature of hydrocele in adults. Herniae in this age group may transilluminate as brightly as hydroceles.

It is commonly taught that unless incarcerated, herniae do not cause symptoms. In older children this is largely true, but in perhaps 80 per cent of infants discomfort is present, as can be judged by listening to the parents who notice a clear improvement following surgery.

Incidence

At birth approximately 95 per cent of infants are said to have a patent processus vaginalis. This figure falls to 40 per cent at one year and 20 per cent at two years. Based on large series of patients, the overall incidence of herniae is one to two per cent, with a preponderance of males to females of four to one. In preterm neonates, the incidence is up to 17 per cent in very premature neonates. Clinically evident bilateral herniae occur in ten per cent, but if the contralateral groin is explored without clinical evidence of a hernia, then nearly 50 per cent are found to have a patent processus vaginalis. Not surprisingly, the younger the child, the higher the incidence of finding a contralateral patency. In boys, right-sided herniae account for 60–70 per cent of cases; 20–25 per cent are left-sided, while 5–15 per cent may be bilateral. Contralateral herniae are found twice as often when the index side is left. Laterality is equal in girls, but a contralateral patent processus is present in six per cent when the index side is right and 19 per cent when it is left.

Only about one in four contralateral patent processus develop a hernia. Therefore, routine contralateral exploration is not indicated. This has been supported by a meta-analysis (Miltenburg et al. 1998). Careful examination will reveal some cases of bilaterality, in which case both groins should be explored. Even with preterm babies, contralateral exploration is no longer deemed mandatory. Methods to detect bilateral patency have included contrast radiography, transperitoneal probing, laparoscopy, pneumoperitoneography and ultrasonography. If laparoscopic inspection is performed, then it must be realized that some deep rings have a fold of peritoneum on the medial aspect. This does not represent a patent processus.

Management

As soon as a child's hernia is detected, he or she should be referred for surgery. Any infant under one year of age, and certainly those under six months, should be seen urgently for fear of incarceration developing. The vast majority of children are best operated on as day cases (Atwell et al. 1973). Examination should confirm the diagnosis whenever possible, although clear evidence from parents or health workers can be accepted. Particular attention must be paid to the opposite side, noting associated pathology such as cryptorchidism.

Particular attention must be given to planning surgery for neonates who were preterm, even after the neonatal period (Kumar et al. 2002), because of their impaired respiratory function in the first year of life. Infants under 44 weeks post-conceptional age (PCA) are at risk of postoperative apnoea, and consideration should be given to postponing surgery until after this age. These risks remain critical up to 52 weeks PCA, and monitoring for 12–24 hours after surgery should be performed even up to 60 weeks PCA. Consideration has to be given to the timing of surgery in the infant who develops a hernia whilst in a special care unit. The predictors of postoperative complications are linked most closely to chronic lung disease rather than prematurity. On occasions, large inguinal herniae may compromise lung function and surgery may improve ventilation. The safest policy is to arrange for surgery to be undertaken immediately before discharge from the baby unit.

Incarcerated herniae

Although incarceration of inguinal herniae may occur at any age in childhood, this complication is most common in the first six months of life, particularly in babies born preterm, even if the hernia presents in later years. In infancy, it is estimated that up to 50 per cent of herniae may present with an episode of incarceration. Regrettably, nearly half of such cases could have been prevented by expeditious surgery.

The clinical features are often insidious in onset, with the baby being non-specifically disturbed. Later, a tender red swelling in the groin becomes obvious, with features of intestinal obstruction. It is an absolute rule that any baby appearing miserable in a non-specific way must be examined with the nappy removed. The differential diagnosis includes testicular torsion and suppurative inguinal lymphadenopathy.

In girls, the ovary may enter the hernia sac and be irreducible without being strangulated. This is a situation that requires expeditious though not emergency surgery, as incarceration or torsion may supervene, either silently or overtly. The management of an infant with an incarcerated hernia is by resuscitation, reduction and repair. Considerable fluid loss may occur within a few hours, in which case intravenous fluids need to be given before any attempt at reduction. To reduce the hernia, the fingers of one hand are placed at the neck of the sac to support it and to prevent the hernia simply being pushed around under the skin (Figure 35.2). Gentle pressure by these fingers may help to reduce some of the oedema. At the same time, the fingers of the opposite hand exert pressure on the lower end of the hernia. If there is any difficulty in performing this reduction, then the patient should be sedated with morphine after ensuring intravenous access.

The organ most at risk of ischaemia is the gonad. Even so, it is less likely to undergo atrophy if reduction can be achieved non-operatively. Once reduced, the hernia should be repaired within a few days for fear of recurrence. The best approach to these herniae is by the preperitoneal route. This avoids having

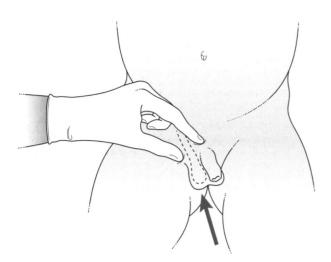

Figure 35.2 *Method of reducing an inguinal hernia.*

to dissect a very friable sac and allows dissection at the very upper end of its neck. Moreover, the cord structures are separated more easily at this level, and full inspection of incarcerated bowel to ensure its viability is possible, even if it reduces back within the peritoneal cavity. In children, it is extremely rare to have to resect bowel, but failure to make adequate inspection has led to deaths. It not true that gangrenous bowel cannot be reduced or that reduction *en masse* never occurs in children. Surgery for incarcerated herniae must be performed by a paediatric surgeon.

Operative techniques

Inguinal herniotomy is one of the most satisfying procedures in surgery and has evolved over the years. The correct procedure is based on knowledge of anatomy, may be technically challenging, and is highly effective, with rare complications. The laparoscopic approach is advocated by some but does carry the risks of laparoscopy. The various procedures described here are planned in the belief that the shutter mechanism of the inguinal canal should not be laid open unless necessary. The procedure that is chosen depends mainly on the patient's age. The operation is performed under general anaesthesia, with local or regional infiltration with local anaesthetic.

LOW APPROACH

This is the classic procedure for children under two years of age when the inguinal canal has no significant length. A transverse incision is made in the lower abdominal skin crease (Figure 35.3a) approximately 2 cm long, just cephalad of where the cord structures can be palpated as they cross the pubic bone. The fat and Scarpa's fascia are divided carefully to minimize bleeding and obviate the use of diathermy in the operation, thus removing risk to the vas. The wound is then retracted caudally, so that the dissection is continued perpendicular to the skin surface to explore the anterior aspect of

the cord as it emerges from the superficial ring. This can be recognized by a shiny bluish colour. The superficial layer is picked up and divided with scissors (Figure 35.3b), and the opening is spread to allow the cremaster to be picked up. This is recognized by its interweaving pinkish fibres (Figure 35.3c). This layer draws with it the internal spermatic fascia and processus vaginalis, so division with scissors must be done with care. Experience alone facilitates recognition of these tissue planes. The cremaster is split open to allow the processus vaginalis to be grasped with a mosquito forcep (Figure 35.3d) and to be drawn up on to the index finger of the left hand for a right-sided hernia or the right hand for a left-sided hernia. The cord structures may then be teased off the sac using the edge of blunt dissecting forceps while the sac is pulled up by the thumb on to the supporting finger, using it like an anvil. Dissection is carried around the sac, never grasping the vas, until a clear plane is seen between the cord and the sac (Figure 35.3e). A mosquito forcep is then placed across the sac, which is divided distally. The sac is dissected to its neck, transfixed with 3-0 polygalactin and divided (Figure 35.3f). There is no need to excise the distal end of the sac. If oozing occurs from the pampiniform plexus, it is best controlled by firm pressure. In most cases, the sac wall is thin enough for simple inspection to reveal that there is no sliding element or abdominal structure such as the Fallopian tube. If there is any doubt, then the sac should be opened, well away from the deep ring, and any contents inspected. The wound is then closed with 4-0 absorbable sutures to the fat and subcuticular layer. Finally, in boys, the correct scrotal placement of the testis is ensured. A similar procedure may be performed using a periscrotal incision, which is thought to be cosmetically superior by some surgeons (Figure 35.4).

The most common difficulties in this operation are due to an inability to recognize the structures involved and failing to keep the dissection perpendicular to the skin, thus wandering off line in the prepubic fat. Once the cremasteric layer has been opened, a well-formed condensation of connective tissue may mimic the sac. Finally, sometimes the dissection around the sac seems to be never-ending. Usually this is due to the surgeon dissecting around the end of a bubonocele; once this is recognized, clearing of the sac is easy.

Sliding herniae present special difficulties. First, the anatomy has to be realized. Quite often, an ovary or fallopian tube may be freed from the sac wall sufficiently to permit simple transfixion of the sac. If not, and where bowel or bladder is involved, then the simplest and most effective procedure is to place a purse-string suture around the external aspect of the neck of the sac and thus invert the sliding viscus at the same time as closing the processus.

HIGH APPROACH

Once there is a significant length to the canal at about two years of age, the above procedure necessitates pulling the sac down the inguinal canal, which is feasible but more traumatic. An alternative is to expose the neck of the sac at the deep

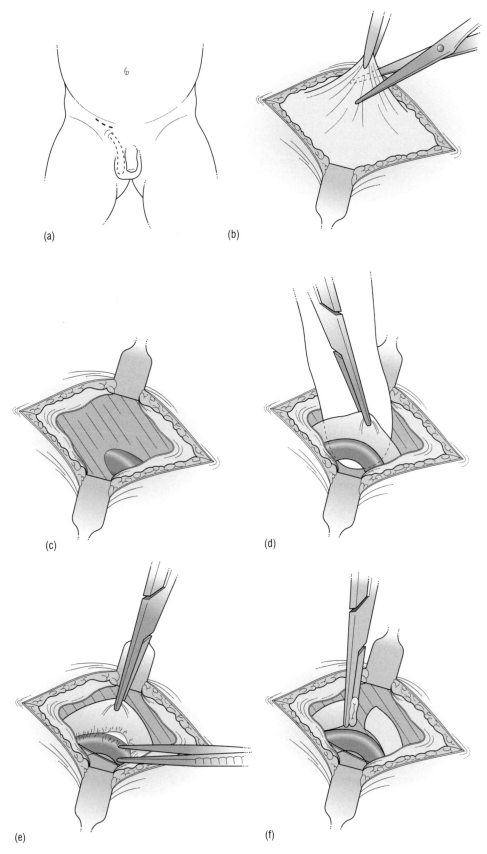

Figure 35.3 *Low approach to inguinal herniotomy. (a) Skin incision. (b) Division of superficial cord coverings. (c) Cremaster muscle seen over cord emerging from superficial inguinal ring. (d) Processus vaginalis being lifted forward, with index finger supporting behind. (e) Processus vaginalis being dissected free from cord. (f) Processus vaginalis transfixed and divided.*

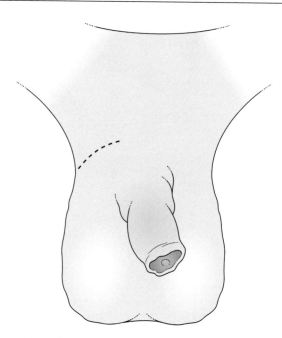

Figure 35.4 *Periscrotal incision for inguinal herniotomy.*

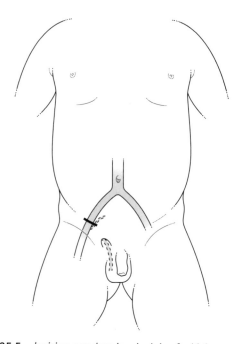

Figure 35.5 *Incision over deep inguinal ring for high approach.*

inguinal ring through a short 'buttonhole' opening in the external oblique but without opening the canal along its full length. This requires accurate placement of the incision and line of dissection. A skin-crease incision 2 cm long is made over the deep ring (Figure 35.5). The external oblique is then incised for 1.0 cm perpendicularly below the skin. Often, the inguinal nerve can be seen through the aponeurosis, which must be opened just caudal to this nerve. The internal oblique muscle is split with mosquito forceps as it becomes the cremaster muscle, the edges being held open by blunt dissecting forceps. The cremaster must be split fully, and likewise the internal spermatic fascia (or transversalis fascia), thus revealing

the cord or round ligament with the hernia sac lying in front of these structures. If it is difficult to lift the sac forwards, then there may be one of three problems. First, the hernia may not be reduced fully. Second, the transversalis fascia may not have been split. Third, the parietal peritoneum may have been grasped in error. If the sac is not found, then usually it is lying on the deep aspect of the lower part of the internal oblique muscle. From this point on, the dissection is similar to the low approach, the wound requiring one suture of 3-0 polygalactin suture to close the external oblique aponeurosis.

PREPERITONEAL APPROACH

This is advocated in particular for incarcerated herniae. However, it is also probably the optimum procedure in infancy and for recurrent herniae. It is a slightly more difficult technique to learn than the two previous procedures, but with experience the dissection of cord structures from the sac is easier. Because the merging of the neck of the sac and parietal peritoneum is in view, there should be virtually no possibility for recurrence. The approach also allows inspection of the posterior wall of the canal, looking for a direct element and the femoral canal. The incision is made in the skin fold, as with the low approach, but it is twice as long (Figure 35.6a). The subcutaneous fat and Scarpa's fascia are divided and then separated cephalad from the external oblique aponeurosis for 2–3 cm. A transverse muscle-splitting incision is then made in the external and internal oblique muscles, often splitting the lateral margin of the rectus sheath (Figure 35.6a). The extraperitoneal plane is then dissected until the neck of the processus vaginalis is defined by blunt dissection. It often lies more medial than at first one might expect; it is recognition of its appearance that requires experience and is key to the operation. The transversalis fascia is then opened in front of the sac and careful dissection continued on either side, working posteriorly until eventually a mosquito forcep can be placed behind the sac. The contents of the hernia must be reduced before this step, otherwise dissection is almost impossible. If there is any question of viability of contained bowel, then the sac is opened at its neck and the bowel inspected. Occasionally, it is necessary to pass an instrument extremely carefully through the deep ring to stretch the inguinal orifices to permit reduction if the hernia is incarcerated. The anterior wall of the sac is grasped and drawn medially. Then the sac is separated from the vas and vessels by dissecting around the lateral side (Figure 35.6b). The supporting mosquito may then be replaced in the plane between the cord and the sac before the sac is cross-clamped (Figure 35.6c), divided and transfixed at its neck with 3-0 polygalactin. If the deep ring is seen to be very wide, then a layer of transversalis fascia can be sutured over it. The muscles are closed with 3-0 polygalactin and the fat and skin with 4-0 suture. Finally, as always, the testes must be seen to be fully descended.

Postoperative care

Most patients can be discharged the same day and are likely to require a mild analgesic for less than 48 hours. Early activity

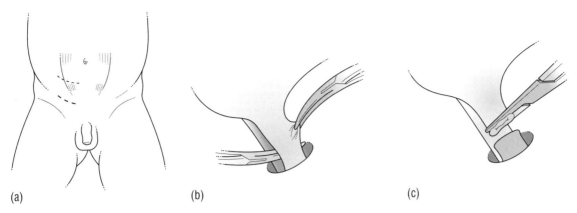

Figure 35.6 *(a) Incision on skin (- - -) for preperitoneal approach and in muscle fascia (----). (b) Dissection behind sac, separating it from cord structures. (c) Sac clamped and divided.*

should not be detrimental to the surgery, but common sense dictates avoidance of contact sports for ten days. In some patients, there may be thickening and bruising of the scrotum, which resolves in one to two weeks. This can be mistaken for an early recurrence with incarceration. Many units arrange for a visit by a district nurse the following day, but the need for this is doubtful. Children should be able to return to school after two to three days, or even sooner.

Complications

RECURRENCE

Large series indicate a low incidence of postoperative problems. Review of national figures in England and Wales revealed an overall recurrence rate of six per cent. However, in areas where it could be identified that all procedures would have been performed in a paediatric surgical unit, the rate was one per cent. At re-exploration, the cause is not usually evident, but laparoscopic inspection may be beneficial in the diagnosis. Hydrocele fluid may collect in the distal end of an incompletely excised sac, but this resolves spontaneously in almost all cases.

INFECTION

Rarely, infection occurs in the superficial layers in sporadic cases. If clusters of infection occur, then theatre management should be reviewed. Deep infection is an occasional complication of using non-absorbable sutures to transfix the sac.

TESTICULAR DAMAGE

Iatrogenic cryptorchidism may occur even when care is taken to ensure that the testis lies in the lower pole of the scrotum at the end of surgery. It has been reported in one per cent of operations. More serious is the small incidence of testicular atrophy. This complication is more common in neonatal herniotomy, and its incidence may be as high as ten per cent. Reduced testicular volume may be detected in ten per cent of older boys. Risk of injury to the vas can be minimized by not using diathermy during the operation; however, as the vas

adherers to the sac wall, it may be divided in about 0.33 per cent of operations, with a similar incidence of injury to the epididymis. Not only does injury to the vas causes obstruction to the passage of sperm, but also there is evidence of increased anti-sperm antibodies in adult life.

HYDROCELES

Basic science

The embryology of hydroceles in the same as for indirect inguinal herniae. In girls, a hydrocele presents as a swelling along the line of the round ligament and is often called a hydrocele of the canal of Nuck. In males, the majority of hydroceles are confined to the tunica vaginalis (Figure 35.1b), but they may be associated with a hernia that is not clinically evident. Commonly, hydroceles first arise following a systemic viral illness or after creation of a peritoneal cerebrospinal fluid (CSF) shunt or establishment of peritoneal dialysis. Hydroceles of the cord (Figure 35.1c) are clinically obvious but can be confused with a rare crossed ectopic testis. The serious differential diagnosis of a hydrocele in the scrotum is a testicular teratoma, which can be partly cystic and, therefore, may transilluminate. Teratomas have been described as feeling like a hydrocele. It is imperative, therefore, that a normal testis can be felt on the posterior wall of a hydrocele sac; if too tense to palpate, then transillumination will reveal its position. It must be remembered that herniae also transilluminate in young children.

Management

In the first year of life, hydroceles resolve spontaneously in over 90 per cent of cases. If very gross, parents often press for surgery; if their requests are acceded to, recurrence is frequent. Under such circumstances, the best action is to wait for resolution. These may well be examples of abdominoscrotal hydroceles, the management of which is controversial. It is possible that if social pressures can be resisted, then an expectant policy leads to resorption in at least some cases.

Hydroceles seldom present in the second year of life. At this age, they could be left alone, but thereafter surgery is advisable as resolution is unlikely. The operative procedure is the same as for herniae, but often the processus vaginalis in the inguinal canal is very narrow and easily missed. It must be traced cephalad until it is seen to widen out at the peritoneum. The best route to identify the processus is the high approach in the majority of children. This ensures transfixion of the sac at its neck. Equally important is to ensure thorough drainage of hydrocele contents, either by passing an instrument such as a mosquito forcep down the distal limb of the processus or by pushing the testis into the lower end of the incision and widely draining it. This is performed because spontaneous reabsorption of the fluid is slow. Recurrence is rare and may require re-exploration; in these cases, the preperitoneal route allows certainty of displaying the relevant anatomy.

FEMORAL HERNIAE

Much less common than inguinal herniae, femoral herniae have an equal sex incidence in children (Al-Shanafey and Giacomantonio 1999). Occasionally, they are secondary to disruption of pelvic anatomy by orthopaedic surgery. The sac may contain any pelvic organ, small bowel or omentum. Incarceration is very infrequent. Clinically, femoral herniae have to be distinguished from inguinal herniae by their inferior and more medial position, and from enlarged lymph nodes. Frequently, the diagnosis is missed and they re-present as recurrence of putative inguinal hernias.

These herniae may be tackled from below at the lower end of the femoral canal. However, it is not always easy to separate the sac from the surrounding fat. The easiest procedure is to use the preperitoneal approach, as described for inguinal herniae, suturing the medial end of the inguinal ligament to the pectinate ligament with a 3-0 polygalactin suture. A compound curved needle facilitates this manoeuvre.

MIDLINE HERNIAE

Umbilical herniae

These are the most common herniae in children. The umbilicus is a scar, so it is not surprising that it contracts, leading to resolution in most cases. This occurs in the first year of life in about 90 per cent of cases, but still there is a significant chance of spontaneous closure of the defect at the age of five years. Parents often fear, needlessly, that the thin sac will rupture, but strangulation is rare. Rupture has been reported in association with cutaneous infection in African countries. The other fear of parents is that the child will be teased, but this depends more often on family attitudes than the opinion of peers. Indications for surgery are rather vague, but some children do seem to have discomfort, which may indicate surgery, and in some social pressures are sufficiently strong to warrant surgery. In the first three months of life, strapping the abdominal wall so as to obturate the hernia can be performed, but this is probably of no real benefit.

Operative repair is quite simple. It is performed under general anaesthesia, with local anaesthetic infiltration for postoperative pain relief. The loose skin is grasped with an Allis forcep and a curved incision made around 50 per cent of the circumference of the defect (Figure 35.7a,b), which must lie within the umbilicus. By a combination of blunt and sharp dissection, the plane around the base of the hernia sac is developed (Figure 35.7c). The skin is then dissected off the sac, but if some peritoneum remains attached, this causes no problem. The lateral ends of the sac are grasped with haemostats and the sac is excised (Figure 35.7d,e). There are no significant vessels to ligate. Any contained omentum must be reduced before closure, which can be performed by a double row of 3-0 polygalactin mounted on a cutting needle (Figure 35.7f). A formal Mayo procedure is not necessary. Before closing the skin, the margin may need to be trimmed if there is gross redundancy and the deep aspect has to be sutured to the line of closure of the hernia sac. To prevent a haematoma forming, the wound is dressed with a pledget in the umbilicus held in place with a folded dressing swab and a 7.5-cm-wide sticking plaster.

Para-umbilical herniae

These are not common in children. They lie just above, or occasionally below, the umbilicus. A para-umbilical hernia can be distinguished from a true umbilical hernia because the latter has a circular orifice, whereas the former has a transverse elliptical orifice. They differ in their outcomes, since para-umbilical herniae seldom, if ever, resolve spontaneously and so are more likely to require repair.

Epigastric herniae

These comprise a small herniation of extraperitoneal fat, single or multiple, in the midline through the linea alba. They lie one-third to one-half the distance from the umbilicus to the xiphisternum. Rarely, they cause pinpoint discomfort related to the lesion, but often parents attribute non-specific abdominal pain to them. Only if necessary should epigastric herniae be operated upon, in which case the protruding fat may be excised or reduced and the hole closed with a single suture. Surgery will exchange a symptom-less small swelling for a permanent scar, which may be quite obvious. We have reviewed our cases not operated upon; at the beginning of teenage years, none of the patients regretted the decision.

Divarication of the recti

This occurs frequently in infants. It is important to know that no action is required, although it can be difficult to reassure parents.

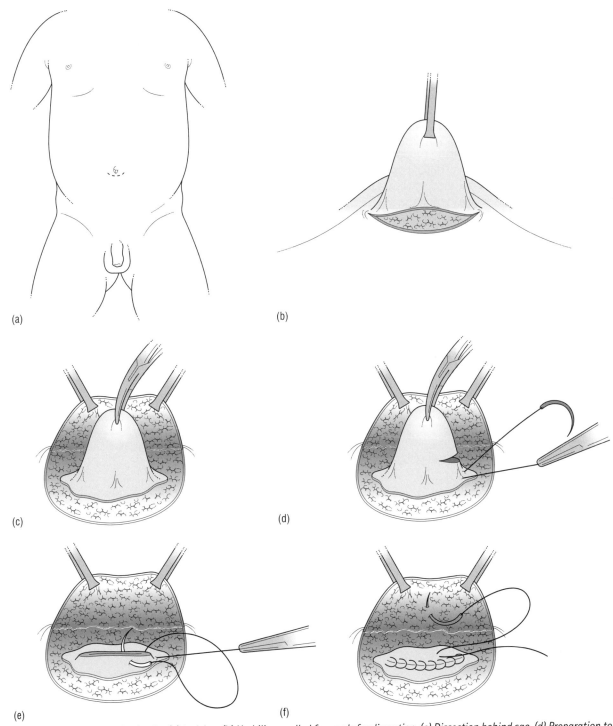

Figure 35.7 *Umbilical herniorrhaphy. (a) Incision. (b) Umbilicus pulled forwards for dissection. (c) Dissection behind sac. (d) Preparation to excise sac. (e) Sac excised and repair started. (f) Repair complete.*

OTHER HERNIAE

Rare herniae of the abdominal wall may occur in children. These include interstitial herniae, Spigelian herniae and lateral abdominal-wall herniae. Interstitial herniae emerge through a peritoneal processus arising close to the deep inguinal ring and contain the ipsilateral testis. They may present at a site similar to a Spigelian hernia or lie closer to the inguinal canal, where their true nature may be mistaken for a simple undescended testis. Spigelian herniae seem to be associated with inguinal hernias. Lateral abdominal-wall herniae may arise through the potential defects in which the latissimus dorsi and external oblique muscles overlap at the iliac crest below or costal margin above. Such herniae also may be associated with neurogenic lesions. The method of repair depends on the local anatomy, but often there is no true sac and mobilization of a flap of muscle or fascia is required.

CLINICAL SCENARIO

A male infant, born at 33 weeks' gestation and weighing 1.0 kg (<2 centile) required ventilation for four days. He was discharged home after three weeks in the special care baby unit. Three days later his parents noticed him to be more irritable, and the next day they saw a swelling in the right groin. They saw their general practitioner, who contacted the paediatric surgical unit, where the baby was seen the following day in the outpatient department. The family was advised that because of the neonatal history, particularly the need for ventilation, it would be safer if surgery was delayed until the baby was 52 weeks' gestational age. His name was entered in the theatre diary for that date and a cot reserved on the neonatal surgical unit. Additionally, the family was warned of the symptoms and signs of incarceration. Three days later at 10.30 p.m., the baby awoke crying and was sick. The parents took off the nappy: they saw that the hernia was larger than before, and touching it made the baby cry more. They took him to the hospital, as instructed previously, where with patience the duty surgeon managed to reduce the hernia. After 36 hours, the baby underwent herniotomy with a caudal anaesthetic and was discharged the following day.

REFERENCES

Al-Shanafey S, Giacomantonio M. Femoral hernia in children. *Journal of Pediatric Surgery* 1999; **34**: 1104–6.

Atwell JD, Burns JMS, Dewar AK, Freeman NV. Paediatric day case surgery. *Lancet* 1973; **2**: 895–7.

Cook BJ, Hasthorpe S, Hutson JM. Fusion of childhood inguinal hernia induced by HGF and CGRP via an epithelialtransition. *Journal of Pediatric Surgery* 2000; **35**: 77–81.

Kumar VH, Clive J, Rosenkrantz TS, Bourque MD, Hussain N. Inguinal hernia in preterm infants (< or = 32-week gestation). *Pediatric Surgery International* 2002; **18**: 147–52.

Miltenburg DM, Nuchtern JG, Jaksic T, Kozinetiz C, Brandt ML. Laparoscopic evaluation of the pediatric inguinal hernia: a meta-analysis. *Journal of Pediatric Surgery* 1998; **33**: 874–9.

Popek EJ. Embryonal remnants in inguinal hernia sacs. *Human Pathology* 1990; **2**: 339–49.

Skinner MA, Grosfeld JL. Inguinal and umbilical hernia repair in infants and children. *Surgical Clinics of North America* 1993; **73**: 439–49.

FURTHER READING

Devlin HB. *Management of Abdominal Hernias.* London: Butterworths, 1988.

Hutson JM, Beasley SW. *Descent of the Testis.* London: Arnold, 1992.

Scorer CG, Farrington GH. *Congenital Deformities of the Testis and Epididymis.* London: Butterworths, 1971.

36

The undescended testis

A BIANCHI

Learning objectives

- To understand the aetiology of the undescended testis.
- To achieve a clear understanding of the clinical evaluation and classification of undescended testes.
- To have a clear concept of the treatment of testicular undescent and an understanding of the different surgical approaches.
- To develop a management plan for the child with testicular undescent based on clinical evaluation, classification and expected outcome.

INTRODUCTION

The testis is an important and relevant organ. The presence, position and function of the testis – or, better still, two testes – are relevant practically and psychologically to the growing child as an 'index of maleness' and to the adolescent/adult and his family in relation to fertility.

Testicular undescent is still not fully understood, and there remains appreciable confusion in the evaluation, classification and management of the undescended testis. As newer surgical modalities develop, it is even more relevant to have a clearer understanding, such that morbidity, e.g. testicular loss, multiple operations and unnecessary loss of fertility are reduced and appropriate management offered in optimal time.

EMBRYOLOGY

Early gonadal differentiation occurs in the urogenital ridge and is regulated by at least two genes, ZFY and SRY, located on the short arm of the Y chromosome. The SRY (sex-determining region of Y) gene encodes for a testis-specific deoxyribonucleic acid (DNA)-binding protein that stimulates development of the embryonic gonad towards a testis. Subsequent hormone production, specifically testosterone and Müllerian inhibiting substance (MIS), by the fetal testis controls a cascade of secondary changes leading to virilization of the basic female external genitalia and influencing the process of testicular descent (Figure 36.1).

Testicular descent is biphasic, with each phase influenced by separate hormones. The transabdominal phase, between the

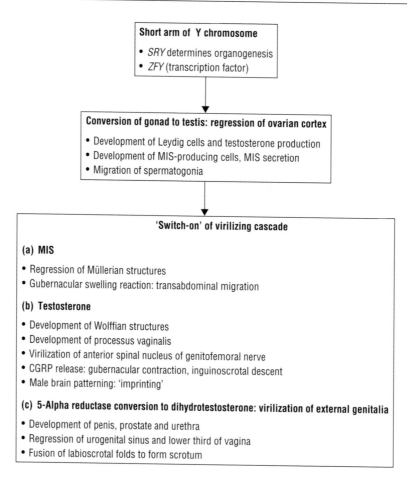

Figure 36.1 *Virilization process.*
CGRP, calcitonin gene-related peptide; MIS, Müllerian inhibiting substance.

urogenital ridge and the internal inguinal ring, is not androgen-dependent. The migratory process is associated with regression of the cranial suspensory ligament, while the gubernacular swelling reaction is associated with thickening and shortening of the gubernaculum, drawing the testis towards the internal inguinal ring. This process occurs only in males and is seen also in patients with complete androgen insensitivity. It is thought to be influenced primarily by insulin 3, aided by MIS, which is probably produced by the Sertoli cells of the developing testis, both having a local action. The final phase of inguinoscrotal descent is androgen-dependent. Ahead of the descending testis, the processus vaginalis develops within the inguinal canal to the scrotum. It is surrounded by the cremaster muscle, which is innervated by the genitofemoral nerve. Androgens produced by the fetal testis act to irreversibly virilize the sensory dorsal root nucleus of the genitofemoral nerve (sexual dimorphism). A neurotransmitter, calcitonin gene-related peptide (CGRP), released through the sensory fibres of the genitofemoral nerve, acts on the CGRP-receptor-rich gubernaculum, inducing strong rhythmic contractions (100/second), which draw the testis through the inguinal canal into the scrotum.

The development of the fetal testis, hormonal secretion and, hence, testicular descent are controlled by the hypothalamo-pituitary-gonadal axis. At four to six weeks after conception,

luteinizing hormone-releasing hormone (LHRH) is detectable in the hypothalamus, indicating the presence of a functioning hypothalamic oscillator in the arcuate nucleus. LHRH stimulates the release from the anterior pituitary of luteinizing hormone (LH) and follicle-stimulating hormone (FSH), which control testicular function and, eventually, male reproduction. Regulation is by a negative-feedback mechanism. Pituitary LH influences Leydig cell function and, hence, testosterone secretion, whereas FSH is involved in the transformation of primordial germ cells into spermatogonia and in the differentiation of Sertoli cells.

TESTICULAR DEVELOPMENT

At term, the seminiferous tubules in the normal testis are filled with gonocytes, spermatogonia and Sertoli cells. Leydig cells are easily identifiable within the interstitial tissue. Accentuated growth during the second to sixth months of postnatal life is associated with a crucial surge in testosterone production and further maturation of the spermatogonia, followed by relative regression until the onset of puberty. Spermatogonia are quantifiable as the tubular fertility index (TFI), which represents the percentage of tubules containing spermatogonia. The TFI rises after the sixth year of life, and by the eighth year spermatocytes appear. Development of a tubular lumen and Sertoli cells is followed by spermatogenesis.

In 1929, Cooper noted that the younger the child and the further the level of testicular descent, the closer to normal was the histology of the undescended testis. It is now considered that the cryptorchid testis contains normal numbers of germ cells and maintains a normal tubular diameter at least up to two years of age. There is then a progressive reduction in the number of germ cells, with failure of maturation of the spermatogonia to form spermatocytes. From the outset, the number of Leydig cells is reduced, with consequent absence of the normal testosterone surge during the first six months of postnatal life. This reduction in Leydig cells may represent a failure of the hypothalamo-pituitary-gonadal axis to stimulate testicular development and, therefore, appropriate hormone production influencing testicular descent. The prepubertal cryptorchid testis typically shows an empty interstitium surrounding small or degenerate tubules containing few or no germ cells.

GENERAL FEATURES

Jackson and colleagues (1986a,b) noted that the true incidence levelled off at 1.58 per cent and remained unchanged. Following ongoing spontaneous descent over the first six months after birth, the true incidence levels off at 1.58 per cent and remains unchanged thereafter. Right-sided undescent (53–58 per cent) is more common than left-sided undescent (42–47 per cent). Bilateral undescended testes occur in 10–25 per cent of all cases of undescent. The incidence is higher in premature babies. There is a family incidence in 14 per cent of cases, reflecting a genetic predisposition. Undescended testes are not uncommon in association with hypospadias and occur as part of undervirilization and other endocrine disorders. There is also an association with abdominal-wall anomalies such as gastroschisis, ectopic bladder, prune belly syndrome and various chromosomal disorders.

The cause of testicular undescent may lie with the testis itself, may relate to a failure of the hypothalamo-pituitary-gonadal axis or may relate to mechanical factors, such as abnormal gubernacular development, e.g. ectopic position, or alteration in intra-abdominal pressure, e.g. prune belly, distended bladder.

When the child is warm and relaxed, the normal testis lies in the lowermost scrotum. During childhood, in response to even minor stimuli, particularly in the supply area of the genitofemoral nerve, the increasingly active cremasteric reflex draws the testis out of the scrotum into the superficial inguinal pouch in the groin. At clinical examination, gentle downward pressure along the inguinal canal overcomes the cremasteric pull, such that the normal retractile testis passes into its most caudal position in the lowermost scrotum, on a demonstrably long spermatic cord, without any tension and

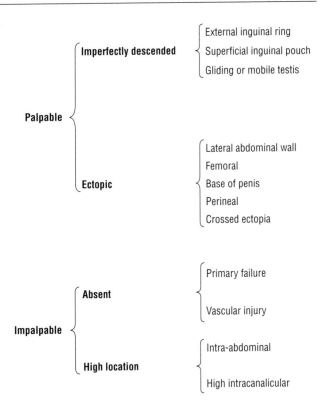

Figure 36.2 *Classification of testicular undescent.*

without discomfort to the child. Normal testicular volume increases steadily from <2 mL up to 11 years of age to 12–14 mL by 15 years of age. Testicular volume and the most caudal testicular position are the only two clinical prognostic indicators as to the normality of the testis and should always be recorded accurately.

The undescended testis can be classified as palpable or impalpable (Figure 36.2). Within the palpable group are the incompletely descended testis, which is held up along the normal pathway of descent, and the ectopic testis lying in any other location. It may be found laterally at the groin, medially at the base of the penis, and even perineally between the scrotum and the anus. Interestingly, ectopic testes are of better quality histologically, tending to suggest a mechanical problem rather than an interruption of hormone-dependent development. Within the spectrum of the incompletely descended testis is the gliding or mobile testis, which descends spontaneously to the high/mid-scrotum but has a short processus vaginalis, such that traction on the testis causes obvious discomfort to the child. Gliding testes are smaller in volume and often are associated with a hypoplastic scrotum. They show histological features of cryptorchidism and classify as undescended testes, requiring the same attention.

Some 15–20 per cent of undescended testes are impalpable, being absent because of primary failure of development or secondary to an antenatal accident, e.g. testicular torsion. More commonly, the testis is present and may be found lying intra-abdominally within the peritoneal cavity at the internal inguinal ring. Some high testes occasionally may be palpable within the inguinal canal but can rarely be manipulated much below the external inguinal ring. Abdominal and high inguinal testes have been reported to contain a high number of germ cells during the first six months after birth but show a progressive loss over subsequent years. Such findings have led Hadziselimovic *et al.* (1975) to regard testicular undescent as a progressive disease process rather than a congenital anomaly, implying the possibility of arresting the process and inducing maturation of spermatogonia by medical treatment.

Testes that have been documented to be in the scrotum at birth but subsequently are found to be undescended are often classified as ascending. The situation may be due to a failure of proportional elongation of the spermatic cord, such that the testis is progressively retracted out of the scrotum by linear body growth. More common is the iatrogenic undescended or rising testis that becomes attached to the inguinal fascia by scar tissue following an inguinal operation, e.g. for hernia or hydrocele, and is then drawn out of the scrotum with body growth. Iatrogenic undescent is different from recurrent or residual undescent, which is due to inadequate mobilization of the testicular vessels and vas at the time of orchidopexy, such that the testis is placed in the scrotum under tension. This situation is often a consequence of an inappropriate choice of surgical procedure for a testis on a short vascular pedicle.

ASSOCIATED PATHOLOGY

Failure of the testis to reach the lowermost scrotal position is associated with persistent patency of the processus vaginalis, often presenting as a hernia or hydrocele. In this respect, the ectopic testis is different in that the processus tends to become obliterated, even though the testis has never been in the scrotum. The undescended testis is abnormally mobile and therefore is more prone to torsion, a process that may also occur antenatally, such that no testicle is present at birth. Blind-ending testicular vessels and vas are evidence of previous testicular presence. D'Agostino *et al.* (1996) reported a 17–25 per cent incidence of epididymotesticular dissociation and epididymal anomalies, which has a major bearing on the incidence of infertility in patients with undescended testes.

Cryptorchidism is characterized by a failure of maturation of the seminiferous tubules with inability to produce sperm. Hadziselimovic *et al.* (1975) and others have reported a relatively normal tubular architecture and high numbers of germ cells in undescended testes at birth. They have noted subsequent failure of maturation and progressive irreversible loss of spermatogonia, particularly after the second year of life. Although primary gonadal failure or hypothalamo-pituitary-gonadal axis dysfunction could be responsible, it would appear that testicular deterioration relates also to the deleterious effect on spermatogenesis of a higher body temperature. Hadziselimovic *et al.* therefore regard testicular undescent as a potentially treatable condition by a combination of medical and surgical therapy. Hutson and Beasley (1992) agree that early transfer of the testis

to a cooler scrotum, soon after the sixth postnatal month, is definitely relevant to preserve spermatogonia.

It has long been accepted that the undescended testis and, to a lesser extent, the contralateral scrotal testis carries a greater content of dysgenetic material, which is most likely responsible for the increased risk of neoplasia. The contralateral scrotal testis carries an increased (five per cent) risk of neoplastic change. Sixty per cent of tumours developing in undescended testes are seminomas presenting at the usual young age for testicular tumours of 20–40 years. The incidence of carcinoma-in-situ is 1.7–2 per cent; it is considered to arise from abnormal gonocytes. The contralateral scrotal testis carries an increased five per cent risk of neoplastic change, such that one in five tumours associated with testicular undescent arises within the contralateral scrotal testis. Long-term follow-up is mandatory for patients with testicular undescent, particularly those who have had unilateral malignancy.

Failure of testicular descent, the absence of testes in the scrotum, and possible infertility cause profound psychological disturbance for both the adolescent patient and his family. The potential impact on body image, gender identity and, hence, self-esteem and personality should not be underestimated. It is especially relevant, therefore, to attempt to preserve both testes and to place them in appropriate scrotal compartments as soon as possible, not only to protect fertility but also to ensure a normal genital appearance from an early age.

The undescended testis usually is capable of relatively normal Leydig cell function and testosterone production, however high its position. Sufficient hormone has usually been present in fetal life to ensure normal male external genital development and 'male' brain imprinting. Patients usually will virilize normally at puberty and develop normal libido and potency.

CONSIDERATIONS IN MANAGEMENT

The term baby continues to show spontaneous testicular descent for the first three to six months of extrauterine life. Surgical transfer to the scrotum therefore is not relevant before the sixth month of life. Subsequently, it becomes increasingly important, in order to limit the irreversible loss of spermatogonia due to exposure to a higher body temperature. Thus, scrotal transfer of the undescended testis is best undertaken as soon as possible after the sixth month of postnatal life. More recently, the absence of the postnatal testosterone surge in children with undescended testes has been regarded as potentially relevant, such that it may be appropriate to offer medical therapy at this time to aid in the maturation of spermatogonia and, hence, fertility. Certainly, all boys should be reviewed at their first birthday, when undescent is pathological and an indication for surgery.

Perhaps the most relevant indication for orchidopexy (scrotal placement of the testis) is to provide normal genitalia from an early age, thus enhancing the bonding process between the parents and their son. The lower scrotal temperature is important for preservation of spermatogonia and for spermatogenesis and may even be associated with a reduced incidence of neoplasia. Coincidental obliteration of the patent processus vaginalis and placement of the testis in an ipsilateral subdartos pouch reduce the risks of hernia and testicular torsion. Even if infertile, the testis has psycho-aesthetic and hormonal values that outweigh the increased but comparatively minor risk of neoplasia. Orchidectomy rarely should be performed before puberty, and then only for the severely dysgenetic, hormonally non-functional testis, in the context of a fully consenting patient mature enough to realize all the possible implications.

CLINICAL APPROACH

- *Palpable testis:* at first examination, the presence, volume, consistency and the most caudal position to which the testis can be brought without discomfort to the child are recorded. Persistent undescent after six months of age is pathological and an indication for early orchidopexy.
- *Impalpable testis:* in view of the low incidence of anorchia, it is always important to attempt to locate an impalpable testis. Laparoscopy constitutes the only definitive investigation, during which the location and anatomical characteristics of the testis, epididymis, vas, testicular vessels and any residual Müllerian structures can be determined bilaterally. Should a testis not be present, it is always relevant to visualize blind-ending testicular vessels, an atretic vas alone being insufficient evidence of an absent testis.

Bilateral impalpable testes are best approached jointly with a paediatric endocrinologist and a geneticist. Low serum LH and FSH levels may indicate hypothalamo-pituitary-gonadal axis dysfunction, whereas a raised testosterone response to intramuscular human chorionic gonadotrophin (HCG) (1500 IU daily for three days, or a single dose of 4500 IU) will confirm the presence of hormonally functional testicular tissue. However, a low or absent testosterone response will not exclude the presence of a severely dysgenetic hormonally inactive gonad carrying a high risk of neoplasia. Laparoscopy, therefore, remains imperative.

Surgical exploration of the inguinal area is disruptive and has been superseded by laparoscopy. The passage of a vas and testicular vascular pedicle through the internal inguinal ring is evidence of previous testicular passage out of the abdomen towards the scrotum. It is debatable as to whether failure to palpate the testis in this area need be followed by surgical exploration, since testicular atrophy is usually total and it is rare to find any residual testicular tissue. However, if there is any clinical doubt, e.g. a chubby child, or if it is considered relevant to allay parental anxiety, then exploration is appropriate. The situation is different if the testis is not palpable following attempted orchidopexy. Testicular atrophy cannot be assumed and groin exploration is mandatory, since often the testis will be found encased in or beneath dense scar tissue.

The management of a child with an impalpable testis will depend on whether one or both testes are impalpable, or whether it is the single remaining testis following natural or iatrogenic loss of the contralateral gonad. It involves an assessment of the following (Figure 36.3):

- presence, location and quality of the testis, vas and epididymis and the testicular vessels;
- age of the child in relation to fertility;
- risk of neoplasia.

There is little role for medical or hormonal treatment for induction of testicular descent. LHRH and HCG therapy have a minor effect in reducing cremasteric contractility and possibly are effective in inducing additional descent of low undescended testes that most likely would have descended spontaneously at puberty. More recently, hormonal induction of maturation of spermatogonia with a combination of LHRH analogues and HCG has been proposed as adjuvant therapy to early orchidopexy to enhance fertility and may become a relevant part of the management plan.

SURGICAL OPTIONS

Surgery remains the mainstay for management of testicular undescent. Orchidopexy remains the appropriate procedure for the palpable testis with adequate vessel and vasal length. The testis is mobilized on its vascular pedicle and on the vas with its intact vessels, also preserving the collateral circulation between the testicular and vasal vessels. Additional vessel length can be obtained by high retroperitoneal dissection towards the origin of the vessels. The processus vaginalis is obliterated high above the internal inguinal ring, and the testis is then passed, without tension, into a subdartos pouch in the ipsilateral scrotum. The conventional approach is undertaken through a skin-crease groin incision, with or without laying open the inguinal canal to reach the internal inguinal ring and the retroperitoneum. The alternative transscrotal approach, described by Bianchi and Squire (1989), satisfies the same criteria but utilizes a more aesthetic single scrotal skin-crease incision and involves less tissue dissection, such that it is more comfortable and better suited to day-case surgery. Complication rates for both approaches are not dissimilar. Those specific to orchidopexy include the following:

- Failure to place the testis in the scrotum, which usually is due to inadequate dissection of the testicular vascular pedicle or inappropriate choice of procedure for a testis on short vessels.
- Recurrence of testicular undescent, which may relate to placement of the testis in the scrotum under tension but also may occur gradually with linear body growth following scar fixation of the spermatic cord to the fascia at the external inguinal ring.

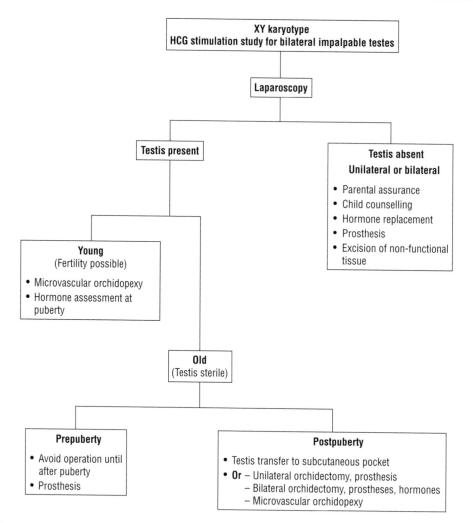

Figure 36.3 *(a) Management of bilateral impalpable testes.*
HCG, human chorionic gonadotrophin.

- Injury to the testicular vessels may lead to atrophy, which rarely occurs spontaneously for intrinsic reasons.
- Vasal and epididymal injury may occur from handling of the epididymis and vas or possibly from interference with their blood supply. Investigation is relevant, since an obstructed or divided vas may be amenable to microsurgical reconstruction.

THE TESTIS ON SHORT VESSELS

High inguinal and intra-abdominal testes represent some 20 per cent of undescended testes. The majority have a short vascular pedicle that will not allow scrotal placement. The presently available surgical options are as follows:

Mutistage orchidopexy

With or without a silastic wrap, this involves at least two operative interventions. The dissection through scar tissue makes vasal and testicular vessel injury more likely. Although occasionally successful, the incidence of failure or testicular loss is considerable.

Fowler–Stephens procedure

Following high retroperitoneal division of the main testicular vessels, the Fowler–Stephens concept relies on the collateral circulation from the vasal vessels for testicular survival. Primary transfer of the testis to the scrotum has been associated with an unacceptably high incidence of testicular atrophy (50–100 per cent). As such, the more widely practised two-stage Fowler–Stephens procedure proposes delayed scrotal transfer of a testis on a stronger collateral circulation, some three to six months after high interruption of the main testicular pedicle, and with no initial testicular mobilization. Vascular interruption is performed at open operation or laparoscopically. Although reduced, the incidence of testicular atrophy is at best 25 per cent and is still considerable. Tsang *et al.* (1993) undertook paternity studies in rats and

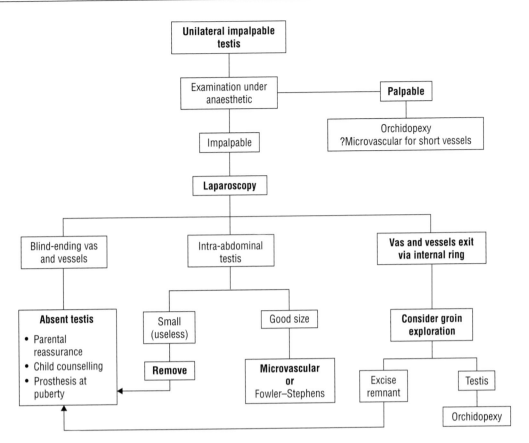

Figure 36.3   *(b) Management of unilateral impalpable testis.*

demonstrated a high incidence of sterility even in surviving testes following the Fowler–Stephens approach.

The testis on a long-loop vas, 'looping' into the scrotum and returning, has been considered ideal for the Fowler–Stephen procedure because of a better-developed collateral circulation from the vasal vessels. Careful clinical observation at the time of surgery demonstrates clearly that this 'favourable' collateral circulation is of no greater benefit, such that the testis on a long-loop vas requires the same considerations for effective scrotal transfer.

Microvascular orchidopexy

It seems relevant, therefore, to attempt to secure a full blood supply at orchidopexy. Once the main testicular pedicle has been divided, and the testis has been passed into the scrotum with vas and vasal vessels intact, the testicular artery and vein are anastomosed to the inferior epigastric vessels, such that a full blood supply is returned to the transferred organ within a warm ischaemia phase of some 60–120 minutes. Microvascular orchidopexy requires specific skills in microvascular surgery. High magnification with an operating microscope is essential, since the various vessel diameters are between 0.3 and 1.2 mm. Wherever possible, both artery and vein should be anastomosed, since the return of a 'normal' circulation is associated

with a 92 per cent testicular survival rate of a hormonally active, psycho-aesthetically acceptable testis in the ipsilateral scrotum, with growth of approximately 75–80 per cent of normal volume at puberty.

Studies in rabbits led Domini *et al.* (1997) to propose the vein-only 'refluo technique', since they noted that the reason for testicular atrophy following the Fowler–Stephens procedure related to insufficient venous drainage, the reduced arterial input being adequate. Paternity studies in rats by Tsang *et al.* (1993) confirmed a higher testicular survival rate and a paternity rate of 75 per cent, compared with the almost normal 85 per cent for full microvascular reconstruction and 12 per cent for the Fowler–Stephens model.

It is the author's opinion that wherever possible (and certainly for bilateral cases), the ideal operation for the intra-abdominal and the high canalicular testis on a short blood supply is the return of a full blood supply by arterial and venous reconstruction within the shortest warm ischaemia time. Failing this, a venous anastomosis alone is likely to give acceptable testicular survival, whereas the Fowler–Stephen procedure should be considered only as a fallback position and in the event of no other possibilities. In such circumstances, it is relevant to consider preserving at least one hormonally active, but sterile, testis in a palpable subcutaneous position in the inguinal area, rather than running the risk of total testicular loss following bilateral Fowler–Stephens procedures. If the contralateral testis is normally descended, then an ipsilateral nubbin is best removed. However, consideration should be given to retaining a hypoplastic or small testis that is potentially hormonally active, placing it in a subcutaneous pouch and possibly considering orchidectomy after puberty is complete.

Of particular note is the child with prune belly syndrome and with testes lying intra-abdominally or intracanalicularly. Undescent is possibly related to a failure of intra-abdominal pressure to assist passage into the inguinal canal and/or possible mechanical displacement of the descending gonad by the large hypotonic urine-filled bladder. Interestingly, these testes often have well-developed vascular pedicles of more than adequate length for tension-free scrotal transfer, and orchidopexy should be considered routinely after the sixth month. Prune belly syndrome carries a high incidence of epididymal and vasal anomalies, which may account for the high incidence of infertility.

ADJUVANT THERAPY

There is no medical treatment for testicular undescent, and early surgery is the only realistic option. For the palpable testis, this is often straightforward day-case surgery, with excellent long-term prospects. The testis on short vessels requires a more complex approach, with microvascular orchidopexy providing a 92 per cent chance of testicular survival. Hormonal manipulation with LHRH analogues and HCG is being proposed as adjuvant therapy to early orchidopexy, with a view to inducing maturation of the spermatogonia and enhancing fertility; this may yet become a relevant part of the management plan.

COUNSELLING

Of particular relevance to testicular undescent and potential testicular loss is the psychological impact on the growing child/young adolescent and his family. Body image and gender identity start early in life and have major implications on the personality and mental wellbeing of the patient and his parents. At every stage in the management the clinician should be sensitive to the need for counselling and reassurance. The offer of early and effective management from the sixth month of life onwards is of major relief to the parents, who can view their son as a 'complete male', and to the child, who develops with normal male genitalia. It is relevant to the child and his family, even at a young age but particularly at puberty, to offer the possibility of testicular prostheses to ensure a normal scrotal appearance. Similarly, the offer of hormonal assessment reassures the family of a likely normal puberty. Children who have lost all testicular tissue will need the services of a specialist paediatric endocrinologist to assist them through puberty and to ensure subsequent potency. For this group in particular, a specialist paediatric team, including surgeon, endocrinologist, geneticist

and counsellor, is of particular relevance. A link with specialist adult services is necessary for eventual transfer of care as the child grows to adulthood. Recent developments in *in vitro* fertilization, including single-sperm fertilization, provide hope for patients with vasal and epididymal anomalies. The compromised testis therefore should be preserved and orchidectomy considered only for neoplasia or the totally non-functional testis.

CONCLUSION

The 60 per cent of undescended testes that are palpable (imperfectly descended or ectopic) in the inguinal area are amenable to tension-free scrotal placement on a full blood supply after six months of age, by conventional or transscrotal orchidopexy, often as day-case procedures. Intraabdominal and high canalicular testes on short vessels require specialist services. Groin exploration is disruptive and has no place in diagnosis. A small proportion of patients will achieve tension-free transfer on a full blood supply by laparoscopic means alone. The majority will require microvascular reconstruction for return of a full blood supply if testicular survival rates are to be maximized. Where microvascular expertise is not available, the two-stage Fowler–Stephens operation is still practised, accepting that the success rate for testicular survival is considerably lower. All forms of orchidopexy are possible after six months of age, and delay is unacceptable because of further loss of spermatogonia. Adjuvant hormonal induction of maturation of spermatogonia may help to enhance fertility and may become relevant practice in future. Orchidectomy is acceptable only for neoplasia and for a demonstrably totally non-functional dysplastic gonad, and even then preferably only in the context of a patient who is mature enough to appreciate fully the consequences of the procedure.

The testis is a relevant organ and is becoming more so with major advances in fertility therapy. Testicular undescent requires a sensitive approach by a specialist paediatric team, which should include a specialist surgeon versed in microvascular reconstruction, a paediatric endocrinologist, a geneticist and specialist counsellors. A link with specialist adult endocrine and fertility services is crucial to ensure cradle-to-grave high-quality care for patients and their families.

CLINICAL SCENARIOS

Case 1

Bilateral undescended testes of 1-mL volume were noted at birth to be palpable in the superficial inguinal pouches in an otherwise normal male at 35 weeks' gestation. There were concomitant patent process presenting as hydroceles. The child was reviewed at six months of age, when the right testis was found to be normally retractile with a fused processus.

The most caudal position for the left testis was high scrotum, and the left hydrocele was still present. A left trans-scrotal orchidopexy was undertaken as a day case before the child's first birthday.

Case 2

A four-year-old boy was referred following failed bilateral conventional orchidopexies. Both testes were noted to have short vascular pedicles. The right testis was palpable at the external ring, but the left could not be definitively identified clinically. An ultrasound scan of the left groin suggested the possible presence of a testis. Groin exploration was planned with time and equipment available to proceed to microvascular orchidopexy. The right testis was mobilized through a trans-scrotal approach and sufficient vascular length was obtained at extended retroperitoneal dissection to place the testis in an ipsilateral subdartos pouch without tension. The left testis was located beneath dense fibrous tissue. The vas and vessels were identified and noted to be intact. After full high mobilization, vessel length was still insufficient to reach the scrotum. A left microvascular orchidopexy was performed. Both testes were in the scrotum and of equal volume two years later.

REFERENCES

Bianchi A, Squire BR. Transscrotal orchidopexy: orchidopexy revised. *Pediatric Surgery International* 1989; **4**: 189–92.

D'Agostino S, Campobasso P, Spata F, Belloli G. Cryptorchidism: anomalies of the secretory ducts and azoospermia. [In Italian.] *Pediatria Medica e Chirurgica* 1996; **18** (5 suppl.): 41–4.

Domini R, Lima M, Domini M. Microvascular autotransplantation of the testis: the 'refluo' technique. *European Journal of Pediatric Surgery* 1997; **7**: 288–91.

Hadziselimovic F, Herzog B, Seguchi H. Surgical correction of cryptorchidism at 2 years: electronmicroscopic and morphometric investigations. *Journal of Pediatric Surgery* 1975; **10**: 19–26.

Hutson JM, Beasley SW. *Descent of the Testis*. London: Arnold, 1992.

Jackson MB, Chilvers C, Pike MC, *et al*. Boys with late descending testes: the source of patients with 'retractile' testes undergoing orchidopexy. *British Medical Journal* 1986a; **293**: 789–90.

Jackson MB, Chilvers C, Pike MC, *et al*. Cryptorchidism: an apparent substantial increase since 1960. *British Medical Journal* 1986b; **293**: 1401–4.

Tsang TM, Bianchi A, Carneiro PMR, Chan YF, McLean J. A study of warm testicular ischaemia and paternity in rats. *Pediatric Surgery International* 1993; **8**: 41–4.

FURTHER READING

Bianchi A. Microvascular orchidopexy for high undescended testes. In Frank JD, Johnson JH (eds). *Operative Paediatric Urology*. Edinburgh: Churchill Livingstone, 1990; pp. 113–22.

De Muinck Keizer-Schrama SMPF, Hazebroek FWJ. The treatment of cryptorchidism: why, how, when. Clinical studies in prepubertal boys. PhD thesis. Rotterdam: Erasmus University, 1986.

Hadziselimovic F, Herzog B, Girard J. Cryptorchidism. *European Journal of Pediatrics* 1987; **146**: S1–68.

Woodhouse CRJ. Undescended testes. In: Woodhouse CRJ (ed). *Long Term Paediatric Urology*. Oxford: Blackwell Scientific, 1991.

Head and neck disorders

BEN HARTLEY

Learning objectives

- To be able to carry out the clinical assessment of child with a neck lump and to know when to investigate.
- To understand the diagnosis and management of neck infections.
- To understand the embryology and surgical principles of thyroglossal and branchial anomalies.
- To understand the classification and management principles of congenital vascular lesions.
- To know when to suspect head and neck malignancy and when to biopsy.

INTRODUCTION

Neck swellings in children are relatively common. The majority are due to reactive lymphadenopathy associated with tonsillitis and other common upper respiratory infections. These are usually self-limiting, but they may progress to cellulitis, suppuration and abscess formation. Chronic infections are less common, but if the swelling persists, then they need to be considered.

Congenital mass lesions may be present at birth, but not infrequently they present in older children. The onset of the swelling may be precipitated by an acute inflammatory episode. These present as central abnormalities (which most commonly are associated with the thyroglossal duct) and lateral branchial anomalies. Congenital vascular lesions are subdivided into two groups: haemangiomas, with a distinctive growth pattern of proliferation and involution, and vascular malformations, which grow with the child.

Among the group of children with common neck swellings are a small number with underlying malignancy. These are most commonly lymphomas and sarcomas. Neuroblastomas and thyroid tumours also should be considered. Squamous carcinoma is rare in children and accounts for only a very small proportion of paediatric head and neck malignancy. For this reason, a child with a neck mass requires a different approach than an adult. It is very important to maintain an index of suspicion for malignancy in all persistent neck swellings in children and to pursue a tissue diagnosis by biopsy (or, less often, by fine-needle aspiration for cytology) when appropriate.

CLINICAL ASSESSMENT OF NECK SWELLING IN CHILDREN

History

- *Duration:* this is important. Swellings that have been present for a few days are likely to represent acute inflammation. After six weeks, a swelling generally is regarded as chronic, and further investigation should be considered. Investigation should be considered earlier than six weeks if there are suspicious clinical features, e.g. rapid enlargement or associated nerve palsies.
- *Size:* very large swellings or swellings that enlarge progressively despite antimicrobial treatment should be considered for further investigation.
- *Age:* most acute lymphadenitis occurs in children older than six months. Swellings occurring at or shortly after birth are likely to be congenital or neoplastic in origin.
- *Associated symptoms:* a preceding upper-respiratory infection is often a feature of inflammatory lymphadenitis. Fever, rhinorrhoea, sore throat and malaise are common. With chronic swellings, enquiries should be made about weight loss, night sweats and swellings elsewhere in the body.
- *Contacts:* enquire about tuberculosis, other infections, and exposure to cats, farm animals and ticks.
- *Medical history:* identify any known illnesses.
- *Family and social history:* identify any familial disease or congenital anomalies and any social factors. If a diagnosis of human immunodeficiency virus (HIV) infection is suspected, then involve a paediatrician with a special interest in infectious diseases.

Examination of the neck

SITE OF THE SWELLING

The site of the swelling within the neck gives important information about the possible aetiology:

Lateral neck swellings

Lymph nodes are distributed throughout the neck, but the most common site is along the superficial and deep cervical chains. The deep cervical chain lies deep to sternomastoid muscle in the upper neck and along its anterior border in the lower neck. Enlarged lymph nodes are the most common cause of lateral neck swellings. The principal differential diagnosis includes congenital anomalies, such as branchial cysts, which may also become acutely inflamed. The differential diagnosis of a lateral neck swelling in a child also includes congenital vascular lesions (haemangiomas and vascular malformations, including lymphatic malformations), benign and malignant neoplasia arising from the neural or connective tissue elements present, and rare secondary metastases.

Central neck swellings

The principal causes of a neck swelling in the central area of the neck around the midline are thyroglossal duct cyst, lymph node and dermoid cyst. It is not uncommon for thyroglossal duct cysts to become acutely inflamed. Less commonly, children can develop inflammatory and neoplastic thyroid disease. Lymphatic malformations occasionally can involve this region.

Parotid swellings

Acute parotitis (mumps) is due to a self-limiting viral infection. Vaccination for measles, mumps and rubella is now reducing the frequency of mumps. Bacterial parotitis may occur in children and may be recurrent; it is usually distinguished from other conditions by its acute painful presentation followed by resolution on antibiotics. Occasionally, chronic inflammatory swelling persists and must be distinguished from neoplasia. Vascular malformations and haemangiomas cause swellings in the parotid region. Magnetic resonance scanning can be very helpful with this differential diagnosis. Occasionally, fine-needle aspiration or biopsy is required to exclude neoplasia. This may be lymphoid or salivary gland in origin. Occasionally, rhabdomyosarcoma or other connective tissue tumours present with a mass in this region.

Submandibular swellings

Enlarged lymph nodes, floor-of-mouth infections, acute sialadenitis and, occasionally, lymphatic vascular malformations or congenital 'plunging' ranula all cause swelling in this region.

Posterior triangle swellings

Most commonly, these are lymph nodes, but branchial anomalies, vascular malformations and, rarely, neoplasia should be considered.

NATURE OF THE SWELLING

Classic signs of acute inflammation may be present, e.g. redness, tenderness and heat. Chronic swellings usually do not show these signs. If abscess formation has occurred, then the clinical sign of fluctuance may be present and the mass may feel cystic. A classical tuberculous abscess lacks the clinical features of acute inflammation ('cold abscess').

HEAD AND NECK EXAMINATION

A careful examination for a source of primary infection should be made. This should include examination of the pharynx, oral cavity, teeth, nose and ears, as well as looking for any cutaneous lesion.

GENERAL EXAMINATION

Fever, tachycardia or rash should be identified. A general examination should include a search for any associated lymphadenopathy and hepatosplenomegaly.

Investigation

The investigation of neck swellings in children is dependent on the clinical assessment. In many cases, no investigation is required. Simple observation of presumed viral infection or antibiotic treatment of bacterial infection with careful clinical follow-up often will result in resolution.

LABORATORY TESTS

See Box 37.1.

If the child is systemically unwell, then a full blood count may demonstrate a neutrophilia consistent with bacterial infection. Occasionally, haematological malignancy may be detected. A monospot test for infectious mononucleosis should be considered. Other serological tests for toxoplasmosis, *Bartonella* (cat-scratch) or cytomegalovirus (CMV) titres should be considered for persistent lymphadenopathy. Mantoux or Heaf tests for tuberculosis may be helpful, particularly in non-immunized children. If the thyroid gland is enlarged, then thyroid function tests and auto-antibody titres should be performed.

RADIOLOGY

See Box 37.2.

There is only a limited place for plain radiographs. Plain films of the chest may be helpful, particularly if tuberculosis

---

Box 37.1 Laboratory investigations

Full blood count
Monospot
Serology: toxoplasmosis, *Bartonella*, cytomegalovirus, HIV
Mantoux or Heaf test

HIV, human immunodeficiency virus.

Box 37.2 Radiology

Plain films, chest, neck: not routine; occasionally helpful for tuberculosis or retropharyngeal abscess

Ultrasound: non-invasive, distinguishes cystic versus solid; provides information regarding lymph-node architecture

CT: may require sedation in children; distinguishes cystic versus solid; gives information regarding architecture of mass and surgical relationships

MRI: usually reserved for persistent soft-tissue masses

CT, computed tomography; MRI, magnetic resonance imaging.

---

is a possibility. Lateral neck films may demonstrate a retropharyngeal mass but are not recommended routinely.

Ultrasound examination of a neck mass is a very useful test. It may provide valuable information without sedation or anaesthesia. Ultrasound will help to determine whether this is cystic or solid lesion. If an abscess is identified, the ultrasound will help in the definition of the anatomical relationships of the abscess and with surgical planning. An experienced ultrasonographer can comment on the internal architecture of lymph nodes and may give rise to a suspicion of malignancy. Computed tomography (CT) scanning may require sedation or even general anaesthesia in small children. Good anatomical detail, however, is provided, and it is helpful in surgical planning. Magnetic resonance imaging (MRI) rarely adds useful information in the case of acute inflammatory lesions, but it is very useful for vascular malformations and salivary-gland and soft-tissue masses.

INFLAMMATORY NECK SWELLINGS

There is a broad differential diagnosis for inflammatory neck swellings in children. The principal causes are listed in Table 37.1.

Specific conditions

VIRAL INFECTIONS

Viral upper-respiratory infections, e.g. with adenovirus, rhinovirus and enterovirus (coxsackie A and B), may cause reactive lymphadenopathy. This is generally self-limiting and of a short duration.

Infectious mononucleosis is caused by Epstein–Barr virus and is frequently associated with cervical lymphadenopathy, which may be massive. Fever, fatigue, malaise and an exudative tonsillitis are characteristic. Other lymphoid tissue, including liver and spleen, may be enlarged. Serological tests, including Monospot and Paul Bunnel, usually confirm the diagnosis. There is a characteristic picture on the blood film with the presence of atypical lymphocytes. In cases where the acute tonsillitis is associated with airway obstruction, steroids are used and intravenous antibiotics given to treat any coexistent bacterial infection. On occasion, endotracheal intubation may be required to protect the airway until the swelling subsides. Cases with hepatosplenomegaly should be managed in cooperation with a paediatrician.

HIV infection is associated with repeated opportunistic infections. The majority of paediatric HIV infections are acquired from the mother by vertical transmission. Acute infection may mimic infectious mononucleosis. Persistent generalized lymphadenopathy including the cervical nodes becomes a feature as the disease progresses. Weight loss and recurrent fevers occur. Following HIV infection, it may be years or decades before the full acquired immune deficiency

Table 37.1 *Inflammatory causes of neck swelling in children*

Infectious disorders	Inflammatory disorders
Viral:	Kawasaki syndrome
Upper respiratory: rhinovirus, adenovirus, enterovirus	Sarcoidosis
Common childhood illnesses: measles, mumps, rubella, varicella	Sinus histiocytosis with massive lymphadenopathy
Infectious mononucleosis	Kikuchi–Fujimoto disease
Cytomegalovirus	PFAPA syndrome
HIV	
Bacterial:	
Acute lymphadenitis: *Streptococcus, Staphylococcus*, less commonly Gram-negative organisms	
Suppurative lymphadenitis with deep or superficial neck abscess: usually pyogenic organisms (*Streptococcus, Staphylococcus*)	
Mycobacterial: tuberculous or 'atypical' mycobacterial	
Other chronic bacterial infections: cat-scratch disease, actinomycosis, brucellosis, tularaemia, bubonic plague, syphilis	
Fungal:	
Histoplasmosis, uncommon fungal infections (immunocompromised host), *Candida, Aspergillus*	
Parasitic:	
Toxoplasmosis, filariasis	

HIV, human immunodeficiency virus; PFAPA, periodic fever, apthous stomatitis, pharyngitis, cervical adenitis.

syndrome (AIDS) develops. There is significant evidence of increased life expectancy with early retroviral treatment. Investigation and management should be in cooperation with a specialist in paediatric infectious diseases.

BACTERIAL INFECTIONS

Acute lymphadenopathy with suppuration

Group A beta-haemolytic *Streptococcus* and *Staphylococcus aureus* are the most common causative organisms for suppuration in the neck. Other bacteria that may be implicated include anaerobes (19 per cent) *Haemophilus influenzae* and *Moraxella catarrhalis* (Brodsky *et al.* 1992).

Cervical abscesses

Bacterial infection within a cervical lymph node may progress to cause local cellulitis and abscess. Occasionally, a solid mass of inflammatory tissue forms due to coalescence of a group of lymph nodes; this is referred to as a phlegmon. The distinction between phlegmon and abscess is important, as abscesses usually require surgical drainage whereas phlegmon settle with intravenous antibiotics. The most important assessment is clinical. Abscesses are tender and usually reddened and exhibit the clinical sign of fluctuance, confirming their cystic nature. Imaging is helpful but not absolute. The choice is between ultrasound and CT scanning. Ultrasound has the advantage of not requiring anaesthesia or sedation and being readily available and inexpensive. CT scanning gives the surgeon more precise anatomical detail with regard to the relationships between the abscess and surrounding structures, particularly the great vessels, which is helpful in planning surgical drainage. Both these tests have an incidence of false-negative findings. If there is strong clinical suspicion of an abscess, then the area should be explored surgically, even if imaging suggests a solid nature to the swelling.

The treatment of neck abscesses is surgical drainage. This may be performed by a neck incision, which is ideal for superficial lesions and the majority of deep cervical abscesses. Some surgeons advocate the intra-oral route for parapharyngeal and retropharyngeal collections.

Mycobacterial infections

There are two groups of mycobacterial infections that involve the neck in children. The distinction between the two is important and can be challenging. The first group comprises infections caused by *Mycobacterium tuberculosis* (TB). The second comprises infections caused by other mycobacteria. Most accurately, the latter are termed non-tuberculous mycobacteria (NTM); commonly, however, they are referred to as atypical mycobacteria. They include *Mycobacterium avium intracellulare*, *Mycobacterium scrofulaceum*, *Mycobacterium fortuitum* and *Mycobacterium haemophilum*.

The usual presentation of mycobacterial neck infections is of a painless, firm, enlarging mass in the neck. In NTM infection, the overlying skin frequently is discoloured. In children with tuberculosis, weight loss, fever and anorexia may be present. There may be associated cough and respiratory symptoms.

The differential diagnosis also includes lymphoma. If a mass lesion persists without developing into an acute abscess or discharging, then it may be necessary to obtain a tissue diagnosis (from either needle-aspiration cytology or open biopsy) to exclude lymphoma. Biopsy specimens are sent for both histopathological examination and microbiology, including staining and culture specific to mycobacterium. The typical histopathological appearances of tuberculosis are of caseating granuloma formation. Acid- and alcohol-fast staining bacilli may be seen. It may, however, not be possible histopathologically to distinguish tuberculous from non-tuberculous mycobacterial infection. Culture of the mycobacterium may take several weeks. In such cases, all patients should be assessed by a paediatrician with a special interest in infectious diseases, as occasionally empirical treatment with anti-tuberculous therapy may be appropriate until the diagnosis is confirmed. A chest X-ray should be carried out to identify features of tuberculosis. A tuberculous skin test is often helpful.

A positive test in a non-immunized population, such as in the USA or children aged under 13 years in most regions of the UK, is highly suggestive of tuberculous infection. Unfortunately, there is an incidence of positive testing with NTM infection, and this test is not absolutely diagnostic for tuberculosis. Genetic probing of the cultured organisms can also be used to try to make the distinction between tuberculous and non-tuberculous mycobacterial infection.

Treatment of non-tuberculous mycobacterial infections
NTM neck infections are chronic and resistant to medical treatment but ultimately self-limiting after a period of around 18 months. If anatomically suitable, they are preferably managed by complete surgical excision of the involved nodes. If this is possible, then the disease can be controlled quickly and further treatment is not necessary. A neat surgical scar results and is preferable to the scarring that occurs if a lesion is treated medically and a fistula forms. Prolonged medical therapy is an alternative. With medical therapy, it is not unusual for the mass to persist for up to 18 months.

If the nodes have been breached by the infection and there has been spread into the surrounding tissue, then there is a risk of skin breakdown and fistula formation. These fistulas often persist for months. Once a fistula has formed, there is a strong pressure to perform surgery, as it is extremely disruptive to the life of an otherwise well child. Curettage has been advocated as a treatment for infection that has spread beyond the lymph nodes and is not amenable to complete excision. This may reduce the duration of the disease, but complete excision is preferable.

Primary medical treatment of non-tuberculous neck masses has been advocated using either macrolide antibiotics based on some *in vitro* experiments or anti-tuberculous therapy. This usually involves prolonged treatment, as the organisms are notoriously resistant to anti-tuberculous therapy.

CONGENITAL HEAD AND NECK MASSES

Thyroglossal abnormalities

Thyroglossal duct cysts are the most common congenital neck swellings in children. They account for 70 per cent of congenital neck abnormalities. They can present at any age but most commonly during the first decade of life.

PRESENTATION AND DIFFERENTIAL DIAGNOSIS

The usual clinical presentation is with an anterior midline neck mass (Figure 37.1) that rises on tongue protrusion. They may be adjacent to the midline, more frequently, on the left. Secondary infection is not uncommon, and they may present with acute inflammation or abscess formation. The principal differential diagnosis is between dermoid cyst and lymph node (both of which are solid). Rarely, a lymphangioma occurs at this location. These are usually multicystic and irregular or

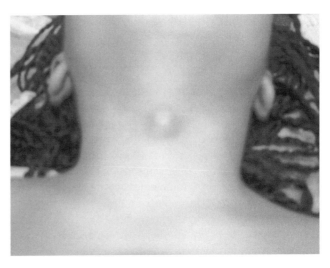

Figure 37.1 *Thyroglossal cyst.*

oval-shaped rather than round. A thyroid mass or unusual neoplasm should be considered in the case of solid lesions.

EMBRYOLOGY

The thyroid anlage appears towards the end of the third week of gestation as an invagination of the endodermal cells on the floor of the primitive pharynx between the tuberculum impar and the copula, which go on to form the tongue. In the adult, this area corresponds to the foramen caecum at the junction of the posterior one-third and anterior two-thirds of the tongue. The thyroid anlage migrates caudally to form a bilobed diverticulum in the neck, which becomes the thyroid gland. The tract forms an epithelial lined tube known as the thyroglossal duct, which atrophies. The duct lies ventral to the hyoid bone but hooks up around the inferior border before descending into the neck.

Histopathological studies of resection specimens have demonstrated that the thyroglossal duct has multiple lateral branches, or arborizations (Pelausa and Forte 1989). It is these lateral branches that underlie the need for a wide surgical approach and explain the relatively high recurrence rates in the literature for excision of thyroglossal duct cysts.

SURGERY

The early operation was a simple incision and drainage procedure. High recurrence rates prompted Schlange in 1893 to propose excision of the cyst and central portion of the hyoid bone, reducing the recurrence rate to approximately 20 per cent. In 1920, Sistrunk concurred with Schlange but counselled against any attempt to locate the thyroglossal duct remnant proximal to the hyoid and advocated removal of a core of tissue from the hyoid bone to the foramen caecum. Although he did not state it at the time, it is clear that in adding this extra component, Sistrunk was excising the lateral branches of the thyroglossal duct into the tongue base. The recurrence rate with this procedure is much lower.

RECURRENCE OF THYROGLOSSAL DUCT CYSTS AND THE NEED FOR WIDER SURGERY

There is wide variation in the range of surgery performed, although the majority of surgeons describe the procedure they perform as the Sistrunk procedure . Surgery is often performed poorly, with an excision of less tissue than advocated in the classical Sistrunk operation. The overall recurrence rates for thyroglossal duct cyst surgery in the larger series in the literature are high (9–26 per cent) (Pelausa and Forte 1989). This has prompted several surgeons to employ wider surgical excisions, with various terminologies but the same principle. Howard and Lund (1986) reported 63 cases treated with an anterior block dissection of the neck with only one recurrence. Other authors have also reported low recurrence rates for wider procedures.

In conclusion, for a primary operation, with the surgeon performing the Sistrunk operation in its classic form (with an excision of the central part of the hyoid and a wide core of tongue muscle above the hyoid and no attempt to identify the tract itself), a recurrence rate in the order of three to five per cent can be expected. The wider operations (anterior or central neck dissection) offer a recurrence rate of zero to two per cent and should be considered for recurrent thyroglossal duct cysts. Some surgeons (including the author) practise wider surgery as a primary operation. Anything less than a classic Sistrunk procedure has an unacceptable recurrence rate.

Lateral head and neck cysts and sinuses

The congenital abnormalities of the lateral part of the head and neck fall into four clinicopathological groups, as follows:

PRE-AURICULAR SINUSES

The external ear forms by fusion of the six auricular hillocks derived from the first and second branchial arches. The common pre-auricular sinus is an abnormality of fusion of the auricular hillocks and is always situated anterior-superior to the tragus. It is frequently bilateral and has multiple branches. An asymptomatic sinus may be noticed after birth. Inflammation and abscess formation in the sinus are not uncommon. Current practice is to perform surgery only if lesions are symptomatic. The traditional sinusectomy approach with injection of methylene blue dye is associated with high recurrence rates, and wider local excisions are now preferred. Pre-auricular sinus should not be confused with first branchial cleft cysts and sinuses (see below). Importantly, surgery for pre-auricular sinuses can be performed without identification of the facial nerve.

SECOND BRANCHIAL CLEFT ABNORMALITIES

These traditionally are referred to as branchial cysts and branchial fistulae. As the second arch mesoderm proliferates, it migrates caudally lateral to the third and fourth arches, towards the epicardial ridge. In doing so, it temporarily creates the cervical sinus, which subsequently is obliterated. The conventional explanation for the formation of branchial cysts is the persistence of the cervical sinus with the formation of a cyst. If the second arch fails to fuse with the epicardial ridge, then an external opening persists, usually along the anterior border of the sternomastoid. The external opening has a tract that follows a course towards the internal second pouch, which forms the tonsillar fossa. The external opening and tract together are commonly referred to as a branchial fistula (although usually this is not a true fistula, as there is rarely a communication between the two epithelial surfaces). Other theories of origin have been suggested for branchial cysts. The most popular alternative is that the cyst develops from degeneration of a lymph node. In support of this theory, there is often a large amount of lymphoid tissue in the cyst, and branchial cysts may present in later life.

Surgical excision of branchial cysts and fistulae involves an excision around any external opening and following the tract, together with any associated cyst, through the structures of the neck to its termination at the pharyngeal wall adjacent to the tonsil.

The child's parents should be warned that more than one surgical incision may be required (a stepladder incision). Unlike in thyroglossal cysts and pre-auricular sinus surgery, recurrence is rare.

FIRST BRANCHIAL CLEFT ABNORMALITIES

These are rare and are regarded as abnormalities of development of the ear canal, which forms from the first branchial cleft. They present as cysts or sinuses around the ear or, occasionally, along the border of the mandible. They may communicate with the ear canal or middle ear structures. A classification was suggested by Work, based on anatomical and histopathological features. In essence, a type 1 lesion presents as a cystic mass and is purely ectodermal, with no relation to the facial nerve. A type 2 lesion presents as a cyst sinus or fistula and may run deep to the facial nerve or its branches. In performing surgery for first branchial cleft anomalies, an incision for a superficial parotidectomy should be performed and the facial nerve identified and preserved.

THIRD AND FOURTH POUCH SINUSES

These lesions are also referred to as pyriform fossa sinuses. There is some discussion as to whether they arise from the third or fourth branchial pouch, as both structures together form part of the pyriform fossa. The clinical presentation is usually of recurrent neck abscesses. A subsequent barium swallow may reveal an internal opening in the pyriform fossa. This can be confirmed by endoscopy (rigid pharyngolaryngoscopy). The lesion is almost invariably on the left side. In the presence of recurrent neck abscesses, consider endoscopy, even if the barium swallow is normal, as radiology can miss the sinus.

Chronic suppuration in the neck around the superior lobe of the thyroid results. Surgical excision involves removal of the infected area, usually together with the superior lobe of the thyroid and identification of the tract, following it to the pyriform fossa mucosa. Endoscopic placement of a catheter in the sinus aids surgical excision.

CONGENITAL VASCULAR LESIONS

Previously, tremendous confusion existed with regard to the classification and treatment of congenital vascular lesions. More recently, a practical classification proposed by Mulliken and Glowacki (1982) has been adopted widely. This divides the lesions into two distinct groups, based on pathophysiology and clinical behaviour.

The two groups are haemangiomas and vascular malformations. The principal clinical difference is that haemangiomas involute spontaneously in the first few years of life, whereas vascular malformations do not; instead, they grow with the child.

Haemangiomas

These lesions form from endothelial cells in the walls of capillaries. They are flat or absent at birth, but in the first few weeks of life they undergo a rapid proliferation. This is apparently in response to secretion of a growth factor known as alpha-fibroblast-derived growth factor. After 9–12 months, they enter a stationary phase without growth before involuting at age three to five years. Involution as late as 12 years has been reported. Cutaneous lesions are often red, as they are superficial and involve the skin (the traditional 'strawberry naevus'). The lesions, however, may be placed more deeply and may not discolour the skin at all.

The conventional approach to haemangiomas is simply to observe the lesion and await spontaneous involution. The exception is those lesions that impinge on function, such as vision or airway, which merit intervention. Haemangiomas often reduce in size when treated with corticosteroids. This effect may be temporary. If treatment is required, then a choice must be made between prolonged steroid treatment and surgical intervention. Prolonged steroid treatment may have major side effects, with weight gain, hypertension and all the features of Cushing syndrome. Surgical excision will leave a scar. There is an emerging role for laser treatment of haemangiomas.

It should be mentioned that although watchful waiting is usually the best management for haemangiomas that do not cause a functional disturbance, i.e. cosmetic lesions, it is increasingly being documented that watchful waiting is associated with significant scar formation due to stretching and then atrophy of the skin and subcutaneous fat, possibly with telangiectasia formation, prompting earlier cosmetic intervention in selected cases.

Vascular malformations

These are almost always present at birth and enlarge slowly by hypertrophy. They neither proliferate nor involute. They are structural abnormalities that exhibit a normal rate of endothelial turnover, enlarging slowly as they child ages.

They are subdivided into low-flow lesions, including venous malformations and lymphatic malformations (also called lymphangiomas and cystic hygromas), and high-flow lesions, which are arteriovenous malformations. MRI is very helpful in distinguishing between the different lesions, with the use of angiography or ultrasound in selected cases. High-flow lesions often are intracranial and managed in conjunction with neurosurgery. Two specific lesions have particular relevance to paediatric surgery: cystic hygromas and venous malformations.

LYMPHATIC MALFORMATIONS (CYSTIC HYGROMAS)

Lymphatic malformations are not uncommon. In the head and neck, they are referred to as cystic hygromas. Surgery for cystic hygromas is complex, as the lesions tend to entangle and adhere to major vessels and nerves of the head and neck. The traditional view has been that they are impossible to excise completely; however, this has not been the author's experience and, with a meticulous comprehensive neck dissection from skull base to clavicle, the majority of lesions can be excised (Figures 37.2 and 37.3). Lesions with extensive tongue involvement are a notable exception. Sclerotherapy remains an alternative, using traditional alcohol-based agents or, more recently, OK432 (a sclerotherapy agent derived from streptococcal antigen; at the time of writing, it was not approved in the USA by the Food and Drug Administration (FDA) for this purpose, but it is now used widely in Europe). Sclerotherapy reactions with massive swelling and abscess formation are not uncommon. Multiple injection treatments may be required to reduce the size of the lesion. Surgery following sclerotherapy is more difficult. For these reasons, it is the author's practice to recommend primary surgical excision for the majority of head and neck cystic hygromas.

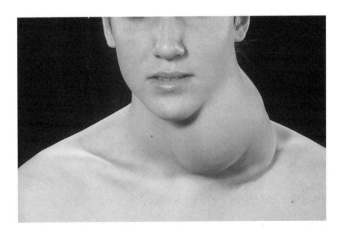

Figure 37.2 *Preoperative cystic hygroma.*

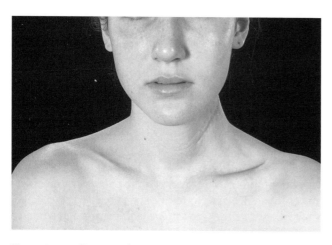

Figure 37.3   *Postoperative cystic hygroma, following extended neck dissection.*

VENOUS MALFORMATIONS

Venous malformations usually cause a bluish swelling that is compressible. If superficial venules are involved, then the term 'venular malformation' may be used. Surgical excision of venous malformations may be associated with massive bleeding and difficult haemostasis. Surgery may be appropriate, but surgeons should be aware that there is a mortality associated with surgery for venous malformations, which often are cosmetic lesions. The use of minimally invasive techniques, such as various types of laser therapy and, occasionally, sclerotherapy, for these lesions has shown some success, and they are best referred to a centre with a special interest.

CONGENITAL MUSCULAR TORTICOLLIS (STERNOMASTOID TUMOUR OF INFANCY)

This is caused by unilateral contracture of the sternocleidomastoid muscle. Fibrosis within the muscle leads to shortening. This tilts the head to the ipsilateral side and rotates the chin to the opposite side.

The deformity may be noticed at or soon after birth. Within the first two weeks of life, a 'fibrous tumour' becomes palpable. The mass persists for about a month and then regresses, leaving contracture. Ultrasound examination confirms the nature of the mass. Treatment is with passive stretching exercises. If this is started within the first three months and carried out regularly, then there is a 90 per cent chance of successful correction. If this management fails, then surgical division of the heads of the muscle is performed, with postoperative splinting and exercises.

DERMOID LESIONS

These lesions contain ectodermal and mesodermal elements and are located around the midline at various sites, including

the nose and neck. Occasionally, they are located around the orbit.

Nasal dermoids usually present as a mass or sinus along the nasal dorsum. These lesions may have an associated tract communicating with the anterior cranial fossa. In this situation, an intracranial approach may be required to excise the lesion completely. All nasal dermoids should have preoperative imaging to identify an intracranial connection. MRI has a higher sensitivity than CT for detecting soft-tissue abnormalities, although CT scanning gives better detail of bony abnormalities. In complex cases, some surgeons would advocate both forms of imaging.

If imaging has excluded an intracranial connection, then the lesion is excised via an external approach. Incisions on the nasal dorsum give poor cosmesis, and the external rhinoplasty approach with a nasal columella incision is preferred. Lesions high in the glabellar region may be unsuitable for an external rhinoplasty approach, and the use of a bicoronal flap should be considered. This does require extensive dissection, and occasionally horizontal ('gull-wing') incision in the glabellar region is preferred.

Lesions with intracranial connection are excised in conjunction with neurosurgery utilizing an intracranial approach. There has been some success with endoscopic intranasal surgery for selected lesions extending from the nose towards the skull base. With these techniques, avoiding a craniotomy (with the associated five per cent risk of postoperative epilepsy) may be possible.

Orbital dermoids constitute five per cent of orbital masses. They appear most commonly in the upper outer quadrant (external angular dermoids). Superficial lesions present with a mass, while deeper lesions may cause proptosis. Treatment is surgical excision.

PAEDIATRIC HEAD AND NECK MALIGNANCY

Cancer is the second largest childhood killer after accidents. An estimated five per cent of primary malignant tumours in childhood occur in the head and neck. However, one in every four paediatric malignancies eventually involves this area.

This is a complex field because of the diverse pathologic nature of the malignancies encountered and because of the close and complex anatomical relationships of the structures of the head and neck. All paediatric malignancy should be managed by a multidisciplinary team. The role of the surgeon remains a very important one, both in diagnosis and in the treatment of selected lesions.

The spectrum of disease is quite different to adult head and neck malignancy. For example, squamous cell carcinoma, which accounts for the vast majority of adult head and neck malignancy, accounts for less than two per cent of paediatric tumours in this part of the body (Cunningham *et al.* 1987).

The most common lesions are lymphomas and sarcomas, which are usually managed with chemotherapy or, occasionally,

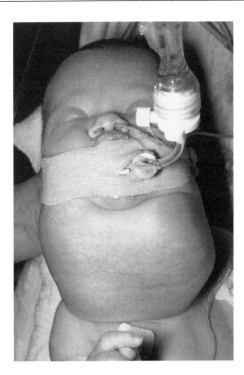

Figure 37.4 *Preoperative teratoma.*

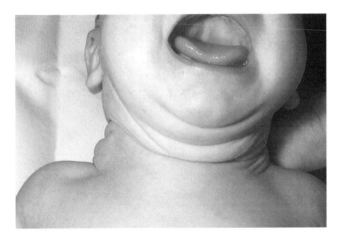

Figure 37.5 *Postoperative teratoma (tracheostomy can be avoided).*

radiotherapy. The surgeon's role in these lesions is to establish an early accurate diagnosis. The principles of awareness of malignancy and the roles of cytology and quality open biopsies are discussed earlier in the section on assessment. Some sarcomas and other tumours are best treated surgically (Figures 37.4 and 37.5) or with combination therapy. A detailed description of the management of these tumours is beyond the scope of this chapter, and a specialist text regarding surgical treatment of head and neck malignancy should be consulted.

CLINICAL SCENARIOS

Case 1

A three-year-old girl presents with a 4-cm left submandibular mass of three weeks' duration and no other symptoms. Ultrasound scan confirms a solid enlarged lymph node adjacent to the submandibular gland. Atypical mycobacterial infection is suspected and confirmed by excision biopsy of the lesion via a submandibular approach.

Case 2

A one-year-old child presents with a 10-cm soft neck mass, which appeared following a mild upper respiratory infection. Examination reveals a soft cystic mass in the lateral neck. Ultrasound confirms multicystic nature. MRI scan defines the exact surgical anatomy. Surgical excision is performed by selective neck dissection, with identification and preservation of all related cranial nerves.

Case 3

A 2-week-old baby presents with a 2-cm firm lateral neck mass and torticollis. Ultrasound confirms a mass within the sternomastoid muscle. Physiotherapy is commenced for three months, with resolution of the mass and torticollis.

REFERENCES

Brodsky L, Belles W, Brody A, *et al.* Needle aspiration of neck abscesses in children. *Clinical Pediatrics* 1992; **31**: 71–6.

Cunningham MJ, Myers EN, Bluestone CD. Malignant tumours of the head and neck in children: a 20 year review. *International Journal of Pediatric Otorhinolaryngology* 1987; **13**: 279.

Howard DJ, Lund VJ. Thyroglossal ducts, cysts and sinuses a recurrent problem. *Annals of the Royal College of Surgeons of England* 1986; **68**: 137–9.

Mulliken JB, Glowacki J. Hemangiomas and vascular malformations in infants and children: a classification based on endothelial characteristics. *Plastic and Reconstructive Surgery* 1982; **69**: 412–22.

Pelausa MEO, Forte VF. Sistrunk re-visited: a 10 year review of revision thyroglossal duct surgery at Toronto's Hospital for Sick Children. *Journal of Otolaryngology* 1989; **18**: 325–33.

FURTHER READING

Bluestone CD, Stool SE, Alper CM, *et al. Paediatric Otolaryngology*, 4th edn. Philadelphia, PA: Saunders, 2002.

Cummings CW, Flint PW, Harker LA. *Paediatric Otolaryngology: Head and Neck Surgery*, 3rd edn. St Louis, MO: Mosby, 2005.

38

Head injury

DOROTHY LANG

Learning objectives

- To know the patterns of head injury in childhood.
- To understand the pathophysiological changes that occur after head injury.
- To understand how to carry out a basic clinical assessment of a head-injured child and to recognize the indications to transfer selected patients to neurosciences or paediatric intensive care.
- To understand the principles of managing raised intracranial pressure.

BACKGROUND

Head injury in children is common. Different patterns and modes of injury are seen in different age groups. Minor head injury usually results in a full recovery: less than one in 800 head-injured children admitted for neurological observations go on to develop serious complications.

CAUSES

Common causes of head injury in children include:

- road traffic accidents (most common cause of death in childhood);
- cycling accidents (20 per cent);
- non-accidental injury (NAI; 25 per cent of all head-injured children under two years of age admitted to hospital);
- falls from domestic furniture, trees, walls, etc.;
- penetrating injury.

Over the past two decades, measures aimed at preventing head injury have gained more attention. Initiatives include specially designed car seats for children and cycle helmets; children who wear a cycle helmet have an 85 per cent reduction in the risk of head injury.

Of recent interest is the concept of genetic vulnerability of the brain to injury. There is evidence to suggest an association between certain patterns of apolipoprotein E (apoE) genotypes and a patient's vulnerability to head injury. This has implications for therapeutic intervention as well as prediction of outcome.

The mortality from serious head injury has been reduced because of improved understanding of the pathophysiology of traumatic brain injury and improvement in neurocritical care.

NEUROPATHOLOGY

Head injury can result in soft-tissue injuries to the head, injury to the skull vault or skull base, and injury to the brain.

Soft-tissue injuries

These are rarely life-threatening. The exception is extensive laceration of the scalp in a small infant, where blood loss and depletion of circulating blood volume may lead to haemodynamic instability and/or circulatory collapse.

Cephalhaematomas

These can be either subgaleal or subperiosteal. The former can occur with or without a linear fracture and may cross suture lines. The infant will have a soft fluctuant mass. Blood transfusion may be required. Haematomas located below the periosteum are usually seen only in newborns, sometimes relating to scalp monitoring or birth trauma. The sutures limit extension of the haematoma. Eighty per cent resorb within two to three weeks, often associated with jaundice due to absorption. They may calcify, but most do not need treatment. Surgery may be required for cosmetic reasons.

Injury to the skull vault

Vault injury may result in a skull fracture. These can be linear or depressed, compound or non-compound. The so-called 'ping-pong ball fracture' may occur in the newborn. In a cosmetically unimportant area, an expectant policy can be adopted. In the frontal region, elevation is required for cosmetic reasons. An extensive linear skull fracture with wide separation of the fracture edges in early childhood and an underlying dural tear may produce a so-called 'growing skull fracture'. This is rare (0.05–0.6 per cent of all skull fractures), but it is important to recognize and treat it. Dural repair and cranioplasty are required.

Damage to the cranio-orbital facial skeleton may produce complex patterns of injury, with aesthetic and functional sequelae.

Skull–base injury

Injury to the skull base is under-diagnosed. Usually, the injury affects the anterior cranial fossa floor (ACF) or the petrous temporal bone. A range of complications may occur, including cerebrospinal fluid (CSF) leak, cranial nerve damage, e.g. anosmia, blindness (if the ACF is affected), hearing loss, vestibular dysfunction and traumatic facial palsy (following temporal bone fractures).

Brain injury

There are a number of ways of classifying brain injury. Clinicians tend to refer to 'minor', 'moderate' and 'severe' head injury. Head injury can be isolated or associated with an extracranial injury. In addition, in the clinical setting, the classification into primary and secondary brain damage is useful.

Primary damage is impact damage. Impact damage includes contusions, haematomas and injury to axons. Secondary injury occurs after the impact. Hypoxia is a major problem within minutes of injury. The brain comprises only two per cent of the body mass but demands 13 per cent of the cardiac output and consumes 20 per cent of the oxygen carried by the blood. Thereafter, secondary injury may occur because of hypoxia, hypotension or raised intracranial pressure (ICP). Furthermore, after brain injury, a complex cascade of neurochemical reactions occurs. Neurotransmitters such as glutamate, calcium and free radicals may be released, and the resultant uncontrolled neuronal activity may lead to cell death.

Brain injury can also be classified according to the imaging findings on computed tomography (CT) scans. Neurosurgeons find this classification useful for diagnosis and treatment as well as for assessing prognosis. Neuropathological studies would tend to indicate that head-injured children sustain similar patterns of brain damage to adults, albeit that age-specific features have been emphasized.

NON-ACCIDENTAL INJURY

In non-accidental head injury, the most common neuropathological findings are skull fractures (36 per cent), subdural haemorrhage (72 per cent) and retinal haemorrhage (71 per cent). The most common cause of death in NAI is raised ICP secondary to brain swelling. Hypoxic brain damage is found in 77 per cent. In general, infants who have sustained NAI typically present with apnoea or respiratory dysfunction, have axonal injury at the craniocervical junction, a skull fracture and subdural haemorrhage; they tend not to have extracranial injuries. By contrast, in older children (over one year of age), extracranial injury, especially abdominal trauma, is more common.

CLINICAL MANAGEMENT

Initial assessment is in the accident and emergency (A&E) department. The vast majority of head-injured children are discharged home under the supervision of a responsible parent or guardian with written advice on re-attendance. A child suspected of sustaining NAI who would otherwise be discharged home should be referred to paediatric services for assessment.

Children with a history of loss of consciousness, vomiting or headache, or a skull fracture, should be admitted to a paediatric service for neurological observation.

Children with moderate or severe head injury and those with multiple injuries and a head injury of any severity should be assessed using advanced trauma life support (ATLS)/paediatric advanced life support (PALS) principles. Airway and cervical spine control, breathing and ventilation, circulatory control and management are emphasized initially. The pupillary responses should be noted and the conscious level assessed using the Glasgow Coma Scale (GCS) (Table 38.1). At this stage, the patient may need to be intubated, sedated and ventilated. Mandatory monitoring includes electrocardiography (ECG), pulse oximetry and blood pressure. Blood gas analysis should be done and ventilation adjusted to ensure normocapnia and a minimum partial pressure of oxygen in the arterial blood (PaO_2) of 90 mmHg. Volume replacement to ensure normovolaemia is required.

The emphasis then shifts to identification of extracranial injuries, pain control and more detailed assessment of neurological function. After resuscitation and assessment, essential investigations should be organized, e.g. C-spine X-ray, CT scan or trauma protocol, provided that full monitoring is in place to detect and treat secondary insults. In paediatric practice, significant brain injury may occur in the absence of a skull fracture; therefore, the threshold for scanning a child is much lower than in adult practice (Figure 38.1).

The impact on the brain of hypoxia and hypotension needs to be understood and applied in practice (Table 38.2).

Children with severe head injury, and those with minor or moderate head injury in association with extracranial injuries, should be transferred to a paediatric intensive care unit (PICU) with access to an on-site neurocritical care unit (NCCU). Transfer should not be carried out until the patient has been resuscitated and is stable. Specialist PICU retrieval teams are often able to transfer such patients. The exception is the child with a CT scan that has identified a surgical lesion, e.g. an acute extradural haematoma (EDH); such children should be transferred without delay by the referring team to a neurosurgical theatre for emergency intervention.

Observation in the paediatric ward includes monitoring of respiratory function, blood pressure, conscious level and neurological signs, including pupils. Observations should be recorded as frequently as necessary on standard head injury observation charts. The GCS score not only reflects the severity

Table 38.1 *Glasgow Coma Scale (GCS)*

	Adult	Child	GCS score
Eye-opening	Spontaneous	Spontaneous	4
	To speech	To sound	3
	To pain	To pain	2
	None	None	1
Verbal response	Oriented	Age-appropriate	5
	Confused	Cries	4
	Monosyllabic	Irritable	3
	Incomprehensible sounds	Lethargic	2
	None	None	1
Motor response	Obeys commands	Age-appropriate	6
	Localizes pain	Localizes pain	5
	Flexion to pain	Flexion to pain	4
	Spastic flexion	Spastic flexion	3
	Extension	Extension	2
	None	None	1

Table 38.2 *Effect of hypoxia and hypotension on outcome of brain injury*

	Patients (*n*)	Dead (%)	Good recovery (%)
Hypoxia and hypotension	5	100	0
Hypotension	12	75	8
Hypoxia	29	59	17
Neither	104	34	34

Source: Gentleman and Jennett (1981).

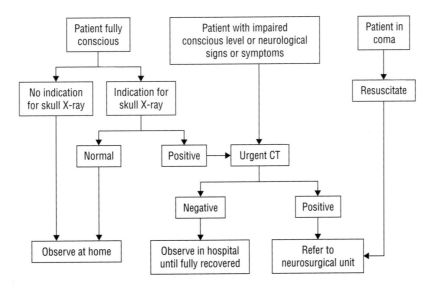

Figure 38.1 *Management of head injuries. A skull X-ray is not needed if a computed tomography (CT) scan is to be done. From Teasdale GM, Murray G, Anderson E, et al. Risks of traumatic intracranial haematoma in children and adults: implications for managing head injuries.* British Medical Journal *1990;* **300***: 363–7.*

of the injury but also has prognostic implications. If CT scanning was done within six hours of injury, then it should be repeated before discharge.

More severely injured children will be managed in a neurosurgical paediatric facility, NCCU or PICU. Initial management tends to be dictated by the CT findings (Table 38.3).

The importance of this classification is also reflected in the fact that the CT findings are strong indicants of outcome. Patients with diffuse brain injury (DBI) and no visible pathology (NVP) have a mortality rate of ten per cent, but the mortality rate is 50 per cent in patients with DBI 4.

GUIDELINES FOR TRANSFER TO REGIONAL NEUROSURGICAL UNIT

In the UK, currently only a small proportion (three to five per cent) of head-injured patients are transferred to a regional neurosurgical unit (NSU) (Table 38.4).

Table 38.3 *Computed tomography (CT) scanning classification in head injury*

Classification	CT findings
DBI	
1	NVP
2	Basal cisterns present: no lesions >25 mL in volume and/or midline shift <5 mm
3	Compressed or absent cisterns, midline shift 0–5 mm and no lesions >25 mL
4	Midline shift >5 mm and no lesion >25 mL
Intracranial mass lesion	
5	Mass lesion not evacuated
6	Mass lesion evacuated

DBI, diffuse brain injury; NVP, no visible pathology.

Table 38.4 *Indications for urgent discussion and possible transfer of a head-injured patient to a neurosurgical unit*

Coma
  GCS less than 9 after resuscitation
  Deteriorating level of consciousness or progressive foca
   neurological deficits
  Fracture of the skull with any of the following:
  Confusion or deteriorating level of consciousness
  Fits or neurological symptoms or signs
Open injury:
  Depressed compound fracture of skull vault
  Base of skull fracture or penetrating injury
Patient fulfils criteria for CT of the head within referring hospital
  but this cannot be performed within a reasonable time (e.g. 2–4 h)
Abnormal CT scan
After neurosurgical opinion on images transferred electronically
Normal CT scan but unsatisfactory progress

GCS, Glasgow Coma Scale; CT, computed tomography.

The patient must be resuscitated and stabilized before transfer, and it is imperative that intensive care is continued during transfer. Transfer of these patients is a major event and requires very careful consideration and detailed preparation. Insults such as hypoxia and hypotension result in increased morbidity and mortality.

MANAGEMENT OF SPECIFIC COMPLICATIONS OF HEAD INJURY

Raised intracranial pressure

ICP monitoring should be carried out only in a NCCU or PICU, where there are on-site neurosurgeons. About 13 per cent of head-injured patients with a normal scan have raised ICP. Indications for ICP monitoring are listed in Box 38.1.

Causes of raised ICP include:

- hypercapnia
- hypoxia
- hyperthermia
- inadequate sedation/analgesia (a frequent cause of elevated ICP, often associated with nursing manoeuvres, e.g. suction).

The following represents a rough guide to the management of raised ICP. Protocols should be agreed and published locally by neurosurgeons, paediatricians and intensivists in referring hospitals and centres treating children with head injury.

In general, ICP should be maintained below 20–25 mmHg in adults and older children. In infants and young children, ICP should be maintained at 5–15 mmHg. A target of 50 mmHg for cerebral perfusion pressure (CPP) is acceptable in young children and infants, but may be safely managed within a range of 30–40 mmHg. Adults and older children (aged over ten years) ideally should have a CPP of 60–70 mmHg. Isolated short-lived spikes of ICP may not need treatment. Protracted spikes of elevated ICP (more than 20 minutes) represent a serious damaging secondary insult with significant implications for outcome.

Box 38.1 Relative indications for intracranial pressure (ICP) monitoring

Coma
Lateralizing neurological signs
CT scan depicting absence of third ventricle and/or basal cisterns
CT scan depicting occult mass lesion
Multiple trauma (treatment for other injuries may adversely affect ICP)
Postoperative, after removal of intradural lesion

CT, computed tomography.

The protocol below should be followed. Simple manoeuvres are followed by more complex strategies. Those marked * are controversial.

1 Remove surgical lesions, e.g. contused brain, haematomas.
2 Elevate head 30–45 degrees* and avoid kinking the neck veins by maintaining central head position.
3 Aim for normovolaemia: use pressors, not fluid boluses, for hypotension.
4 To correct hypovolaemia, use small fluid boluses (1–2 ml/kg of 3% saline). NB: monitor serum osmolarity and avoid 3% saline if osmolarity if over 305 mosm/L.
5 In general, aim for normocapnia. Hypocapnia may be indicated (25–30 mmHg*).
6 If ICP is elevated despite sedation, use osmotic therapy.
7 Mannitol/furosemide (frusemide).
8 Steroids*.
9 Treat hyperglycaemia.
10 Trial paralytic agents.
11 Use external ventricular drain (EVD) to drain CSF.
12 Consider barbiturate coma.
13 In cases with refractory raised ICP and no new surgical lesions, consider decompressive craniectomy.

Depressed skull fracture

SIMPLE DEPRESSED SKULL FRACTURE

If the depression is cosmetically significant, then the depressed fragments can be elevated. Other indications for surgery include mass effect from the fragments or an associated intracranial haematoma. In the midline or over venous sinuses, surgical elevation should be avoided because of the risk of life-threatening haemorrhage.

COMPOUND DEPRESSED OR COMMINUTED SKULL FRACTURE

First aid consists of wound closure after thorough cleaning and removal of foreign bodies. In the absence of a dural tear, this may suffice. Definitive surgery should be carried out as soon as possible if there is a suspected dural laceration, intracranial haematoma or moderate to severe wound contamination. Wound drains should not be used, in order to minimize the risk of infection.

A depressed fracture may be complicated by meningitis or an intracerebral abscess and epilepsy (up to 30 per cent).

Haematoma

EXTRADURAL HAEMATOMA

EDH occurs in 0.5 per cent of head-injured patients admitted to hospital. It may complicate a relatively mild injury. Most patients are under the age of 20 years; it is rare after the age of 40 years. In infants, EDH is rare because of vault pliability and dural adhesion at the site of the sutures. The large head size of the infant relative to the body mass means that the volume of the extradural space is large in relation to the blood volume. Hypovolaemia or circulatory collapse may be the primary presenting feature with an infantile EDH. In an adult or older child, the dura becomes separated from the skull immediately below the point of impact and/or fracture, and a clot of blood develops. Bleeding may be arterial or venous.

In classic cases, after a brief loss of consciousness the patient recovers consciousness, only to subsequently deteriorate – the so-called 'lucid interval'. Intervention before coma, a unilateral dilated pupil, hemiparesis, slow pulse and rise in blood pressure is mandatory if serious morbidity and mortality are to be avoided.

The haematoma must be removed by a neurosurgeon within two hours of the first sign of deterioration. The maximum mortality rate for EDH is ten per cent or less, and many neurosurgeons believe that mortality should approach zero.

ACUTE SUBDURAL HAEMATOMA

Acute subdural haematomas (SDHs) are relatively common. They occur in all age groups. They are associated with significant impact damage and morbidity, and mortality is higher than with extradural haematoma. In general, acute SDH is associated with severe brain damage, which is often frontal or temporal – the so-called 'burst lobe'. SDH may also occur if bridging veins are damaged by acceleration/deceleration or rotational injury.

Acute SDH may also occur in patients with coagulopathy or taking anticoagulants, including aspirin and anti-inflammatories.

In about 15–20 per cent of patients, acute SDH is bilateral. About 50 per cent are associated with a skull fracture. In the vast majority of cases, evacuation is indicated. A poor prognosis is usual because of the associated brain damage. The mortality rate is often over 50 per cent, with an associated high morbidity.

TRAUMATIC INTRACEREBRAL HAEMORRHAGE

This may result from cerebral contusions or a penetrating injury. Serial CT scans have shown that after 24–72 hours, these haematomas are commonly surrounded by an area of oedema and/or ischaemia. Increasing mass effect will lead to a rise in ICP and a decrease in CPP and, ultimately, cerebral blood flow. Although surgical removal of the mass will reduce ICP and therefore secondary insults, ischaemic neuronal damage will result in neurological deficits.

Extra-axial fluid collections in children

Causes of extra-axial fluid collections in children include:

- benign subdural collections
- cerebral atrophy

- 'external hydrocephalus'
- acute subdural haematoma (blood may appear to be low-density if the haematocrit is low).

Benign subdural collections are best referred to as extra-axial collections, as it can be difficult to decide whether they are subdural or subarachnoid. They may result from peri-natal trauma and are more usual in term infants. Intervention is not usually needed.

Symptomatic extra-axial collections may require burr-hole evacuation or installation of a subdural-peritoneal shunt.

Cerebrospinal fluid leaks

A traumatic CSF leaks occurs in about two per cent of closed and nine per cent of penetrating head injuries. A traumatic CSF leak usually appears within the first 48 hours after injury, but it can appear several years later. The severity of the head injury has little if any correlation with the occurrence of a leak.

CSF leak via the nose (rhinorrhoea) is the most common. CSF is clear, tastes salty and does not cause excoriation of the skin. The fluid can be confirmed as CSF by using glucose test strips. In doubtful cases, beta-2-transferrin assays can be done. Beta-2-transferrin is present in CSF but is absent in tears, saliva and nasal secretions. Rhinorrhoea usually stops within one week. The risk of meningitis is around five to ten per cent. The cumulative risk of meningitis in patients with an unre-paired basal dural tear is more than 80 per cent at 20 years. All skull-base fractures should be discussed with a neurosur-geon, as repair may be required. CSF otorrhoea (via the ear) usually stops spontaneously within three weeks, and surgery is required only for persistent leaks.

In the acute phase, conscious patients are nursed head up to reduce the intracranial CSF pressure. There is no evidence to support the use of prophylactic antibiotics.

Bone-windowed CT scans using 2-mm slices in both axial and coronal planes will localize the vast majority of skull-base fistulae. Examination with intrathecal contrast may be required but is only of value in patients with an active CSF leak.

Traumatic aerocele

Air may enter the skull after basal fractures and is usually readily visible on brow-up lateral skull X-rays. The air may be subarachnoid, subdural, intraventricular or intracerebral. Urgent decompression may be required if the aerocele is responsible for a clinical deterioration, but usually a delayed dural repair is required after the patient has recovered from the acute effects of the head injury.

Craniofacial repair

Management of a severe cranio-orbitofacial injury is complex and requires a multidisciplinary approach. Initially, emphasis is focused on the brain injury. Thereafter, the best strategy is a single-stage craniofacial repair. Definitive repair needs to be preceded by CT in axial and coronal planes to visualize frac-tures of the anterior cranial fossa, orbit, skull base and facial skeleton. Three-dimensional CT scans are particularly useful in some complex cases.

Post-traumatic epilepsy

The overall incidence of post-traumatic epilepsy is about three to five per cent. Seizures can occur early (within one week) or late. The risk of late seizures after a mild head injury (no skull fractures and post-traumatic amnesia of less than 30 minutes) is 0.1 per cent after one year and 0.6 per cent after five years.

Post-concussion syndrome

Post-concussion syndrome is characterized by a plethora of symptoms without objective neurological signs that occur after head injury. In the vast majority of cases, the head injury is minor and the cause of the symptoms remains unclear. It is unusual in children but it may present in older children. Careful evaluation and expert involvement of neuropsychol-ogists and educational psychologists is required.

REHABILITATION

Multidisciplinary early rehabilitation is mandatory if poten-tial for recovery is to be realized. The heterogeneous nature of recovery from brain injury is yet to be understood clearly. Motivation, cognitive and behavioural problems in patients with brain injury seem to be a biological issue that is affected by pre-existing cognitive and social skills.

OUTCOME

The development of the Glasgow Outcome Scale (Table 38.5) has been important not only in assessing the individual patient but also in allowing comparison of a variety of treatment options. There are a number of predictors of outcome after severe head injury, including GCS score after resuscitation, pupillary responses, age, ICP and intracranial diagnosis on CT scanning. After severe head injury, overall mortality at six months is 36 per cent in patients looked after in an experi-enced NSU. In non-specialist units, mortality following head injury may vary from 43 per cent less than expected to more than 52 per cent greater than expected. These differences are explained largely by variation in outcome in patients with a low risk of death and not in the high-risk group of patients. There is, therefore, a compelling argument that neurosurgi-cal assessment and supervision are as important for the less severely injured patient as in the severely injured patient. Unfortunately, neurocritical care is under-resourced.

Table 38.5 *Glasgow Outcome Scale*

1	Good recovery: resumption of normal life despite minor deficits
2	Moderate disability (independent but disabled)
3	Severe disability (conscious but dependent)
4	Vegetative state: unresponsive and speechless; after two or three weeks, may open eyes and have sleep/wake cycles
5	Dead

REFERENCE

Gentleman D, Jennett B. Hazards of inter-hospital transfer of comatose head injured patients. *Lancet* 1981; **ii**: 853.

FURTHER READING

American College of Surgeons. *Advanced Trauma Life Support Course Manual*. Washington, DC: American College of Surgeons, 1993.

Brain Trauma Foundation, American Association of Neurological Surgeons, Joint Section on Neurotrauma and Critical Care. Guidelines for the management of severe head injury. *Journal of Neurotrauma* 1996; **13**: 641–734.

Jennett B. *Epilepsy after Non-missile Head Injuries*. London: Heinemann, 1975.

Jennett B, Bond M. Assessment of outcome after severe brain damage. *Lancet* 1975; **i**: 480–84.

Maas AI, Dearden M, Teasdale GM, *et al.* EBIC guidelines for management of severe head injury in adults. European Brain Injury Consortium. *Acta Neurochirurgica* 1997; **139**: 286–94.

Neuroanaesthesia Society of Great Britain and Ireland and the Association of Anaesthetists of Great Britain and Ireland. *Recommendations for the Transfer of Patients with Acute Head Injuries to Neurosurgical Units*. London: Neuroanaesthesia Society of Great Britain and Ireland and the Association of Anaesthetists of Great Britain and Ireland, 1996.

Teasdale GM, Nicoll JAR, Murray G, Fiddes M. Association of apolipoprotein E polymorphism with outcome after head injury. *Lancet* 1997; **350**: 1069–71.

Thermal and chemical burns

HUGH MARTIN

Learning objectives

- To understand the local and systemic effects of burns.
- To be able to assess a child who has been burnt.
- To be able to initiate appropriate management of a child with a burn.
- To be able to determine which children need specialized burn care.
- To understand the principles of physical and emotional rehabilitation of the burnt child.

INTRODUCTION

Burns are one of the most common accidents likely to befall a child. Thermal or chemical injury to the skin sets up a progression of local and systemic effects. Larger burns produce systemic effects, which, in the extreme, are one of the most devastating but potentially recoverable injuries that a human can sustain. The psychosocial background from which the patient comes often has a major contributing influence on the cause of the burn and will shape the way in which the child and his or her family reacts to the burn. In the long term, the quality of the emotional recovery is equally important as the physical recovery. Except for small straightforward burns, treatment is best given by a multidisciplinary group, the burns team.

RELEVANT BASIC SCIENCE

Zones of injury

Jackson (1953) described the model that is a key element in understanding burn injury. When thermal or chemical injury to the skin is sustained, three zones of injury are created (Figure 39.1):

- *Zone of coagulative necrosis* is the tissue that becomes necrotic at the time of the burn incident. If skin cells are subject to temperatures of 44 °C or higher, then metabolic processes are disturbed. Higher temperatures lead to rapid death. Thus, the depth of this zone is

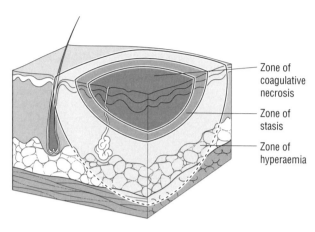

Figure 39.1   *Jacksons's zones of injury.*

governed by the temperature of the injuring agent and the length of exposure.

- *Zone of stasis* is immediately adjacent to the zone of coagulative necrosis. It is a zone of severe inflammation, in which blood flow through the microcirculation slows progressively and then ceases altogether. This causes progressive necrosis, so the burn wound deepens over the 12–24 hours after the incident. Treatment can modify the changes in this zone, while diminished perfusion (due to local or systemic factors) can deepen it.
- *Zone of hyperaemia* lies outside the zone of stasis. Inflammation is less severe, so there is no progression to necrosis unless other deleterious factors (such as desiccation or infection) supervene. The outer (deep) boundary of this zone is diffuse. If more than 20–25 per cent of body surface area (BSA) is burned, then the production of inflammatory mediators is such that the whole body undergoes the changes seen in the zone of hyperaemia in smaller burns. Fluid, electrolyte and protein losses occur in this zone, clinically evident as oedema. Large burns, therefore, cause hypovolaemic shock.

The mechanisms by which these changes occur are complex. A very wide variety of mediators have been identified as being involved. Burns involving more than 25 per cent BSA have a profound systemic effect on every organ system, particularly the neurohumoral control of metabolism, the immune system and the gastrointestinal tract. Thus, a patient with large burns has a systemic injury best treated in a specialized unit.

Depth of a burn

The depth to which necrosis occurs is of great importance to both treatment and outcome. Most burns are not of even depth but are heterogeneous.

Microscopically, necrosis can extend from the epidermis down to deeper tissues, even bone. Numerical categorization ('degrees') has largely been replaced by description: epithelial, superficial partial thickness (extending into the superficial

dermis), deep partial thickness (extending into the deep dermis), and full thickness (full depth of epidermis and dermis are necrotic). As far as outcome is concerned, if the majority of the dermis has been destroyed, then healing will be slow and scarring almost invariable.

Macroscopically, the appearance varies with the depth, the time since burning and the treatment given.

The practical assessment required is to determine whether the burn will heal without significant scarring, so that decisions about treatment can be made.

Children have thin skin, so relatively small amounts of heat will cause a deep burn. Fluid at 60 °C will cause a deep burn in one second in most areas, so a spilt cup of tea or coffee can cause a serious injury.

Natural history

Untreated, a burn can undergo healing if there are epithelial elements still viable under the necrotic surface. Sweat glands and hair follicles can supply epithelial cells, which will migrate across the burn at the junction of viable and non-viable tissue (epithelialization). If necrosis extends only into the superficial dermis, then this process will take less than two weeks, and in the long term scarring is rare. If necrosis involves the deep dermis, then even though a few epithelial remnants survive, epithelialization is slow (more than three weeks) and scarring is probable. Practically speaking, these are deep burns. Many children's burns lie in the difficult group that will take between two and three weeks to heal, with variable amounts of scarring (intermediate burns).

Colonization of a burn is inevitable, unless active measures to exclude bacteria are taken. In the absence of clinical infection, they cause the dead surface tissue (eschar) to separate from the underlying viable tissue.

Once epithelialization is complete, variable amounts of fibrous tissue may form (scar). This can be much thicker than the original dermis (hypertrophic scar). In some individuals, proliferation of fibrous tissue is very exuberant, forming a thick plaque that is larger in extent than the area originally injured (keloid).

Scar tissue undergoes maturation in most individuals. While keloid does not, even severely hypertrophic scars tend to become paler, flatter and softer over one to years after injury. However, as the tissue evolves, it tends to shorten, creating contractures.

Scar rules:

- All scars shorten.
- Comfort leads to contractures.

INCIDENCE

Toddlers and preschool children make up the majority of children with burns in most countries. These children are mobile and inquisitive, but lacking in reality-based judgement.

Scalds make up the overwhelming majority at this age. Spill scalds, such as pulling down containers of hot water (cups, kettles, pans) or being in the way when an adult spills hot water, soup or cooking fluid, are the most common. Immersion scalds tend to be deeper and more extensive. Clothing can act as a reservoir of hot fluid.

Flame burns are more common in older children. There is a strong male preponderance, because a large proportion of these burns involve risk-taking behaviour. House fires contribute a variable number, largely dependent on whether wood is a commonly used building material, whether smoke alarms are commonly used, and whether cooking on open fires is widespread.

Chemical cutaneous burns (excluding oesophageal burns) are relatively rare in children, making up less than one per cent in most developed countries.

NON–ACCIDENTAL INJURY

Burning is one of the most common forms of non-accidental injury (NAI). While some children are burnt by deliberate acts, such as cigarette burns and immersion scalds, a larger group of children are burnt by adult neglect. The borderline between a momentary lapse of protection (i.e. accident) and persistent neglect (child at risk) is difficult to draw (Andronicus et al. 1998).

Judging which incidents have been deliberate acts of harm can be difficult. Although patterns of injury may help to raise suspicion, usually a full assessment of the circumstances of the incident and the family are necessary before reaching that conclusion. A false accusation of NAI is extremely injurious to the family and interferes with treatment. Making an assessment of neglect is even more difficult. Such assessments should be made by a burns team in which there are individuals experienced in the emotional causes and effects of burns.

ASSESSMENT

The severity of the impact of a burn on a child depends largely on its area, expressed as a percentage of the body surface. The depth and the site of the burn are important, as are any pre-existing conditions and concomitant trauma.

Area is best assessed by marking out the limits of the burn on a body outline chart. This is done most accurately at the bedside, constantly referring back to the patient as the three-dimensional original is transcribed to two dimensions. Faint erythema can be ignored. Once a picture of the area has been obtained, the percentage of the total BSA can be calculated using the 'rule of nines', modified for children. For small burns, the palmar surface of the patient's hand (the 'paw-print') is almost one per cent of BSA at all ages (Figure 39.2).

Depth is much more difficult to assess. The appearance of a burn changes dramatically over the first two to five days. Frequently, the history can give a good idea of how deep the burn is likely to be, as it gives a guide as to the temperature and duration of exposure.

The most valid assessment is based on blood supply. If the deep dermal plexus is intact, then healing is likely. This can be detected by the response to pressure (blanching and refilling) early after the event. By days three to five, clinical assessment begins to become more accurate, but there are still quite a large number of children whose burns can only be assessed finally at 10–12 days. Attempts to measure viability by instruments have largely proved too difficult or too inaccurate, with the exception of the laser Doppler flowmeter, which has been shown to have high accuracy, but only more than 48 hours after the burn.

Classically, epithelial burns are dry, pink and painful (sunburn). Superficial dermal burns are blistered and moist, with a pink, blanching base. Deep dermal burns are darker or mottled and do not blanch with pressure. Full-thickness burns are pale and waxy or translucent and amber-coloured. The ability of the patient to distinguish pinprick from touch over the burn is not of practical use in children. If the burn involves special areas (face, respiratory system, hands, genitalia, perineum, feet), then management must be modified. Care of the wound and indications for operation differ in all these areas, so transfer to a burns unit is recommended.

Major concomitant trauma should be detected when the trauma 'ABCs' are applied.

FIRST AID

The progression of the depth of the burn can be modified by appropriate first aid.

Stopping the burning process is the first step. If the patient is on fire, 'stop, drop and roll'. For scalds, remove the hot fluid, including removing soaked clothing. If cold water is at hand, then the clothing may be cooled more quickly by applying liberal amounts of cool fluid if the child is struggling. Chemicals should be brushed (powders) or washed (liquids) off. They should then be diluted by prolonged irrigation.

Next, cool the burned surface. Use water at 8–25 °C. The optimal temperature is not known but is probably around 15 °C. Start as soon as possible. Some benefit is probably achieved up to three hours after injury. After this, the inflammatory cascade is unstoppable. Continue for at least 20 minutes, but longer if possible. As children have a large surface/mass ratio, hypothermia can be a serious problem. Warming the environment to tropical temperatures (28–31 °C) while continuing cooling is ideal. If this is not possible, wrap the child warmly. Laying water-soaked cloths on the burn is of limited use, as the cloths warm rapidly to near-body temperature. Flow or spray water on the burn if the body part cannot be immersed. Cooling the wound gives excellent analgesia, probably because production of inflammatory cytokines is suppressed.

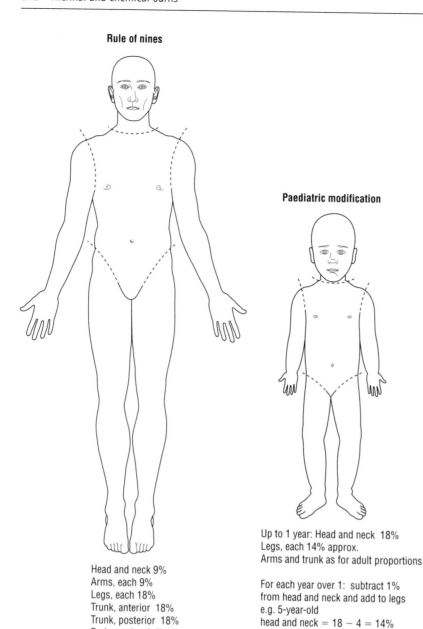

Rule of nines

Paediatric modification

Head and neck 9%
Arms, each 9%
Legs, each 18%
Trunk, anterior 18%
Trunk, posterior 18%
Perineum/genitalia 1%

Up to 1 year: Head and neck 18%
Legs, each 14% approx.
Arms and trunk as for adult proportions

For each year over 1: subtract 1%
from head and neck and add to legs
e.g. 5-year-old
head and neck = 18 − 4 = 14%
Each leg = 14 + 4/2 = 16%

Figure 39.2 *Rule of nines. Estimation of surface area of skin in adult compared with child.*
Area of head and neck = 18% − (age of child − 1).
Area of each lower limb = 14% + [(age of child − 1)/2].
By ten years of age, body proportions are adult. Ignore fractions of 1%.

EARLY TREATMENT

The initial treatment is aimed at minimizing complications and getting the patient to appropriate care. Major burns and burns associated with multi-trauma are complex issues and are dealt with in courses such as advanced trauma life support and emergency management of severe burns.

Inhalation injury takes one of three forms. Systemic intoxication by carbon monoxide occurs when the patient is confined in a space with a fire. It may be associated with hydrogen cyanide inhalation and hypoxia. Oxygen given by facemask or endotracheal tube is the treatment. Hyperbaric oxygen is used, but its effectiveness is anecdotal.

Upper-airway burns are thermal. The upper airway is an efficient heat-exchange mechanism, so inhalation of hot gases affects the mucosa and causes swelling. Respiratory obstruction usually commences as oedema increases, four to eight hours after injury.

Lower-respiratory (infraglottic) injury is due to smoke particles dissolving in the moist lining of the respiratory tract to produce a variety of injurious chemicals. The process takes days to become clinically evident.

Fluid resuscitation is needed for children with greater than eight to ten per cent BSA burns. Traditionally, this is given intravenously as Hartmann's solution or normal saline with 5 mmol/L of potassium. Initial volumes are calculated by the formulae given in Box 39.1.

Oral resuscitation is gaining acceptance and can be used in burns of up to 20–25 per cent BSA, providing that the

Box 39.1 Fluid resuscitation

Volume to be given in 24 hours = weight of patient ×
% BSA burned × 3 or 4

Plan to give half of the calculated volume in the first eight hours after the burn and the remaining half in the next 16 hours.

For children under 30 kg, add standard maintenance containing some glucose.

Adjust the volume to maintain a urinary output of approximately 1 mL/kg/h (range 0.5–2 mL/kg/h). An IDC is needed if the burn is greater than 12–15 per cent BSA.

A lower output almost invariably requires more fluid (150 per cent of planned volume in next hour). A greater output signifies excessive fluid intake and creates excessive oedema, unless haem pigment in the urine is present, in which case volumes of 2–4 mL/kg/h are needed.

BSA, body surface area; IDC, indwelling catheter.

child is not vomiting or in transit. The oral route can be used to supply maintenance requirements. Enteral nourishment diminishes the gastrointestinal effects of burns.

WOUND CARE

The burned area is washed with dilute chlorhexidine or saline to remove foreign material and dead keratin. The treatment of blisters is controversial: in the first few hours, it may be valuable to aspirate them with a fine needle, but later they are probably best left alone. The wound should then be covered with a dressing. This should be an antibacterial dressing, the standard being silver sulfadiazine with chlorhexidine. Burns judged to be superficial may be covered with semipermeable membrane dressings, which are designed to remove excess water and exudate but prevent desiccation so can be left intact for a number of days. Some contain antibacterials, such as colloidal silver.

If the burn is circumferential, then the unyielding nature of the eschar can cause sufficient compression to occlude venous return, and then arterial supply, as the limb swells. All circumferentially burned limbs must be elevated and the circulation observed. If, when elevated, there is venous congestion, or if capillary refill (nail pressure and release) is over two seconds, then division of the eschar (escharotomy) probably is needed. Discussion with a burns unit is essential.

LATER CARE

The continuing care of the patient with a major burn is beyond the scope of this text. It is the purview of a specialized burns unit.

Smaller burns treated initially with an antibacterial should have daily dressing change, with cleaning of the burn wound. This requires analgesia (oral premedication with or without nitrous oxide or midazolam). If healing is not evident in seven to ten days, or if initial appearances indicate a deep burn, then excision and split skin grafting must be considered. Once it is evident that grafting is necessary, operation should be performed as soon as is practicable.

Chemical burns

Water or saline lavage should be continued for several hours. With the notable exception of hydrogen fluoride (HF) burns, no attempt to neutralize chemicals should be made. HF burns require calcium, topically, by local injection, regionally or systemically. Aggressive excision of contaminated tissue should be considered if the HF solution was highly concentrated.

Alkalis tend to penetrate deeply, and so corneal burns with these types of agent are particularly serious. Household cleaners, e.g. drain-cleaning fluid, and cement are the agents usually involved.

Volatile hydrocarbons, e.g. petrol and paint thinner, penetrate the skin because they are lipid-soluble. Like many chemical burns, the ill effects are often manifest 12–24 hours after exposure.

TRANSFER

Transfer criteria are as follows:

- Adults: deep burns of ten per cent or greater BSA.
- Children: deep burns of five per cent or greater BSA.
- Burns to the face, hands, feet or perineum.
- Suspected inhalation injury.
- Limb burns that are circumferential or involve the flexor surfaces over joints.
- Burns and serious pre-existing disease.
- Burns with concomitant major trauma.
- Suspected child abuse or neglect.
- Chemical or electrical burns.

These criteria must be interpreted with reference to the level of expertise available locally. A decision as to where the patient can best be treated can be made in a telephone consultation with a burns unit.

EMOTIONAL CARE

The emotional impact of a burn is not proportional to the size or severity of the injury. While all families of patients who are transferred to a burns unit should have psychosocial assessment and continuing treatment, surgeons should be alert to the possibility of serious emotional disturbance in the families of children who sustain small burns that are properly cared for outside a burns unit. Previous family tensions may be exacerbated. Guilt is invariable. Blame between partners may be destructive. Giving time for families to express their feelings and sympathetic acceptance of negative emotion can assist recovery greatly.

Referral to a burns unit for psychosocial reasons is valid. Any suspicion that the child is 'at risk' is sufficient and is legally mandatory in many countries. Later, such referral may be needed if emotional problems become evident after wound healing. Children and their families may need help from time to time for decades after the injury.

LONG-TERM CARE

Just as emotional rehabilitation may be needed for years, treatment of scars may be prolonged. Early after healing (grafting or spontaneous healing that takes more than two weeks), scar treatment is essential. Stretching the scar with exercises and splinting to maintain the full range of movement, and pressure, are the mainstays of treatment. Other topical agents can be used. Treatment should continue until scar maturity is obviously progressing, as evident by decreasing vascularity and rigidity of the scar.

Surgical revision may be on a functional or cosmetic basis. The surgeon should aim to restore full function. Cosmetic indications are less clear, and the possibility of worsening the appearance must be borne in mind. Apart from simple procedures, such surgery is best done by those trained and experienced in this field.

CLINICAL SCENARIOS

Case 1 (Figures 39.3 and 39.4)

CLINICAL DETAILS

This toddler was in the kitchen when her mother answered the telephone on the other side of the room. The child pulled a saucepan of hot water down on herself, it having been placed on the stove so that the handle projected out from the front of the stove. Her mother immediately took the child to the bathroom, removing the soaked clothing on the way, and ran cold water over the burnt area for ten minutes. Then she sat the child in the bath, with a blanket around the child's shoulders, so she could sponge cold water over the area before taking her to the local hospital. Good blanching and capillary refill were present over all the pink area, with only a very small patch that was darker, and blanched less, near the right nipple. Antibacterial dressings were applied. Spontaneous healing occurred, with epithelialization being completed at day 12–14. The small dark red area was the last to area heal. There was no significant long-term scarring, but the deepest area had some permanent thinning of the dermis.

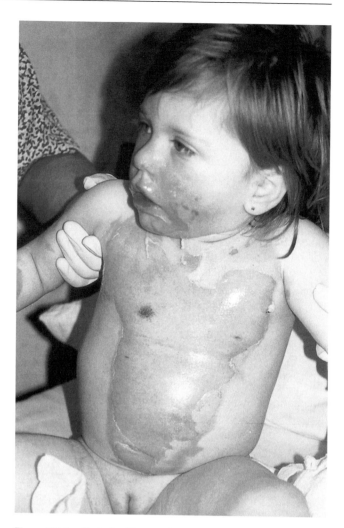

Figure 39.3 *Typical spill scald, four hours after injury. See also Colour Plate 6.*

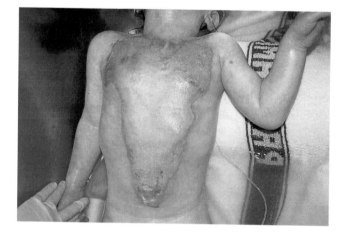

Figure 39.4 *Same patient as in Figure 39.3, seven days after injury. See also Colour Plate 7.*

LEARNING POINTS

- Spill scalds in toddlers are the most common paediatric burn injury.

- Kitchens and bathrooms are the most frequent places where such injuries occur.
- Events are so quick that the presence of adults in the vicinity does not necessarily protect the child.
- Awareness of dangers around the house can lead to effective preventive measures, with dramatic reduction in the incidence of such burns.
- Correct first aid is simple, but hypothermia must be avoided.
- Assessment of depth early after the injury is difficult, but the presence of intact circulation is the best guide.
- Burns are rarely of uniform depth.
- Marked changes in appearance occur in the first days after injury.
- Good first aid and provision of an optimal environment for healing will allow many scald burns to heal spontaneously.
- Scarring is unlikely if a burn heals within 14 days.

Case 2

CLINICAL DETAILS

This ten-year-old girl went to stop a group of boys kicking a flaming tennis ball, which they had filled with spirits (alcohol). The ball exploded as she approached them, injuring only her. She was wearing a light cotton top, denim jeans and a leather belt. She rolled on the ground to extinguish the flames. Both legs were burnt circumferentially from the feet to the upper thighs, and all required grafting. The girl wore compression garments for over 12 months. Surgically, the result was 'good', but the scars are obvious and permanent.

LEARNING POINTS

- Boys playing with flammable fluid or engaging in other risk-taking activities are the most common causes of burns in older children.
- Correct first aid for flame burns starts with extinguishing the fire.
- Burns are usually heterogeneous.
- Early assessment of depth is often difficult.
- The majority of flame burns require grafting.
- Once the whole thickness of the skin is destroyed, permanent scarring is inevitable.
- What surgeons consider satisfactory may still be far from normal.

Case 3 (Figures 39.5–39.8)

CLINICAL DETAILS

This six-year-old girl was playing with her mother's cigarette lighter after locking herself in the car, delaying rescue. She sustained burns to the trunk and limbs totalling 30 per cent BSA. The burn of the right upper limb (depicted) was almost

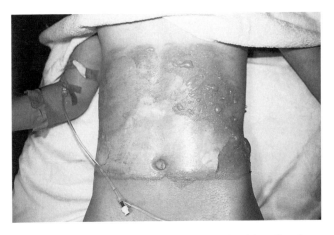

Figure 39.5 *Flame burn of trunk, four hours after injury. See also Colour Plate 8.*

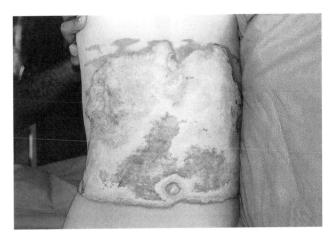

Figure 39.6 *Same patient as in Figure 39.5, six days after injury. See also Colour Plate 9.*

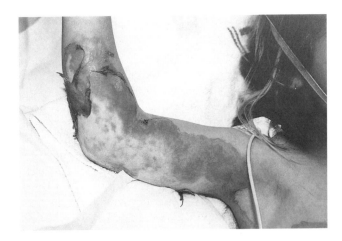

Figure 39.7 *Flame burn six hours after injury. Child semi-recumbent, with head of bed raised and arm elevated. See also Colour Plate 10.*

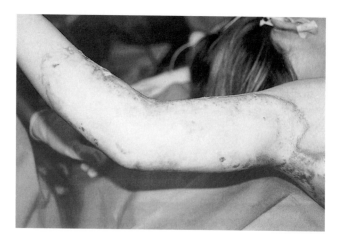

Figure 39.8   *Same patient as in Figure 39.7, two days after injury. Child anaesthetized for operation. See also Colour Plate 11.*

circumferential. All burnt areas needed grafting. The right posterior axillary fold was tight, but splinting and scar therapy successfully avoided the need for surgical scar release in the medium term (two years). Her mother's initial intense guilt was resolved successfully by frequent contact with the members of the unit responsible for emotional care, and her parenting skills, e.g. ability to be supportive but apply appropriate limits to the child's behaviour, improved compared with the premorbid level.

LEARNING POINTS

- Note strap of oxygen mask, oxygen administration being a routine part of the resuscitation of major burns (as for all major trauma).

- Elevation of arm to reduce oedema and minimize need for escharotomy.
- Central pale area clearly deep at presentation, but surrounding brick-red zone becoming more obviously deep in 48 hours.
- Early excision and wound closure as soon as demarcation of that which needs to be grafted is clear.
- Splinting areas that are at risk of contracture formation in the overcorrected position should start on day one and be followed by intensive physiotherapy to reduce the need for secondary procedures.
- Management of the emotional effects of a burn, on the child and the family, are as important as the physical treatment.
- The burn injury is a crisis that may give an opportunity for premorbid psychosocial pathology to be addressed, sometimes with long-term benefit to the whole family.

REFERENCES

Andronicus M, Oates RK, Peat J, Spalding S, Martin HCO. Non-accidental burns in children. *Burns* 1998; **24**: 552–8.
Jackson DM. The diagnosis of the depth of burning. *British Journal of Surgery* 1953; **40**: 588–96.

FURTHER READING

Herndon DN. *Total Burn Care*. Philadelphia, PA: WB Saunders, 1996.

40

Hydrocephalus and spina bifida

PAUL CHUMAS AND ATUL TYAGI

Learning objectives

- To understand the embryological and anatomical bases of hydrocephalus and spina bifida.
- To know the presenting features, investigations and treatment options for these conditions.
- To appreciate the functional outcomes related to these conditions.

HYDROCEPHALUS

Definition

Hydrocephalus is a descriptive term implying a mismatch between cerebrospinal fluid (CSF) production and absorption. This usually manifests itself by dilation of the ventricular system; in turn, this is often associated with an increase in intracranial pressure (ICP). Virtually all cases of hydrocephalus are secondary to obstruction. Classically, the site of this obstruction is used to describe the type of hydrocephalus: *communicating hydrocephalus* indicates a problem with absorption, while *non-communicating hydrocephalus* indicates an obstruction to CSF flow at some point between the site of production and the site of absorption. The generally accepted view is that the CSF circulates by bulk flow, from the choroid plexus (production) to the pacchionian granulations (absorption).

Incidence

Hydrocephalus is the most common neurosurgical condition treated in the paediatric age range. The incidence of congenital and infantile hydrocephalus is between 0.48 and 0.81 per 1000 births (live and still). In one trial, the median corrected age of patients at the time of first shunt surgery was 55 days. Table 40.1 shows the underlying causative aetiology and symptoms and signs before the first shunt insertion in a typical cohort of paediatric patients. The causes of the hydrocephalus in underdeveloped countries are likely to differ from these, with infection and spina bifida being more common.

Treatment options

NON-SURGICAL TREATMENT

Diuretics (furosemide (frusemide), acetazolamide) and steroids are known to decrease CSF production. Diuretics are still used frequently in neonatal patients with post-haemorrhagic hydrocephalus (PHH), despite reports of side effects such as acidosis, CO_2 retention and electrolyte disturbance and a multicentre study showing no benefit. Just as the use of diuretics would appear to be futile, so the use of regular lumbar punctures should probably be abandoned, as it is ineffective and carries a risk of introducing infection. Repeated ventricular taps risk not only infection but also the development of 'puncture porencephaly' and are inadvisable.

Table 40.1 *Causes and presenting signs and symptoms of hydrocephalus (based on Drake et al. 1998)*

Cause/symptom/sign	Incidence (%)
Hydrocephalus cause	
Intraventricular haemorrhage	28.1
Myelomeningocele	15.8
Tumour	10.5
Aqueduct stenosis	5.3
CSF infection	5.3
Head injury	0
Two or more causes	10.5
Other	13.2
Unknown	11.4
Symptom	
Headache	15.0
Nausea or vomiting	22.0
Irritability	25.9
Lethargy	18.2
New seizures or change in seizure pattern	9.7
Diplopia	6.7
Fever	0.9
Delayed developmental milestones	21.3
Worsening school performance	3.9
Sign	
Papilloedema	7.7
Bulging fontanelle	72.5
Increased head circumference	80.0
Decreased level of consciousness	10.6
Nuchal rigidity	0.9
Sixth nerve palsy	5.5
Loss of upward gaze	14.4
Hemiparesis	0.9
Other focal neurological deficit	12.4
Delayed developmental milestones	24.5
Cutaneous signs of occult spinal dysraphism	2.6
Other positive physical finding	4.3

CSF, cerebrospinal fluid.

PHH is decreasing in frequency with better general perinatal care. Intraventricular fibrinolytic treatment has also been used in an attempt to prevent permanent obstruction of the CSF pathways in PHH, but studies to date have not been encouraging. In passing, it should be noted that the CSF protein concentration *per se* is of no consequence with regard to the timing of surgical intervention, but the degree of cellular debris may well be.

SURGICAL TREATMENT

Surgical drainage of CSF appears to date from the time of Hippocrates. Virtually every cavity has been tried, including the subdural space, the subarachnoid space, the subcutaneous tissues of the scalp, the paranasal sinuses, the thoracic duct, the pleura, the peritoneum, the gallbladder, the ureters and the bloodstream. Initially, the atrium was the preferred site for placement of the distal catheter, but atrial shunts have a unique

set of complications, including endocarditis and glomerulonephritis. The peritoneum is now the favoured site for the distal catheter, unless there are problems with absorption or abdominal sepsis. Lumbar peritoneal shunts are used rarely for the treatment of hydrocephalus in children and have been associated with the development of scoliosis and cerebellar tonsillar herniation.

The modern era of shunting started in the 1950s, with the realization that a one-way valve was required and that silicone tubing was the best material for use in manufacture.

Shunts

Although the results for treating hydrocephalus were far superior following the introduction of shunts, it soon became apparent that shunts had their limitations. In particular, it became clear that all shunts malfunction in three ways: infection, mechanical failure and functional failure.

Shunt infection Although single-institution studies have reported infection rates of less than one per cent, most studies have reported rates of the order of five to ten per cent (significantly higher than this in the neonatal period). The role of antibiotic prophylaxis has been studied by meta-analysis, and antibiotic cover is recommended. Most shunt infections occur in the first six months after operation. The most common organisms are staphylococci (*S. epidermidis* 40 per cent, *S. aureus* 20 per cent). Other species that have been noted include coryneforms, streptococci, enterococci, aerobic Gram-negative rods and yeasts. Most shunt infections are a result of contamination with the patient's own skin flora, which underlines the need for meticulous attention to surgical technique. Unfortunately, once a shunt is infected, it is almost always necessary to remove the shunt and insert a temporary external ventricular drain. Antibiotic treatment alone is sometimes effective in the treatment of infection by *Streptococcus* and *Haemophilus* species. Apart from the practical problems associated with the treatment of shunt infection, it has been shown that there is an increase in the development of loculated CSF compartments, impaired intellectual outcome and death after shunt infection (Chumas *et al.* 2001).

Mechanical failure The use of Kaplan–Meier curves to display shunt survival has led to a far greater understanding of shunt failure. Virtually all the studies to date have shown an exponential curve, with approximately 40 per cent of shunts failing (including infection) in the first year and then approximately five per cent per year (Figure 40.1). Over 50 per cent of first shunt failures are due to obstruction, with the vast majority of these occurring at the ventricular catheter. This is almost certainly a consequence of the fact that all shunts overdrain, so the ventricular catheter comes to lie against the ependyma and choroid plexus of the ventricle; these tissues can then become incorporated into, and block the holes at the end of, the catheter. Although it is reassuring to see collapsed ventricles on a scan, this is probably not ideal for long-term shunt functioning. Very occasionally, patients develop slit-ventricle syndrome, with transient symptoms of raised ICP in

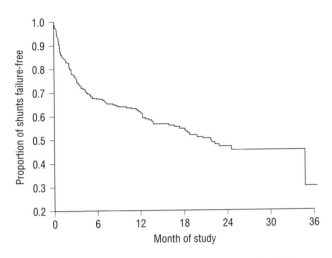

Figure 40.1 *Kaplan–Meier curve showing shunt survival (from Drake et al. 1998).*

the setting of a scan that shows small or non-existent ventricles. Although poorly understood, it would appear that these children lose their CSF buffering reserve and are susceptible to episodes of raised pressure in situations that normally would be of no consequence. This can be a difficult management problem, sometimes requiring formal ICP monitoring to make the diagnosis. Although there are various treatment options, such as altering the shunt valve, adding an antisiphon device and skull expansion (e.g. subtemporal decompression), this remains one of the most testing conditions to treat in paediatric neurosurgery.

Other shunt malfunctions include fracturing of the tubing (the cause of approximately 15 per cent of primary shunt malfunctions), migration of part or all of the shunt (7.5 per cent) and problems with overdrainage (seven per cent).

Functional failure   Most cases of functional failure relate to overdrainage. The underlying problem is one of siphoning from the ventricle to the level of the distal tube (over 1 m in an adult). This overdrainage can result in subdural haematoma, low-pressure symptoms (postural headache, nausea) and craniosynostosis. Studies have shown that in normal subjects, initially the ICP decreases on going from the horizontal to the vertical position and then stabilizes (after approximately 30-degrees elevation) at -5 to $+5\,cmH_2O$. In contrast, in asymptomatic patients with shunts, there is a rapid near-linear fall in ICP, with consistently negative upright pressures (-15 to $-35\,cmH_2O$). What is perhaps more surprising, therefore, is that not all patients with shunts suffer with symptoms of overdrainage. In patients with persistent symptoms, it is possible to alter the valve or include an antisiphon device in series with the valve. Again, formal ICP monitoring may be of use in confirming the diagnosis.

There has only been one randomized trial comparing shunt valves. This found no significant difference between three types of shunt. This is despite the quite different profiles of each shunt type on bench testing and on testing *in vivo*.

Using sophisticated statistical techniques, Tuli *et al.* (2000) reported on the risk factors for repeated shunt failures. They found that the failure time from the first procedure was an important predictor for all future failures, with a hazard ratio of 1.5 times for subsequent shunt failures if the original shunt failed within six months of insertion compared with those that failed later than six months. Likewise, patients younger than 40 weeks' gestation and between 40 weeks and one year of age had hazard ratios of 2.49 and 1.77, respectively, compared with patients older than one year at the time of initial shunt insertion. In this study, certain causes of hydrocephalus (intraventricular haemorrhage, post-meningitis, tumour) were significant causative factors in recurrent shunt failure. Concurrent surgical procedure was also noted to increase shunt failure.

THIRD VENTRICULOSTOMY

Open third ventriculostomy (literally, making a hole to connect the third ventricle with the subarachnoid space) was first reported in the 1920s by Dandy, but it was associated with a significant mortality rate. After this, percutaneous third ventriculostomy techniques were utilized, but these also had relatively high rates of mortality and morbidity. Although Mixter performed the first endoscopic procedure in 1923, it has been over the past two decades that endoscopic third ventriculostomy (ETV) has grown in popularity as an alternative to shunt placement for patients with triventricular (obstructive) hydrocephalus. This popularity has been partly a response to the problems associated with shunts, but it is also due partly to the improvement in optical technology. An additional factor is that endoscopic procedures are aesthetically pleasing, to both the surgeon and the patient.

ETV entails entering the lateral ventricle, passage through the foramen of Monro (Figure 40.2a), identification of the mamillary bodies, and then perforation of the floor of the third ventricle, just anterior to the bifurcation of the basilar artery (Figure 40.2b).

However aesthetically appealing, there is no point in performing a third ventriculostomy if the absorptive capacity is abnormal. Unfortunately, there is no easy and reliable method of determining absorptive capacity.

A number of recent studies have described 'success' rates with ETV of 49–100 per cent. However, most of these studies have been descriptive and the outcome measures vague. Nonetheless, there appears to be some conformity from these studies, with most showing approximately 70 per cent of patients with aqueduct stenosis requiring no further surgical intervention. Controversy, however, remains over the success rate of the procedure in children under one year of age.

Gradually, the complication rate associated with ETV is becoming manifest. Failure to complete the procedure for technical reasons has been reported in up to 26 per cent of patients. The main complication is haemorrhage secondary to vascular damage. Other reported complications include death, cardiac arrest, diabetes insipidus, inappropriate secretion of

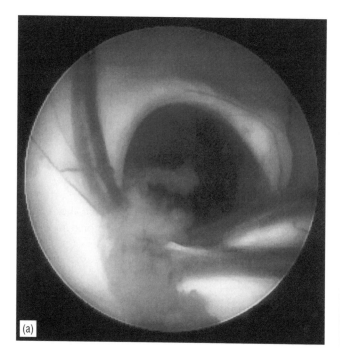

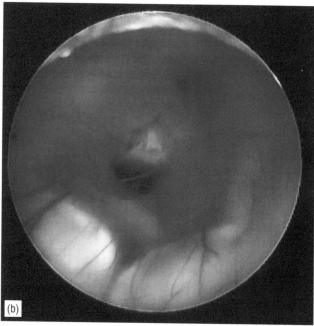

Figure 40.2 *(a) Endoscopic view of the foramen of Monro. (b) Floor of the third ventricle, showing the mamillary bodies inferiorly and the infundibular recess superiorly, with the stoma in the middle, in front of the basilar artery bifurcation.*

antidiuretic hormone (ADH), subdural haematoma, meningitis and cerebral infarction. As the potential operative risks with third ventriculostomy are greater than with shunting, careful patient selection is paramount.

Outcome for hydrocephalus

The natural history for untreated hydrocephalus is poor, with 50 per cent of children dying before three years of age, and only 20–23 per cent of patients reaching adult life. Of these survivors, only 38 per cent are of normal intelligence. Considering the frequency with which shunts are inserted, it is somewhat depressing that better outcome data are still unavailable. Although the actual surgical mortality rate is low, the ten-year mortality rate for non-tumoral hydrocephalus is of the order of 5–15 per cent. A significant number of these deaths are avoidable and attributable to delay in diagnosis and treatment of shunt malfunction. Most patients will have neurological deficits (60 per cent motor deficits, 25 per cent visual or auditory deficits).

Routine obstetric sonography has shown that the diameter of the atrium of the fetal lateral ventricle is of some prognostic value. If the atrium measures 11–15 mm, then the child has a 21 per cent chance of developmental delay; if this measurement is greater than 15 mm, then the risk of developmental delay is over 50 per cent. It is, however, important to compare the ventricular measurement with the head circumference in order to differentiate between fetal hydrocephalus and cerebral atrophy. Likewise, the finding of multiple central nervous system and/or extracranial abnormalities is of considerable prognostic value. Interestingly, once the child is born, there is no correlation between cognitive outcome and thickness of cerebral mantle (unless the latter is less than 2 cm).

EPILEPSY

Most series of non-tumoral hydrocephalic patients have reported an overall rate of epilepsy of approximately 30 per cent. Most authors have found a correlation between the cause of the hydrocephalus and the incidence of epilepsy, with spina bifida carrying a low risk (seven per cent), cerebral malformations and intraventricular haemorrhage carrying a moderate risk (approximately 30 per cent), and infection carrying a high risk (50 per cent). Changes in seizure pattern may represent shunt malfunction. Perhaps more important is the need to distinguish between 'hydrocephalic attacks' (decerebrate posturing secondary to raised ICP) and epilepsy.

FUNCTIONAL OUTCOME

Many factors correlate with the final functional and intellectual outcome in children with hydrocephalus, including birth weight, degree of prematurity, presence of structural brain abnormalities, epilepsy, visual and hearing impairment, and other congenital abnormalities. Overall, approximately 50–55 per cent of shunted hydrocephalic children will achieve an IQ of greater than 80, with verbal cognitive skills being superior to non-verbal skills. Not surprisingly, epilepsy appears to be an important predictor for poor intellectual outcome in shunted hydrocephalic children, with an IQ over 90 being seen in 66 per cent of children without epilepsy compared with 24 per cent of children with epilepsy. Studies looking at outcome post-schooling are virtually non-existent. One study has shown that two-thirds of children followed through to adulthood were socially independent but living at home with their parents. A further 16 per cent have left home and are living either alone or with a partner.

SPINA BIFIDA

The term 'spina bifida' includes developmental abnormalities that vary from incomplete fusion of the vertebral arch with normal intraspinal structures to myelomeningocele (MMC), consisting of an open neural-tube defect (NTD). These abnormalities are classified by the presence or absence of skin cover into spin bifida operta (open) and occulta (closed), respectively.

Embryology

The spinal cord as far caudal as the second sacral spinal cord segment forms from the ectodermal cells that lie above the notochord in the first three weeks of fetal development (neurulation). The notochord induces the formation of the neural plate, which then rolls up to form the neural tube. The superficial ectoderm separates from the neural tube and forms the skin. Mesoderm migrates between the neural tube and the skin to form the tissues surrounding the spinal column. Disturbance in this period results in anomalies such as MMC, lipomyelomeningocele and dermal sinuses.

The distal end of the spinal cord forms from the caudal cell mass, which undergoes canalization to form the initial conus medullaris. The distal portion undergoes involution to form the filum terminale. The process of involution is termed 'retrogressive differentiation'. Abnormalities of retrogressive differentiation result in anomalies such as thickened filum terminale and lipoma of the filum terminale.

At completion, the spinal cord extends to the coccygeal level. Because of differential growth between the spinal column and the spinal cord, the spinal cord ascends and the conus comes to lie at L2–3 at birth. By two months of age, it lies in the adult position at L1–2.

Myelomeningocele

The non-closure theory proposes that MMCs are the result of a primary failure of the neural tube to close. Neural-tube closure is dependent on a variety of embryonic processes, and disruption of any of these may lead to a failure of neurulation. Both the location and the length of the un-neurulated segment determine the nature and severity of the resultant malformations. A failure of caudal neurulation results in an MMC. A portion of the neural tube fails to close and the neural fold remains attached to the cutaneous ectoderm. A part of the neural plate (placode) is thus exposed on the dorsal surface.

AETIOLOGY

Both genetic and environmental factors appear to play a role in the aetiology of MMC. Nutritional deficiency states have been suggested as aetiological factors. The supplementation of folic acid 0.4 mg/day before conception and through early pregnancy appears to reduce the occurrence of spina bifida in high-risk and first-time pregnancies by as much as 72 per cent. Taking carbamazepine and valproic acid increases the risk of having a child with MMC by one to two per cent.

EPIDEMIOLOGY

The incidence of MMC has declined over the past decades from one to two per 1000 live births before 1980 to 3.2 per 10 000 live births in 1992 in the USA. The true incidence of MMC in England and Wales, including cases diagnosed prenatally and aborted, has fallen from 215 per 100 000 in 1972 to 38 per 100 000 in 1991. The reasons for this decline are multifactorial and include improved maternal nutrition, availability of antenatal screening and vitamin supplementation. The incidence of MMC is higher in females and Caucasians (particularly in the UK and Ireland). Indian and eastern Mediterranean populations also appear to have a higher risk of NTD. In North America, the risk of having a child with spina bifida is 0.05 per cent, and the risk of a subsequent child being affected is five per cent. Genetic counselling therefore should be offered to all parents with affected children and, eventually, to the patient.

ANTENATAL DETECTION

Maternal serum alpha-fetoprotein level assay is an effective way of screening the fetus for an open NTD. Antenatal ultrasound in experienced hands also is very accurate. Antenatally, MMC may be picked up on ultrasound as early as 12 weeks (by the 'banana and lemon' sign, the splayed cerebellum resembling a banana and the anterior part of the skull resembling a lemon). These cranial abnormalities are visible earlier than the spinal defects.

CLINICAL FINDINGS

MMC is evident as a lesion on the back neural tissue (the placode) with an arachnoid sac (Figure 40.3). The placode may be elevated or flush with the skin. The lumbar and sacral regions are the most common sites, followed by the thoracic and cervical regions. CSF may leak from the MMC. A full fontanelle (a sign of hydrocephalus) may be present at birth or become evident in up to 80–90 per cent of children. Neurological deficits depend upon the level involved and include limb weakness and orthopaedic abnormalities (e.g. clubfeet, hip dislocations) and sphincter involvement. All patients have Chiari II malformation (descent of the cerebellar vermis through the foramen magnum); in a small number of patients, this may cause bulbar dysfunction requiring surgical decompression (a largely cervical procedure as the posterior fossa is small and there is usually a low-lying torcular). Cardiac or urogenital abnormalities also may be encountered. The neonate with

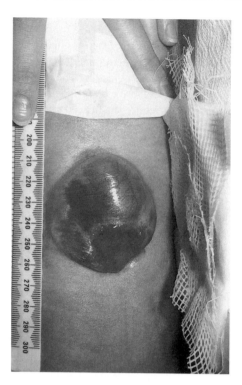

Figure 40.3 *Myelomeningocele, with the neural placode exposed inferiorly.*

MMC should be assessed in the postoperative period by paediatric surgical, orthopaedic and urology teams. Attention to bladder function and early intermittent catheterization can reduce urinary tract damage.

INVESTIGATIONS

Ultrasound is helpful in identifying hydrocephalus, defining the anatomy of the lower spinal cord and assessing the bladder and renal system. Plain X-rays will reveal bifid posterior arches at the affected level and any associated vertebral anomalies, e.g. hemi-vertebrae, fusion.

TREATMENT

Antenatal counselling

Many parents on hearing that their unborn child has spina bifida will opt for termination of the pregnancy. However, the outlook for children with low spinal lesions is much better than for those with high lesions, and ultrasound is becoming more accurate with regard to the size, level and type of lesion present. Many of the long-term data on outcome for children with spina bifida are from the era before prenatal diagnosis and relate to all degrees of severity. There is a paucity of accurate long-term follow-up data for children with low lesions.

The parents should be made aware that 80 per cent of children with MMC will survive the first two to five years. The majority ($\geqslant$80 per cent) will have normal intelligence (IQ > 70), although 75 per cent have learning difficulties, the most common problems being with concentration, short-term memory, organizational skills, hand/eye coordination

and motivation. Although 85 per cent will walk with or without some form of assistance, many children capable of walking with aids such as calipers will opt to use wheelchairs as they get older. Therapeutic interventions may be needed for hydrocephalus, neurogenic bladder and bowel, and orthopaedic deformities. Only six per cent of children will have totally normal bladder function. There is some evidence that birth by caesarean section is associated with improved neurological outcome, due to less damage to the exposed neural tissue.

Intrauterine surgery

Closure of MMC has been carried out *in utero*. At present, the benefit appears to be limited to a reduction in the incidence of hydrocephalus and the reversal of established hindbrain herniation, rather than preservation of spinal cord function.

Postnatal management

Conservative management of children with spina bifida previously was practised to select out and avoid operating on babies with severe deficits. With advances in prenatal imaging, the decision to terminate or continue with the pregnancy has usually been made both by the parents and by the medical team before delivery. Conservative management may be indicated in the rare situation in which there are multiple congenital abnormalities/defects that are felt to be incompatible with long-term survival. The majority of babies born with spina bifida are now treated within 72 hours of birth.

After delivery, the lesion is covered with a wet sterile saline-soaked gauze or plastic wrap. The neonate is positioned in the lateral or prone position to avoid direct pressure on the exposed placode. Closure is usually carried out within 72 hours of birth, in order to reduce the risk of ventriculitis.

The aim of surgery is cover the exposed spinal cord and surround it in CSF. The placode is dissected from the arachnoid/skin junction. The last normal lamina is exposed just above the placode and the dura is identified. Any excess skin tissue is removed from the neural placode under magnification. The spinal cord can then be converted into a tube by placing pia-arachnoid sutures to approximate the lateral edges. The dura is closed over, followed by the lumbosacral fascia, subcutaneous tissue and skin. Plastic procedures may be required to cover large defects. If hydrocephalus develops, then it may be treated either at the time of closure of the MMC or as a separate procedure. Options include insertion of a shunt and third ventriculostomy. Complications of CSF leak and wound dehiscence need to be managed aggressively in order to avoid ventriculitis.

FOLLOW-UP

Children with MMC require long-term neurosurgical, orthopaedic and urological/bowel follow-up into adult life.

Closed dysraphic states

These vary from inconsequential failure of fusion of the posterior vertebral arch (seen on X-ray in 20–30 per cent of the population at L5 or S1) through to complex congenital abnormalities. The lesion may be identified by spinal cutaneous changes (e.g. dimples, sinus tracts, hypertrichosis, deviation of the natal cleft, capillary haemangiomas lipomas) or development of a neurological, urological or orthopaedic problem.

The natural history of these conditions is far from clear, but most neonates appear neurologically intact at birth. Herein lies the dilemma of their treatment: does the subsequent development of an abnormality signify true neurological deterioration or merely the developmental unmasking of an innate problem, e.g. continence?

INVESTIGATION

X-rays of the affected area may show hemi-vertebrae, fused vertebrae, absent spinous processes, widening of the interpedicular distance, scoliosis and kyphosis.

Ultrasound can identify the position of the spinal cord, tethering and intraspinal mass lesions, but its use is limited up to six months of age. Ultrasound is helpful in picking up abnormalities in the urogenital tract at presentation and gives valuable information on the state of the bladder and kidneys during follow-up.

Magnetic resonance imaging (MRI) is the diagnostic modality of choice for investigation of dysraphic lesions. Information can be obtained about the level of termination of the spinal cord, and the anatomy of the spinal cord, nerve roots and filum terminale.

Urodynamics is important in monitoring urological function.

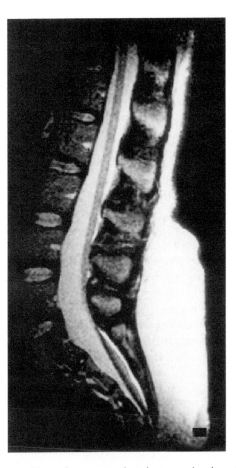

Figure 40.4 *Magnetic resonance imaging scan, showing a low termination of the spinal cord and a thickened filum terminale.*

PATHOLOGY

The dysraphic states result in tethering of the spinal cord. Experimental studies have suggested that the lumbosacral cord and the cauda equina are the most sensitive to stretch, and this may initiate metabolic, vascular and conduction changes. Common intraspinal abnormalities encountered include the following:

Filum terminale abnormalities
The filum may be thickened (>2 mm on axial MRI) (Figure 40.4) or have a lipoma within it. These tend to be truly occult and can be normal findings in up to five per cent of adults in the presence of a normal level of cord termination. Some, however, can be associated with a low-lying conus medullaris and can tether the spinal cord. They may occur in association with other congenital anomalies, e.g. anorectal malformations. These abnormalities may present with late-onset symptoms, such as leg pain and sphincter disturbance. Treatment consists of sectioning the filum (Figure 40.5).

Lipomyelomeningocele
Spinal lipomas are thought to arise when the cutaneous ectoderm separates prematurely from the neural plate before neural-fold fusion. The surrounding mesenchyme ingresses between the neural tube and the overlying cutaneous ectoderm

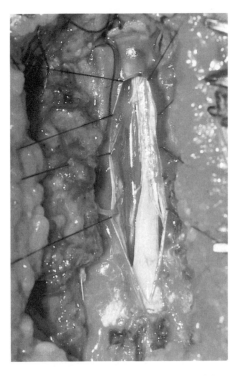

Figure 40.5 *Intraoperative exposure intradurally of the terminal spinal cord and a filum terminale thickened and infiltrated with fat.*

to gain access to the ependymal surface of the developing neural tube. This contact may result in the mesenchyme being induced to form fat rather than dura. This is the most common of the closed dysraphic conditions (one in 4000 births). The abnormality consists of a fibrolipomatous mass extending from the subcutaneous region through the dura into the spinal cord (Figure 40.6). The conus medullaris is usually affected, although other parts of the spinal cord can be involved.

The treatment of symptomatic lesions consists of resection of the subcutaneous and intraspinal lipoma along with release of the spinal cord from the lipoma. Surgical untethering can stabilize spinal deformity, reverse motor and sensory changes, and result in relief of back and leg pain. Once established, however, bladder malfunction improves in a very small proportion of patients, most of whose symptoms stabilize.

The treatment of asymptomatic patients is controversial. The American literature is in favour of prophylactic untethering to prevent the onset of neurological and urological deficits. The French experience, however, suggests that a high proportion of patients undergoing prophylactic operations still deteriorate and require further surgery. The benefit of prophylactic untethering remains unproven. Most centres in the UK monitor these patients closely and intervene surgically if deterioration occurs.

Diastematomyelia

Split cord malformations are thought to be anomalies arising from disorders of gastrulation. The term implies splitting of the spinal cord over one or more segments. The split may be around a bony spur or a fibrocartilaginous septum, which arise from the posterior aspect of the vertebral body and become continuous with the lamina (Figure 40.7). The two hemi-cords usually unite below the split. The spur or an associated thickened filum terminale can result in traction on the spinal cord, leading to neurological signs. Diastematomyelia also may be associated with MMC and other dysraphic states.

Treatment consists of excision of the spur passing through the split spinal cord, with reconstitution of the two dural sacs into one, with division of the filum terminale if it is felt to be tethering the spinal cord.

Dermal sinus

Dermal sinuses are thought to arise from incorrect separation of the neuroectoderm from the cutaneous ectoderm, allowing a portion of cutaneous ectoderm to lie between the neural tube and the skin. This remnant can result in dermal sinus tracts or intraspinal epidermoid/dermoid tumours. The sinus usually consists of one or more pinpoint holes in the lumbar or sacral area. These track through the subcutaneous tissue and can end at the dura or enter intradurally and may attach to the conus. Dermal sinuses can both tether the spinal cord and act as a source of bacterial contamination of the spinal canal, leading to meningitis and intraspinal abscesses. Dermal sinuses may occur alongside intraspinal dermoid and epidermoid tumours.

Small dermal pits within the natal cleft are seen commonly in infants and may be referred to as 'post-anal dimples' or pits.

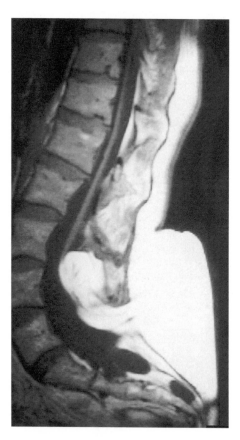

Figure 40.6 *Magnetic resonance imaging scan, showing the cord terminating in a lipoma that extends into the subcutaneous fatty lump through a dural and bony defect.*

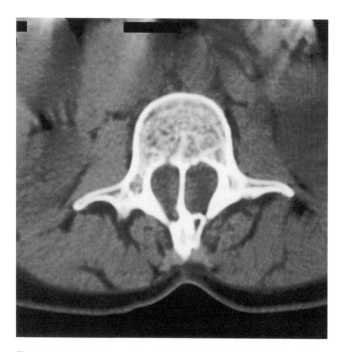

Figure 40.7 *Axial computed tomography scan of the lumbar spine, demonstrating the bony spur in the midline separating the spinal canal into two.*

Such pits can be ignored if they are within the natal cleft and there is no associated abnormal natal cleft asymmetry. Pits above the natal cleft or associated with asymmetry require spinal MRI. If this confirms a dermal sinus, then it should be treated as soon as possible, because of the infective risks posed by it. Treatment consists of excision of the entire tract.

Caudal agenesis

This term covers a group of caudal malformations in which there is a partial or complete absence of a variable number of lumbar and/or sacral vertebrae, together with the corresponding regions of the caudal neural tube. The vertebral anomalies include agenesis, hemi-vertebrae and fused vertebrae. The distal spinal cord ends in a dysplastic glial nodule. Associated limb anomalies are common, as are visceral malformations, including intestinal malformations (tracheo-oesophageal fistula, Meckel's diverticulum, cloacal exstrophy, omphalocele, malrotation) and urogenital malformations (renal agenesis, horseshoe kidney, ureteral and bladder duplications, anomalies of external genitalia).

Congenital malformations arising from abnormalities of the caudal embryo include VATER (vertebral anomalies, anal imperforation, tracheo-oesophageal fistula, renal and radial anomalies) syndrome and OEIS (omphalocele, cloacal exstrophy, imperforate anus, spinal anomalies) syndrome. In the more severe types, the entire sacrum may be missing and the spinal cord may end in a club-shaped lower end. Lower-sacral anomalies are associated with low-lying cords, which may be tethered and may require surgical untethering. All patients with congenital caudal abnormalities should be referred for neurosurgical assessment.

CLINICAL SCENARIO

A 19-year-old prima gravida who had not taken folate supplementation was referred for a neurosurgical consultation, having had an ultrasound scan (and subsequent MRI) at 18 weeks that had shown a lumbosacral spina bifida associated with marginal ventricular enlargement. After a lengthy discussion, the mother elected to continue the pregnancy. Serial ultrasound showed the hydrocephalus to increase to a moderate level and then to stabilize. An elective caesarean section was performed at 38 weeks. Examination of the child revealed a large open lumbar defect leaking CSF. The head circumference

was on the ninetieth percentile. In the lower limbs, there were bilateral rocker-bottom feet and equino varus deformities. Formal limb charting revealed good movements at the hip and knee but limited movements at the ankle. Orthopaedic and urological referrals were initiated, and ultrasound examination was performed of the head, spine and bladder. A subsequent MRI scan confirmed the moderate hydrocephalus, tectal beaking and Chiari II abnormality within the cranium and showed that the MMC was associated with a terminal syrinx.

After further discussions with the family, the child underwent closure of the MMC. In view of the size of the defect, plastic surgical input was requested, and the skin was closed using transposition flaps. Postoperatively, the child was nursed prone. A small CSF leak was stopped by additional skin sutures. By the fourth day postoperatively, the head circumference had crossed to the ninety-eighth percentile and the fontanelle was full. In view of the anatomy (large massa intermedia), it was felt that third ventriculostomy was not feasible and a ventriculoperitoneal shunt was inserted. The mother was taught to catheterize the child, and the family was allowed home on day 12.

REFERENCES

Chumas PD, Tyagi A, Livingston J. Hydrocephalus: what's new? *Archives of Disease in Childhood: Fetal and Neonatal Edition* 2001; **85**: 149–54.

Drake JM, Kestle JRW, Milner R, *et al.* Randomized trial of cerebrospinal fluid shunt valve design in pediatric hydrocephalus. *Neurosurgery* 1998; **43**: 294–305.

Tuli S, Drake JM, Lawless J, *et al.* Risk factors for repeated cerebrospinal shunt failures in pediatric patients with hydrocephalus. *Journal of Neurosurgery* 2000; **92**: 31–8.

FURTHER READING

Chumas PD. The role of surgery in asymptomatic lumbosacral spinal lipomas. *British Journal of Neurosurgery* 2000; **14**: 301.

Drake JM, Sainte-Rose C. *The Shunt Book.* New York: Blackwell Scientific, 1995.

McLone D. Care of the neonate with a myelomeningocele. *Neurosurgical Clinics of North America* 1998; **9**: 111–20.

Pang D. *Disorders of the Pediatric Spine.* New York: Raven Press, 1995.

Part 5

Oncology

41

Neonatal tumours, including haemangioma and lymphangioma

SIMON N HUDDART

Learning objectives

- To understand the types of neonatal tumour.
- To appreciate the different presentations and imaging of neonatal tumours.
- To understand the relevant embryology and basic science.
- To be able to describe the surgical techniques required and the role of a multidisciplinary approach.

INTRODUCTION

Neonatal tumours are rare: only 2.6 per cent of tumours in children occur in this age range. Of these tumours, 30–40 per cent are malignant. However, some tumours that look malignant histologically may act in a benign fashion, and some benign tumours may prove to be fatal because of their anatomical position, e.g. epignathus. The neonatal death rate from malignancy in the USA has been estimated at one per 6.4 million live births, but this is probably an underestimate, as sacrococcygeal teratomas (SCTs) were not included. A study in Denmark showed an incidence of 2.4 per 100 000 births, with the most common tumour being neuroblastoma (26 per cent) (Borch *et al.* 1994). Retinoblastoma, neuroblastoma and Wilms tumour have the best prognoses. Overall survival is around 45–55 per cent.

As experience of such tumours is limited, the neonate should be referred to a specialist centre for treatment. Many such tumours can now be identified on antenatal ultrasound scan, and the parents can be counselled before birth and appropriate arrangements made for postnatal care. The presence of a tumour identified on prenatal ultrasonography may influence obstetric management. For example, a very large sacrococcygeal tumour may require caesarean delivery, while an obstructing epignathus or cervical teratoma may require *ex utero* intrapartum treatment (EXIT; see below).

Important family medical history, e.g. Li–Fraumeni syndrome or retinoblastoma, has been found in 16 per cent of cases, and 15 per cent have associated congenital abnormalities (Parkes *et al.* 1994).

Several studies have shown the incidence of neonatal tumours to be increasing.

This chapter does not cover the very rare neonatal leukaemias or intracranial tumours.

RELEVANT BASIC SCIENCE

The average blood volume for a neonate is around 80 mL/kg, so in a 3-kg baby with a total blood volume of 240 mL, loss of

24 mL represents a significant bleed. Large tumours such as SCTs may cause high-output cardiac failure or hydrops fetalis *in utero* and may require specific surgical techniques to avoid lethal blood loss during surgery. Both aprotinin and cardiopulmonary bypass have been utilized to enable excision of huge tumours. In addition, the fluid requirements based on preoperative weight may need to be adjusted following surgery.

The glomerular filtration rate is relatively low at birth and does not reach an adult level until the child is two years of age. The dosage of chemotherapy regimens must, therefore, be adjusted carefully to take this into consideration. Body weight rather than surface area should be used to calculate chemotherapy doses, and the drugs should be started at reduced levels, increasing as tolerated.

Radiotherapy is almost never required for neonates and should be avoided if possible, as neonates are extremely sensitive to its side effects, such as asymmetrical growth, scoliosis and intellectual impairment. In addition, thyroid malignancy following neonatal radiation exposure has been described. Tangential-beam radiotherapy in low doses has been described as treatment for the huge hepatomegaly of stage IV-S neuroblastoma, when splinting of the diaphragm threatens respiration.

Surgical excision must be precise to avoid collateral damage, and the effects of surgery and resultant scarring should be planned with long-term growth in mind. Following surgery for SCT, up to 29 per cent of children may have a neuropathic bladder (Malone *et al.* 1990). It is uncertain whether this is due to the tumour bulk preoperatively or damage due to surgery. The majority of malignant neonatal tumours respond well to chemotherapy, and mutilating surgery should be avoided.

Alpha-fetoprotein (AFP) is a single-chain glycoprotein produced by the fetal liver, bowel and yolk sac. The peak synthesis occurs at the fifteenth week of gestation, but the fetal levels fall rapidly in the third trimester. In the neonate, physiological AFP levels are at their highest at birth, and then decline along a logarithmic curve to attain a normal level (<10 ng/mL) by eight months of age.

Malignant teratomas and yolk-sac tumours cause raised levels of AFP in children. After successful removal of an AFP-producing tumour, the AFP level falls gradually, with a half-life of five days, to normal. An AFP level that rises from normal after tumour resection is a sensitive measure of tumour recurrence.

Maternal therapeutic drug use during pregnancy has been associated with neonatal malignancies, but the relatively small numbers have precluded accurate study. Amongst the drugs incriminated are phenytoin (neuroblastoma), paracetamol (sarcomas), antibiotics (leukaemias), petroleum (hepatoblastoma) and dicycloverine (dicyclomine) (teratomas).

PRESENTATION

Antenatal ultrasonography can identify tumours such as teratomas, neuroblastomas and lymphangiomas. The antenatal diagnosis of a lymphangioma of the neck may necessitate amniocentesis because of an association with chromosomal abnormalities. Poor swallowing by the fetus due to a neck teratoma can cause maternal polyhydramnios. Massive tumours can cause high-output cardiac failure and subsequent hydrops fetalis.

Postnatally, abdominal tumours present because of palpation by the midwife, doctor or parent. Mediastinal teratomas present as respiratory distress confirmed by chest radiology. Another common presentation is of non-specific malaise, failure to thrive or poor feeding, with the lesion visible on subsequent imaging. Stage IV-S neuroblastomas may present with the 'blueberry-muffin' baby appearance of multifocal bruised skin lesions. Stage IV neuroblastoma is rare in neonates but can present with periorbital bruising ('panda-eye sign'), which can be misdiagnosed as child abuse.

HISTOLOGICAL TYPES

Neonatal tumours present as germ-cell tumours (46 per cent), neuroblastomas (15 per cent), retinoblastomas (17 per cent), soft-tissue tumours (eight per cent) and others (14 per cent).

Teratomas

The primordial germ cells develop in the yolk sac of the fetus at about three weeks' gestation. From here, they migrate along the dorsal mesentery of the hindgut to the genital ridges, arriving at six weeks' gestation at the gonads. Germ-cell tumours may arise in the gonads; or, if there is aberrant migration of these totipotential cells, tumours can arise in sites corresponding to the migratory route: retroperitoneum (dorsal mesentery), sacrococcygeal area, neck, mediastinum or pineal gland. Teratomas arise from these pluripotential cells and are composed of tissue from all three germinal layers (Box 41.1).

Box 41.1 Histopathological classification of germ–cell tumours (after Dehner 1986)

Germinoma:
    A: intratubular germ-cell neoplasia
    B: invasive (dysgerminoma, seminoma)
Teratoma:
    A: mature/benign
    B: immature
    C: malignant (teratoma plus one or more
       malignant elements)
Embryonal carcinoma (adult type)
Endodermal sinus tumour (yolk-sac tumour)
Choriocarcinoma
Gonadoblastoma

SACROCOCCYGEAL TERATOMA

Forty-seven per cent of teratomas arise in the sacrococcygeal region, and SCTs are the most common neonatal tumours, with an incidence of one in 40 000 live births. The ratio of boys to girls is one to four.

When the diagnosis has been made prenatally, serial ultrasound measurements of the tumour should be taken, with a view to performing elective early caesarean delivery if the tumour threatens dystocia (tumour size >5 cm at 32 weeks' gestation) or if there are signs of hydrops. Rupture of a large tumour at birth can cause sudden death due to haemorrhage.

Serum AFP and human chorionic gonadotrophin (HCG) should be measured as baseline investigations, although levels will be elevated (compared with adult levels) for the first 6–12 months. Magnetic resonance imaging (MRI) is the best imaging technique for these tumours.

Altman et al. (1974) described four subgroups of tumour in a study of 398 patients. The most common site was predominantly external (type 1: 46 per cent), followed by external with significant intrapelvic component (type 2: 35 per cent), external, pelvic and significant intra-abdominal intrusion (type 3: nine per cent), and entirely presacral or abdominal (type 4: ten per cent). As expected, there may be a delayed diagnosis of type 4 tumours, where symptoms may be attributed erroneously to constipation or perianal abscess.

Although the majority of neonatal SCTs are benign, malignant teratomas and yolk-sac tumours occur in ten per cent of affected neonates and up to 67 per cent of affected infants. Surgery therefore should be carried out within a few days of birth.

Currarino et al. (1981) described a triad of congenital anorectal stenosis, anterior sacral defect and presacral mass. In the majority of cases, the presacral mass has been a teratoma, although anterior meningoceles and dermoid cysts have been reported. A tethered cord may be present in 18 per cent of cases.

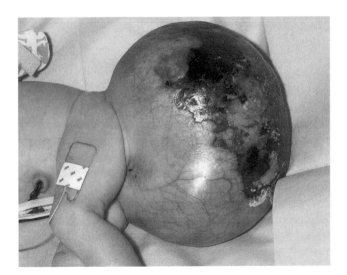

Figure 41.1 *Large sacrococcygeal teratoma.*

Primary treatment is surgical resection, with coccygectomy. Classically, surgery is performed through a chevron incision, although the author favours the aesthetics of a midline incision and has not encountered difficulty with resection (Figure 41.1). A combined abdominoperineal approach may be required for removal, and very large tumours may require ligation of the median sacral vessels early in the procedure. Frozen section can be used to ensure that margins are clear, but mature teratoma can be difficult to distinguish from normal tissue. The aims of surgery are non-mutilating complete resection with preservation of sacral plexus nerves and an acceptable scar.

Postoperatively, children should be followed up with two- to three-monthly AFP measurements for at least 48 months. Up to 29 per cent of children suffer neuropathy of bladder or bowel function, although it is not known whether this is the result of the presence of the tumour or a consequence of the excision surgery. At review, symptoms of bladder dysfunction should be actively sought, and renal tract ultrasound and uroflowmetry performed, with urodynamic studies being undertaken if these are abnormal.

A recurrence rate of up to 14 per cent is reported. However, chemotherapy for recurrence is often successful. For malignant tumours, chemotherapy with carboplatin, etoposide and bleomycin (JEB) is almost universally successful, so mutilating surgery should be avoided (Mann et al. 1998).

The differential diagnosis of a sacral mass includes a lipomeningocele (usually posterior to the sacrum; does not displace the rectal gas shadow on a lateral radiograph) or an anterior meningocele. In the latter, rectal digital pressure causes bulging of the fontanelle.

HEAD AND NECK TERATOMAS/EPIGNATHUS

Only two per cent of teratomas originate in the head and neck. However, despite their usually benign histology, they can be lethal by virtue of airway obstruction. They may arise in the mouth (tongue or palatal fossa), skull/facial skeleton or neck. Teratomas of the tongue are very rare and can be associated with cleft palates in 25 per cent of cases. Large oropharyngeal tumours may interfere with fetal swallowing and cause maternal polyhydramnios.

The EXIT procedure may be required for nasopharyngeal and cervical tumours. This procedure consists of securing the airway of the fetus partially delivered and still connected with the placenta. This technique leaves an intact fetoplacental circulation for up to 60 minutes and guarantees normal fetal oxygenation while fetal airway patency is secured. The EXIT procedure is indicated whenever fetal airways can be compromised at birth, i.e. when oropharyngeal masses, laryngeal atresia, cystic hygroma or goitre are encountered during prenatal ultrasound.

Surgical excision is the prime treatment for these benign tumours, but due consideration should be given to the cosmetic results of head and neck surgery. Thyroid and parathyroid function should be checked after excision of neck teratomas.

GONADAL TERATOMAS

The primary diagnosis of an enlarged testis at this age would be neonatal torsion. However, germ-cell tumours of the testis can occur rarely, and these require a high inguinal orchidectomy. Histology varies from mature teratoma to malignant yolk-sac tumour. Essentially, treatment for stage one is surgery alone, but advanced stages of malignancy require chemotherapy, which is almost always successful.

Childhood ovarian teratomas occur mainly in early adolescence, but ovarian cysts may be diagnosed antenatally. Clearly, the vast majority of these will be benign, but the thrust of management is to identify those that may not be. Sequential ultrasound scanning commencing in the neonatal period and combined with serum tumour markers will identify malignant elements. A conservative approach can be used for simple cysts less than 5 cm in diameter. Larger cysts and cysts with solid elements or septae should be excised to avoid the risk of torsion or to remove the very rare cases of teratoma. It is often possible to preserve some ipsilateral ovarian tissue during resection.

GASTRIC TERATOMAS

Gastric teratomas comprise less than one per cent of teratomas. Ninety per cent occur in males, and the majority are benign. A gastric teratoma usually presents as an abdominal mass, associated with vomiting or gastrointestinal bleeding. Roentgenography shows a large soft-tissue mass, often with calcification and occasionally teeth or bone visible. Complete surgical excision is usually possible and is curative.

MEDIASTINAL TERATOMAS

A teratoma of the anterior mediastinum may present antenatally, incidentally on a chest X-ray or following investigation for respiratory distress. Computed tomography (CT) and MRI (Figure 41.2) demonstrate the extent of the tumour and indicate appropriate surgical approach. Total surgical excision with appropriate oncological follow-up is required.

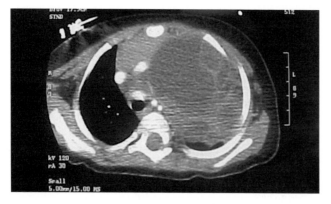

Figure 41.2 *Magnetic resonance imaging scan, showing a large anterior mediastinal mature teratoma in a neonate with respiratory distress.*

These tumours can be approached via lateral thoracotomy or midline sternotomy, as appropriate.

NEUROBLASTOMA

Neuroblastoma in neonates may present as an adrenal mass detected on antenatal ultrasound scan, or as hepatomegaly secondary to stage IV-S disease. Infiltration of the liver by metastatic neuroblastoma or leukaemia is a more common cause of hepatomegaly than primary hepatic tumours. In addition, neuroblastomas can present with Horner syndrome (apical thoracic disease) or opsomyoclonus (dancing eye syndrome), both of which carry a very good prognosis.

The prognosis of neuroblastoma detected before one year of age is excellent, particularly in patients whose disease is detected by screening. In some institutions, patients with stage I or II neuroblastoma detected by screening have been observed closely without any treatment. Most showed tumour regression or maturation and are surviving without tumour resection. Resection of neonatal neuroblastoma sometimes is complicated by vascular accidents, resulting in vanishing kidney or intestinal infarction. The role of surgery in the treatment of neonatal stage I or II neuroblastoma therefore is becoming controversial.

Evans *et al.* (1971) described stage IV-S of neuroblastoma, which behaves in an unusual fashion. The infant usually has a small abdominal or adrenal primary tumour and widespread metastatic disease, with bone marrow, liver and/or skin involvement. The prognosis is paradoxically good for such children, and 80 per cent will resolve spontaneously without aggressive chemotherapy. Surgery may be required to excise the primary tumour after regression. If the infant presents with massive hepatomegaly, then the development of an abdominal compartment syndrome may require releasing incisions in the abdominal wall, which will allow the child to survive for the two or three months necessary for the hepatomegaly to resolve.

Some five per cent of children with neuroblastoma present with signs and symptoms of spinal-cord compression due to dumbbell tumours. Surgery to the tumour and cord decompression by laminectomy may be required in addition to chemotherapy and/or radiotherapy. Sequelae of ongoing paralysis or scoliosis occur in 40 per cent of survivors, and some authors have advocated chemotherapy alone to avoid this risk.

Advanced stage III and IV neuroblastomas account for only five per cent of cases diagnosed in the neonatal period. In view of the serious risk of renal vascular damage following surgery, surgery should be limited to diagnostic biopsy only before planned treatment with a specialist oncologist.

Overall survival for a neonate diagnosed with neuroblastoma is 91 per cent (100 per cent for stages I, II and III; 81 per cent for stage IV-S; 50 per cent for stage IV).

Renal tumours

Renal tumours are rare in this age group, and non-malignant causes of a mass such as hydronephrosis or multicystic kidney should be considered. When they do occur, Wilms tumours usually have a good prognosis when treated by surgery alone.

Congenital mesoblastic nephromas (CMNs, Bolande's tumours) are more common than Wilms tumours in the neonatal period. They may be diagnosed antenatally on ultrasound scanning. They have been described as causing polyhydramnios. Postnatally, a mass can be felt. Often, they are the cause of hypertension. Ultrasound examination usually shows a well-delineated round tumour with inhomogeneous echo texture and equal or increased echogenicity in comparison to the liver. They often enclose small cysts, but they seldom have metastases or calcifications.

Early nephrectomy is curative for the majority, although metastatic tumours have been described (usually to the brain), for which chemotherapy (vincristine) has a good effect. The description of a t(12;15)(p13;q25) chromosomal translocation in both cellular CMN and congenital infantile fibrosarcoma suggests that these entities have a common pathogenesis.

Neonatal liver tumours

Although 60 per cent of childhood hepatoblastomas occur in the first year of life, diagnosis in a neonate is rare. Surgical resection may be required but carries significant morbidity.

Hepatic haemangiomas are rare benign vascular tumours that manifest as asymptomatic liver masses or with high-output cardiac failure, anaemia or consumptive coagulopathy. Cutaneous haemangioma may give a clue to the diagnosis. Rarely, resection or vessel embolization to reduce arteriovenous shunting may be required.

Cardiac tumours

Very rarely, rhabdomyosarcomas, haemangiomas and teratomas may cause heart failure in a neonate or be diagnosed on antenatal ultrasonography. Cardiac myomas have not been described in neonates.

Soft-tissue sarcoma

The most common tumours are those of fibrous tissue: the fibromatoses (infantile fibromatosis and myofibromatosis) and fibrosarcoma. These tumours occur particularly in the head, neck and extremities and may be locally aggressive, requiring radical surgery, but they seldom metastasize.

Rhabdomyosarcomas are rare in neonates, as are haemangiopericytomas, undifferentiated sarcomas and leiomyosarcomas. Treatment is much the same as for older children, but the prognosis appears to be very poor for rhabdomyosarcomas, with all six babies diagnosed in a study in Toronto dying of the disease within 16 months.

Retinoblastoma

Seven per cent of retinoblastomas present at birth, usually with leucocoria (white or yellow retinal reflex), heterochromia iridis or strabismus. In addition, screening of babies with a family history can electively diagnose retinoblastoma. Most cases are due to spontaneous mutation of the retinoma gene on chromosome 13, although multifocal or bilateral retinoblastomas are usually due to an inherited genetic defect (Knudson's two-hit hypothesis). Treatment is by chemotherapy, local cryosurgery or laser surgery, radioactive plaques or external beam irradiation. Enucleation is required rarely in eyes already blinded by the tumour.

Vascular malformations

Vascular lesions have been classified into haemangiomas (endothelial hyperplasia) and vascular malformations characterized by errors of vascular morphogenesis (Table 41.1).

Haemangiomas are benign neoplasms that proliferate rapidly in infancy and involute in early childhood. The majority of these require no treatment other than reassurance, but large lesions that interfere with sight or respiration, and very disfiguring lesions, may be reduced with corticosteroids or interferon alfa-2a.

Vascular malformations are not tumours but errors of vessel (arterial, venous, capillary or lymphatic) formation.

LYMPHANGIOMA: CYSTIC HYGROMA

Cystic hygroma is a congenital malformation of the lymphatic system appearing as a single or multiloculated fluid-filled cavity, most often in the cervical region. The malformation is believed to arise from failure of the lymphatic system to communicate with the venous nuchal system. When discovered before 30 weeks' gestation, it is associated with chromosomal abnormality in 70 per cent of fetuses, often leading to spontaneous or therapeutic abortion. This seems especially true for Turner syndrome (the largest aetiological group associated with cystic hygroma) and the lethal multiple pterygium

Table 41.1 *Mulliken and Glowacki's (1982) biological classification of vascular lesions*

Classification	Former terminology
Haemangioma	Angioma
Single malformation:	
Capillary	Port-wine stain
Arterial	
Venous	
Lymphatic	Cystic hygroma, lymphangioma
Combined malformation:	
Arteriovenous	
Capillary-venous-lymphatic	Klippel–Trénaunay
Capillary arteriovenous	Parkes Weber
Combined	Sturge–Weber

syndromes. Down syndrome may be diagnosed antenatally in this way. Sometimes, the lesion progresses to fetal hydrops, causing fetal death.

However, when appearing after the thirtieth week of gestation, cystic hygroma has a more benign course and is not associated with chromosomal abnormalities.

Around 60 per cent of cystic hygromas are visible at birth, and 90 per cent appear before the child has reached his or her second birthday. MRI is the imaging of choice and often shows a lesion that is more extensive than that seen on ultrasonography.

Lymphangiomas develop early embryologically and do not follow tissue planes, making complete surgical excision challenging. Good results can be obtained with injections of bleomycin, OK432 or triamcinolone (10 mg/kg) repeated at intervals. Mutilating surgery should be avoided.

HAEMANGIOMAS

Haemangiomas are present in one to two per cent at birth but may appear in the first few weeks of life; the incidence is ten per cent at one year of age. They grow by cellular proliferation, and their hallmark is rapid neonatal growth. Spontaneous regression begins when the infant is six to ten months old, but it may continue until eight to ten years of age. Half involute by the time the child reaches his or her fifth birthday. Spontaneous regression leaves superior cosmesis, and surgery should be avoided in most instances. Surgical care frequently consists of reassuring parents that the lesion will regress.

However, large haemangiomas may be associated with consumptive coagulopathy (Kasabach–Merritt phenomenon) or high-output cardiac failure. The use of systemic corticosteroids and/or interferon alfa and, in some cases, embolization or surgical resection may be required.

Rarely, the lesions interfere with sight, respiration or feeding, and active treatment is required.

VASCULAR MALFORMATIONS

Vascular malformations are present at birth, although they may not become clinically evident until later, and do not regress. They are seen in 0.5 per cent of neonates. They grow at the same rate as the child and may require treatment to improve cosmesis. Doppler flow ultrasonography and MRI are useful to distinguish slow-flow and fast-flow lesions and to document the full extent of the lesion, which is often far in excess of what the surface markings would suggest.

For the majority of malformations, surgical excision is adequate, but this may need to be repeated. In addition, compression garments, laser therapy, embolization, and bleomycin or OK452 injection may be required. Capillary malformations may signal a more complex underlying lesion, such as Klippel–Trénaunay syndrome, Parkes Weber syndrome, proteus syndrome, phacomatosis pigmentovascularis or Sturge–Weber syndrome.

The more aggressive and rare vascular tumours, kaposiform haemangioendothelioma and tufted angioma, are often associated with thrombocytopenia and coagulopathy and are less responsive to pharmacological therapy.

CONCLUSION

Tumours in neonates require specialist care from paediatric oncologists, surgeons, neonatologists, radiologists and anaesthetists. These tumours are rare and do not behave like tumours in older children or adults. Surgery is curative in many cases, but mutilating operations should be avoided. The long-term sequelae of surgery, chemotherapy and radiotherapy should be monitored and taken into account during treatment. All such tumours should be entered into a tumour registry.

CLINICAL SCENARIOS

Case 1

A sacrococcygeal teratoma was diagnosed antenatally and confirmed at birth. The girl was delivered vaginally without difficulty. Preoperative imaging included ultrasound scanning and MRI. These showed a large multicystic teratoma extending into the pelvis (Altman type 3), together with an enlarged bladder. Preoperative alpha-fetoprotein levels were 100 000 IU – normal for a neonate. At one week of age, she underwent a combined abdominoperineal resection of the tumour, including coccygectomy. She made a rapid recovery and was followed up in the regional oncology department with bimonthly AFP measurement. Her AFP levels fell as expected towards the normal level of below 10 IU and have remained normal. At three years of age she is well, but she is awaiting urodynamic studies as there are some features of mild bladder neuropathy.

Case 2

An antenatal ultrasound scan showed a mass replacing the left adrenal gland. The postnatal diagnosis lay between adrenal haemorrhage and neuroblastoma. Raised urinary catecholamine levels confirmed the latter diagnosis. Further imaging revealed multifocal liver metastases and a positive bone-marrow aspiration. Chemotherapy was given for stage IV-S disease, as the liver enlargement was causing respiratory embarrassment. After one cycle, positive-pressure ventilation and tangential-beam radiotherapy or an abdominal wall patch were considered. However, the child's condition stabilized and he is now well, off therapy. After four cycles of chemotherapy, a left adrenalectomy was performed without incident.

Case 3

A right cervical cystic hygroma was diagnosed at 12 weeks' gestation. Chorionic villous sampling was undertaken, which confirmed normal 46,XX chromosomes. After delivery, a large right parotid cystic hygroma was present, which showed retropharyngeal extension on MRI scanning. A subtotal excision was performed when the infant was aged six months. Surgery was limited by extension of the mass around the facial nerves and great vessels. Two injections of bleomycin have since been performed under ultrasound control, with limited effect. The child is now 18 months old.

Case 4

The mother of a two-week-old girl reported that a discoloured spot above the infant's right eye began to enlarge. When seen at one month of age, this was diagnosed clinically as a haemangioma, and a conservative approach was undertaken. The child, who is now three years old, has been reviewed regularly to reassure her mother and to ensure that the haemangioma does not encroach to threaten the child's vision. Recently, the mass has started to decrease in size, with a characteristic central pallor. It is expected to diminish completely within the year, with excellent eventual cosmesis and little residual scarring.

REFERENCES

Altman RP, Randolph JG, Lilly JR. Sacrococcygeal teratomas. American Academy of Pediatric Surgical Section Survey. *Journal of Pediatric Surgery* 1974; **9**: 691.

Borch K, Jacobsen T, Olsen JH, Hirsch FR, Hertz H. Neonatal cancer in Denmark 1943–1985. *Ugeskrift for Laeger* 1994; **156**: 176–9.

Currarino G, Coln D, Votteler T. Triad of anorectal, sacral and presacral anomalies. *American Journal of Roentgenology* 1981; **137**: 395–8.

Dehner L. *Paediatric Surgical Pathology*, 2nd edn. Baltimore, MD: Williams & Wilkins, 1986.

Evans AE, D'Angio GJ, Randolph JG. A proposed staging for children with neuroblastoma. *Cancer* 1971; **27**: 374.

Malone PS, Spitz L, Keily EM, *et al.* The functional sequelae of sacrococcygeal teratoma. *Journal of Pediatric Surgery* 1990; **25**: 679–80.

Mann JR, Raafat F, Robinson K, *et al.* The UKCCSG Germ cell tumour studies: improving outcome for children with malignant extracranial non-gonadal tumours – carboplatin, etoposide and bleomycin are effective and less toxic than previous regimens. *Medical and Pediatric Oncology* 1998; **30**: 217–27.

Mulliken JB, Glowacki J. Haemangiomas and vascular malformations in children: a classification based on endothelial characteristics. *Plastic and Reconstructive Surgery* 1982; **69**: 412–22.

Parkes SE, Muir KR, Southern L, *et al.* Neonatal tumours: a thirty year population based study. *Medical and Pediatric Oncology* 1994; **22**: 309–17.

42

Wilms tumour

RICHARD SPICER

Learning objectives

- To understand the history, differing international strategies and rationale for multimodal therapy of Wilms tumour.
- To recognize common modes of presentation of Wilms tumour.
- To understand how the paediatric surgeon must liaise with colleagues in paediatric oncology, radiology and pathology in the management of Wilms tumour.
- To know the principles of safe surgical management of Wilms tumour.

INTRODUCTION AND HISTORY

Max Wilms (1867–1918), Professor of Surgery in Heidelberg, described the tumour that still bears his name in 1899. It is, therefore, incorrect to write 'Wilm's tumour' or 'Wilm tumour'. 'Wilms tumour' is correct, but 'Wilms' tumour' is acceptable.

Wilms tumour (WT, nephroblastoma) is the most common renal tumour of childhood and the second most common intra-abdominal malignancy after neuroblastoma. Approximately 100 new cases per year are diagnosed in Great Britain and Ireland and treated according to UK Children's Cancer Study Group (UKCCSG) protocols. The incidence is higher in black children than in white children. Historically, less than 20 per cent of children with Wilms tumour were cured in the era when surgery was the only treatment. The introduction of radiotherapy and chemotherapy improved survival rates. However, with modern multimodal therapy, long-term survival rates of 90 per cent are achievable, and even in patients with metastatic disease, 70 per cent can achieve long-term cure.

There are international philosophical differences in the approach to treatment. In the USA, surgery is still the preferred initial treatment, but in France and many other European countries, it has for many years been routine to give all patients preoperative chemotherapy. A UK clinical trial (UKW3) that ran from 1991 to 2001 aimed to compare these strategies in a randomized multicentre study and reached the following important conclusions regarding the advantages of systematic neo-adjuvant therapy:

- It reduces the incidence of intraoperative rupture from 15 to zero per cent. This is important, because ruptured tumours mandate abdominal radiotherapy, which carries a serious risk of adverse late effects in young children (Figure 42.1).
- Operative blood loss is reduced.
- It increases the proportion of stage I tumours and reduces the proportion of stage III tumours, thus reducing the burden of therapy (chemotherapy and radiotherapy).

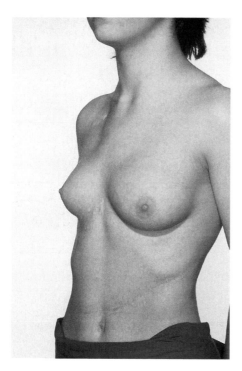

Figure 42.1 *Breast hypoplasia due to previous radiotherapy for right Wilms tumour.*

The current UK trial (WT 2002–01) therefore mandates preoperative chemotherapy for the majority of patients.

BASIC SCIENCE

The typical nephroblastoma is histologically 'triphasic', with blastemal, stromal and tubular elements. Anaplastic elements are known to be associated with higher clinical stage and a less favourable outcome. The so-called 'bone-metastasizing Wilms tumour' is actually a sarcoma and also has a worse prognosis.

Other factors known to be associated with a worse outcome include *p53* mutation and allele loss at 1p and/or 16q.

Although most children with Wilms tumour have no associated congenital anomalies, there are some rare syndromes known to carry a high risk of Wilms tumour. These include:

- Beckwith–Wiedemann syndrome;
- hemi-hypertrophy;
- WAGR syndrome (Wilms tumour, aniridia, genitourinary anomalies, mental retardation);
- Denys–Drash syndrome (nephrotic syndrome and ambiguous genitalia).

In addition, some Wilms tumour families have been identified, and studies of these families and the syndromic patients have led to interesting insight into the genetics and oncogenesis of Wilms tumour. A Wilms tumour gene (*WT1*) has been identified on chromosome 11p13, but this is not associated with most cases; in some, it may arise as a sporadic mutation.

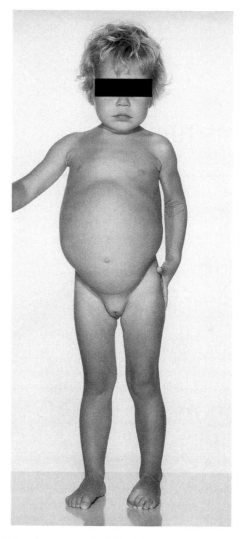

Figure 42.2 *Asymptomatic child with abdominal mass due to bilateral Wilms tumours.*

It is thought that Wilms tumour arises from fetal undifferentiated metanephric blastema via an intermediate histological entity called nephrogenic rests, which are an incidental finding in one per cent of neonatal autopsies. As the incidence of Wilms tumour is one in 10 000 children, the implication is that only one per cent of children with nephrogenic rests progress to develop Wilms tumour. The clinical situation in which a child has multiple small renal lesions that have not yet progressed to be Wilms tumour, is known as 'nephroblastomatosis'.

CLINICAL PRESENTATION

The child typically is aged between three and five years and is found to have an asymptomatic abdominal mass (Figure 42.2). Other presenting features may include:

- haematuria (15 per cent);
- abdominal pain (ten per cent);
- fever (20 per cent).

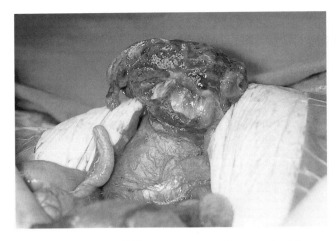

Figure 42.3 *Ruptured Wilms tumour presenting as acute abdomen.*

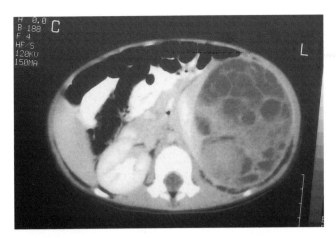

Figure 42.4 *Typical computed tomography scan appearance of a left Wilms tumour. Note the solid and cystic elements.*

Hypertension occurs in ten per cent of patients and may be a significant clinical problem. In some cases, this can be shown to be due to elevated serum renin.

In the child presenting with abdominal pain, it is important to look for peritonism and a falling haemoglobin level, as some children may present with rupture or bleeding into the tumour (Figure 42.3).

DIFFERENTIAL DIAGNOSIS

Benign renal masses usually can be distinguished radiologically. Of particular importance is xanthogranulomatous pyelonephritis (XGP). Associated fever, pyuria, anaemia and leucocytosis indicate XGP, and an experienced paediatric radiologist usually can distinguish this condition from Wilms tumour on ultrasound. Contralateral renal hypertrophy is usual in XGP.

Other malignancies occur at extremes of age, i.e. mesoblastic nephroma in the neonate and renal-cell carcinoma in the older child.

Renal rhabdoid tumour has a poor prognosis and may be suspected on imaging and proved by biopsy.

Neuroblastoma may be confused with Wilms tumour, but elevated urinary catecholamines are usually discriminatory.

IMAGING

As indicated above, imaging by an experienced paediatric radiologist is crucial to successful management.

If calcification is seen on *plain abdominal X-ray*, then the tumour is more likely to be neuroblastoma than Wilms tumour. *Chest X-ray* (postero-anterior and lateral) should be done in all cases. Computed tomography (CT) scanning is necessary if metastases are suspected.

Ultrasound in experienced hands is highly accurate in defining the primary tumour. It is also useful for detecting liver metastases or extension and, in particular, tumour extension along the renal vein into the inferior vena cava. The radiologist must measure three dimensions to allow an estimate of volume and facilitate measurement of shrinkage after chemotherapy.

Echocardiography is complementary in demonstrating whether venous tumour thrombus extends to the right atrium.

CT scanning (Figure 42.4) is not essential to the management of Wilms tumour in developing countries with limited facilities. Indeed, it was not done commonly in the UK until relatively recently. The scan should always be done with intravenous contrast. Indications for CT scanning are:

- the possibility of small pulmonary metastases: it is essential that no child being treated under the current UK protocol is allocated to stage I unless a chest CT scan has been done;
- to confirm that the contralateral kidney is normal: the alternative is to surgically mobilize and examine all surfaces of the contralateral kidney, but abdominal CT scan has been shown to be more accurate and is now recommended for UK patients;
- if the tumour is thought to be non-resectable ('inoperable'): CT scanning may help in making this decision.

Magnetic resonance imaging (MRI) is not indicated often, but it may be useful in two specific situations:

- intracaval tumour extension (Figure 42.5)
- nephroblastomatosis

Arteriography is useful for preoperative planning in patients with a solitary kidney, bilateral tumours or a tumour in a horseshoe kidney.

Isotope renography ^{99m}-Tc-dimercaptosuccinic acid (DMSA) scan may be helpful in the preoperative planning of bilateral tumours.

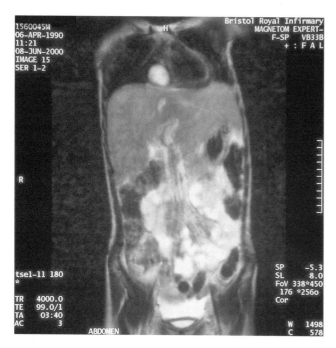

Figure 42.5 *Magnetic resonance imaging scan, showing tumour extension along the renal vein and up the inferior vena cava to the right atrium.*

STAGING AND RISK STRATIFICATION

Different national groups use different staging systems. The UK staging system is summarized below:

Stage I: tumour confined to the kidney and completely resected.

Stage II: tumour extends beyond the kidney but is completely resected.

Stage III: any one of the following:
– incomplete tumour resection;
– tumour in abdominal lymph nodes;
– tumour rupture (preoperative or intraoperative);
– peritoneal spread;
– open biopsy (not needle biopsy).

Stage IV: metastatic disease (usually pulmonary).

Stage V: bilateral renal tumours.

In previous UK protocols, the intensity of chemotherapy was related mainly to stage. In the current study, the situation is much more complicated, since the majority of tumours are pretreated with chemotherapy; the paediatric pathologist then has to examine the nephrectomy specimen and allocate the patient to a histological risk group, which is then used, in conjunction with stage, to determine the intensity of chemotherapy. Completely necrotic tumour is deemed to indicate a low risk. There is a new concept of 'regressive tumour', which is defined as more than two-thirds of the tumour being necrotic; most of these will fall into the intermediate-risk group. A heavy responsibility falls on the pathologist, who allocates a patient

Table 42.1 *Risk stratification for tumours treated with pre-nephrectomy chemotherapy*

Low-risk tumours	Intermediate-risk tumours	High-risk tumours
Mesoblastic nephroma	Nephroblastoma, epithelial type	Nephroblastoma, blastemal type
Cystic partially differentiated nephroblastoma	Nephroblastoma, stromal type	Nephroblastoma, diffuse anaplasia
Completely necrotic nephroblastoma	Nephroblastoma, mixed type	Clear-cell sarcoma of kidney
	Nephroblastoma, regressive type	Rhabdoid tumour of kidney
	Nephroblastoma, focal anaplasia	

to low risk (implying minimal chemotherapy and a high risk of relapse if this judgement is erroneous) or high risk (with the implication of a heavy burden of therapy and increased likelihood of adverse late effects). As there is a shortage in the UK of skilled paediatric pathologists, and some centres may lack the necessary expertise, it is a mandatory requirement that the histological specimens are sent for urgent central review by an expert panel in any patient who is allocated to the low-risk or high-risk group.

A further complexity is that UK pathologists have been accustomed to seeing nephrectomy specimens that are not pretreated, and difficult judgements have to be made as to whether resection margins or lymph nodes show evidence of treated tumour (e.g. necrosis, macrophages), which would upgrade the patient to stage III.

Histological risk stratification is summarized in Table 42.1.

CHEMOTHERAPY

All patients have chemotherapy before surgery, unless there are indications for primary surgery, e.g. doubt in diagnosis, rupture, cystic tumours, age under six months. Except in the case of stages IV and V tumours, this chemotherapy is as follows:

- Vincristine 1.5 mg/m² weekly for four weeks.
- Dactinomycin 45 μg/kg × 2 doses (weeks one and three).

As indicated above, the decision regarding further postoperative chemotherapy is based on stage and histological risk group (Table 42.2).

Stage IV disease

The three-drug regime is given for six weeks, with nephrectomy being carried out at seven weeks. If nephrectomy is impossible or metastases are persistent, then there are further recommendations for treatment, but these are beyond the scope of this chapter.

Table 42.2 *Chemotherapy*

Risk	Stage I	Stage II	Stage III
Low	No further treatment	Vincristine + dactinomycin, 4 months	Vincristine + dactinomycin, 4 months
Intermediate	Vincristine + dactinomycin, 4 weeks	Randomized, three drugs *v.* two drugs	Randomized, three drugs *v.* two drugs
High	Vincristine + dactinomycin + doxorubicin, 4 months	Etoposide + carboplatin + cyclophosphamide + doxorubicin, 6 months	As for stage II, high risk

The randomized study for stages II and III intermediate risk is designed to determine whether the addition of doxorubicin (a cardiotoxic drug) improves survival of these patients.

Abdominal radiotherapy is added for high-risk stage II and III patients.

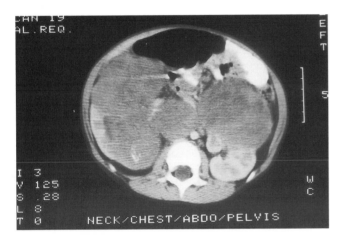

Figure 42.6 *Computed tomography scan in a case of bilateral (stage V) Wilms tumour.*

Stage V disease (Figure 42.6)

Two-drug treatment is given initially to minimize nephrotoxicity. Thereafter, treatment is individualized, according to response.

Nephroblastomatosis

Two-drug treatment is given for 12 months.

SURGERY

As mentioned above, UK practice has now moved towards routine preoperative chemotherapy, with nephrectomy being carried out at five to six weeks. Immediate surgery is indicated in the following situations:

- ruptured tumour at presentation (emergency);

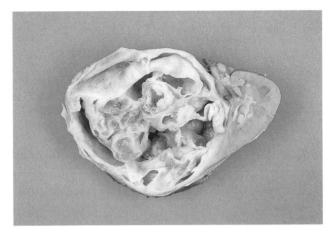

Figure 42.7 *Cystic partially differentiated nephroblastoma. Such tumours should be treated by immediate nephrectomy and should not be biopsied.*

- largely cystic tumour (not possible to biopsy, relatively insensitive to chemotherapy) (see Figure 42.7);
- doubt in diagnosis, despite needle biopsy;
- infants under six months of age (likelihood of mesoblastic nephroma, increased difficulties in chemotherapy).

Biopsy

This is a controversial topic, since in France and many other European countries the diagnosis is made on clinical and imaging information only, with a high diagnostic accuracy. However, since approximately five per cent of patients do turn out to have a malignancy other than Wilms tumour, and one per cent have benign disease despite high-quality imaging, the current UK study recommends needle biopsy before chemotherapy. The following points should be noted:

- All inoperable and stage IV tumours should be biopsied.
- Cystic tumours should not be biopsied (Figure 42.7).
- Open biopsy should be done rarely (and renders the patient stage III).
- Fine-needle aspiration cytology is not appropriate.
- A 14- or 16-gauge spring-loaded cutting-core biopsy needle should be used.
- Ultrasound guidance should be used.
- A posterior retroperitoneal approach is ideal. If the biopsy is transperitoneal, then the track should be marked and excised at the time of nephrectomy.
- One to three cores should be taken and the tissue delivered fresh, not fixed, to the pathologist.
- The main purpose of the biopsy is to exclude other diagnoses. Non-diagnostic biopsies should not be repeated, and chemotherapy should not be delayed.

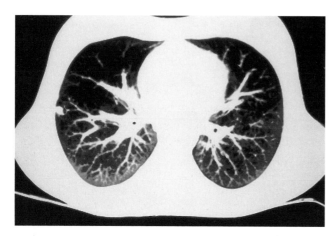

Figure 42.8 *Computed tomography scan, showing pulmonary metastasis from Wilms tumour.*

Nephrectomy

This is always performed via a generous transverse upper-abdominal supraumbilical incision, never via the loin. The first step is usually to mobilize the colon from the tumour. In right-sided tumours, the duodenum should be identified and dissected from the tumour.

The subsequent steps in dissection may vary according to the particular anatomical situation, but the following principles should be borne in mind:

- Dissection should be delicate: clumsy handling may rupture the tumour.
- It is helpful to identify and divide the ureter and gonadal vessels early and then dissect upwards, towards the renal hilum.
- The ureter does not need to be dissected down to the bladder (cf. adult urothelial carcinoma). It should be ligated at the pelvic brim.
- Sharp dissection and bipolar diathermy should be used to dissect along the aorta and inferior vena cava towards the hilum. At the same time, four hilar and para-aortic lymph nodes should be sampled for staging purposes and placed in formalin. N.B. Large nodes may be free of tumour, and small nodes may contain tumour.
- The renal artery should be ligated before the renal vein to avoid sequestration of blood within the tumour, congestion and rupture. This can be achieved either by slinging and retracting the vein or by rotating the kidney medially and identifying the artery posteriorly.
- Other structures that must be dissected from the tumour during mobilization include the diaphragm, posterior abdominal wall, liver and adrenal gland.
- If normal kidney adjoins the adrenal, as in a lower-pole tumour, then the gland may be preserved. The adrenal gland has a very rich blood supply, and adrenal vessels must be secured carefully and individually if the gland is being removed with the kidney.

- Before dividing the renal vein, it should be inspected carefully and vascular clamps applied so that any tumour extension can be seen and extracted.
- The tumour and kidney should be removed *en bloc* and received fresh by the pathologist.
- Haemostasis should be absolute, and drains should not be used.

Intracaval extension

This should always have been identified by preoperative imaging. If the extension is infrahepatic, it can be extracted safely by cavotomy alone. If intrahepatic or intra-atrial, the operation should be planned with a paediatric cardiac surgeon and cardiopulmonary bypass must be available.

Partial nephrectomy

This should be reserved for bilateral tumours and tumours in a solitary kidney.

Some surgeons in non-UK centres have done partial nephrectomy for unilateral tumours, but the evidence from large multicentre studies is that:

- partial nephrectomy is feasible in less than five per cent of cases;
- there is a 20 per cent local recurrence rate.

Metastases

Occasionally, pulmonary or hepatic metastases persisting after chemotherapy may be localized and surgically curable.

Surgical complications

Prolonged ileus and ileal intussusception may occur postoperatively.

Surgical mortality should be less than one per cent; the most common reason is delayed management of late adhesive obstruction. Historically, deaths occurred from haemorrhage and tumour embolus.

OUTCOME

Treatment-related deaths are more commonly due to chemotherapy and/or radiotherapy than surgery.

Relapsed patients can often be salvaged by appropriate therapy. Expected long-term survival is as follows:

Stage I: 90–95 per cent.
Stage II: 80–90 per cent.
Stage III: 80–85 per cent.

Stage IV: 70–75 per cent.
Stage V: 80–85 per cent.

Survival beyond three years from diagnosis usually equates with long-term cure.

There are theoretical concerns in the long term about hyperperfusion injury in children who have had nephrectomy, but in practice this seems to be restricted to the small minority of patients with aniridia or nephroblastomatosis.

The UKCCSG currently recommends the following life-long follow-up:

- annual blood pressure measurement;
- five-yearly serum creatinine;
- annual early-morning urine for protein/creatinine ratio.

CLINICAL SCENARIOS

Case 1

In 1995, an asymptomatic 2.5-year-old boy was found, by his mother whilst drying him after a bath, to have an abdominal mass. Clinical examination confirmed a right renal mass. Abdominal ultrasound showed a solid mass replacing most of the right kidney. Chest X-ray was normal.

Under the then current UK Wilms Tumour Study (UKW3), he was randomized to immediate surgery and had an uneventful right nephrectomy. Lymph nodes were free of tumour and histology showed a triphasic nephroblastoma confined to the kidney and excised completely (stage I).

He received ten weekly intravenous injections of vincristine, with minimal side effects, and he remains well eight years later.

Case 2

A five-year-old boy developed acute right-sided abdominal pain. A clinical diagnosis of acute appendicitis was made, and he proceeded to removal of a normal appendix. Postoperatively, his pain persisted. Clinical examination revealed a right upper quadrant mass. His haemoglobin, which had been 10.9 g before his appendicectomy, fell to 8.2 g.

Ultrasound confirmed a solid mass arising from the upper pole of the right kidney, with echogenic areas suggesting haemorrhage into the tumour. No lung lesions were detected on CT.

Needle biopsy showed cells 'compatible with but not diagnostic of nephroblastoma'. He proceeded to vincristine and actinomycin pretreatment and had a nephrectomy seven weeks later. Histology showed blastemal nephroblastoma and tumour in hilar and para-aortic nodes. He is currently receiving four-drug chemotherapy via a double-lumen cuffed central venous catheter and has been assessed for abdominal radiotherapy.

Case 3

A seven-year-old girl had been unwell for several months with abdominal and chest pain, dyspnoea and fatigue. Eventually, an abdominal mass was detected, and ultrasound and CT scanning confirmed a large mass replacing the left kidney. Chest X-ray showed multiple pulmonary metastases. Doppler ultrasound demonstrated intracaval tumour; echocardiography demonstrated that this extended to, and filled, the right atrium. Needle biopsy confirmed nephroblastoma. She was treated with multi-agent chemotherapy and her symptoms improved. The pulmonary metastases disappeared after eight weeks, but the intra-atrial extension persisted although somewhat reduced in size.

At 20 weeks, left nephrectomy was accomplished, the incision being extended to a median sternotomy through which the paediatric cardiac surgeon established cardiopulmonary bypass. By a joint approach, the caval and atrial tumour was extracted.

She completed chemotherapy, and abdominal and pulmonary radiotherapy were given.

She is free of disease two years later but has demonstrable cardiomyopathy due to a combination of doxorubicin and radiotherapy.

SUMMARY

Wilms tumour is one of the great success stories of paediatric oncology, but maximal long-term survival, with minimal late effects, can be achieved only by a multidisciplinary team working within a major regional paediatric oncology centre. Improvements in treatment protocols can be achieved only by large national or international collaborative studies. There is no place for the occasional practitioner.

FURTHER READING

International Society of Paediatric Oncology Nephroblastoma Clinical Trial and Study SIOP WT 2001. Published as UKCCSG Protocol No. WT 2002-02 by United Kingdom Children's Cancer Study Group. www.ukccsg.org

Pritchard-Jones K. Controversies and advances in the management of Wilms' tumour. *Archives of Disease in Childhood* 2002; **87**: 238–40.

Spicer RD, Frank JD. Wilms tumour. In: Frank JD, Gearhart JP, Snyder HM (eds). *Operative Paediatric Urology*, 2nd edn. London: Churchill Livingstone, 2002; pp. 245–57.

43

Neuroblastoma

EDWARD KIELY

Learning points

- To understand that biochemical and molecular markers enable the diagnosis and prognosis to be refined.
- To understand that surgical excision is based upon a vascular dissection.
- To understand that surgical excision may result in significant morbidity.
- To understand that abdominal tumours may be managed differently from those within the thorax.

INTRODUCTION

Neuroblastoma is the most common abdominal malignancy of childhood and constitutes about six to ten per cent of all types of childhood cancer. The cause is unknown and the incidence of the disease has not changed over many years. There is a slight male preponderance.

Until recent years, the outlook was very poor, with an overall mortality from the disease of 80–90 per cent. With the advent of a systematic approach to diagnosis and management, roughly 50 per cent of affected children will now survive this disease.

PATHOLOGY

The tumour arises from sympathetic neuroblasts originally derived from the neural crest. In early fetal life, sympathetic neuroblasts migrate to the sympathetic ganglia and to the adrenal medulla, as well as to other perivascular collections of sympathetic cells, predominantly around the aorta.

In patients whose disease is progressive, local extension with vascular encasement occurs with metastases to lymph nodes, bone, bone marrow, liver and skin.

On histological examination, the immature neuroblasts appear as sheets of dark-blue nuclei with scanty cytoplasm set in a delicate vascular stroma. More differentiated areas show the presence of ganglion cells with a more abundant stroma.

The histological appearance correlates with the biological behaviour of the tumour; accordingly, histological grading systems are used to define tumours with more aggressive behaviour. Of the different systems available, the International Neuroblastoma Pathology Classification is probably the most widely used. Using this classification, neuroblastomas may be graded into favourable or unfavourable groups on the basis of haematoxylin and eosin stained sections.

Neuroblastomas arise predominantly in the adrenal gland (40–60 per cent of the total), other abdominal sites (20 per cent), mediastinum (ten per cent), pelvis (two to six per cent) and neck (less than two per cent). Locally advanced or metastatic disease is already present in about 70 per cent of affected children at the time of diagnosis. Disease is localized in about 25 per cent; five to ten per cent of patients have the unusual metastatic disease found early in life known as stage 4S disease.

SCREENING

Because neuroblastomas frequently secrete raised levels of catecholamines, the breakdown products of these may be detected in the urine. The main break down product is vanillylmandelic acid (VMA), and raised levels of urinary VMA are detected in about 85 per cent of all neuroblastomas. As a consequence, screening programmes have been evaluated in different countries using estimation of urinary VMA during the first year of life.

A national screening programme has been in operation in Japan for some years, and pilot studies also have been undertaken in other countries. The findings have been consistent: increased numbers of children with neuroblastoma are diagnosed. The tumours detected on screening are predominantly low-stage tumours with good biological profiles. The number of children presenting with advanced disease, however, has not altered, suggesting that many of the tumours detected by screening would have resolved spontaneously.

STAGING

Staging systems are used to stratify treatment and to allow comparison between different modes of treatment. The most commonly applied system in use at present is the International Neuroblastoma Staging System (INSS) (Table 43.1).

Table 43.1 *International Neuroblastoma Staging System (INSS)*

Stage	Definition
1	Localized tumour with complete gross excision, with or without microscopic residual disease; representative ipsilateral lymph nodes negative for tumour microscopically (nodes attached to and removed with the primary tumour may be positive).
2A	Localized tumour with incomplete gross excision; representative ipsilateral non-adherent lymph nodes negative for tumour microscopically.
2B	Localized tumour with or without complete gross excision, with ipsilateral non-adherent lymph nodes positive for tumour. Enlarged contralateral lymph nodes must be negative microscopically.
3	Unresectable unilateral tumour, infiltrating across the midline,* with or without regional lymph node involvement; *or* localized unilateral tumour with contralateral regional lymph node involvement; *or* midline tumour with bilateral extension by infiltration (unresectable) or by lymph node involvement.
4	Any primary tumour with dissemination to distant lymph nodes, bone, bone marrow, liver, or other organs (except as defined for Stage 4S).
4S	Localized primary tumour (as defined for stage 1, 2A or 2B), with dissemination limited to skin, liver and bone marrow[†] (limited to infants younger than 1 year).

*The midline is defined as the vertebral column. Tumours originating on one side and crossing the midline must infiltrate to or beyond the opposite side of the vertebral column.

[†] Marrow involvement in stage 4S should be minimal (i.e. $<10\%$ of total nucleated cells identified as malignant on bone marrow biopsy or on marrow aspirate). More extensive marrow involvement would be considered to be stage 4. The *meta*-iodobenzylguanidine scan (if performed) should be negative in the marrow.

BIOCHEMICAL MARKERS

Three biochemical markers are commonly estimated, and the levels at diagnosis have prognostic implications. These include ferritin, lactate dehydrogenase (LDH) and neuron-specific enolase (NSE). Patients with high levels of these markers (ferritin > 142 ng/mL, LDH > 1500 IU/mL, NSE > 100 ng/mL) have a significantly worse outcome despite treatment.

MOLECULAR MARKERS

A substantial number of molecular markers of disease activity and disease behaviour have been defined for neuroblastoma. These include *MYCN* amplification, gain of 17q, deletion of 1p, DNA-ploidy, *CD44* expression and *TRKA* expression.

MYCN amplification (more than ten copies) is associated with advanced stage at diagnosis and with disease progression. It is associated with a worse outcome, regardless of age and stage of diagnosis.

Gain of 17q is the most common chromosomal alteration in neuroblastoma (over 50 per cent of patients) and is associated with a worse outcome. Deletion of the short arm of chromosome 1 (1p deletion) is also known to be associated with a more aggressive tumour and a worse outcome.

Diploid or near-diploid DNA content is associated with a lower survival rate. *CD44* expression generally is associated with lower-stage disease and a better outcome. The proto-oncogene *TRKA* is expressed in most patients with neuroblastoma, and high levels correlate with a better outcome.

PRESENTATION

A small number (less than five per cent) of tumours are detected on antenatal ultrasound. Antenatally diagnosed tumours tend to be low-stage tumours with good biology.

For the majority of children, insidious presentation with vague symptomatology is the rule. Malaise, fever, weight loss, sweating and bone pain are not unusual. Abdominal examination in such a child may reveal a hard, craggy abdominal mass.

In children with stage 4S disease, the presence of skin nodules or progressive abdominal enlargement may call attention to the underlying problem.

DIAGNOSIS

The diagnosis is suspected on the basis of the history, physical findings and imaging. The diagnosis is confirmed by urinary VMA estimation and evaluation of biopsy specimens. Biopsy is considered mandatory for evaluation of tumour biology in order to further stratify treatment. Needle biopsies normally give sufficient material for diagnosis and for evaluation of biological factors.

In all cases, bone-marrow aspiration and bone trephine are evaluated.

In addition to the molecular and biochemical markers of disease, the usual blood parameters are also measured.

IMAGING

Plain radiographs and ultrasound examination are often useful. However, cross-sectional imaging by computed tomography (CT) or magnetic resonance imaging (MRI) is essential to delineate the anatomy of the tumour. In addition, bone scanning and *meta*-iodobenzylguanidine (MIBG) scanning are essential to demonstrate distal disease.

TREATMENT

Optimal treatment is provided by a coordinated approach involving paediatric oncologists, surgeons, pathologists, radiologists and radiotherapists and experienced ward staff. For children with stage 1 or 2 disease, surgery alone may be sufficient. It is not essential to achieve complete macroscopic clearance in these children, as minor residual disease is usually stable.

Initial chemotherapy is mandatory for children with stage 3 or 4 disease. Immediate surgery for those with locally advanced disease is markedly more difficult and unsatisfactory.

In some children with stage 4S disease, no treatment is necessary and the disease resolves spontaneously. Treatment, however, is required in the face of relentless hepatomegaly. This is generally a feature in young infants, and treatment should not be delayed once there is any suggestion of respiratory compromise. Early recourse to chemotherapy is advised under these circumstances.

Chemotherapy protocols change on a frequent basis. Combination chemotherapy may include cyclophosphamide, vincristine, cisplatin, carboplatin, doxorubicin and etoposide, among others. In addition, myelo-ablative therapy may be used, with subsequent bone-marrow transplantation.

SURGERY

Complete or near-complete resection is usually possible. However, as vascular encasement is the rule, all the vessels that traverse the tumour must be dissected free before any tumour removal is undertaken. Once the vascular anatomy has been displayed, tumour removal is straightforward.

Different methods are used to display the vessels, including the use of ultrasonic dissectors, but knife dissection is still regarded as the gold standard. Since demonstration of the vascular tree is the only safe way to remove a neuroblastoma, there will be children in whom complete resection is impossible. Nevertheless, it is agreed within the UK Childrens Cancer Study Group (UKCCSG) that complete resection is the stated aim of surgery. Partial resection should be avoided, and surgeons who are unwilling to undertake such extensive vascular dissections are advised to refer patients to those who are willing to attempt complete macroscopic removal.

The risks related to the surgery are thus those that flow from an extensive dissection of the vascular tree. In arterial dissection, the natural plane of cleavage is between the adventitial and medial layers. Small punctures into the arterial lumen are relatively commonplace and can be controlled with a carefully placed vascular suture. Inadvertent transection of major aortic branches is a recognized complication of the surgery when the aorta is enclosed in a dense tumour that entirely obscures the origin of the vessels. Vascular division may be impossible to repair, resulting in visceral loss. Such potential consequences of attempted resection must be disclosed during the consent procedure. Venous dissection may be more difficult than arterial dissection, due to thinner vessel walls. The site of bleeding from venous breaches is also more difficult to define, as blood tends to well up from the wound rather than spurt out as a jet from a defined point on the vessel.

The extensive dissection of para-aortic lymphatic channels inevitably causes substantial perioperative lymphatic leakage. This can result in abdominal distension within a few days or weeks of tumour resection. Such distension is usually managed conservatively, but if the abdominal distension becomes symptomatic, then a peritoneovenous shunt (e.g. Denver shunt) can be placed.

Thoracic neuroblastoma

This deserves a separate mention because of its different symptomatology and management. Sited on the sympathetic chain within the thorax, the posterior mediastinal mass is often diagnosed incidentally during chest radiography. Alternatively, sympathetic involvement may lead to presentation with an ipsilateral Horner syndrome. If the thoracic tumour has extended into the spinal canal, then cord compression may lead to long-tract signs.

Thoracic neuroblastomas may have differentiated into ganglioneuroblastomas or ganglioneuromas by the time of diagnosis. There is evidence that this process of differentiation may result in a stable mature mass that may merit treatment only on the basis of local symptoms rather than malignant potential. The knowledge of the possibility of this maturation, combined with proximity to the great vessels at the apex of the thoracic cavity, makes the decision to perform resection less certain.

Therefore, whilst the majority of abdominal tumours will undergo an attempted resection following chemotherapy, thoracic tumours are approached in a more pragmatic fashion.

RESULTS

Tumours detected antenatally have a favourable biological profile, and survival is in excess of 90 per cent for these children. Children presenting under the age of 12 months have a better outcome, independent of tumour stage and biological profile. The reasons for this are unclear.

The presence of *MYCN* amplification is associated with a worse outlook, regardless of age and stage. Survival rates as low as ten per cent are sometimes reported for those with advanced disease and *MYCN* amplification. In one study, gain of 17q showed 30 per cent compared with 86 per cent survival at five years in children without this abnormality. 1p deletion was associated with a four-year survival of 32 per cent in one study, compared with 76 per cent survival for those without the abnormality. When associated with *MYCN* amplification, four-year survival was seven per cent.

Currently, patients who present with stage 1 or 2 disease have survival rates in excess of 90 per cent. Those with stage 3 disease have survival rates of about 70 per cent if complete resection has been possible. Survival is about 25–30 per cent for those with stage 4 disease.

CONCLUSION

Overall, there is still a substantial mortality for children who develop a neuroblastoma. At the time of writing, the increased understanding of this tumours biology has not translated into an improved outlook for these children.

CLINICAL SCENARIO

A three-year-old girl presents with a three-week history of malaise, lethargy, general irritability and weight loss. In the past week, she has developed a limp. Examination confirms a pale thin child with mild abdominal distension and a central irregular abdominal mass, which is fixed. Urinary VMA level is elevated and plain abdominal X-rays show specks of calcification centrally in the upper abdomen. Ultrasound shows a heterogeneous mass. CT scan confirms the presence of a large central abdominal mass overlying the aorta and displacing the inferior vena cava to the right. The coeliac axis and superior mesenteric vessels are embedded in tumour. At its maximal dimension, the tumour measures 17 cm. Bone-marrow aspirates and trephines are normal and show no evidence of tumour. Tumour biopsy shows the appearances of undifferentiated neuroblastoma. Molecular biology confirms *MYCN* amplification. Bone scan is normal and MIBG scan shows uptake in the primary tumour only.

On the basis of these findings, the child is treated as having a poor-risk stage 3 neuroblastoma and is commenced on chemotherapy.

Restaging at two months shows that the primary tumour has shrunk to a remarkable degree. Surgery was planned at three months but was deferred because of multiple episodes of fever associated with neutropenia. The final delay was because of slow recovery of the platelet count.

At operation, a substantial lump was encountered overlying the upper abdominal aorta. Tumour clearance was achieved, and histology showed live neuroblastoma in a predominantly fibrotic stroma.

She developed moderately severe abdominal distension in the postoperative period. After two weeks, it was clear that she had problematic ascites. Treatment with a low-fat diet initially and subsequent total parenteral nutrition did not resolve the problem, and finally a peritoneovenous shunt was required to resolve the problem. The shunt was clearly blocked 12 months later and was removed without recurrence of ascites. Seven years on from her treatment, she remains well.

FURTHER READING

Brodeur GM, Castleberry RP. Neuroblastoma. In: Pizzo PA, Poplack DG (eds). *Principles and Practice of Pediatric Oncology*, 5th edn. Philadelphia, PA: Lippincott-Raven, in press.

Kiely EM. Neuroblastoma. In: Ashcraft K (ed.). *Paediatric Surgery*, 4th edn. Philadelphia, PA: WB Saunders, 2004; pp. 933–49.

Maris JM, Matthay KK. Molecular biology of neuroblastoma. *Journal of Clinical Oncology* 1999; **17**: 2264–79.

Shimada H, Umehara S, Monobe BY, *et al.* International Neuroblastoma Pathology Classification for prognostic evaluation of patients with peripheral neuroblastic tumours: a report from the Children's Cancer Group. *Cancer* 2001; **92**: 2451–61.

44

Rhabdomyosarcoma

JOHN M HUTSON AND LARA KITTERINGHAM

Learning objectives

- To understand the histological types and possible presentations of rhabdomyosarcoma.
- To understand the recent thoughts on aetiology and molecular biology associated with rhabdomyosarcomas.
- To know the investigations required for clinical staging of rhabdomyosarcomas.
- To understand the principles of the various treatment modalities and to be aware of the current therapy regimes, in particular to appreciate that surgery is only a part of therapy.
- To know the outcome and potential complications of the more common types of rhabdomyosarcoma.

INTRODUCTION

Rhabdomyosarcoma (Greek *rhabdo*, 'rod'; *mys*, 'muscle'; *sarkos*, 'flesh') is a primary malignancy in children and adolescents that arises from embryonic mesenchyme, with the potential to differentiate into skeletal muscle. Wiener first described it in 1854, but it was not until the 1950s that the first series was reported, and Horn and Enterline described their histological classification, which is still used widely today.

Rhabdomyosarcoma is the most common soft-tissue sarcoma of childhood and represents the third most common solid malignancy in this age group, after neuroblastoma and Wilms tumour. Rhabdomyosarcoma accounts for four to eight per cent of all malignant disease and 5–15 per cent of all solid malignancies of childhood. The male/female ratio is three to two, with an increased incidence in Caucasians compared with non-Caucasians (ratio four to three).

Rhabdomyosarcoma can occur at any age in childhood, but is it associated more commonly with a bimodal frequency, with the early peak between two and five years and the late peak between 15 and 19 years of age. Six per cent of tumours occur during infancy, and half will be discovered before five years of age. Rhabdomyosarcoma may appear in almost any part of the body, including tissues that do not usually contain striated muscle. They have been reported as primary tumours in every part of the body, except the brain (Table 44.1).

Table 44.1 *Distribution of primary tumour sites in the body*

Site of rhabdomyosarcoma	Patients (%)
Head and neck	35
Genitourinary	26
Limb	19
Other	20

AETIOLOGY

The cause of rhabdomyosarcoma is unknown but thought to be multifactorial, with congenital, environmental and genetic factors being influential.

Rhabdomyosarcoma is known to occur with increased frequency in patients with neurofibromatosis type 1, fetal alcohol syndrome, basal cell nevus syndrome and Beckwith–Wiedemann syndrome.

Many environmental factors have been implicated in the causation of rhabdomyosarcoma, either in conjunction with or independent of genetic risk factors, such as chlorinated phenoxy herbicides, marijuana, cocaine, maternal alcohol ingestion, maternal exposure to radiation and maternal history of stillbirth. Also, some animal studies have suggested a link between rhabdomyosarcoma and viral illness.

The Li–Fraumeni syndrome is an autosomal dominant cancer syndrome in which there is a significantly increased risk of rhabdomyosarcomas and other sarcomas, premenopausal breast carcinoma and other types of carcinomas (brain tumours, adrenal carcinoma, leukaemia) in affected relations. This risk has been associated with certain germ-line mutations in the tumour suppressor gene *p53* located on the short arm of chromosome 17, a phenomenon seen in a number of other malignancies. The *p53* gene controls cellular deoxyribonucleic acid (DNA) damage during cell proliferation, and, therefore, a defect in its function can lead to abnormal cell proliferation. Independent of Li–Fraumeni syndrome, ten per cent of patients with rhabdomyosarcoma have mutations of the *p53* gene.

MOLECULAR BIOLOGY

Embryonal and alveolar tumours can be identified by characteristic structural chromosomal changes. Embryonal tumours have a loss of heterozygosity on the long arm of chromosome 11, so that the paternal DNA appears duplicated with the maternal DNA absent. This is a locus where the insulin growth factor II (*IGF-II*) gene resides, leading to an overexpression of this gene. IGF-II has been shown to stimulate the growth of rhabdomyosarcoma, whereas the blockade of this factor using monoclonal antibodies will inhibit tumour growth both *in vitro* and *in vivo*.

Alveolar rhabdomyosarcomas characteristically have a 2,13 translocation (t[2;13][q35;q14]). This results in the juxtaposition of the *PAX3* gene from chromosome 2 to chromosome 13. The *PAX3* gene is involved in transcription regulation and is moved to a site close to *FKHR*, which is part of the forkhead family of transcription factors. This translocation can be identified by polymerase chain reaction (PCR) and thus can be used to diagnose alveolar rhabdomyosarcoma.

The ploidy of rhabdomyosarcoma cells has been shown to have prognostic significance. In patients with unresectable rhabdomyosarcoma, the presence of a diploid tumour cell line was associated with a dismal prognosis (no survivors), whereas patients with hyperdiploid tumours had a good survival rate (83 per cent). Hyperdiploid tumours were exclusively of the embryonal type. Near-tetraploidy was associated with alveolar histology.

PATHOLOGY

Macroscopic features are not particularly distinguishing, except for the grape-like clusters arising from a hollow viscus that denotes a sarcoma botryoides (Figure 44.1). The remaining tumours are usually firm, nodular and varying in size. They have a tendency to form a pseudo-capsule, although microscopic evaluation reveals that the tumour infiltrates beyond the pseudo-capsule, requiring a wide resection for complete tumour removal. There is often a mild inflammatory reaction around the tumour, which may make it difficult to distinguish the tumour.

Histologically, it is classified within the category of small, round, blue-cell tumours, which also includes neuroblastoma, Ewing's sarcoma, small-cell osteogenic sarcoma, non-Hodgkin's lymphoma and leukaemia (Figure 44.2). This may make it difficult to distinguish between these tumours with light microscopy alone. Electron microscopy may be required to reveal the Z-bands associated with actin–myosin bundles, and more complex biochemical staining may be needed for the muscle proteins actin, myosin, desmin and myoD that rhabdomyosarcomas may express.

The first classification of rhabdomyosarcoma was in 1958 by Horn and Enterline, who proposed four different pathological types:

- embryonal
- botryoid
- alveolar
- pleomorphic.

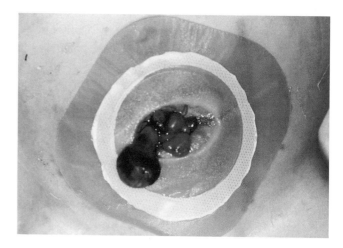

Figure 44.1 *Bladder rhabdomyosarcoma growing out of a vesicostomy despite chemotherapy.*

This was the standard pathological nomenclature used for rhabdomyosarcomas for several decades and has been used by the Intergroup Rhabdomyosarcoma Study (IRS) since its inception. However, many other classification schemes have been proposed, each with its own advantages and limitations. A universal system was described in an international collaborative effort among paediatric pathologists in 1994. The Horn and Enterline system was modified by ascribing prognostic significance to each histological type (Table 44.2).

Embryonal tumours

The most common type of tumour is embryonal, accounting for 50 per cent of all newly diagnosed tumours, 80 per cent of genitourinary tumours, 60 per cent of head and neck tumours and about 50 per cent of tumours at other sites (not including the trunk and perineum).

It has an intermediate prognosis, compared with the botryoid and spindle-cell variants, which are both classed as subvariants of the embryonal rhabdomyosarcoma but have a favourable prognosis.

Alveolar tumours

This is the second most common type and usually occurs in older children and adults. They account for 20 per cent of

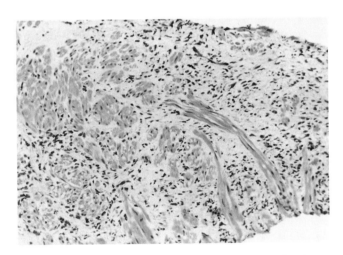

Figure 44.2 *Histology of prostatic rhabdomyosarcoma, showing small dark cells interspersed with differentiated muscle fibres.*

Table 44.2 *International rhabdomyosarcoma pathological classification*

Histological classification	5-year survival (%)
Favourable prognosis: botryoid, spindle-cell	90
Intermediate prognosis: embryonal, pleomorphic (rare)	65–75
Poor prognosis: alveolar (including solid variant), undifferentiated	40–55

rhabdomyosarcomas seen in children and arise mainly from the extremities, trunk and perineum. A subtype of alveolar rhabdomyosarcoma is the solid alveolar rhabdomyosarcoma, which lacks any intercellular stroma.

Pleomorphic tumours

These are rare tumours representing one per cent of rhabdomyosarcomas in childhood. They are seen mainly on the trunk and extremities.

Undifferentiated tumours

About 10–20 per cent of tumours are so undifferentiated that it is difficult to classify them. They are made up of small primitive round cells that can often resemble Ewing's sarcoma; the difference is that they arise from soft tissue rather than bone. However, with immunohistochemistry, undifferentiated tumours frequently can be identified as rhabdomyosarcomas.

INVESTIGATIONS

The aim of the investigations is to determine the histological variant and primary site of the tumour as well as the extent of the disease. Basic haematological tests, including full blood count, clotting, serum electrolytes, creatinine and liver function, should be performed. Creatinine kinase levels are sometimes raised, which may aid the diagnosis. No other serum markers are available. Standard urinalysis is required to exclude concurrent urinary tract infection if bladder tumours are suspected.

Imaging is required to identify the organ of origin, to identify both local and metastatic spread and to assess the surgical management options. Also, tumour response can be monitored once treatment is initiated.

Initial imaging is usually ultrasound. However, once a tumour is confirmed, cross-sectional imaging of the primary site is required (Figure 44.3). This should be performed with intravenous contrast, taking care to record measurements of the tumour in at least two directions. There is controversy as to whether computed tomography (CT) or magnetic resonance imaging (MRI) is the better modality. There is little difference in terms of diagnostic accuracy between CT and MRI, although CT may be superior in assessing abdominal lymphadenopathy. However, most radiologists prefer MRI due to the lack of ionizing radiation and its multiplanar capabilities. The disadvantages of MRI are that oedema following radiotherapy can be misinterpreted as residual disease in up to 20 per cent of cases, and on T2-weighted images urine images brightly, which can obscure tumour in the bladder wall. In real terms, the most important thing is not necessarily which modality is best but to ensure consistent imaging. The same modality should be used to follow the tumour response to therapy.

Biopsy for tissue diagnosis can be obtained by percutaneous, core or open biopsies. These have the potential problems of providing inadequate amounts of tissue for evaluation and needle-track seeding in the case of percutaneous or core biopsies and are more invasive in the open case. They should be sited carefully so that the needle track can be incorporated in the surgical excision.

Endoscopy, if appropriate, can further delineate the extent of the tumour and allows tissue biopsy. This has the advantage of eliminating the risk of needle-track seeding and is less invasive than an open biopsy.

Assessment of metastases

A chest X-ray, bone-marrow aspirate, chest CT and, if possible, spiral CT (as this is superior in detecting lung lesions) should be performed to detect metastases. Bone scanning is controversial, as it has a high false-negative rate and identifies lesions in only four per cent of patients. Therefore, some clinicians recommend a bone scan only for patients with bone symptoms and/or patients whose tumours have unfavourable histology.

CLINICAL STAGING

Clinical staging allows different treatment regimens to be used for different extents of disease and comparison of treatment and outcome within and among institutions. The two main study groups of rhabdomyosarcomas – the IRS and the International Society of Paediatric Oncology – have, unfortunately, staged rhabdomyosarcoma using two different systems (Tables 44.3 and 44.4).

The IRS group uses a post-surgical clinical classification. The advantages of the TNM (tumour, node, metastasis) system are that it provides pretreatment staging and it takes into account the site of the tumour. Its disadvantages are that it can be difficult to accurately identify tumour-positive nodes on imaging and to differentiate them from inflammatory

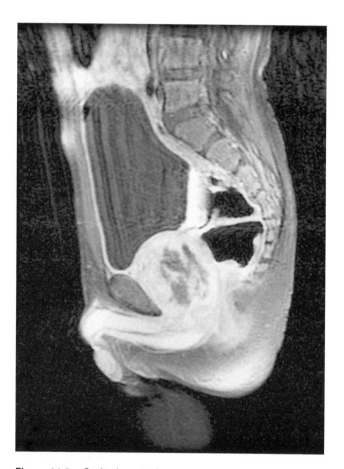

Figure 44.3 *Sagittal magnetic resonance imaging section, showing prostatic rhabdomyosarcoma pushing the bladder upwards and compressing the rectum.*

Table 44.4 *Intergroup Rhabdomyosarcoma Study Group clinical staging classification*

Group	Residual tumour after resection
1	No gross or microscopic residual tumour
2a	Microscopic residual tumour, no positive nodes
2b	Positive nodes, no residual tumour
2c	Microscopic residual tumour and positive nodes
3	Gross residual tumour
4	Distant metastases

Table 44.3 *TNM pretreatment staging classification of patients with rhabdomyosarcoma in the Intergroup Rhabdomyosarcoma Study (IRS) IV*

Stage	Site	Tumour size	Regional nodes	Metastasis
I	Orbit, head and neck (superficial), genitourinary (non-B)	a or b	$N_0 N_1$ or N	M_0
II	Bladder/prostate, extremity, trunk, parameningeal, other	a	N_0 or N	M_0
III	Bladder/prostate	b	N_1	M_0
	Extremity, trunk, parameningeal		$N_0 N_1$ or N	
IV	All	a or b	Any N	M_1

nodes, leading to errors in pretreatment staging. The TNM system currently is being evaluated in IRS-IV.

RHABDOMYOSARCOMA STUDY GROUPS

Intergroup Rhabdomyosarcoma Study

As a result of several pioneering studies using single and then combination chemotherapeutic agents, the severe debilitating radical surgery, and the low numbers of children with rhabdomyosarcoma, the Children's Cancer Group (CCG) and the Children's Oncology Group (COG) collaborated on a multidisciplinary study, the IRS. The IRS was established in 1972, and eligible patients from CCG and COG institutions have been enrolled in the four major protocol studies. Between 686 and 1062 patients have been entered in each full study.

The IRS studies current treatment protocols, with the aims of streamlining treatment to reduce complications without reducing long-term survival. For example, IRS-I showed that radiotherapy provided no benefit for group 1 patients (Table 44.4), and this was confirmed in IRS-II. IRS-II also showed that cyclophosphamide therapy for group 1 or 2 patients was not necessary, hence reducing the potential side effects (e.g. haemorrhagic cystitis, bladder fibrosis), and showed that repetitive-pulse therapy (monthly for two years) was better than pulse therapy for group 3 patients.

IRS-III staged patients based on their histology and tumour site as well as clinical group to test whether tumours with a more unfavourable histology in group 1 and 2 patients required more intensive therapy than those with favourable histology. It also studied more intensive new drug regimes to improve the survival rates of patients in groups 3 and 4.

At the time of writing, IRS-IV is still ongoing and is evaluating split-course, accelerated hyperfractionated radiation therapies for higher tumour kill with fewer late side effects; a preoperative TNM staging system; and comparison of cyclophosphamide versus ifosfamide versus ifosfamide and etoposide. It is also evaluating rank ordering of induction drug doublets (vincristine/melphalan versus ifosfamide/etoposide versus ifosfamide/doxorubicin) and the role of new agents such as topotecan (which inhibits the enzyme topoisomerase), paclitaxel and docetaxel (which blocks cell cycling).

IRS-V is planning to assess the use of genetics in predicting relapses, leading to a more judicious use of therapy. This will include DNA-ploidy, cytogenetic staging, molecular genetics and tumour biology studies.

Malignant Mesenchymal Tumour Committee (MMT 95 study)

This is an alternative study group to IRS. Their aim is to use more intensive primary chemotherapy, with restriction of local therapy (surgery or radiotherapy), in an attempt to reduce late functional and cosmetic sequelae, while maintaining satisfactory overall survival.

TREATMENT

Treatment of rhabdomyosarcoma involves three modalities: surgery, radiotherapy and chemotherapy. All three, or a selection of the three in differing orders, may be required (Figure 44.4).

Principles of surgery in treatment

A surgical biopsy may be required for diagnosis.

There is no need for surgery if complete remission occurs following chemotherapy. However, surgery can help to achieve complete remission in 50 per cent of patients who have had only a partial response to chemotherapy. Debulking procedures have no benefit in the management of these tumours, and in fact large tumours should be shrunk with neoadjuvant chemotherapy first. Wide local excision of the tumour, with emphasis on organ preservation, should be performed wherever possible, although radical surgery maybe required if there is unresponsive primary disease and local recurrence.

Principles of radiation

Radiation should be restricted to patients with residual or metastatic disease. The suggested radiation field is 2 cm beyond the tumour margin and the dose between 40 and 60 Gy, which is not altered for histological type, tumour size or the patient's age. Hyperfractionated radiotherapy and brachytherapy are being investigated.

Principles of chemotherapy

Neoadjuvant and adjuvant chemotherapy have been shown to be beneficial. The current standard regime is either intensive vincristine and dactinomycin (VA) or pulsed vincristine, dactinomycin and cyclophosphamide (VAC), although these regimes will be customized based on the clinical group, histological type and site of the tumour.

TREATMENT-RELATED COMPLICATIONS

There are a large number of potential complications secondary to rhabdomyosarcoma treatment with each of the modalities. Cardiomyopathy can occur, particularly following therapy with anthracycline drugs, e.g. doxorubicin. Pulmonary dysfunction is possible due to either (i) radiation (adolescents develop pulmonary fibrosis, whereas children appear to get impaired growth of both the lung and chest wall) or (ii) chemotherapy agents, such as bleomycin, cyclophosphamide

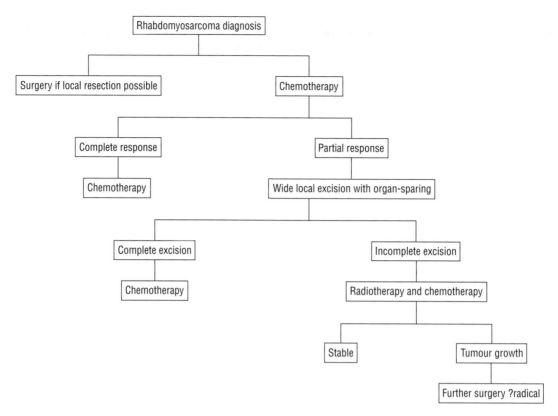

Figure 44.4 *Algorithm for management of rhabdomyosarcoma.*

and methotrexate. Potential gastrointestinal complications include oesophageal strictures, chronic enteritis, perforation and fistula formation secondary to radiation.

Gonadal dysfunction is dependent on age, pubertal status at time of treatment, dose of radiation, and dose and type of chemotherapy. Male germ cells are very sensitive to alkylating agents and radiation therapy, whereas Leydig cells are more resistant. Ovaries are generally very resistant to chemotherapy, particularly before puberty. However, ovarian failure can still occur with high doses, so brachytherapy and ovarian transposition will reduce the incidence of ovarian failure in pelvic rhabdomyosarcoma. The risk of congenital anomalies in offspring is no higher than in the general population. However, spontaneous abortion, premature labour and low-birth-weight babies are more common.

There are a wide range of potential renal complications, including chronic renal failure secondary to chemotherapy agents, e.g. cisplatin, methotrexate, ifosfamide and cyclophosphamide. Ureteric strictures and chronic bladder dysfunction leading to urinary incontinence, fistulae and urethral strictures can occur up to 20 years after radiation. Haemorrhagic cystitis occurs in ten per cent of patients receiving radiation, and increases to 30 per cent of patients if chemotherapy such as cyclophosphamide, bleomycin or cisplatin is added. There is a significantly increased risk of bladder carcinoma following use of cyclophosphamide, and a 3–12 per cent incidence of developing a second cancer within the first 20 years of the initial cancer diagnosis. Alkylating agents and

epipodophyllotoxins are linked with leukaemias, while irradiation causes solid tumours.

Finally, radical surgery can be severely debilitating, resulting in significantly reduced quality of life.

OUTCOME

Overall five-year disease-free survival of children with rhabdomyosarcoma is about 65 per cent, as reported by IRS-III. However, metastatic disease is still a problem, with a low survival rate. As there is a high risk of late complications, long-term follow-up is required. Surgery should be utilized initially only if the primary tumour is small and easily resectable without mutilation. Otherwise, chemotherapy should be employed first, with surgery reserved for incomplete or non-responsive cases.

CLINICAL SCENARIOS

Case 1

A two-year-old girl presented with a ten-day history of a mass protruding from the vagina. Examination revealed a 5-cm purple mass at the introitus. Examination under anaesthesia revealed a polypoid mass arising from the upper third of the

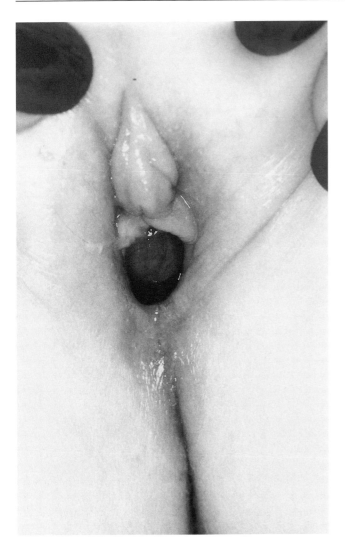

Figure 44.5 *Sarcoma botryoides arising from upper vagina.*

vagina, with normal urethra and rectum (Figure 44.5). Biopsies revealed an embryonal rhabdomyosarcoma.

Chest X-ray, CT of the lung, bone scan and bone-marrow aspirate were all negative. CT of the pelvis showed the mass to be confined to the vagina and consistent with a stage III tumour. Subsequent treatment consisted of chemotherapy (VAC and cisplatinum/etoposide (VP-16)), with almost complete response, and brachytherapy with iridium rods following laparoscopic ovarian relocation. Complications included radiation proctitis, treated with laser ablation, and vaginal

stenosis requiring dilation 11 years later. During dilation, a hole was made in the bladder, which was treated with drainage and hyperbaric oxygen therapy. A resultant vesicovaginal fistula was repaired operatively with vaginal replacement by a pedicle colonic graft and vascularized perineal skin flaps.

Case 2

A six-month-old boy presented with macroscopic haematuria. Micturating cystourethrogram confirmed a botryoid lesion at the bladder base, with endoscopic biopsy confirming the diagnosis. After preoperative chemotherapy, the bladder neck and prostatic urethra were excised with primary anastomosis. Brachytherapy was used, with control of local disease. At four to five years of age, neurofibromatosis (NF-1) was diagnosed when pigmentation began to appear in the scar. Late stricture in the urethra led to bladder augmentation and Mitroffanof stoma. The boy remains under NF-1 surveillance ten years later. Loss of sexual function remains an issue.

Case 3

An 11-year old boy presented with a painless lump in the scrotum, consistent with a tumour. No metastases were identified on imaging. He underwent radical orchidectomy and para-aortic lymph node sampling, which revealed a rhabdomyosarcoma with one tiny secondary in the nodes. Because of this, he had adjuvant irradiation therapy and is disease-free more than five years later.

FURTHER READING

Filipas D. Surgery for urogenital rhabdomyosarcoma. *Current Opinion in Urology* 2001; **11**: 563–5.

McDowell HP. Update on childhood rhabdomyosarcoma. *Archives of Disease in Childhood* 2003; **88**: 354–7.

Raney RB. Soft-tissue sarcoma in childhood and adolescence. *Current Oncology Reports* 2002; **4**: 291–8.

Xia SJ, Pressey JG, Barr FG. Molecular pathogenesis of rhabdomyosarcoma. *Cancer Biology and Therapy* 2002; **1**: 97–104.

45

Germ-cell tumours

GORDON A MacKINLAY AND CLAIRE CLARK

Learning objectives

- To understand the basic sciences of germ-cell tumours.
- To be able to differentiate between the different types of germ-cell tumour and tumour sites.
- To understand the management of germ-cell tumours.

INTRODUCTION

Germ-cell tumours (GCTs) are a rare group of tumours that arise from primitive germ cells. They are a heterogeneous group of tumours containing both malignant and benign subtypes and with the potential to differentiate along several disparate lines. They can occur within the gonads and at extragonadal sites.

Three to five children per one million will develop a GCT. They account for three per cent of all neoplasms under the age of 15 years. Between 25 and 30 per cent of GCTs are malignant. The incidence of extragonadal GCT varies with gender: girls are more likely to develop sacrococcygeal tumours, while boys are more likely to develop intracranial and mediastinal tumours. Malignant germ-cell tumours (MGCTs) are more common in boys than girls. There is evidence that the incidence of GCTs are increasing, but the reason for this is unknown (Stringer *et al.* 1998; Hawkins 1990; Palmer *et al.* 2003; Dos Santos Siva *et al.* 1999).

PATHOGENESIS

Primitive germ cells migrate from the allantois in the extra-embryonic yolk sac to the genital ridge on the posterior abdominal wall of the embryo. GCTs can arise in genital sites or, if mistakes in migration occur, anywhere in the midline, e.g. the mediastinum, the brain and the sacrococcygeal area (Palmer *et al.* 2003).

CLINICAL ASSOCIATIONS

GCTs can be associated with many clinical conditions (Table 45.1) (Hawkins 1990).

CLASSIFICATION

Due to the totipotential nature of germ cells, the type of tumour depends on the state of differentiation at the time of neoplastic change. GCTs can be classified as:

- teratomas
- germinomas (pure GCTs)
- embryonal tumours
- endodermal sinus tumours (yolk-sac tumours)
- choriocarcinomas
- mixed germ-cell tumours.

Table 45.1 *Clinical conditions associated with germ-cell tumours (GCTs)*

Condtion	Association with GCT
Pyloric stenosis	Four-fold increased risk of developing any GCT
Familial cancer syndromes, e.g. Li–Fraumeni	Increased risk of developing any GCT
Monozygotic twinning	Sacrococcygeal teratoma
Schinzel–Giedion syndrome	Malignant sacrococcygeal teratoma
Trisomy 8, Klinefelter XXY	Malignant mediastinal and CNS GCT
Russell–Silver syndrome (males only)	Seminoma
Maldescended or undescended testes	Five- to ten-fold increased risk of developing GCT
Intersex, Turner syndrome (XO), sacral agenesis	Gonadoblastoma/germinoma
Aniridia–Wilms tumour association	

CNS, central nervous system.

Figure 45.1 represents a proposed pathway for the development of GCT.

Teratomas

Teratomas (teratomata) are the most common childhood GCT. They are defined as tumours containing tissue derived from endo-, meso- and ectoderm. They can be divided as follows:

- *Mature*: these tumours are benign, well-encapsulated and frequently cystic in nature. They may contain mature neuronal tissue, pancreas, lung and prostate. They account for 80 per cent of teratomas.
- *Immature*: these tumours contain immature tissue. They are graded according to the amount of immature neuroectodermal embryonal tissue present. The behaviour of these tumours is unpredictable. The higher the grade, the more likely is its behaviour to be malignant (Heifetz *et al.* 1998).
- *Malignant*: these are teratomas that are frankly malignant. Those containing squamous cell carcinomas and adenocarcinomas tend to occur only in adults (Palmer *et al.* 2003).

Germinomas

Germinomas account for 15 per cent of all GCTs. They are encapsulated, solid, grey-pink tumours with a rubber consistency and with small foci of necrosis and haemorrhage. They are referred to as dysgerminomas in the ovary, seminomas in

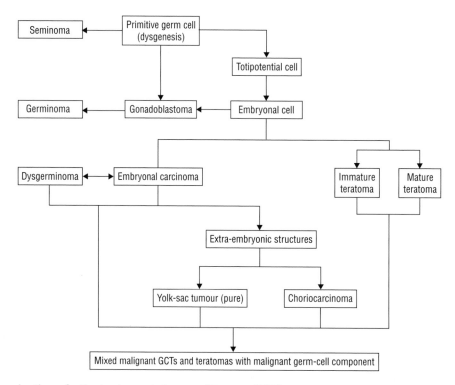

Figure 45.1 *Proposed pathway for the development of germ-cell tumours (GCTs).*

the testes and germinomas in extragonadal sites. Germinomas are pure GCTs, because malignant transformation occurs before differentiation. They tend to be less aggressive malignant tumours (Hawkins 1990; Palmer *et al.* 2003).

Embryonal tumours

These are poorly differentiated anaplastic tumours with extensive necrosis. They tend to occur as part of a mixed GCT in the gonads or mediastinum (Hawkins 1990; Palmer *et al.* 2003).

Endodermal sinus tumours

These are also known as yolk-sac tumours. They are generally encapsulated tumours composed of friable pale grey mucoid tissue with necrosis and haemorrhage. They are less aggressive tumours (Hawkins 1990; Palmer *et al.* 2003).

Choriocarcinomas

These are highly malignant tumours. Fortunately, they are rare in childhood. Choriocarcinomas can be fetal or maternal tumours that have metastasized to the baby. They tend to be very friable and haemorrhagic.

Mixed germ-cell tumours

These are tumours that contain two or more GCT subtypes.

TUMOUR MARKERS AND BIOLOGY

Tumour biology is different in adult tumours and childhood tumours. In adults, there is a cytogenetic change with a gain of chromosome 12p. 12p is also seen in adolescent GCT, but it is seen rarely in infants (Palmer *et al.* 2003; Bussey *et al.* 1999).

GCTs secrete alpha-fetoprotein (AFP) and beta-human chorionic gonadotrophin (HCG). Levels of these substances can be used, therefore, for diagnosis, to gauge response to treatment and for post-treatment surveillance.

AFP is a glycoprotein produced by the endoderm of the yolk sac, immature hepatocytes and intestinal cells. The concentration at birth is high, falling to adult levels of < 12 ng/mL by one year of age. The half-life of AFP is five to seven days. An isolated elevated AFP in infants can be difficult to assess, as AFP can also be elevated in hepatic malignancy and post-gastrointestinal surgery (Stringer *et al.* 1998; Hawkins 1990; Palmer *et al.* 2003). A very high level of AFP at the time of diagnosis of GCT is a powerful predicator of poor outcome (Heifetz *et al.* 1998).

Beta-HCG is a glycoprotein made up of two polypeptide chains: the alpha- and beta-subunits. The alpha subunit is the same as that in follicle-stimulating hormone (FSH), luteinizing hormone (LH) and thyroid-stimulating hormone (TSH). The alpha subunit is specific to HCG. HCG is produced by the syncytiotrophoblasts of the placenta and is markedly elevated in choriocarcinoma. Some germinomas secrete HCG if they contain syncytiotrophoblastic giant cells. Due to the similarity of the alpha-subunit of beta-HCG with LH, a cross-reaction between the two may cause GCT to present with precocious puberty. HCG has a half-life of 12–24 hours (Hawkins 1990; Von-Eyben 2003).

TUMOUR SITES AND CLINICAL PRESENTATION

The clinical presentation of GCT depends on the site of origin.

Gonadal tumours

OVARIAN TUMOURS

The ovary is the second most common site for GCTs (30 per cent of all GCTs) (Figure 45.2). Ovarian GCTs are mostly benign mature cystic teratomas. They tend to present in adolescence with abdominal distension or a palpable mass or abdominal pain due to rupture or torsion. Staging can be by the system shown in Table 45.2 or the TNM (tumour, node, metastasis) staging system (Table 45.3).

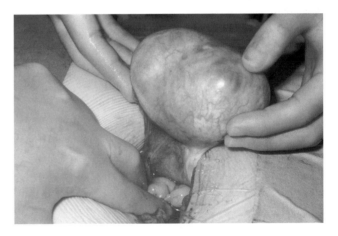

Figure 45.2 *Ovarian teratoma in a ten-year-old.*

Table 45.2 *POG/CCG staging system for ovarian germ-cell tumours*

Stage	Description
1	Limited to the ovaries
2	Microscopic residual or positive lymph nodes and negative peritoneal washings
3	Gross residual, positive lymph nodes, positive peritoneal washings
4	Distant metastases

Table 45.3 *TNM staging can be used for all extracranial germ-cell tumours*

Stage	Clinical	Post-surgical
1	Tumour <5 cm, no adenopathy, no metastases	PSI: tumour without local regional extension, completely removed, no metastases
2	Tumour >5 cm, no adenopathy, no metastases	PSII: tumour with local regional extension, with or without lymph-node involvement, completely removed, no metastases
3	Tumour of any size, locoregional extension and/or lymph-node involvement, no metastases	PSIII: tumour with local regional extension, with no metastases, incompletely removed PSIIIa: microscopic residual PSIIIb: macroscopic residual
4	Metastatic tumour including distant lymph nodes (lumbar aortic are locoregional for testicular tumours)	PSIV: tumour with distant metastases

Table 45.4 *Altman's classification of sacrococcygeal teratomas*

Type	Proportion of sacrococcygeal teratomas (%)	Description
I	47	Tumour mainly external, minimal presacral component
II	35	Tumour mainly external but with some intrapelvic extension
III	8	External tumour with intrapelvic and intra-abdominal extension
IV	10	No external presentation; only intra-hepatic and intra-abdominal tumour; patients tend to be late presenters with poorer prognosis

reduces the incidence of subsequent malignancy, although hopefully subsequent malignancy will be recognized earlier. Staging is similar to that in ovarian GCT (Stringer *et al.* 1998; Hawkins 1990; Palmer *et al.* 2003; Von-Eyben 2003; Dos Santos Siva 1999).

Extragonadal tumours

SACROCOCCYGEAL TUMOURS

The sacrococcyx is the most common site for GCTs in both sexes, with sacrococcygeal GCTs accounting for 40 per cent of all GCTs. It is three times more common in females. It occurs in one in 35 000 live births. Between 75 and 80 per cent are benign mature teratomas; 5–15 per cent are immature. The most common malignant tumour at this site is an endodermal sinus tumour, which occurs more frequently in males. These tumours present antenatally with hydrops fetalis or obstructed labour due to the size of the tumour, or postnatally with a sacral mass and functional problems of the bowel, bladder and lower limbs. Staging is by the TNM staging (Table 45.3) or Altman's classification (Table 45.4) (Stringer *et al.* 1998; Hawkins 1990; Palmer *et al.* 2003).

Ten per cent of neonatally detected and treated sacrococcygeal teratomas (Figure 45.4) will recur as malignant GCTs within three years. Therefore, regular tumour assay follow-up is essential (Hawkins 1993).

MEDIASTINAL TUMOURS

Mediastinal GCTs account for six to ten per cent of all GCTs. The mediastinum is the second most common extragonadal site for GCTs. Mediastinal GCTs tend to occur in the anterior mediastinum. There is an increased risk in patients with Klinefelter syndrome. Patients present with symptoms of airway compression such as cough, wheeze and dyspnoea, heart failure and precocious puberty due to aberrant hormone production. Chest X-ray usually shows a calcification. Mediastinal tumours tend to have a worse prognosis than gonadal or sacrococcygeal tumours of similar pathology, due to difficult surgical access (Hawkins 1990).

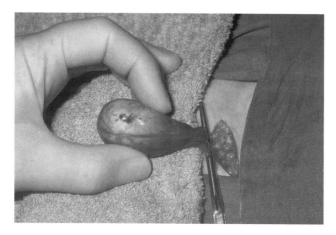

Figure 45.3 *Endodermal sinus tumour in an infant. A soft clamp is across the cord and a biopsy is taken for frozen section.*

Mature ovarian teratomas sometimes are associated with peritoneal implants. These are mature glial cells. They do not alter the prognosis, but they may require further surgical resection if they increase in size (Hawkins 1990; Palmer *et al.* 2003).

TESTICULAR TUMOURS

Testicular GCTs account for seven to ten per cent of all GCTs. Eighty per cent of testicular GCTs are malignant. They tend to be endodermal sinus tumours (Figure 45.3). There are two incidence age peaks at under five years and at adolescence. Testicular GCT presents with a painless scrotal mass, torsion or due to metastasis. There is an increased risk of testicular GCT in boys with undescended testes. Orchidopexy will make the surveillance easier; however, there is no evidence that this

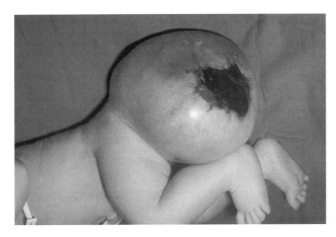

Figure 45.4 *Sacrococcygeal teratoma.*

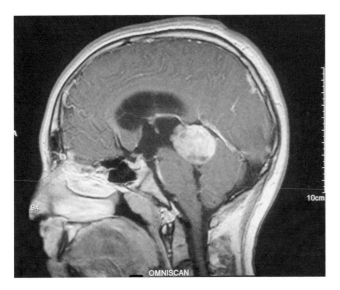

Figure 45.5 *Intracranial germ-cell tumour seen in pineal region on magnetic resonance imaging scan.*

RETROPERITONEAL TUMOURS

Retroperitoneal tumours account for two to three per cent of GCTs. They occur most commonly in children under the age of two years. They tend to present with an abdominal mass.

OTHER EXTRAGONADAL TUMOURS

Extragonadal GCTs can also occur in the liver, bile duct, head and neck, pelvis, abdominal wall, prostate gland and vagina. Vaginal GCTs present with bleeding and should be considered (with the differential diagnoses of rhabdomyosarcoma botryoides and clear-cell carcinoma) in all prepubertal girls who present with this symptom (Rescorla *et al.* 2003). Head and neck GCTs are usually benign and present at birth (Hawkins 1990).

Intracranial germ-cell tumours

Intracranial GCTs (Figure 45.5) account for six to ten per cent of all GCTs. They are more common in males than females.

They tend to present between the ages of 6 and 14 years. Intracranial GCTs tend to be midline in pineal or suprasellar sites. They present with increased intracranial pressure or with neuroendocrine symptoms. Visual-field problems can arise due to chiasmatic involvement with pineal tumours. Intracranial GCTs are mostly germinomas. Histologically, they are similar to extracranial GCTs, but their prognosis is poorer, due to their difficult position for surgery. They require intensive chemotherapy and radiotherapy (Hawkins 1990; Nicholson *et al.* 2002).

INVESTIGATIONS

GCT should be suspected in any child who presents with a midline mass. Initial investigations should include blood sampling for AFP and beta-HCG. Radiology of the tumour site includes computed tomography (CT), magnetic resonance imaging (MRI), chest X-ray and bone scans, and examination of bone marrow to look for metastases in malignant disease.

Intracranial GCT require cerebrospinal fluid (CSF) and blood sampling for tumour markers and imaging of head and spine. The diagnosis of intracranial malignant GCT is made on tumour markers and radiology, rather than biopsy, due to the unacceptable risk of surgical complications (Nicholson *et al.* 2002).

MANAGEMENT

The management of GCT is dependent on the site, size and histology of the tumour.

Surgery

Surgery is the mainstay treatment of benign GCT. If the tumour is confined to an area with no metastases, and it can be surgically removed without danger to the major organs, then it should be completely excised. This is most commonly the case in gonadal and neonatal tumours. Retroperitoneal lymph-node sampling in malignant gonadal GCT is no longer advised because the associated morbidity is high, and chemotherapy can control the disease effectively. In ovarian immature teratomas with peritoneal seeding at the time of surgery, the nodules should be sampled, followed by close observation with imaging and a second-look laparotomy and excision if they progress (Marina *et al.* 1999).

Mature and immature sacrococcygeal teratomas need to be completely excised with the coccyx to prevent recurrence. Despite this, ten per cent can recur as malignant GCTs. Tumour surveillance with regular tumour marker assays need to be carried out for three years (Heifetz *et al.* 1998; Marina *et al.* 1999).

Tumours that cannot be surgically resected (excluding intracranial malignant GCTs) should be biopsied. If there is elevation of tumour markers and typically radiological features, then a diagnosis of GCT can be made without tumour resection. When a GCT has been resected as a whole and the histology is malignant, then postoperative staging with CT scans of the chest and abdomen, bone scans and bone aspiration must be performed.

Chemotherapy

The survival of patients with malignant GCT before the introduction of cisplatin therapy was poor, with nearly 100 per cent mortality. Recent trials from the US Children's Oncology Group using a combination of bleomycin, etoposide and cisplatin (BEP or PEB), in four cycles for stage 1 or 2 extragonadal and stage 2 testicular tumours, and four to six cycles for all other malignant GCTs, has increased the five-year event-free survival (EFS) to 80 per cent (90 per cent for gonadal tumours, 73 per cent for extragonadal tumours) (Giller *et al.* 1998). The UK Children's Cancer Study Group (UKCCSG) has used high-dose carboplatin, which is less oto- and nephrotoxic than cisplatin, with etoposide and bleomycin (JEB). Children received the number of cycles required to normalize tumour markers, plus two more cycles. The five-year EFS was 100 per cent for testicular tumours, 91 per cent for ovarian tumours, 86 per cent for sacrococcygeal tumours, 80 per cent for vaginal/uterine tumours and 75 per cent for mediastinal tumours. The overall survival rate was 91 per cent, which is comparable to BEP (Mann *et al.* 2000).

Current UK recommendations for malignant GCT are as follows:

Stage I: surgical resection, weekly tumour markers until normalization for age, then four- to six-weekly intervals for three years following diagnosis. Chemotherapy (JEB) is given if markers do not normalize or if they rise again, even if the tumour is not radiologically evident. Twenty-five per cent of this group will require chemotherapy. Prognosis is excellent, with 100 per cent EFS.

Stages II–IV: biopsy or incomplete resection followed by chemotherapy of JEB for four to six cycles, followed by surgical resection of residual tumour. Long-term tumour follow-up. Salvage chemotherapy includes cisplatin, ifosfamide and vinblastine (VIP) for recurrent tumours.

Radiotherapy

Radiotherapy has little role in the first-line treatment of extracranial malignant GCTs, but it may have a role in relapsed patients. Intracranial germinoma can be cured in 90 per cent of cases with craniospinal radiotherapy. This can also be achieved with focal radiotherapy followed by chemotherapy of carboplatin, ifosfamide and etoposide. The International Society of Paediatric Oncology (SIOP) is currently doing a trial that is based on this combined with an increase in the radiotherapy field to include the ventricles, where relapse most commonly occurs. Non-germinomatous GCTs have a poorer outcome than germinomas. SIOP currently advises four cycles of cisplatin, etoposide and ifosfamide (PEI) followed by focal radiotherapy in this group. Two-thirds of these patients will be cured (Nicholson *et al.* 2002).

FOLLOW-UP

The length of follow-up is dependent on the histology of the GCT. Mature teratomas require three years of regular follow-up. Malignant GCTs require long-term follow-up with tumour markers and clinical examination. The clinician needs to be vigilant in detecting recurrence of tumour and the consequences of previous chemotherapy and radiotherapy such as acute myeloblastic leukaemia, hearing loss, panhypopituitarism and cognitive impairment.

CLINICAL SCENARIO

A 15-month-old boy is referred from the Middle East, with bilateral hydronephrosis. He was born with an obvious external sacrococcygeal teratoma (SCT), which had been excised at birth. During his surgery, torrential haemorrhage had been encountered and had proved very difficult to control. His complete radiology record reveals that during his work-up for the excisional surgery, an ultrasound scan revealed that the teratoma had extended into the pelvic outlet but bowel gas had prevented delineation of the proximal extent of the tumour.

Postoperative plain radiology had not demonstrated residual disease and had shown normal sacrococcygeal architecture.

His outpatient follow-up, consisting of rectal examination and AFP, had discontinued at four months, having had two attendances with normal findings.

This child may have a recurrence of his SCT, because his primary surgery omitted excision of the coccyx. It is likely that the recurrent mass has impinged on the posterior aspect of the bladder, causing bilateral ureterohydronephrosis. Since the significance of coccygeal excision has been recognized, the recurrence rate in SCT has fallen dramatically.

A residual mass in the anterior sacral space is less likely, although it is possible that intraoperative bleeding may have hampered the direct vision necessary to excise the superior component. However, provided the plane of dissection is maintained, it would be unusual to fail to remove solid contiguous tumour elements.

If cross-sectional imaging had been used preoperatively, then a substantial intrapelvic component may have been revealed, and this should have led to an intravenous contrast phase. This may have revealed an enlarged median sacral vessel, which was probably responsible for the significant intraoperative haemorrhage. Suspecting the presence of an enlarged median sacral artery, establishing its existence, and then performing a laparotomy and ligation of the artery before turning the patient over for definitive SCT excision can avoid this dangerous situation.

Follow-up for SCT should be performed for at least three years, although some surgeons advocate five years. The normal falling AFP in infants does not reach its nadir until four months and is a sensitive sign of malignant transformation in any residual or recurrent tumour.

REFERENCES

Bussey KJ, Lawce J, Olson SB, *et al.* Chromosome abnormalities of 81 paediatric germ cell tumours: sex-, age-, site and histopathology-related differences. A Children's Cancer Group Study. *Genes, Chromosomes and Cancer* 1999; **25**: 134–46.

Dos Santos Siva J, Siveralaw AJ, Stiller CA, Reid A. Incidence of testicular germ-cell malignancies in England and Wales: trends in children compared with adults. *International Journal of Cancer* 1999; **83**: 630–34.

Giller R, Cushing B, Lauer S, *et al.* Comparison of high-dose or standard dose cisplatin with etoposide and bleomycin (HDPEB vs PEB) in children with stage III and IV malignant germ cell tumours (MGCT) at gonadal primary sites: a Pediatric Intergroup trial (POG9049/CCG8882). *Proceedings of the American Society of Clinical Oncology* 1998; **17**: 525a.

Hawkins E. Pathology of germ cell tumours in children. *Critical Reviews in Oncology/Hematology* 1990; **10**: 165–79.

Hawkins E. Occult malignancy in neonatal sacrococcgeal teratomas. A Report from a Combined Pediatric Oncology Group and Children's Cancer Group Study. *American Journal of Pediatric Hematology/Oncology* 1993; **15**: 406–9.

Heifetz S, Cushing B, Giller R, *et al.* Immature teratomas in children: pathological considerations. A Report From the Combined Pediatric Oncology Group/Children's Cancer Group. *American Journal of Surgical Pathology* 1998; **22**: 1115–24.

Mann JR, Raafat K, Robinson J, *et al.* The United Kingdom Children's Cancer Study Group's second germ cell tumour study: carboplatin, etoposide, and bleomycin are effective treatment for children with malignant germ cell tumours, with acceptable toxicity. *Journal of Clinical Oncology* 2000; **18**: 3809–18.

Marina NM, Cushing B, Giller R, *et al.* Complete surgical excision is effective treatment for children immature teratomas with or without malignancies: a Paediatric Oncology Group/Children's Cancer Group Intergroup study. *Journal of Clinical Oncology* 1999; **17**: 2137–43.

Nicholson JC, Punt J, Hale J, Saran F, Calamitus G. Neurosurgical management of paediatric germ cell tumours of the CNS: a multi-disciplinary team approach for the new millennium. *British Journal of Neurosurgery* 2002; **16**: 93–5.

Palmer RD, Nicholson JC, Hale JP. Management of germ cell tumours in childhood. *Current Paediatrics* 2003; **13**: 213–20.

Rescorla F, Billmire D, Vincur C, *et al.* The effect of neoadjuvant chemotherapy and surgery in children with malignant germ cell tumours of the genital region: a Pediatric Intergroup trial. *Journal of Pediatric Surgery* 2003; **38**: 910–12.

Stringer MD, Oldham KT, Mouriquand PDE, Howard RE. *Pediatric Surgery and Urology: Long Term Outcomes.* London: WB Saunders, 1998.

Von-Eyben FE. Laboratory markers and germ cell tumours. *Critical Reviews in Clinical Laboratory Sciences* 2003; **40**: 377–427.

46

Liver tumours

MARK DAVENPORT AND TOM CLARNETTE

Learning objectives

- To understand the differential diagnosis of liver lesions in childhood.
- To gain a working knowledge of common liver tumours.
- To understand the diagnostic work-up of a child with an abdominal mass.
- To gain a basic understanding of the segmental anatomy of the liver.

INTRODUCTION

Neoplastic liver masses may occur in children, but they are uncommon. Figure 46.1 illustrates a simplified classification of the nature of the lesions that can present as liver masses. The most common benign lesions are typically of vascular origin, are usually incidental and may not need specific treatment. Malignant liver tumours make up only two per cent of all cancers in the USA, the UK and Western Europe in this age group. There are two related but distinct malignant variants that occur with any degree of regularity: hepatoblastoma (HB) and hepatocellular carcinoma (HCC). HB is similar in its behaviour, relationship to genetic anomalies and good

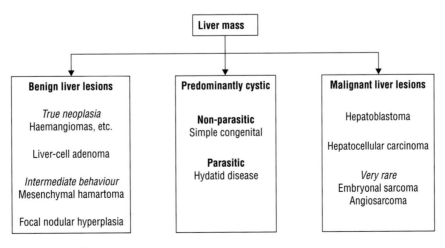

Figure 46.1 *Practical classification of liver masses.*

response to treatment to other 'embryonal' tumours such as nephroblastoma. HCC is similar to its counterpart in adults, typically arising in abnormal livers and associated with a poor prognosis.

BENIGN LIVER TUMOURS AND CYSTS

Hepatic vascular tumours (haemangiomas and haemangioendotheliomas)

Cavernous haemangiomas are usually solitary, unilobar and of variable size. Histologically, these tumours consist of large vascular channels lined with immature endothelial cells. Most present either as an abdominal mass or as an incidental finding. They are not usually associated with any arteriovenous shunting or platelet trapping (see below), and therefore the child has no other systemic manifestations. The diagnosis may be confirmed by ultrasonography and Doppler imaging, which will show the haemangiomas as hypoechoic lesions. Hepatic arteriography or contrast-enhanced computed tomography (CT) imaging will confirm the vascular nature of these tumours. A tissue diagnosis is not always necessary, and percutaneous needle biopsy is definitely contraindicated because of the risk of bleeding. The necessity for specific treatment such as resection or arterial ligation will depend on the symptoms (e.g. abdominal pain) and mode of presentation. Large solitary tumours should be resected, as there is a small risk of spontaneous rupture and catastrophic intraperitoneal bleeding.

Haemangioendotheliomas (HAEs) may be isolated or multiple and can replace up to 80 per cent of liver volume. The clinical presentation is variable and depends on the size of the lesions. HAEs are characterized by rapid arteriovenous shunting through the vascular channels, leading to a raised cardiac output and a vascular 'steal' syndrome. There is enlargement of the hepatic arteries and a recirculation of blood back to the right heart, which leads to overt cardiac failure. Hepatomegaly also contributes to respiratory problems, and a proportion of patients will need ventilatory support. Pooling of blood within the abnormal vascular channels may also be responsible for a presentation of thrombocytopenia due to platelet trapping, accompanied by anaemia and a consumption coagulopathy (Kasabach–Merritt syndrome). The diagnosis should be established, as for cavernous haemangiomas, with ultrasound, Doppler imaging, contrast CT and arteriography.

A variety of medical treatments have been used in HAE, including corticosteroids and, most recently, interferon alfa, although the efficacy, particularly of corticosteroids, is still unclear. Interferon alfa has a defined role in the treatment of life-threatening haemangiomas in sites other than the liver, although the experience of its use in liver haemangiomas has been much less extensive. Both modalities have an effect on angiomatous tissue but require a period of several weeks to induce involution.

Surgical intervention is required for life-threatening lesions and involves either hepatic lobectomy if the lesion is unilobar or ligation of the hepatic artery if the lesion is bilobar and multiple (Davenport et al. 1995). The key to its success is that the hepatic artery preferentially supplies HAE tissue and, therefore, ligation causes a selective ischaemia, which reduces the vascular shunt and prompts spontaneous involution. The same effect can be achieved by selective embolization by an interventional radiologist.

Mesenchymal hamartoma

Mesenchymal hamartomas are the second most common benign liver tumours after haemangiomas. The majority of lesions present in the first year of life, although antenatal presentation is sometimes reported. The characteristic features are of a large solid and/or multicystic mass arising from the right lobe of liver. Despite its size, it is typically asymptomatic, although occasionally pain is reported due to haemorrhage into a cyst. Histologically, the lesions are derived from mesenchymal elements, with pronounced mucinous characteristics. Bile-duct elements are also seen within the walls of the cystic spaces. Although essentially these are benign lesions, there are isolated reports of sarcomatous degeneration.

Biochemical liver function tests and alpha-fetoprotein (AFP) are usually normal. Abdominal ultrasound and CT or magnetic resonance imaging (MRI) scans show a mixed solid and cystic mass that is often well-demarcated from the surrounding tissue. Sometimes this has an almost pedunculated appearance. Excision of the tumour is recommended in most cases.

Focal nodular hyperplasia

Focal nodular hyperplasia (FNH) is a benign liver tumour typically associated with young adult females using the oral contraceptive pill. However, it can be seen at any stage of childhood and beyond.

FNH has been associated with a number of conditions in childhood. Presentation in children is usually as a barely symptomatic mass, although it may be first detected as an incidental finding on imaging for other indications. In children, the tumours are usually solitary; in young adult females, there may be small multiple tumours. Investigations reveal normal liver function tests and AFP levels. MRI scanning is proving superior to abdominal ultrasound and CT in distinguishing FNH from other focal liver tumours such as hepatic adenomas. The radiological hallmark is of a hypervascular area surrounding a central hypovascular 'scar'. If diagnostic doubt persists, then percutaneous needle biopsy should be performed, although most can simply be treated by formal resection. An expectant policy with ultrasound surveillance is, however, reasonable in the absence of diagnostic doubt or symptoms.

Hepatic adenoma

Hepatic adenomas are rare tumours in childhood. In young adult females, the association of hepatic adenomas and oral contraceptive use has been established. In younger children, adenomas may be associated with conditions such as glycogen storage disease and mucopolysaccharidosis or with the administration of exogenous oestrogens or androgens. Clinical presentation ranges from an asymptomatic abdominal mass to more acute presentation with abdominal pain secondary to rapid enlargement of the tumour or haemorrhage into the tumour. AFP and biochemical liver function tests typically are normal. Imaging reveals a solid, usually solitary, tumour that can be difficult to differentiate from its malignant counterpart. Percutaneous needle biopsy may be helpful in establishing the diagnosis and planning resectional treatment. Complete surgical excision because of the propensity to cause symptoms and the small but definite risk of malignant transformation is recommended.

Simple non-parasitic parenchymal cysts

Congenital cysts of the liver are being reported with increasing frequency, presumably due to the widespread use of ultrasonography. These cysts, which may be unilocular or multilocular, are thought to arise from aberrant bile-duct development. The cysts may be intra-hepatic, partially extra-hepatic or even pedunculated. Presentation can occur at any age throughout childhood, most commonly as an asymptomatic abdominal mass. Antenatal presentation is also being reported with increasing frequency. Complications are uncommon but may include cyst rupture or internal haemorrhage. Ultrasound and CT define accurately the structure and position of the cyst in relation to the liver in most cases. Diagnostic doubt can arise in the case of a large pedunculated cyst, where the differential diagnosis may include other causes of intra-abdominal cystic swellings. Connection to the biliary tree can be established or refuted by radionuclide scanning, without recourse to direct aspiration. The optimal management is surgical excision of the cyst, as aspiration alone is associated with recurrence. Management must, however, be tailored to the size of the cyst and the presence of symptoms. For instance, a formal hepatic resection of a small intra-hepatic cyst may not be justified.

Parasitic cysts

Hydatid disease is caused by infection with the cestode parasites *Echinococcus granulosus* and *E. multilocularis*. It is an endemic problem in certain areas of the world where sheep grazing is predominant, e.g. the Mediterranean littoral, Australia and New Zealand. Hydatid cysts commonly develop within the liver, particularly in the right lobe. Although this is mainly a disease of adults, hydatid cysts can be seen in children as young as five years of age. However, at this age, the cysts are largely asymptomatic and uncomplicated. Symptoms may arise if there is secondary infection of the cyst, rupture of the cyst into the peritoneal cavity, or obstruction of the extra-hepatic bile ducts. A specific enzyme-linked immunosorbent assay (ELISA) has replaced the older Casoni skin test as the first-line investigation. Imaging with ultrasound and CT may be diagnostic if daughter cysts or discarded capsular lining are detected within the cyst ('water-lily sign'). Treatment is indicated for larger (>5 cm) and all symptomatic cysts. A preliminary course of treatment using antiscolicidal agents such as albendazole or mebendazole is usually tolerated well in children and may be curative for smaller cysts. Excisional surgery with intraoperative precautions to avoid peritoneal spillage is required for larger cysts and any complications.

MALIGNANT LIVER TUMOURS

Introduction

Approximately 60 per cent of malignant tumours in this age group are HB, and about 25 per cent are HCC. The remainder are distinctly unusual, such as embryonal sarcomas and angiosarcomas. Both HB and HCC have a predilection for boys over girls (two to one), but with a completely different age at presentation. HB occurs in the first three years of life, while HCC merges into its adult counterpart during adolescence.

HB is associated with a number of underlying conditions, such as Beckwith–Wiedemann syndrome, hemi-hypertrophy, familial adenomatous polyposis, fetal alcohol syndrome and maternal gonadotrophin use. HCC typically develops in children with pre-existing liver disease, such as chronic hepatitis, tyrosinosis, glycogen storage disease and biliary atresia (Perilongo and Shafford 1999).

HCC but not HB has a pronounced geographical variation caused by endemic hepatitis B. Therefore, the incidence of HCC in Japan and East Asia is many times that in western countries. Interestingly, this can change: the introduction of universal hepatitis B vaccination in Taiwan in the 1980s and 1990s was associated with a huge reduction in adolescent HCC.

Pathology

HBs arise from the right lobe of the liver in about 75 per cent of cases and may be bilobar in about 30 per cent. The gross appearance of HB is that of a lobulated tumour, with a variegated cut surface, areas of necrosis, areas of haemorrhage and a pseudo-capsule of compressed liver parenchyma.

The histological classification of HB is confusing, and there are numerous subtypes. Essentially, there are two main divisions: pure epithelial and mixed epithelial/mesenchymal. The former can be then be subdivided into fetal, embryonal and macrotrabecular (i.e. resembling overt HCC). The latter can be subdivided depending on whether it has tissue that resembles non-liver structures such as neural or endocrine tissue ('teratoid'), or whether it has cartilaginous or osteoid features ('non-teratoid'). Finally, there is a separate category of poorly differentiated HB, which is termed 'small-cell undifferentiated' (or anaplastic) and which bears some resemblance to other aggressive extra-hepatic tumours, such as Ewing's sarcoma.

Extra-hepatic metastasis may be present in 10–20 per cent of cases at presentation, with the most common site being the lung. Other less common sites include the portal and para-aortic lymph nodes, bone and brain.

HCC has many less favourable pathological features. In HCC, bilobar involvement with multicentric nodules or diffuse involvement is common, resulting in a majority of non-resectable tumours at presentation. In addition, a small but significant percentage of patients with HCC have a primary liver disease that potentially limits the amount of liver tissue that can be resected.

Clinical features

The most common presentation of HB is that of a well child with a large abdominal mass. Children with advanced disease may also present with loss of weight, anorexia and irritability. Less common presentations include acute abdomen resulting from tumour rupture, jaundice and, rarely, isosexual precocity. This latter feature occurs in those tumours able to secrete beta-human chorionic gonadotrophin (HCG) in addition to AFP. Some degree of osteopenia is present in up to a third of cases and results from a poorly defined disturbance in calcium metabolism. Older children with HCC may have additional symptoms and signs related to their pre-existing chronic liver disease.

Investigations

The investigations for a child suspected of having a hepatic tumour follow the same principles as for any child with an abdominal mass. Full blood count may reveal anaemia indicative of advanced disease and occasionally thrombocytosis. Coagulation studies are clearly important if needle biopsy or surgical intervention is being considered. Biochemical liver function tests may be abnormal, but this depends principally on the size of the tumour or, in advanced cases, whether the biliary system has been obstructed.

Serum AFP is the most valuable laboratory test for both the diagnosis and the monitoring of the response to treatment. AFP synthesis occurs initially in the yolk sac and liver but, by 11 weeks' gestation, exclusively in the liver. Its function is comparable to that of albumin in fetal life and has a half-life of six to seven days. Its levels peak at about 14 weeks' gestation and then decline to adult levels at about one year of age. AFP levels are grossly elevated in 70–90 per cent of patients with HB and about 50 per cent of children with HCC.

Imaging

The initial diagnostic imaging invariably will be ultrasonography, which will demonstrate whether the tumour is cystic or solid, whether it is homogeneous or heterogeneous, whether it is unifocal or multifocal, and whether there are other intra-abdominal masses suggestive of it being a secondary tumour.

More detailed imaging is done using CT and MRI, either individually or in combination. HBs typically are large unilobar heterogeneous lesions that may exhibit calcification. About 10–20 per cent of HCCs are multifocal at presentation.

The key diagnostic elements that need to be ascertained from imaging are the tumour's relationship with the portal and hepatic veins in order to determine the potential for resectability. Central tumours with involvement of the portal vein may be unresectable, whatever their size. Similarly, tumours arising adjacent to the hepatic venous confluence can make operative tumour clearance impossible.

The International Society of Paediatric Oncology (SIOP) has introduced a staging system based on pre-intervention assessment and the location of the tumour (PRETEXT staging). In this, the liver is divided into four sectors: the lateral and medial sectors of the left hemi-liver and the anterior and posterior sectors of the right hemi-liver. Groups I–IV are based on the stage and nature of involvement of the tumour and are illustrated in Figure 46.2.

Management

Long-term survival in children with malignant liver tumours is not possible, except in rare cases, without complete resection of the primary tumour. However, only about 50 per cent of HB and less than 30 per cent of HCC are technically resectable at presentation. Therefore, other modalities of therapy, such as chemotherapy, have a crucial role (Stringer et al. 1995).

There are two differing approaches to the treatment of, particularly, HB. The current European (including the UK) approach requires a confirmatory CT scan or ultrasound-guided needle biopsy and then immediate enrolment into a chemotherapy regimen for all except small lateral tumours. A radiological re-evaluation is done following two to three courses of chemotherapy, and a decision is then made about surgical resectability.

The North American approach is to perform an initial laparotomy, which determines the tumour resectability. Resection then occurs or, if deemed unresectable, an open biopsy for confirmatory histology is taken followed by a course of chemotherapy.

The chief advantage of the European approach is that at presentation, up to 50 per cent are probably unresectable but can be made resectable following chemotherapy. This facilitates effective tumour clearance and reduces residual disease. As the operation technically is easier in the post-chemotherapy tumour, there is a reduction of morbidity due to an overaggressive surgical approach. However, advocates of the American approach would argue that some completely excised tumours with favourable histology (i.e. pure fetal histology) do not need any further adjuvant treatment and

Three adjoining sectors FREE

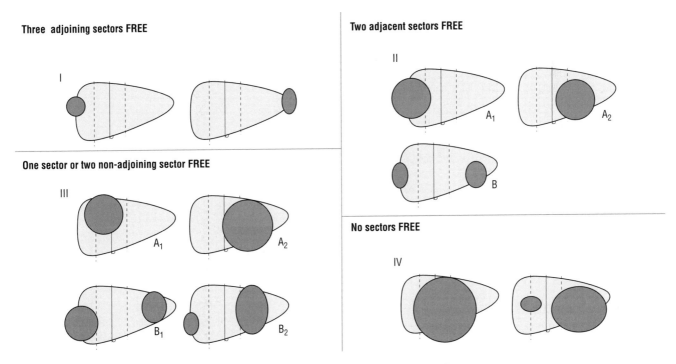

One sector or two non-adjoining sector FREE

Two adjacent sectors FREE

No sectors FREE

Figure 46.2 *International Society of Paediatric Oncology pretreatment staging of malignant liver tumours.*
FREE, free from tumour.

therefore are being over-treated if subjected to a typical chemotherapy regimen. This approach also avoids the theoretical complications of percutaneous needle biopsy, such as abdominal-wall seeding and tumour rupture and bleeding.

Current effective chemotherapeutic agents used in European studies include cisplatin (or carboplatin) and doxorubicin (combined as the cisplatin and doxorubicin (PLADO) regimen). In American studies, these, together with combinations of ifosfamide, vincristine, amifostine and 5-fluoruracil, for more advanced stages or unfavourable histology, are used. A combination of preoperative chemotherapy and resectional surgery can achieve long-term survival in 80–90 per cent of children with HB.

HCC is much less responsive to chemotherapy. Because of its multicentric origin in some cases, the potential benefits of preoperative chemotherapy are less certain. Nevertheless, the same principles of chemotherapy followed by surgical excision apply.

A further treatment option that has been applied recently, especially for unresectable or multicentric HB, is that of total hepatectomy and liver transplantation (Srinivasan *et al.* 2002).

RELEVANT BASIC SCIENCE

Modern surgery of the liver is dependent on a detailed understanding of its segmental anatomy. This knowledge,

combined with improvement in imaging techniques, allows the surgeon to predict accurately the location of vascular structures within the liver and reduce unnecessary complications due to inadvertent vascular or biliary injury.

Morphological anatomy

The human liver is divided by the falciform ligament into a larger right lobe and a smaller left lobe. Within the right lobe lies a smaller lobe, the quadrate lobe, which lies between the bed of the gallbladder and the falciform ligament. More posteriorly is the caudate lobe, which abuts the intra-hepatic vena cava. The gallbladder lies in a depression within the inferior surface of the right lobe and connects via the cystic duct to the common hepatic duct to form the common bile duct. Vascular (portal vein and hepatic arteries) structures enter, and biliary structures leave, the liver via the porta hepatis. Parenchymal venous drainage is typically via three hepatic veins into the inferior vena cava at the level of the diaphragm.

Segmental anatomy

As the right and left portal veins are similar in size and blood flow, it was soon realized that the above anatomical description does not define accurately the true functional nature of the liver. Thus, ligation of either the right or the left portal veins

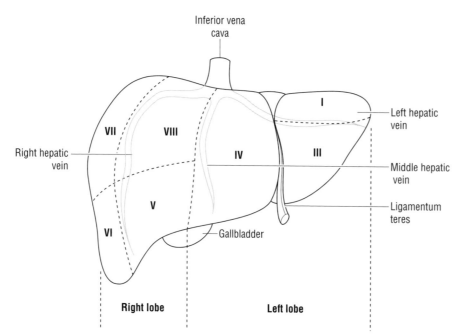

Figure 46.3 *Segmental anatomy of the liver.*

and corresponding arteries shows that the principal plane of the liver is actually unmarked on the surface but runs from the region of the gallbladder bed towards the confluence of the left and middle hepatic veins. Further studies then defined so-called 'liver segments' (Figure 46.3), with defined portal venous and hepatic arterial branches, and these became the smallest surgical units of the liver that could be excised independently without compromising adjacent segments. There are eight such segments, each with an assigned Roman numeral. It should be clear that segments II, III and IV comprise the functional left liver, while segments V, VI, VII and VIII comprise the functional right liver. Segment I (corresponding to the anatomical caudate lobe) has branches from both right and left portal veins and hepatic arteries and has a separate venous drainage via multiple small veins directly into the cava.

Surgical terminology

Removal of the functional right liver (segments V–VIII) or left liver (segments II–IV) is termed a 'partial or hemi-hepatectomy'. Removal of segments II and III (the anatomical left lobe) is termed a 'left lateral segmentectomy' (or, more recently, 'sectionectomy'). Either right or left hemi-hepatectomy can be extended to remove the adjacent segments of the contralateral hemi-liver. For example, an extended right hepatectomy (or right trisectionectomy) would remove all the liver segments up to the falciform ligament, leaving only segments I, II and III. About 80 per cent of the liver mass may be removed without inducing liver failure, and within one to two months the preoperative functioning liver mass should be restored due to regeneration.

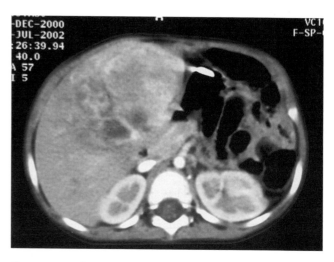

Figure 46.4 *Computed tomography scan of a 18-month-old girl with a mass in the right lobe of the liver (arrowed).*

CLINICAL SCENARIOS

Case 1

An 18-month-old girl presented with an asymptomatic abdominal mass in the upper abdomen. Examination revealed an otherwise well child, with a mass in the right upper quadrant extending to the umbilicus. Full blood count and liver function tests were normal. Serum AFP was elevated (140 000 IU/L). Plain abdominal radiograph showed a mass in the right upper quadrant with no calcification. Abdominal ultrasound was suggestive of a solid lesion arising from the liver. CT scan confirmed the presence of a solid lesion

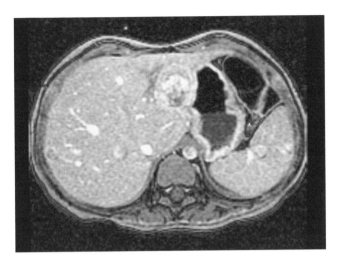

Figure 46.5 *Magnetic resonance imaging scan of a two-year-old girl with a liver mass in the left lobe of the liver (arrowed).*

occupying most of the left lobe of the liver (Figure 46.4). Percutaneous needle biopsy showed HB. Three courses of chemotherapy reduced the tumour size. A left hemi-hepatectomy (segments II, III and IV) was then performed. Three further courses of chemotherapy were given postoperatively. There has been no recurrence after two years.

Case 2

In a two-year-old girl with Beckwith–Weidemann syndrome, a lesion in the left lobe of the liver was detected on routine ultrasound screening. CT and MRI scanning (Figure 46.5)

confirmed the presence of a lesion in segments II and III of the liver. AFP was slightly raised. Percutaneous needle biopsy was suggestive of FNH, and an expectant policy followed. Over subsequent months, the lesion increased in size and AFP levels rose further. A left lateral segmentectomy (segments II and III) was performed. Histology confirmed this as HB arising in areas of FNH.

REFERENCES

Davenport M, Hansen L, Heaton ND, Howard ER. Haemangioendothelioma of the liver in infants. *Journal of Pediatric Surgery* 1995; **30**: 44–8.

Perilongo G, Shafford EA. Liver tumours. *European Journal of Cancer* 1999; **35**: 953–9.

Srinivasan P, McCall J, Pritchard J, *et al.* Orthotopic liver transplantation for unresectable hepatoblastoma. *Transplantation* 2002; **74**: 652–5.

Stringer MD, Hennayake S, Howard ER, *et al.* Improved outcome for children with hepatoblastoma. *British Journal of Surgery* 1995; **82**: 386–91.

FURTHER READING

Carachi R, Azmy A, Grosfeld JL. *The Surgery of Childhood Tumors.* London: Arnold, 1999.

Howard ER, Stringer MD, Colombani PM. *Surgery of the Liver, Bile Ducts and Pancreas in Children*, 2nd edn. London: Arnold, 2002.

Kelly DA. *Diseases of the Liver and Biliary System in Children.* Oxford: Blackwell, 1999.

47

Miscellaneous: lumps, bumps and lymphadenopathy

ISABELLA E MOORE

Learning objectives

- To understand the types of the most common skin conditions in childhood (bumps).
- To understand the types of the most common soft-tissue lesions in childhood (lumps).
- To become aware of the association of some of the bumps and lumps with inherited genetic disorders.
- To become aware of the importance of cytogenetic investigations in malignancies (soft-tissue tumours and lymphomas).

LUMPS

Introduction

In general, the types of soft-tissue tumour that occur in childhood are different from those diagnosed in adults. Many soft-tissue lesions seen in children represent malformations or hamartomas (an abnormal mixture of tissues normally present at that site); for example, vascular lesions such as lymphangiomas are considered as hamartomatous in nature. The remaining lesions represent neoplasms; these can be subdivided into benign neoplasms (e.g. neurofibromas), intermediate or low-grade malignancies (e.g. plexiform fibrohistiocytic tumours) and frankly malignant neoplasms (e.g. rhabdomyosarcomas, primitive neuroectodermal tumours). Vascular lesions (haemangiomas, lymphangiomas) are discussed in Chapter 41.

Relevant basic science and general pathological considerations

A large proportion of soft-tissue neoplasms in children arise in the soft tissues of the head and neck and the genitourinary tract. In adults, the predominant sites are peripheral soft tissues (limbs). Approximately 30 per cent of soft-tissue lesions in children are vascular in nature, followed by tumours showing features of myofibroblasts/histiocytes (24 per cent), neurogenic tumours (15 per cent), tumours with myogenic differentiation (e.g. rhabdomyosarcoma) (14 per cent) and tumours with fat differentiation (six per cent) (Coffin et al. 1997).

The histological appearances of soft-tissue neoplasms do not necessarily reflect their origins. A neoplasm composed of cells that look like skeletal muscle cells (rhabdomyosarcoma) arises not from the skeletal muscle but from the undifferentiated mesenchymal cell, which in this particular tumour tends to show skeletal muscle differentiation. Similarly, a synovial sarcoma arises not from the synovium but from the undifferentiated mesenchymal cell.

The large majority of soft-tissue neoplasms occur sporadically and do not have syndromic or familial associations. However, there are occasional tumours that may lead to a diagnosis of a particular genetic condition, and many such conditions have a high risk of recurrence in the family (autosomal dominant inheritance pattern). For example, fibromatosis may be associated with Gardner syndrome, characterized by the development of multiple tumours, including osteomas of the skull, epidermoid cysts and fibromas, and multiple polyposis, predisposing to carcinoma of the colon. Fetal rhabdomyomas (benign tumours showing skeletal muscle differentiation) may occur in the background of Gorlin–Goltz syndrome, known as a basal-cell naevus syndrome. Some types of neurofibroma (so-called plexiform neurofibromas) may lead to the diagnosis of neurofibromatosis, an autosomal dominant condition with a high risk of development of various malignant neoplasms.

Children with Li–Fraumeni cancer syndrome, another autosomal dominant syndrome and characterized by a mutation in the *p53* tumour suppressor gene, are at particular risk of developing carcinomas of the adrenal gland, breast and colon, and also glial neoplasms and childhood sarcomas, such as rhabdomyosarcoma.

Investigations and diagnosis

A pathological diagnosis is usually established on an incisional biopsy of the lesion, although in small superficial masses an excisional biopsy may be justified. Some intermediate-grade neoplasms may be treated by primary excision.

Biopsies of deep-seated lesions are difficult and may require ultrasound-guided needle biopsy. Occasionally, it may be necessary to request intraoperative frozen section to confirm the presence of diagnostic material in the removed sample.

The amount of diagnostic tissue available becomes a critical factor guiding the pathologist as to which ancillary investigations to consider. Many such investigations may be invaluable in assisting the pathologist in the diagnosis of difficult cases.

With advances in our understanding of the molecular basis of neoplasms, cytogenetic methods of identification of a particular translocation play an increasingly important part in the diagnostic process. These new diagnostic techniques require unfixed (fresh) biopsy tissue transported promptly to the cytogenetics laboratory in a sterile tissue-culture medium. Therefore, it is increasingly important that a pathologist is contacted and the requirements discussed before the biopsy is considered.

The unfixed tissue biopsy is transported rapidly to the pathology laboratory, where triaging of the sample is undertaken. The important decision has to be made by a pathologist as to how much tissue should be fixed and processed routinely for histology and whether there is enough tissue to submit for standard metaphase cytogenetics, to snap freeze for *in situ* hybridization or to send a small sample for electron microscopy. The same principles apply when dealing with a lymph-node biopsy for suspected lymphoma.

Virtually all malignant, and many benign, soft-tissue neoplasms show clonal chromosome aberrations. These chromosomal rearrangements, usually translocations, are expressed in shorthand as follows: t(11;22) indicates a reciprocal exchange of the genetic material between two different chromosome arms, in this case chromosomes 11 and 22. Some of these translocations are so characteristic for particular tumours that they can be used as important adjuncts to diagnosis. Translocation t(11;22) is characteristic for Ewing's

sarcoma and primitive neuroectodermal tumour (PNET); translocation t(2;13) is typical for the alveolar variant of rhabdomyosarcoma; and lipoblastomas frequently show rearrangement of the long arm of chromosome 8 (8q).

In situ hybridization is a relatively new method of molecular cytogenetics in which specific deoxyribonucleic acid (DNA) probes can be applied to cell nuclei on paraffin sections to show all of the above-mentioned chromosomal abnormalities. Fluorescence is used in the process of visualization of abnormalities, hence the term 'fluorescence *in situ* hybridization' (FISH).

The application of immunocytochemistry revolutionized the diagnosis of soft-tissue neoplasms, allowing the pathologist to assess the functional phenotype of the cells making up the lesion in question. A large number of monoclonal antibodies are available and aid the pathologist in the process of identification of the immunophenotype of the lesion. Immunocytochemistry is applied to tissues fixed in formalin and processed in a routine fashion.

Fibrous tumours specific to childhood

There are a few fibrous lesions occurring in children that do not have counterparts in adult life. They may pose diagnostic problems, as frequently they display rapid growth, but this does not necessarily indicate malignant behaviour. Among the more common of these lesions are fibrous hamartoma of infancy, infantile digital fibromatosis and infantile myofibromatosis. All of these lesions are benign and cured by local excision. Another important lesion, seen predominantly in childhood but occasionally diagnosed in adults, is myofibroblastic tumour, also known as pseudo-tumour.

FIBROUS HAMARTOMA OF INFANCY

This lesion usually presents in the first two years of life. In up to 25 per cent of cases, it may be identified at birth. Boys are affected two to three times more often than girls (Weiss and Goldblum 2001). The mass usually shows an initial phase of rapid growth followed by slower growth up to the age of five years. It does not cease growth spontaneously. The areas involved include axillary folds, upper arms, thighs, inguinal and pubic regions, shoulders and back. The lesion seldom ever occurs on the hands and feet. It usually presents as an ill-defined mobile mass, 3–5 cm in diameter, and not attached to the superficial muscle. Virtually all cases are solitary. There is no evidence of any specific association. The lesion is composed of three distinct components: strands of fibrous tissue, loose myxoid areas and mature fat (Figure 47.1). Only 16 per cent recur locally if not completely excised. As the name implies, this is a benign, probably hamartomatous lesion that can be cured by local excision.

INFANTILE DIGITAL FIBROMATOSIS

Almost all of these lesions are diagnosed in the first three years of life. Thirty per cent of cases are present at birth. The fingers

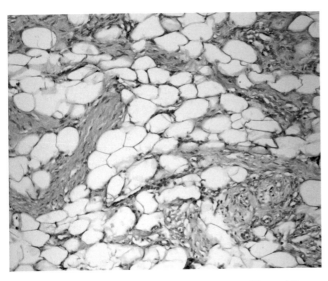

Figure 47.1 *High-power view showing a mixture of fat and fibrous strands in fibrous hamartoma of infancy. See also Colour Plate 12.*

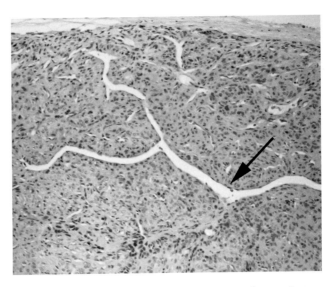

Figure 47.3 *Spindle myofibroblasts present in a solitary variant of infantile myofibromatosis. Arrow indicates a prominent vessel. See also Colour Plate 14.*

INFANTILE MYOFIBROMATOSIS

This is one of the most common fibrous tumours in infancy. It occurs in the first decade, with 88 per cent being diagnosed in the first two years of life and more than half of the tumours presenting at birth or shortly after. There are three distinct patterns of presentation:

* *Solitary lesion*: this is the most common presentation. Seventy per cent present in boys, usually as a nodular mass in the skin or muscle of the head and neck region, the upper extremities and trunk and, rarely, the skeleton. The term 'myofibroblastoma' is often applied to solitary lesions.
* *Multicentric variant*: this is more common in girls, with involvement of the skin, soft tissues, bone and muscle. Occasionally, there are up to 50–100 nodules.
* *Generalized form*: there is visceral involvement (heart, lungs, gastrointestinal tract) in 75 per cent, leading to death due to respiratory distress or gastrointestinal dysfunction.

There may be a familial occurrence, with autosomal dominant and recessive inheritance patterns. Macroscopically, the lesions show a lobulated fibrous appearance, with a haemorrhagic, necrotic and often calcified centre. The lesions may regress spontaneously. They are composed of spindle myofibroblasts (Figure 47.3). The treatment of choice is local excision. Solitary and multicentric variants have an excellent prognosis, with a recurrence risk of less than ten per cent.

Myofibromatosis should not be confused with neurofibromatosis, which affects older children, with 50 per cent of cases having a history of familial involvement and with the evidence of multiple café-au-lait spots.

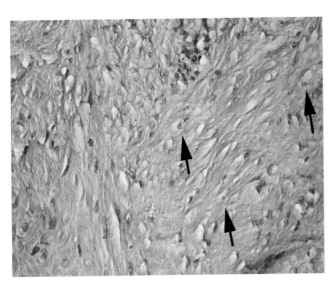

Figure 47.2 *High-power view of infantile digital fibromatosis, with arrows indicating the presence of typical intracytoplasmic inclusions. See also Colour Plate 13.*

(sides or dorsum of the distal or middle phalangeal joints) are affected more frequently than the toes. The thumb is rarely affected. The lesion presents as a non-tender, firm, skin-coloured nodule. Occasionally, there may be associated flexion deformities of the joints. The lesions can be single or multiple. It has been suggested that trauma may predispose to the development of this condition. The characteristic microscopic feature is the presence of red inclusions in the cytoplasm of spindle myofibroblasts (cells combining the features of fibroblasts and contractile muscle cells) (Figure 47.2). These lesions have a marked tendency for local recurrence (60 per cent). Because of the high rate of spontaneous regression, a conservative approach (watch and wait) is advocated. Deformities and contractures may require surgical correction.

INFLAMMATORY MYOFIBROBLASTIC TUMOUR

Inflammatory myofibroblastic tumour (IMT), also composed of myofibroblasts, was previously known as 'pseudo-tumour'.

Since its clonal nature has been established, it is now recognized as a true benign neoplasm with a potential for aggressive local behaviour.

IMT involves the soft tissues and viscera of children and young adults. It has been described in every anatomical location, but by far the most common location is the mesentery and omentum. The presenting symptoms depend on the location of the tumour. In some patients, there may be systemic manifestations such as fever, night sweats, weight loss, raised erythrocyte sedimentation rate (ESR), anaemia and thrombocytosis. These tumours may grow to a large size, particularly in the retroperitoneum and abdominal cavity. Histologically, the tumour may resemble granulation tissue or fibromatosis or look like a scar tissue. Treatment of choice is surgical resection, with re-resection of recurrences, which have been reported in 25 per cent of cases. Intra-abdominal cases behave more aggressively than lesions elsewhere.

Neurogenic tumours

Neurogenic tumours constitute up to 16 per cent of soft-tissue tumours in children. Neurofibroma is the most common benign neurogenic tumour. The most common malignant neurogenic tumour in the paediatric age range is PNET.

NEUROFIBROMA

Neurofibromas are frequently multiple, vary in size and occur in the form of soft, compressible, sometimes pedunculated lesions on any body surfaces. They are composed of spindle Schwann cells and collagen. A variant of neurofibroma known as plexiform neurofibroma is a hallmark for neurofibromatosis, an autosomal dominant abnormality of the neural crest and its mesenchyme. Neurofibromatosis is a common disease, affecting one in 2500–3000 live births. Plexiform neurofibromas are often large and poorly defined, with 'worm-like' thickenings growing along the peripheral nerve. A diagnosis of two or more neurofibromas in a child under ten years of age, or the presence of a single plexiform neurofibroma, is almost pathognomonic for neurofibromatosis. This condition is caused by mutations in the *NF1* gene, encoding for the protein neurofibromin, the function of which has not been determined. The typical clinical features include café-au-lait spots, freckling in the axillary or inguinal region, iris hamartomas known as Lisch nodules, and a variety of benign (cortical fibromas in the bones) and malignant (malignant nerve-sheath tumours, gliomas, leukaemias, malignant soft-tissue sarcomas) tumours. The unusual presentation in a child may include a generalized polyneuropathy or infantile gangrene due to vascular changes seen in neurofibromatosis. Bone defects, spine deformities and growth anomalies of the limbs, with pseudo-arthroses, can all represent early manifestations of the disease. A rapid enlargement or pain in the pre-existing neurofibroma, and particularly in deep lesions, may herald malignant change. It is estimated that the

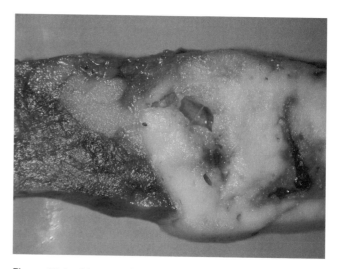

Figure 47.4 *Macroscopical appearance of a primitive neuro-ectodermal tumour occurring in the soft tissues of the subcutis. Note the white firm fibrous appearance in the tumour. See also Colour Plate 15.*

incidence of malignant transformation varies between two and 29 per cent. Patients who have had the disease for many years are at greatest risk.

PERIPHERAL PRIMITIVE NEUROECTODERMAL TUMOUR

This is one of the more common malignant neurogenic tumours in children. The median age varies between 14 and 22 years; only 14 per cent occur in children under five years of age. The most common sites include the chest wall, paraspinal region, extremities and head and neck. Internal organs, except for the kidney, are not commonly involved. The tumour can grow to a large size and may display a lobulated, multinodular appearance, frequently with areas of haemorrhage or necrosis (Figure 47.4). Microscopical appearances typically show a neoplasm composed of sheaths of small blue cells expressing neural markers. PNET is related closely to Ewing's sarcoma, the two conditions forming opposite ends of a clinical spectrum. These tumours share the same chromosomal translocation, t(11;22). The differential diagnosis of such a neoplasm includes other small blue-cell tumours of childhood: neuroblastoma, rhabdomyosarcoma and lymphoma. PNET is a highly aggressive tumour with a very poor prognosis. Most patients die within two to three years following diagnosis. Treatment modalities include surgery combined with chemotherapy and high-dose radiation therapy.

Adipose tumours

Lipomas, the most frequent benign adipose tissue tumours in adults, are relatively uncommon in children. Lipoblastomas are seen in the first five years of life, while liposarcoma is extremely rare in the first two decades of life.

LIPOBLASTOMA

This neoplasm occurs almost exclusively in infancy and early childhood, with 90 per cent of lesions being diagnosed before the age of three years. It presents as a rapidly growing soft-tissue mass, usually on the extremities but also in the mediastinum, retroperitoneum, scrotum, mesentery and head and neck. The term 'lipoblastoma' is applied to circumscribed lesions, while a more diffuse growth pattern justifies the term 'lipoblastomatosis'. The tumour is usually soft and lobulated and can be well-encapsulated. It is related to the embryonic white fat and shows a variable degree of differentiation towards mature fat.

Abnormalities of chromosome 8 are a common feature. The tumour has an excellent prognosis, and complete but conservative local excision is sufficient. The recurrence risk is 14 per cent, usually after incomplete initial excision.

BUMPS

Introduction

This section deals with localized nodular but superficial dermal lesions and swellings, unscientifically designated as 'bumps'. Particular attention is paid to lesions that can mimic malignancies or can be associated with a predisposition to the development of malignancy.

Inflammatory lesions

Lesions such as granuloma annulare and rheumatic and rheumatoid nodules represent so-called necrobiotic granulomas, in which a principal histological feature is a focus of necrotic collagen surrounded by inflammatory histiocytic cells.

GRANULOMA ANNULARE

This is the most common type of necrobiotic granuloma in children. It usually presents as a firm annular (semicircular or circular) papule on the distal extremity. There is no pain or erythema. A two-to-one male predominance, with a mean age of four years, is reported. Spontaneous resolution occurs in 50 per cent of cases; in 30 per cent, the lesion can recur (Dehner 1987). Deep granuloma annulare is a distinct lesion represented by firm painless nodules, frequently larger than 2 cm in diameter, in the pretibial compartments, on the dorsa of the feet and, occasionally, in the periorbital and occipital regions. The lesions can be multiple and have a tendency for multiple recurrences and spontaneous regression. A low-grade, slow-growing but malignant soft-tissue sarcoma known as epithelioid sarcoma can mimic deep granuloma annulare. This tumour classically presents in the deep soft tissues of the forearm in adolescents.

RHEUMATIC AND RHEUMATOID NODULES

Neither rheumatic nor rheumatoid nodules are common. They usually occur in the close proximity of major joints. The rheumatic nodules tend to be smaller, appear for no longer than four to six days and occur late in the course of rheumatic fever. They are usually firm, painless and mobile. Rheumatoid nodules develop late in the course of rheumatoid arthritis and in only five to six per cent of children suffering from juvenile rheumatoid arthritis. These lesions can show almost identical histological appearances to those seen in deep granuloma annulare.

Hamartomatous lesions

HAMARTOMATOUS POLYPS

The term 'hamartoma' describes an abnormal mixture of tissues normally present at a particular location and growing at a rate comparable to that of the host.

Skin tags in adults are represented by fibroepithelial polyps, which are uncommon in children. Skin tags in childhood usually represent hamartomatous polyps. These polypoid growths are covered by skin with its appendages, and with the core composed of a mixture of connective tissue, fat and smooth muscle. Accessory structures such as auricles or digits are considered as hamartomatous in origin. In the accessory auricle, the fibrous core will contain cartilage; in the accessory digit, the presence of bone will be documented.

NAEVUS SEBACEOUS

Naevus sebaceous can be present at birth (50 per cent of cases), mainly on the scalp and neck, in the form of verruca-like hyperpigmented small papules. The lesions undergo progressive changes in their appearances. Sebaceous glands are not as apparent in children as they are in adult lesions. The presence of apocrine sweat glands is a characteristic feature in mature lesions. Naevus sebaceous predisposes to basal-cell carcinoma in ten per cent of cases.

Other hamartomatous lesions to consider in the paediatric age range include connective tissue naevi, with the overgrowth of specific mesenchymal dermal elements (e.g. fat in naevus lipomatosus, collagen in collagen naevus), and a lesion known as 'adenoma sebaceum', representing one of the clinical manifestations of tuberous sclerosis. Adenoma sebaceum presents as a reddish papule or nodule related to the distribution of the trigeminal nerve, although usually sparing the skin of the upper lip and forehead. Histologically, these lesions represent angiofibromas, composed of fibroblasts and dilated blood vessels, and are identified in up to 90 per cent of cases. It is debated as to whether these lesions are true neoplasms or hamartomas. Similar fibrous nodules, periungual fibromas, can be seen around the nail beds. Changes in the skin pigmentation and café-au-lait spots appear to be more common dermal manifestations of tuberous sclerosis than these hamartomatous proliferations. The classical triad of tuberous sclerosis includes adenoma sebaceum, mental retardation and seizures. In 50 per cent of patients, a shagreen patch (raised plaque of thickened slightly pigmented skin) in the lumbosacral region may be seen. Benign tumours also can be detected in the internal organs, including the brain (gliomas), heart (rhabdomyomas) and kidney (angiomyolipomas). Tuberous sclerosis is an autosomal dominant condition, with the majority of cases representing a new mutation. The incidence is one in 20 000–30 000 live births.

Epidermal cysts

A large number of superficial bumps in children are cystic in nature, with squamous epithelial cysts occurring most commonly (approximately 60 per cent).

Cysts lined by squamous epithelium containing the keratohyaline layer and filled with keratin in the centre are termed epidermal or keratinous cysts. In children, such cysts are usually represented by dermoid cysts, which show skin appendages in the cyst wall. They usually present between the ages of three and ten years. The most common location is the face (eyebrow, nose) and scalp, where occasionally such cysts can produce lytic defects in the underlying bone. Dermoid cysts may be found anywhere along the lines of embryonic closure.

Epidermoid cysts are not as common in children compared with adults. Typically, they are lined by the squamous epithelium devoid of skin appendages. They can occur on any body surface; the most common locations are the face, neck and trunk. Both cyst types can rupture, producing an exuberant inflammatory reaction to the keratinous content. In patients presenting with multiple epidermoid cysts, Gardner syndrome should be considered.

Cutaneus polyps

A polypoid lesion at the umbilicus, the so-called 'umbilical granuloma', represents a remnant of an omphalo-enteric duct with islands of enteric epithelium communicating with the skin surface, frequently with associated inflammation, ulceration and granulation tissue formation, and leading to a polypoid lesion simulating a pyogenic granuloma.

The term 'pyogenic granuloma' describes a type of dermal capillary haemangioma. Macroscopically, this is a solitary polypoid nodule with ulceration of the surface and formation of exuberant granulation tissue overlying the deep lesion of a capillary haemangioma, composed of a lobulated arrangement of endothelial cells forming small vascular channels.

Histiocytic proliferations

Histiocytic proliferations, or histiocytoses, encompass proliferations of cells forming a mononuclear phagocytic system. The two most common types – benign juvenile xanthogranuloma

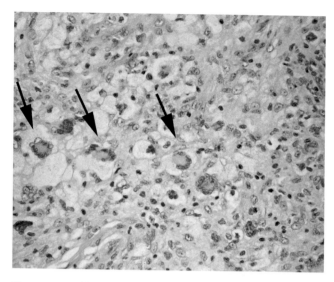

Figure 47.5 *Numerous Touton giant cells (arrows) typical of infantile xanthogranuloma. See also Colour Plate 16.*

and Langerhans cell histiocytosis (derived from a subset of histiocytes known as dendritic cells) – are mentioned here.

Juvenile xanthogranuloma is a prototypic benign histiocytic lesion of childhood and adolescence. It is composed of histiocytes, eosinophils and typical giant cells, with a ring of nuclei known as Touton giant cells (Figure 47.5).

In 60 per cent of cases, the lesions are multifocal. In a small proportion of patients, the lesions present at birth. The most common sites are the head and neck (up to 75 per cent of cases), followed by the trunk and extremities. Extracutaneous involvement has been described in five per cent of cases, particularly in the skeletal muscle and paravertebral soft tissues but also in the eye, lung, heart and liver. Ocular involvement can lead to glaucoma. Lesions usually present as yellow or reddish nodules, either solitary or in clusters. The most important feature is spontaneous regression of the lesions. The exact nature of this lesion has not been established, as it is unclear whether this is an unusual proliferative (in response to a viral infection) or true neoplastic process. It is important that this benign lesion is differentiated from the cutaneous form of Langerhans cell histiocytosis, which probably represents a neoplastic process.

Skin involvement may be part of a progressive diffuse multisystem involvement with a poor prognosis (Letterer–Siwe disease) or a solitary nodular involvement of the skin that is self-limiting and has good prognosis. Langerhans cells have different immunophenotype compared with the histiocytes in juvenile xanthogranuloma.

Epidermal tumours

Adnexal tumours are not common in children. One of the more common benign tumours arising from the hair matrix is pilomatrixoma (also known as a calcifying epithelioma of Malherbe). These lesions are usually diagnosed in children under ten years of age. The most common sites are the face, neck and upper extremities. In two to three per cent of cases, pilomatrixomas are multiple. The lesions are usually hard on palpation, well-circumscribed, up to 4 cm in diameter and located in the dermis or subcutaneous tissue. Calcification is a common feature. The tumours are composed of proliferating basaloid cells, transforming into ghost cells. Recurrence is unusual, even after incomplete excision.

LYMPHADENOPATHY

Introduction

The reasons for lymph-node enlargement in children are somewhat different to those in adults. In the group of reactive inflammatory conditions, specific infections such as atypical mycobacterial infection are common, while malignant lymphadenopathy in children is more commonly due to a lymphoma rather than a metastatic carcinoma.

Reactive inflammatory conditions

Infectious mononucleosis caused by the Epstein–Barr virus (EBV) is common in older children and young adults. This is a benign, self-limiting lymphoproliferative disease presenting with fever, generalized lymphadenopathy, sore throat and splenomegaly. The lymph nodes involved usually include the posterior cervical, axillary and groin nodes. Histologically worrisome immunoblastic reaction in the paracortex of the lymph nodes can be seen in this disease, although lymph nodes are rarely subjected to a biopsy. Appropriate serological investigations usually establish a correct diagnosis. In difficult cases in which the histological diagnosis is uncertain, the use of specific probes for a viral genome may be required.

Cat-scratch disease can lead to a localized lymphadenopathy. In such cases, there are foci of stellate abscesses with palisading histiocytes seen in the lymph nodes. These are caused by infection with the organisms *Afipia felis* or *Rochalimaea henselae*, which can be demonstrated by special silver-staining techniques.

Toxoplasma gondii is an obligatory intracellular organism, usually causing subclinical infection or mild lymphadenopathy in non-compromised hosts. Severe infection can occur in fetuses *in utero* and in immunocompromised patients. Humans can develop toxoplasmosis by eating undercooked pork or lamb infected with *T. gondii* cysts or food contaminated by cat faeces containing oocysts. Cervical lymphadenopathy is the usual feature. Infection with *T. gondii* produces hyperplasia of both B-cell and T-cell areas. The characteristic histological feature is clusters of pale epithelioid macrophages. The diagnosis of toxoplasmosis should be confirmed by positive serology or by culture of a fresh lymph node. Changes similar to those seen in toxoplasmosis can occur in persistent generalized lymphadenopathy due to human immunodeficiency virus (HIV) infection.

Mycobacterial lymphadenopathy in developed countries is due mainly to infection with atypical mycobacteria. The most common infection is *Mycobacterium avium intracellulare* (70 per cent of cases), followed by *M. scrofulaceum*. In 80 per cent of cases, the infection occurs in children between one and five years of age. It usually affects the cervical nodes. Microscopic examination shows areas of caseous necrosis surrounded by macrophages and giant cells. Occasionally, bacilli can be demonstrated by special stains. The site of the lesions, the age of the patient and the clinical history usually point to the diagnosis of atypical mycobacterial infection; however, confirmation by culture of fresh nodal tissue is recommended. Treatment consists of surgical excision of the abnormal node. Lymphadenopathy due to infection with *M. tuberculosis* may show almost identical histological appearances and should be considered first in children from developing countries. Confirmed infection with *M. tuberculosis* requires anti-tuberculous therapy.

Malignant conditions presenting with lymphadenopathy

Metastatic carcinomas are not a common cause of malignant lymphadenopathy in childhood, where non-Hodgkin's lymphoma (NHL; mainly in younger children) and Hodgkin's lymphoma (HL; usually in older children) predominate.

HODGKIN'S LYMPHOMA

All types of HL share similar features: raised lymph nodes, usually of the cervical region, in young adults, and, on histological examination, the presence of characteristic large cells designated as Reed–Sternberg (RS) cells. HLs are subdivided into two main categories: nodular lymphocyte-predominant HL (a B-cell neoplasm involving cervical, axillary or inguinal lymph nodes and presenting mainly in adults) and classic HL, which is subdivided further into four major types: nodular sclerosis, mixed cellularity, lymphocyte-rich and lymphocyte-depleted. Approximately ten per cent of cases of HL occur in children, at an average age of ten years. The most common type is nodular sclerosis (66 per cent of cases) (Gray and Smith 1995). Accurate diagnosis of HL in children can be difficult, as a number of florid lymphoproliferative benign reactions in the lymph nodes (e.g. EBV infection, toxoplasmosis) can mimic HL. The lymphadenopathy is usually localized to one to two nodal areas. Mediastinal involvement frequently is seen in the nodular sclerosis variant. Fever, night sweats and weight loss are present in 40 per cent of patients. It is believed that RS cells are derived from the germinal centre mature B-cells. Conventional cytogenetic studies confirm aneuploidy of RS cells, while comparative genomic hybridization shows subtle gains or losses of the genetic material on a number of different chromosomes (2, 4, 9, 12). The stage of the disease is an important prognostic factor, but with modern chemo- and radiotherapy the large majority of cases of HL are curable.

Table 47.1 *Main differences between non-Hodgkin's lymphoma in children and adults (adapted from Stocker and Dehner 2001)*

Children	Adults
Usually extranodal	Usually nodal
Rapid growth	Slower growth
Rarely follicular	Often follicular
Often leukaemic	Rarely leukaemic

NON-HODGKIN'S LYMPHOMA

The clinical features and types of NHL in children differ significantly from those in adults (Table 47.1).

The most common types of NHL in adults – lymphocytic and follicular lymphomas – are very rare in children, who most frequently suffer from malignant lymphoblastic lymphoma (T-cell or B-cell), malignant B-cell lymphoma of Burkitt's type, and large-cell anaplastic lymphoma.

The most common type is T-cell lymphoblastic lymphoma (85–90 per cent of lymphoblastic lymphomas), which usually occurs in boys and presents with an anterior mediastinal mass or lymphadenopathy. In half of the cases, there is involvement of the blood or bone marrow. After appropriate chemotherapy, 75 per cent of cases achieve lasting remission. B-cell lymphoblastic lymphoma is uncommon and can present with lymphadenopathy or extranodal involvement, usually of the intra-abdominal organs (spleen, liver). Various cytogenetic abnormalities (mainly translocations) have been reported in lymphoblastic lymphomas; some of these are of prognostic importance.

CLINICAL SCENARIO

A four-year-old girl presented with a three-month history of a rapidly enlarging lump present over the third toe of the right foot. The child was otherwise well, with no generalized symptoms. As the diagnosis was uncertain, an incisional biopsy was carried out and a wedge of tissue adherent to the extensor tendon was removed. Macroscopically, the slice of tissue appeared white and slightly gelatinous.

Histological examination showed an appearance of an infantile myofibromatosis. Four months later, the lesion was completely excised, with an ellipse of overlying skin. The histological appearance was identical to that seen in the initial biopsy. However, because the lesion was seen at the resection margin, the patient required close follow-up. Three years later, no recurrence was detected.

REFERENCES

Coffin CM. Fibroblastic-myofibroblastic tumors. In: Coffin CM, Dehner LP, O'Shea PA (eds). *Pediatric Soft Tissue Tumors*. Baltimore, MD: Williams & Wilkins, 1997; pp. 133–78.

Dehner LP. Skin and supporting adnexae. In: Dehner LP. *Paediatric Surgical Pathology*. Baltimore, MD: Williams & Wilkins, 1987; pp. 22–42.

Gray ES, Smith N. Haemopoietic system. In: Gray ES, Smith N. *Paediatric Surgical Pathology*. Edinburgh: Churchill Livingstone, 1995; pp. 113–37.

Stocker JT, Dehner LP. *Pediatric Pathology*. Philadelphia, PA: Lippincott Williams & Wilkins, 2001.

Weiss SW, Goldblum JR. Fibrous tumors of infancy and childhood. In: Weiss SW, Goldblum JR. *Soft Tissue Tumors*. St Louis, MO: Mosby, 2001; pp. 347–408.

FURTHER READING

Brunning RD, Borowitz M, Matures E, *et al*. Precursor B lymphoblastic leukaemia/lymphoblastic lymphoma. In: Jaffe ES, Harris NL, Stein H, Vardiman JW (eds). *Pathology and Genetics of Haematopoietic and Lymphoid Tissues*. Lyon: IARC Press, 2001; pp. 111–17.

Dehner LP. Some general considerations about the clinicopathologic aspects of soft tissue tumours. In: Coffin CM, Dehner LP, O'Shea PA (eds). *Pediatric Soft Tissue Tumors*. Baltimore, MD: Williams & Wilkins, 1997; pp. 1–14.

Kraus MD, Hess JL, Zutter MM. The lymph nodes, spleen and thymus. In: Stocker JT, Dehner LP (eds). *Pediatric Pathology*. Philadelphia, PA: Lippincott Williams & Wilkins, 2001; pp. 1104–11.

Stein H. Hodgkin lymphomas: introduction. In: Jaffe ES, Harris NL, Stein H, Vardiman JW (eds). *Pathology and Genetics of Haematopoietic and Lymphoid Tissues*. Lyon: IARC Press, 2001; pp. 237–53.

Part 6

Urology

48

Nephrogenesis and developmental and genetic disorders of the urogenital tract

ALEXANDER J HOWIE

Learning objectives

- To know the main features of development of the kidney and urinary tract.
- To be able to define and understand the clinical significance of renal agenesis, renal hypoplasia, renal dysplasia, renal aplasia, renal ectopia and renal fusion.
- To know the gene types important in development of the urinary tract and the most important genetic disorders associated with urinary tract abnormalities.
- To understand the genetic background, clinical features and associations of the different types of cystic disease of the kidney.

NEPHROGENESIS

On each side of the body, two embryonic tissues contribute to the human kidney, the ureteric bud and the metanephric blastema (Figure 48.1).

The ureteric bud is a tubular outgrowth from the caudal end of the mesonephric duct, also called the Wolffian duct, near its entry into the cloaca. The part of the mesonephric duct caudal to the ureteric bud becomes incorporated into the wall of the ventral part of the cloaca, the urogenital sinus, which will later become the bladder and urethra. The mesonephric duct and ureter eventually have separate openings, with the ureteric opening cranial and lateral to that of the mesonephric duct. The mesonephric duct later becomes the epididymis, vas deferens, seminal vesicle and ejaculatory duct in the male but degenerates in the female. The female genital tract develops from the paramesonephric duct, also called the Müllerian duct, which grows alongside the mesonephric duct but later degenerates in the male.

The ureteric bud grows into a mass of undifferentiated mesodermal cells, the metanephric blastema, on the posterior abdominal wall of the fetus. This is the caudal part of the nephrogenic cord, which from its cranial end had earlier developed successively into the pronephros and mesonephros, both drained by the mesonephric duct.

For development of the kidney, there is reciprocal induction between the two embryonic tissues. This means that the ureteric bud is induced to proliferate and branch by the metanephric blastema and the tip of a branch induces cells of the metanephric blastema to proliferate, aggregate and form a vesicle that elongates into an S-shaped body. One end of this is attached to the branch of the ureteric bud, and the lumen becomes continuous between the two structures. This part of the 'S' grows down towards the medulla to become the

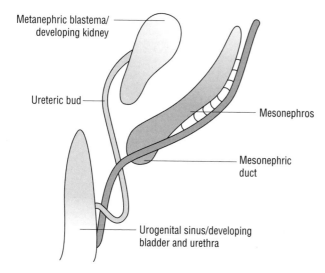

Figure 48.1 *Diagram of early renal development. The ureteric bud arose from the mesonephric duct but now has a separate opening into the urogenital sinus. The ureteric bud has grown into the metanephric blastema and the developing kidney has ascended.*

loop of Henle and the proximal tubule. The other part of the 'S' develops into the glomerulus and always retains its attachment to its own loop of Henle at the macula densa. The ureteric bud forms the collecting ducts, calyces, pelvis and ureter. Cells of the metanephric blastema that are not induced to differentiate into the S-shaped body undergo programmed cell death, known as apoptosis.

The ureteric bud arises during the fifth week of gestation. Nephrons begin to form in the eighth week and new ones are added outside these as the branches of the ureteric bud extend towards the periphery of the kidney, called the nephrogenic zone. By the thirty-sixth week, all nephrons that will be formed have appeared. The developing kidney has a lobulated surface that usually becomes smooth in the first year after birth. Occasionally, fetal lobulation persists for many years after birth.

During development, the kidney remains retroperitoneal but ascends from its initial sacral position to a level roughly between the twelfth thoracic vertebra and the third lumbar vertebra, reaching this point by the eighth week of gestation. The arterial supply is taken from increasingly higher levels of the aorta as the kidney ascends. The hilum, where the pelvi-ureteric system emerges from the kidney, initially is anterior but rotates during development to a more medial position.

DEVELOPMENTAL DISORDERS OF THE KIDNEY

Introduction

The development of the urinary tract is complex. Consequently, developmental disorders are common and are present in about one in ten neonates. Many of these abnormalities are of little significance; however, urinary tract malformation is still the most common cause of chronic renal failure in young children. Renal malformation is nearly always associated with disorders elsewhere in the urinary tract.

Surgery is rarely necessary in developmental disorders of the kidney, unless complications such as reflux nephropathy or hydronephrosis have arisen, but developmental disorders may be found by chance during investigation of other problems, such as congenital abnormalities, particularly of the lower urinary tract and genital tract.

Renal agenesis, hypoplasia, dysplasia and aplasia

Agenesis, complete failure of development of a kidney, is due to failure of development of the ureteric bud, and so the ureter as well as the kidney is missing. There is often maldevelopment of other structures, particularly in the genital tract.

Unilateral agenesis is more common than bilateral agenesis. It is seen in about one in 1000 births, is equally common in males and females, and usually is asymptomatic and found only on investigation of other congenital abnormalities that are frequently associated with unilateral agenesis. Males often have disorders such as maldescent of the testis or absence of the vas deferens on the same side as the absent kidney; females often have a unicornuate or bicornuate uterus. The surviving kidney has compensatory enlargement, unless there are other abnormalities of the urinary tract, particularly vesicoureteric reflux.

Bilateral agenesis is seen in about one in 7000 births. It is more common in boys than girls. The condition is lethal and causes stillbirth or early postnatal death. There are usually widespread developmental disorders, particularly of the lower urinary tract and genital tract, such as hypoplastic or atretic bladder and bilateral absence of epididymis, vas deferens and seminal vesicle.

There is no urine production by the fetus if there is a severe disorder of renal development such as bilateral agenesis, and so there is only a small volume of amniotic fluid (oligohydramnios). The lungs fail to develop normally. This is because amniotic fluid normally enters the fetal lungs and is necessary for their development. Oligohydramnios also allows compression of the fetus and produces deformities of the face, called Potter facies, after Edith L Potter, who described the features. These features include flattened nose, wide-set eyes, low-set ears and receding chin. There are also deformities of limbs and growth retardation.

Renal hypoplasia is the condition in which there is a small kidney not due to an acquired disease such as reflux nephropathy and without evidence of renal dysplasia. Although small, the kidney is otherwise normally differentiated. When the strict definition is used, renal hypoplasia is rare, usually bilateral and not usually associated with other disorders of the urinary tract, but it may be associated with enlargement of glomeruli and tubules if there are fewer of these than normal, in which case the term 'oligomeganephronia' is used.

In renal dysplasia, there is abnormal differentiation of the metanephric blastema, usually due to a disorder of the ureteric

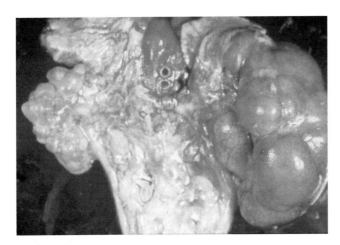

Figure 48.2   *Renal dysplasia. The right kidney shows complete multicystic dysplasia. The left kidney is not affected so severely, but the upper pole in particular is malformed by dysplasia.*

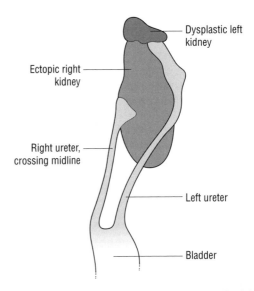

Figure 48.3   *Diagram of crossed fused ectopic kidney. Both kidneys are on the same side of the body and are fused, but the ureters enter the bladder on different sides. The left/upper kidney is dysplastic.*

bud. This developmental meaning of the word 'dysplasia' contrasts with its frequent use in pathology to mean a preneoplastic disorder of tissues. Renal dysplasia can be unilateral or bilateral, may affect part or all of a kidney, may be associated with formation of renal cysts (fluid-filled cavities), can produce a large, small or normal-sized kidney, and may give a distorted renal shape (Figure 48.2). Renal dysplasia is nearly always associated with other abnormalities of the urinary tract in the ureter, bladder or urethra.

In affected parts of the kidney, the medulla is abnormally shaped and contains only a few primitive ducts lined by columnar cells, sometimes ciliated, and surrounded by rings of connective tissue, including smooth-muscle cells. The overlying cortex is also abnormal and contains immature glomeruli and tubules, sometimes with nodules of cartilage.

Renal dysplasia is usually a consequence of either obstruction of the developing ureteric bud and its branches or vesicoureteric reflux into these structures. The abnormal development of the ureteric bud leads to failure of normal induction and development of structures derived from the metanephric blastema. Examples of conditions often associated with renal dysplasia are duplex ureters, in which at least one of the double ureters has an ectopic insertion into the bladder (invariably the upper moiety ureter) and may be obstructed or have vesicoureteric reflux (invariably the lower moiety ureter), and posterior urethral valves, in which vesicoureteric reflux is common (either uni- or bilateral). There is also a likelihood that a few examples of renal dysplasia are due to disorders primarily of the metanephric blastema rather than of the ureteric bud.

Renal dysplasia of any extent is common; it is seen in about one in 50 autopsies in children. The severest form, bilateral dysplasia with or without cysts, is seen in about one in 7000 births. Like bilateral renal agenesis, this produces external abnormalities in the fetus, such as the Potter facies. Areas of renal dysplasia are commonly seen in kidneys removed from children with reflux nephropathy.

Renal aplasia means an extremely small kidney with a ureter, unlike renal agenesis, in which there is no ureter. This is a severe form of renal dysplasia rather than of renal hypoplasia.

Renal ectopia and fusion

Ectopia is a condition in which the kidney is permanently positioned away from its normal site. This can be either simple, in which the kidney and ureter are on the same side of the body as the insertion of the ureter into the bladder, or crossed, in which the ureter crosses the midline and the kidney is on the opposite side of the body to the insertion of the ureter into the bladder. Fusion is a condition in which there is junction of two kidneys whose ureters are inserted on different sides of the bladder (Figure 48.3).

Renal fusion is not the same as renal duplication, in which there is duplication of the ureter and renal pelvis to different extents, and in which there may be a single but duplex kidney, or even two separate kidneys on one side of the body. In duplication, if there are two ureters, then these are inserted on the same side of the bladder, although at least one of the ureters has an ectopic site of insertion. Duplication to any extent is common and affects about one in 20 people, but it is of little clinical significance in most of these.

Simple ectopic kidneys are usually in the pelvis, have malrotation with the hilum anteriorly, may not have the typical kidney shape, and have an anomalous blood supply. These are found in about one in 1000 births and are often associated with skeletal abnormalities. A crossed ectopic kidney almost always has fusion to the other kidney. This is found in about one in 8000 births. There is often renal dysplasia in both simple and crossed ectopic kidneys.

The most common type of renal fusion is the horseshoe kidney, in which the lower poles are fused across the midline. Horseshoe kidneys almost always are ectopic, are in the pelvis, and have malrotation, with the hilum anteriorly on both sides. These patients often have hydronephrosis. Horseshoe kidney is found in about one in 200 children at autopsy, but this is because there are often associated abnormalities, and the prevalence is much less in the rest of the population.

GENETICS OF URINARY TRACT ABNORMALITIES

Introduction

Many genes have roles in the normal development of the urinary tract, in functions such as signalling, proliferation, apoptosis, cell survival by protection against apoptosis, differentiation and morphogenesis (the formation of three-dimensional structures). The main groups comprise genes for transcription factors, growth factors and adhesion molecules.

TRANSCRIPTION FACTOR GENES

Transcription factors are proteins that bind to deoxyribonucleic acid (DNA) and control the expression of other genes, causing either enhanced expression or suppression. An important transcription factor gene in early renal development is Wilms tumour suppressor gene, *WT1*. This is expressed in cells of the metanephric blastema especially after induction by the ureteric bud. *WT1* is mutated and ineffective in a few examples of sporadic nephroblastoma (Wilms tumour) and in all nephroblastomas in Denys–Drash syndrome, in which there is a glomerular disorder and abnormal development of the gonads. Nephroblastomas are neoplasms of the metanephric blastema with only rudimentary differentiation into nephrons.

A transcription factor gene that *WT1* controls is *Pax2*. Induced metanephric blastema and tips of branches of the ureteric bud express *Pax2*, and this probably prevents apoptosis. There is then downregulation by *WT1*, so that expression of *Pax2* declines in the S-shaped body, allowing tubular formation to occur by apoptosis.

GROWTH FACTOR GENES AND GROWTH FACTOR RECEPTOR GENES

Growth factors are proteins that bind to receptors on the cell surface and lead to events such as proliferation. Many growth factors and their receptors are important in the development of the metanephric blastema and ureteric bud and in the interactions between them.

A gene controlled by *WT1* is insulin-like growth factor 2, *IGF-2*. *IGF-2* promotes proliferation and is expressed in the uninduced metanephric blastema, but it is downregulated when *WT1* is expressed strongly. Lack of suppression of this growth factor may be one explanation for transformation of the metanephric blastema into nephroblastoma.

Several growth factors are produced by cells of the induced metanephric blastema and act on receptors on the tips of the ureteric bud to stimulate branching. These include hepatocyte growth factor (HGF), whose receptor is the tyrosine kinase Met, encoded by the gene *c-met*, and glial cell-derived neurotropic factor (GDNF), whose receptor is the tyrosine kinase Ret, encoded by the gene *c-ret*.

ADHESION MOLECULES AND CONNECTIVE TISSUE PROTEINS

Adhesion molecules are proteins that allow cells to adhere either to each other or to matrix. Neural cell-adhesion molecule (NCAM) is expressed on uninduced cells of the metanephric blastema and is replaced by E-cadherin as epithelial structures of the nephron develop. Intracellular intermediate filaments also change from vimentin to cytokeratins during this process.

Several structural proteins appear in the connective tissue matrix around cells of the developing nephron, including collagen type 4, fibronectin, laminins and proteoglycans. These contribute to the formation of basement membranes. Enzymes that degrade connective tissue components are also necessary for the normal development of the kidney. These include matrix metalloproteinases and plasminogen activators.

Integrins are transmembrane proteins that bind to ligands on cells or matrix components, such as laminins and collagen type 4. The intracytoplasmic parts of integrins interact with cytoskeletal proteins and can also act as signal transducers similar to the functions of intracytoplasmic parts of growth factor receptors. Different integrins are expressed at various stages in the developing kidney and have an important role in nephrogenesis.

Important syndromes

The genetic bases of most urinary tract abnormalities are not known. It is likely that more than one genetic disorder can produce apparently identical structural changes. Conversely, a single genetic disorder can result in more than one malformation, and several different developmental abnormalities of the kidney may be found in the same family. For example, unilateral renal agenesis, bilateral renal agenesis, and unilateral renal agenesis with dysplasia of the solitary kidney (sometimes called renal adysplasia) may be found in different members of the same family, when the condition is known as 'hereditary renal adysplasia'.

Not all renal malformations are due to genetic disorders. Teratogens, including vitamin A, glucose, angiotensin-converting enzyme inhibitors, ethanol and thalidomide, can affect renal development. Development can also be abnormal due to mechanical disorders of urinary drainage, namely reflux and obstruction, although sometimes these disorders may themselves be genetic, e.g. vesicoureteric reflux is frequently familial, with autosomal dominant inheritance.

Renal malformation is common in syndromes with malformation of multiple organs, although these syndromes are rare and the genetic abnormality is known in only a few of these. The most common finding is renal dysplasia, often with cysts. Many such syndromes have been described, and some of the better understood disorders are mentioned here.

There is a disorder due to heterozygous mutations of Pax2, a transcription factor important in nephrogenesis. In renal-coloboma syndrome, there is vesicoureteric reflux with renal maldevelopment, associated with blindness.

The gene *KAL* is on the X chromosome and encodes an adhesion protein. Male hemizygotes with *KAL* mutations develop Kallmann syndrome, in which there is anosmia, hypogonadism due to lack of gonadotrophins, and unilateral renal agenesis.

Abnormalities, including renal agenesis, renal dysplasia and vesicoureteric reflux, are common in branchio-oto-renal syndrome, an autosomal dominant disorder associated with deafness, cysts of the neck and pre-auricular pits. This is due to mutations of the gene *EYA1*, probably important in protection of cells against apoptosis.

There is an abnormality of the receptor for fibroblast growth factor 2 (FGF-2) in Apert syndrome, an autosomal dominant disorder with cranial disorders, syndactyly and renal cystic dysplasia.

In Zellweger syndrome, an autosomal recessive disorder of a peroxisomal protein, there are cranial and other skeletal abnormalities, nervous system malformation, hepatic fibrosis and cystic dysplastic kidneys.

In asphyxiating thoracic dystrophy of Jeune, which is autosomal recessive, there are skeletal deformities caused by chondrodystrophy, with renal dysplasia or other renal abnormalities.

In Beckwith–Wiedemann syndrome, often a sporadic disorder, there are enlarged organs, including macroglossia and large kidneys, hemi-hypertrophy and umbilical hernia. Various other renal abnormalities are found, such as medullary sponge kidney and nephroblastoma.

RENAL CYSTIC DISEASES

Cysts are common in the kidney. There are many causes, but the mechanism of formation of cysts is almost always proliferation of the lining cells with secretion of fluid into the lumen, often because the sodium pump, sodium-potassium-adenosine triphosphatase, is on the apical surface of the cells lining the cysts, rather than on the basolateral surface as in normal cells. Another postulated mechanism is obstruction of tubules, but this would cause stretching, thinning and disruption of lining cells, and this is hardly ever seen. The pressure in most cysts is not higher than the pressure in normal tubules.

Surgery is rarely required in cystic disorders in children.

Autosomal dominant polycystic kidney disease

Autosomal dominant polycystic kidney disease (ADPKD) is the most important cystic disorder of the kidney, because it is a common cause of chronic renal failure, although this is in adults, not children. It affects about one in 1000 people, but it is the cause of renal failure in up to one in ten people on renal replacement therapy, depending on the age group studied. Almost always, when the term 'polycystic kidney' is used without qualification, then ADPKD is meant.

There are two recognized genetic forms, with other as yet unrecognized forms. The most common form, seen in 85 per cent of cases, is ADPKD1. The genetic locus is on chromosome 16 and codes for a protein called polycystin-1. This is a transmembrane protein on primary cilia and regulates intracellular calcium levels. The other recognized form is ADPKD2, whose genetic locus is on chromosome 4.

Usually, the kidneys are apparently normal at birth and in childhood, but there is progressive development of cysts and enlargement of the kidneys with age. The kidneys are symmetrical, with marked distortion by cysts of various sizes in all parts of the kidney, including the glomeruli. Both the cortex and the medulla are affected (Figure 48.4). The ureters are normal. Nephrectomy may be necessary in adults if the kidneys are so large that other organs are compressed.

Several other abnormalities may be associated with the renal disorder, particularly in adults. These include cysts in the liver and pancreas, berry aneurysms on cerebral arteries, diverticular disease of the colon and mitral valve prolapse.

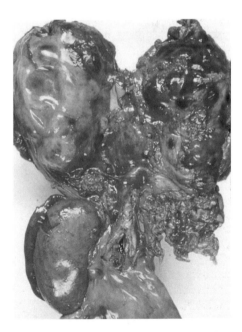

Figure 48.4 *Autosomal dominant polycystic kidney disease. Both kidneys are large and replaced by cysts. There has been a renal transplant.*

Autosomal recessive polycystic kidney disease

Autosomal recessive polycystic kidney disease (ARPKD) is at least ten times less common than ADPKD. The main association is with congenital hepatic fibrosis, a progressive fibrosing disorder of portal tracts associated with malformation of intrahepatic bile ducts. The severity of the renal disease is roughly inverse to that of the liver disease. Severe renal disease usually causes stillbirth or death in infancy, while mild renal disease is associated with presentation in late childhood or adult life, with portal hypertension as a complication of the fibrosis of portal tracts. Stillborn children have the same external features, including the Potter facies, as those with bilateral renal agenesis and other severe disorders of renal development. Siblings with ARPKD do not necessarily have the same severity of the renal abnormalities or present at the same age with the same features.

The relevant gene is on chromosome 6 and codes for a protein called polyductin (or fibrocystin), which is inserted in the cell membrane.

In the severe form, the kidneys are enlarged and symmetrical but, unlike the kidneys in ADPKD, they retain their kidney shape and do not have gross cysts. There are uniformly dilated collecting ducts that appear as tubular structures running radially through the cortex (Figure 48.5). The ureters are normal. Surgery on the kidney is hardly ever necessary in ARPKD.

Juvenile nephronophthisis and medullary cystic disease

These conditions are so similar that they are regarded as aspects of the same disease complex, sometimes called uraemic medullary cystic disease. Both disorders can be produced by more than one genetic abnormality. The kidneys are symmetrical and small and have a variable number of

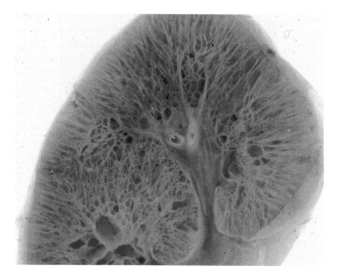

Figure 48.5 *Autosomal recessive polycystic kidney disease. There are dilated collecting ducts that appear as radially dilated tubular structures rather than as cysts.*

small cysts at the corticomedullary junction derived from collecting ducts. The cortex has chronic damage, which is progressive. This group of conditions is one of the most common causes of chronic renal failure in childhood, accounting for about one in six children with chronic renal failure. Males and females are affected equally.

There are autosomal recessive forms (usually in children; called juvenile nephronophthisis), autosomal dominant forms (usually in adults; called medullary cystic kidney disease) and apparently sporadic forms in children without a family history of renal disease. The most common autosomal recessive form is a disorder of the protein nephrocystin. One autosomal dominant form is a disorder of uromodulin (Tamm Horsfall protein).

Medullary sponge kidney

This differs from the juvenile nephronophthisis/medullary cystic disease complex in several ways. The cysts are dilated collecting ducts in medullary papillae rather than at the corticomedullary junction. There is usually no development of chronic damage in the renal cortex, and the disease is usually asymptomatic, unless there are obstructive or infective complications of the stones that frequently form in the dilated ducts.

Medullary sponge kidney affects about one in 5000 people. It is mostly sporadic, but there are associations with Beckwith–Wiedemann syndrome and congenital hemihypertrophy. Surgery may be required for treatment of stones or their complications.

Multicystic renal dysplasia

Dysplastic kidneys occasionally have multiple cysts (Figure 48.2), sometimes with marked enlargement. The cysts can change with time and may disappear, even in the fetus. The ureter is present but has atresia, meaning that the lumen is obliterated for a variable length. The pelvicalyceal system is usually missing. Multicystic renal dysplasia is more often unilateral than bilateral; if unilateral, it is often associated with abnormalities of the contralateral ureter, such as stenosis or duplication. Unilateral multicystic renal dysplasia is found in about one in 5000 births.

Diffuse cystic dysplasia has similarities to multicystic renal dysplasia but is always bilateral, usually has many small cysts, is accompanied by patent ureters without urinary tract obstruction, and is part of inherited syndromes with multiple abnormalities. The most common of these is Meckel syndrome, an autosomal recessive condition with polydactyly, microcephaly, biliary dysgenesis and many other disorders.

Other types of renal cysts

Cystic dilation of the Bowman's capsule of the glomeruli may be called glomerulocystic disease if there is no other abnormality. This is not a single condition. Most children with this have ADPKD. Others have a wide range of recognized and unrecognized genetic or sporadic disorders.

Multiple renal cysts occur in tuberous sclerosis in association with multiple angiomyolipomas of the kidney, often in childhood, and in von Hippel–Lindau syndrome in association with multiple renal cell carcinomas, although the cysts and carcinomas usually are not detected until adult life.

Multiple cysts usually develop in the kidneys of people, including children, on any type of dialysis for a few years, irrespective of the cause of the renal failure. This acquired renal cystic disease may be associated with development of renal cell carcinomas. Nephrectomy may be necessary if there is bleeding from cysts or if a carcinoma is suspected or known to have developed.

Multilocular cysts are rare cystic neoplasms of the kidney. They are usually benign, although a few may contain areas of malignant nephroblastomatous tissue. Nephroblastomas, or Wilms tumours, may themselves be cystic.

Diverticula of the pelvicalyceal system are probably congenital and may be due to either maldevelopment of branches of the ureteric bud or acquired obstruction or reflux after the pelvis has formed. These can appear as pelvicalyceal or pyelocalyceal cysts, are usually single, and are often found by chance. However, they may be symptomatic if complicated by development of infection or stones.

Non-neoplastic cysts in the kidney, usually called simple cysts, are common in adults but rare in children.

FURTHER READING

Bernstein J, Gilbert-Barness E. Congenital malformations of the kidney. In: Tisher CC, Brenner BM (eds). *Renal Pathology with Clinical and Functional Correlations*, 2nd edn. Philadelphia, PA: JB Lippincott, 1994; pp. 1355–86.

Risdon RA, Woolf AS. Development of the kidney. In: Jennette CJ, Olson JL, Schwartz MM, Silva FG (eds). *Heptinstall's Pathology of the Kidney*, 5th edn. Philadelphia, PA: Lippincott-Raven, 1998; pp. 67–84.

Welling LW, Grantham JJ. Cystic diseases of the kidney. In: Tisher CC, Brenner BM (eds). *Renal Pathology with Clinical and Functional Correlations*, 2nd edn. Philadelphia, PA: JB Lippincott, 1994; pp. 1312–54.

49

Radiological imaging of the urinary tract

JOANNA FAIRHURST AND VALERIE LEWINGTON

Learning objectives

- To understand the indications for, and limitations of, available imaging techniques.
- To identify the normal developmental changes in imaging characteristics of the urinary tract.
- To recognize the imaging features of common disorders of the urinary system.
- To be able to assess the most appropriate diagnostic pathway for a given clinical problem relating to the urinary tract.

IMAGING TECHNIQUES

Ultrasound

Imaging has a pivotal role in the diagnosis and management of the majority of conditions affecting the paediatric urinary tract. Of the various imaging techniques available, ultrasound is ideally suited to delineating the child's kidneys and bladder, and this examination has become the initial imaging method of choice. Recent technical advances, such as improved power Doppler imaging, harmonic and compound imaging, and the introduction of ultrasound contrast agents, have expanded the potential of ultrasound in this area.

Renal-tract ultrasound should always start with examination of the bladder. In babies, the sensation of gel (even if warmed) combined with the pressure of the transducer frequently induces voiding, and hence the best chance to evaluate a distended bladder is when scanning starts. Bladder shape and wall thickness are assessed, together with any intravesical lesions. The ureters may be visible behind the bladder and should be assessed for diameter and peristalsis. Ureteric jets may be seen with greyscale imaging but often are better appreciated with colour Doppler, useful in assessing obstruction and, occasionally, in documenting reflux. The distended bladder

may also be used as an acoustic 'window' through which to review pelvic structures. In newborn girls, the uterus and ovaries are frequently seen well, owing to stimulation by maternal hormones. Next, the kidneys should be scanned in the supine position: the upper poles are sometimes seen better with the patient supine, and the course of any dilated ureters can be followed more easily than when the patient is prone. Overall, however, the kidneys are best seen with the child lying prone, as the intervening subcutaneous tissues and muscles interfere far less with image quality than in the adult. Here it is important to document renal position, size, outline, overall parenchymal echogenicity and architecture, as well as the presence of any duplication, calculi or focal lesion. The degree of any hydronephrosis should be assessed by measuring the anteroposterior diameter of the renal pelvis and of any dilated calyces. These measurements are more reproducible and accurate if obtained in the prone position, and this allows progress to be determined on sequential scans. Cortical thickness may also be measured if this appears reduced.

Some centres advocate the use of ultrasound contrast agents in the investigation of vesicoureteric reflux. This technique involves catheterizing the patient and injecting an agent that induces microbubbles in saline. These bubbles are visible in the bladder as it is filled and can be identified in the pelvicalyceal systems if reflux occurs. Both kidneys are scanned during bladder filling and also during voiding. Whilst this examination has the advantage of avoiding exposure to radiation, it remains less sensitive than conventional micturating cystogram in detecting reflux, and it is time-consuming.

The normal neonatal kidney differs in sonographic appearance from that in the older child and adult. Overall cortical echogenicity is increased, such that the cortex is equally or more echogenic compared with the adjacent liver. This means that the echo-poor pyramids are accentuated and can be mistaken for dilated calyces by staff unfamiliar with this appearance. The renal outline is lobulated, and again this can be misinterpreted as scarring. Renal sinus fat, which gives an echogenic central kidney in the older child, is sparse in the neonate, and hence the kidney appears rather featureless. It is important to remember that in the first 48 hours after birth, the infant is relatively dehydrated and has a low glomerular filtration rate (GFR). This may mask any obstruction, as the collecting systems may not appear dilated. If obstruction has been suspected on antenatal ultrasound, then postnatal scanning should be repeated after a week if initially normal.

In the older child, renal ultrasound reveals a smooth outline and a well-defined corticomedullary junction, with relatively hypoechoic pyramids, an echogenic sinus and hilum, and variably bright arcuate arteries.

High-frequency linear probes can be used to examine the testes. Harmonic and compound imaging is of particular use in this field, providing exquisite detail of testicular echotexture and allowing the detection of subtle intratesticular lesions. The main indications for testicular scanning in boys include the assessment of scrotal masses, the detection of undescended or ectopic testes and the evaluation of the painful testis. Technical improvements in colour Doppler imaging, particularly its sensitivity, have increased the specificity of ultrasound for the detection of testicular torsion. However, this must be interpreted with caution, because apparently normal vascularity does not exclude ischaemia, while lack of detection of flow in the neonatal or infant testis does not necessarily indicate testicular torsion. Increased flow, however, is a good indicator of inflammation, and the diagnosis of epididymo-orchitis can be made more reliably.

Micturating cystourethrography

Micturating cystourethrography (MCUG) remains the method of choice for imaging the urethra and for evaluating vesicoureteric reflux (VUR) at initial presentation. As this is a relatively invasive procedure, other techniques such as indirect isotope cystography (see later) are advocated in the follow-up of reflux, but the greater degree of anatomic detail provided by MCUG is required for primary assessment. Preparation for MCUG includes prophylactic antibiotics, particularly in children being investigated for urinary tract infection (UTI). A catheter (usually a 6F or 8F feeding tube) is inserted into the bladder, and water-soluble contrast agent containing iodine at a concentration of 100 mg/mL is instilled

either by slow hand-injection or by gravity-filling from a bottle suspended above the X-ray table. Bladder shape and wall characteristics are assessed by intermittent screening during filling. Voiding images are obtained ideally in the lateral/oblique projection, with views of the vesicoureteric junctions and images of the entire urethra in boys. Post-void cross-kidney view is also crucial to detect subtle intermittent reflux extending to the pelvicalyceal systems.

As the gonads are included in the field of view during MCUG, it is important that dose-minimizing techniques are employed for the procedure. Modern fluoroscopic equipment utilizes a pulsed system, in which intermittent bursts of radiation are used to build up an image, rather than a continuous stream of X-rays. This significantly reduces the overall patient dose, as does the use of special filters added to the X-ray tube, which absorb parts of the X-ray spectrum that do not contribute to the image but do add to the overall dose acquired by the patient. Other crucial dose-reducing methods include accurate collimation to expose only the area of interest, intermittent rather than continuous screening, and the use of frame-grabbed (low-dose) images, in which a certain amount of detail is sacrificed but an image of diagnostic quality is still produced. If these procedures are followed, then it is possible to achieve a diagnostic examination of high quality at approximately half the total effective dose absorbed during radio-isotope cystography.

Intravenous urography

Once a very common diagnostic technique in urinary tract imaging, the intravenous urogram (IVU) has largely been supplanted by ultrasound for many indications. IVU is now reserved primarily for stone disease and for delineation of complicated duplex systems or other congenital anomalies (Figure 49.1). A control film covering the kidneys, ureters and bladder should be obtained before injection of intravenous contrast if stones are suspected. Non-ionic low-osmolar contrast agents are used routinely nowadays; these are pharmaceuticals that contain iodine, a dense element visible on X-ray, at a concentration of between 120 and 370 mg/mL, and an osmolality ranging between 290 and 700 mosmol/kg. They are considerably safer than the previously used high-osmolality agents and have fewer reported side effects. Contrast reactions, however, do still occur; these include minor effects such as flushing, which is seen in up to ten per cent of patients, and major reactions such as laryngeal oedema, bronchospasm and circulatory collapse, which occur in approximately one in 20 000 patients. The sequence of post-injection films is tailored to the problem being investigated. Although bowel clearance and starvation are no longer advocated in preparation for an IVU, delineation of the kidneys is often improved if the child has a fizzy drink immediately after injection; this distends the stomach with air and displaces overlying bowel, allowing a clear view of the renal area. Images are obtained in both the supine and the prone positions, with the renal pelves and ureters best seen when prone. Tomography is rarely necessary.

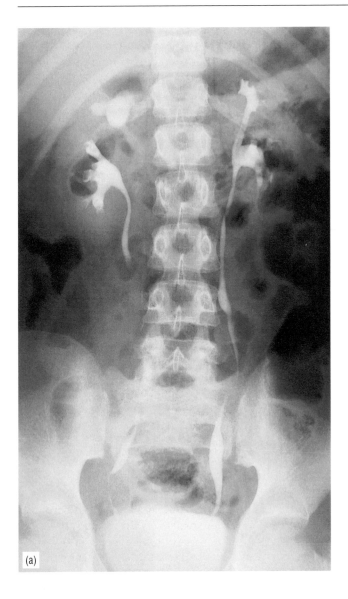

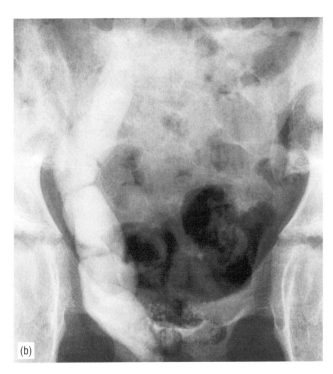

(a)

(b)

Figure 49.1 *(a) Intravenous urogram, showing a right duplex kidney with poorly functioning distorted upper moiety. (b) Retrograde ureterogram, showing the ectopic dilated upper moiety ureter, which inserts into the vagina.*

Computed tomography

The main indications for computed tomography (CT) in the investigation of urinary tract disease are trauma, renal or bladder masses and, recently, in urolithiasis. Choice of parameters for scanning in trauma or tumour is dependent on the size of the patient, but in general pre-contrast images are not required, and images after intravenous contrast injection can be acquired with a pitch of 1.5 and a slice thickness of 5–7 mm. In trauma, it is crucial to document perfusion of both kidneys as well as to assess injury to perirenal structures and other organs. For tumours, the contralateral kidney must be reviewed carefully for evidence of tumour involvement. Although inferior vena cava thrombus may be visualized, this is often better assessed with ultrasound.

The use of CT in urolithiasis is well established in adults, but it has had more limited use in children, both because of the radiation burden associated with CT and because renal, bladder and ureteric stones are identified more reliably with ultrasound in children than in adults. Ultrasound should remain the first investigation is suspected stone disease, but non-contrast CT should now be considered alongside IVU as the next step. Diagnostic accuracy using conventional CT parameters in spiral or multislice scanning is at least equal to IVU, but the radiation burden is greater. It is yet to be determined whether low-dose scanning techniques will be sufficiently discriminatory to replace the IVU in routine practice.

Magnetic resonance imaging

Magnetic resonance imaging (MRI) is now firmly established as a primary imaging modality in renal tumours. It allows assessment of the relationship of the tumour to adjacent structures, vascular involvement, lymphadenopathy and the presence of additional renal tumours, both ipsi- and contralateral (Figure 49.2). In this latter respect, however, ultrasound is complementary, as small peripheral tumours may be seen better with ultrasound than with MRI. MRI has the added benefit of multiplanar presentation, which can act as a roadmap for surgical procedure. The assessment of pulmonary metastases is not currently possible with MRI, and chest CT remains a necessary component of tumour staging.

The technique of magnetic resonance urography allows delineation of the pelvicalyceal systems and ureters without the need for contrast injection. This has been shown to be of particular use in complex duplex systems, especially in demonstrating a poorly functioning upper moiety and in showing the site of ectopic ureteric insertion. Improvements in scanning capabilities already allow accurate functional information to be obtained from dynamic gadolinium-enhanced studies, and current research is directed towards reducing scanning time and improving image resolution. Eventually, this may allow MRI to replace isotope renography and IVU, although currently both financial considerations and the need for sedation in younger patients make this of limited practical application.

Genitography

In suspected intersex or ambiguous genitalia, or where there is a common perineal opening, water-soluble contrast agents can be injected under fluoroscopic control to delineate the anatomy. A catheter initially is introduced into the urethra or urogenital sinus and advanced into the bladder. Contrast may reflux into the vagina, or a second catheter may need to be manipulated behind the first to enter the vagina. This examination can be used to document the presence of a vagina and cervical impression, to evaluate the length of the urogenital sinus and to demonstrate accurately the complex anatomy of a cloacal malformation (Figure 49.3).

Interventional uroradiology

The most commonly performed interventional uroradiological procedure is renal biopsy. Ultrasound guidance depicts

the kidney position, the distance from the skin surface and the required site and angle of entry of the biopsy needle. Scanning during the procedure allows visualization of the biopsy needle and afterwards can assess complications such as haematoma or urine leakage. Similar information is required during percutaneous nephrostomy placement, and this is often achieved by a combination of ultrasound and fluoroscopic guidance. CT guidance is particularly useful for nephrostomy insertion in patients where access is difficult. A variety of drainage systems are available, and the interventional technique must be tailored to the size of patient and his or her individual pathology. Indications for percutaneous nephrostomy include drainage of obstructed systems where endoscopic drainage procedures are not possible, particularly in infected systems. Antegrade insertion of ureteric stents and balloon dilation of strictures are well-accepted radiological procedures. Balloon dilation of pelviureteric junction obstruction is still under scrutiny, and its efficacy is not proven. All of these techniques require either local anaesthesia and sedation, or general anaesthetic.

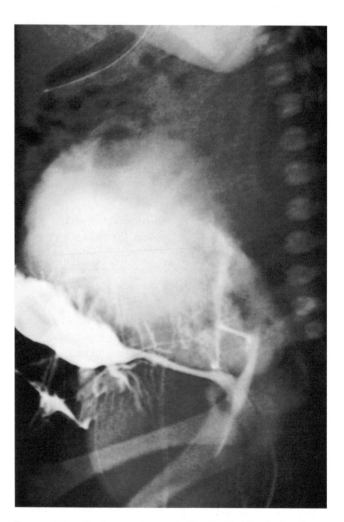

Figure 49.3 *Genitogram demonstrating the bladder displaced anteriorly by a grossly distended uterus, which fills via two fistulae, from the elongated urethra and from the cloaca.*

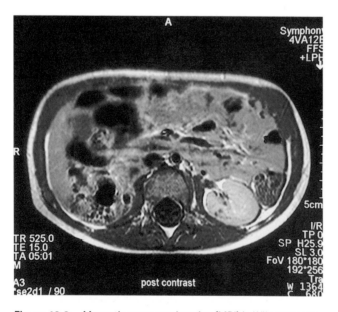

Figure 49.2 *Magnetic resonance imaging (MRI) in Wilms tumour. T1-weighted axial MRI post-gadolinium enhancement, showing several low-signal foci in the left kidney. There has been a right nephrectomy. Biopsy confirmed nephroblastomatosis.*

Percutaneous abscess or urinoma drainage is technically similar to nephrostomy placement and can be undertaken under ultrasound or CT control. Arterial embolization of bleeding renal vessels, tumours and arteriovenous malformations using coils, balloons or gelfoam is a specialized interventional technique available in some centres.

Nuclear medicine imaging

In contrast to the structural approach described above, nuclear medicine imaging demonstrates renal function and the physiological changes that occur in response to renal pathology. Isotope imaging relies upon the selection of a tracer molecule that targets the organ of interest. This is labelled using a gamma-emitting radionuclide, which allows the kinetics and biodistribution of the tracer molecule to be mapped *in vivo* using a gamma camera. Apart from initial venepuncture, radionuclide imaging is non-invasive and delivers a low whole-body radiation absorbed dose. The application of anaesthetic cream is advised routinely in paediatric practice, while distraction techniques reduce the likelihood of movement artefacts.

As function usually changes before structure in response to disease processes, radionuclide techniques are sensitive for the detection of early pathology. The major disadvantage is limited anatomical resolution. Radionuclide scintigraphy is therefore complementary to, but does not duplicate the information gained from, anatomical imaging. Radionuclide renal scintigraphy (renography) falls into two main categories:

- Static imaging examines renal morphology using radio-labelled dimercaptosuccinic acid (^{99m}Tc-DMSA), which is specifically absorbed by the proximal renal tubules, accumulating in the renal cortex.
- Dynamic renography demonstrates renal drainage using pharmaceuticals that are excreted by glomerular filtration and/or tubular secretion. Historically, agents such as ^{131}I-hippuran and ^{99m}Tc-diethylenetriamine-pentacetic acid (DTPA) were used, but these have been largely replaced in paediatric practice by technetium-labelled trimercaptotriglycine (^{99m}Tc-MAG$_3$).

Visual interpretation of both static and dynamic renograms is enhanced by digital data processing, which allows the function of each kidney to be quantified.

STATIC RENAL CORTICAL SCINTIGRAPHY: DMSA IMAGING

^{99m}Tc-DMSA imaging is regarded as the reference method for detecting renal parenchymal damage. The main indications are the investigation of UTI, to detect acute pyelonephritis or permanent scarring and to identify children who are at risk of long-term complications. The high specificity of renal tubular uptake allows imaging even in severe renal insufficiency. Other indications include accurate measurement of relative renal function, investigation of abnormal renal morphology such as agenesis and renal ectopia/fusion, evaluation of multicystic/dysplastic disease, assessment of renal viability

following trauma and investigation of renovascular disease. ^{99m}Tc-DMSA imaging is sometimes performed before biopsy to select the appropriate kidney for histological examination and to confirm the presence of contralateral functioning renal tissue. No specific preparation is required, although the child should be well hydrated. ^{99m}Tc-DMSA is injected intravenously, followed by gamma camera imaging two to four hours later. Anterior, posterior and posterior oblique images are usually acquired. Anterior pelvic images are advisable where renal ectopia is suspected or following renal transplantation. Tomographic imaging is feasible in cooperative older children but requires long imaging times. In practice, the potential advantages of improved anatomical resolution are often cancelled out by movement distortion.

Patterns of uptake on ^{99m}Tc-DMSA imaging of normal kidneys are well defined, with smooth outlines and generally homogeneous cortical uptake, except over the renal pelvis. An example of a normal ^{99m}Tc-DMSA study is shown in Figure 49.4. The cortex is usually distinguishable from the renal medulla, and sometimes prominent columns of Bertin are discernible as linear areas of relatively increased activity radiating from the cortex into the medulla. The spleen commonly produces a linear impression in the superolateral aspect of the left upper pole. Fetal lobulation may result in cortical indentation, but, in contrast to renal scarring, the cortical thickness is well preserved. Computer analysis assesses relative renal function, i.e. the contribution of each kidney to overall GFR as a percentage of injected activity.

The normal range for each kidney is 50 ± 5 per cent. Examples are given of a duplex kidney with obstructed upper moiety (Figure 49.5) and a horseshoe kidney (Figure 49.6).

DYNAMIC RENOGRAPHY: ^{99m}TC-DTPA OR ^{99m}TC-MAG$_3$ RENOGRAPHY

The main indication for dynamic renography is the assessment of renal drainage and, particularly, discrimination between renal dilation and outflow obstruction. It is of considerable value in assessing undiagnosed renal pain and in post-pyeloplasty surveillance. The agent of choice is ^{99m}Tc-MAG$_3$, which is excreted by tubular secretion. The high extraction efficiency results in optimal image quality, even in neonates and children with impaired renal function. Patients should be well hydrated and should void immediately before commencing the study. Imaging can be undertaken with the patient lying supine or seated erect immediately in front of the gamma camera. The tracer is administered as a rapid intravenous bolus followed by a saline flush. Imaging commences immediately, and data are acquired dynamically for 20–30 minutes. Dilation and outflow obstruction are distinguished by recording the response to an intravenous diuretic challenge (furosemide (frusemide) 0.5 mg/kg to a maximum of 20 mg). The timing of diuretic administration varies between protocols, but it is essential that administration is standardized within an individual imaging department to ensure that consecutive studies in the same patient are comparable.

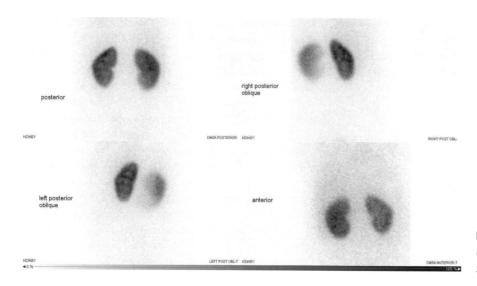

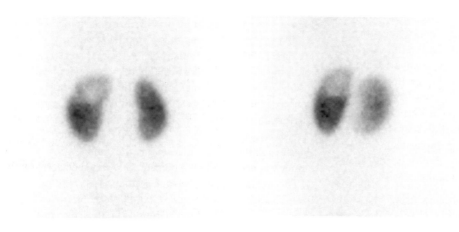

Figure 49.4   *Normal radio-labelled dimercaptosuccinic acid (^{99m}Tc-DMSA) study.*

Figure 49.5   *Radio-labelled dimercaptosuccinic acid (^{99m}Tc-DMSA) study, showing left duplex kidney with obstructed upper moiety.*

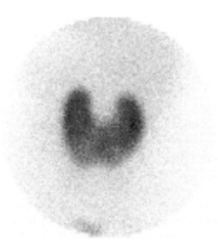

Figure 49.6   *Radio-labelled dimercaptosuccinic acid (^{99m}Tc-DMSA study): anterior image of horseshoe kidney.*

On completion of the dynamic study, a static post-micturition image is essential to assess the completeness of bladder emptying. Voiding may also improve drainage of the upper renal tracts in high-pressure systems. Renal drainage in capacious collecting systems is often influenced by gravity. If

the study has been undertaken in the supine position, then a change of posture followed by a delayed image up to 60 minutes after tracer administration is invaluable to assess drainage under normal physiological conditions. This is particularly useful postoperatively, e.g. following pyeloplasty. In North America, urinary bladder catheterization is undertaken routinely before renography to ensure bladder emptying, but this practice is less common in Europe.

Data interpretation relies on visual inspection of the images acquired and on computer analysis of the stored data. Time–activity curves are generated, which allow the relative function of each kidney to be measured. The transit times for movement of tracer through the renal cortex and pelvis can be estimated by drawing computerized regions of interest over the areas concerned. This is more difficult in children, where cortical thickness is low compared with in adults, particularly in the context of scarring or calyceal dilation. Examples of a normal ^{99m}Tc-MAG$_3$ dynamic renogram and a time–activity curve are given in Figure 49.7.

SPECIAL CONSIDERATIONS: RENAL MATURATION

The neonatal kidney has a full adult complement of nephrons, and subsequent growth occurs by hyperplasia. The GFR,

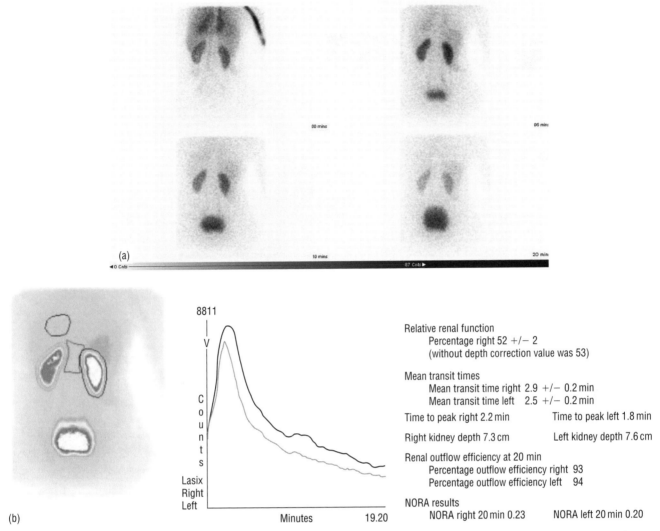

Figure 49.7   *Normal technetium-labelled trimercaptotriglycine (*^{99m}*Tc-MAG$_3$) study. (a) Composite posterior images at 0, 5, 10 and 20 minutes after injection. (b) Time–activity curves for right and left kidneys, showing normal uptake and clearance.*

corrected for body surface area, rises from approximately 30 mL/min at birth to around 84 mL/min (80 per cent of adult values) at age two years and reaches maturity by puberty. Tubular immaturity leads to relatively poor renal uptake of ^{99m}Tc-DMSA in the neonatal period, and imaging should be deferred, where possible, until at least three months of age. ^{99m}Tc-MAG$_3$ is highly protein bound *in vivo*, ensuring high plasma concentrations compared with ^{99m}Tc-DTPA. Taken with the higher extraction efficiency, ^{99m}Tc-MAG$_3$ offers a higher signal-to-noise ratio in early infancy. Where possible, dynamic renography should be delayed until four to six weeks of age, when some renal maturation should have occurred.

INDIRECT RADIONUCLIDE CYSTOGRAM

Indirect radionuclide cystography (IRC) is a useful non-invasive technique for assessing VUR and bladder function under normal physiological conditions and can be performed easily in any child who is toilet-trained. The technique is valid but more time-consuming in younger children. Imaging is usually undertaken 30–60 minutes after a conventional ^{99m}Tc-MAG$_3$ renogram. The child stands or sits erect with his or her back to the gamma camera. Dynamic images of the bladder and kidneys are acquired as the child voids. The sensitivity and specificity of ^{99m}Tc-DTPA IRC are quoted as 74 and 90 per cent, respectively; higher sensitivities are reported for ^{99m}Tc-MAG$_3$. The voided urine volume and activity can be measured and used to calculate full and residual bladder volume, maximum urine flow and reflux.

Diuretic administration may reduce the sensitivity of IRC. Where dynamic renography is performed to assess both upper tract drainage and reflux, the most important objective of the examination should be clarified before commencing the dynamic study, and diuretic prescription planned accordingly. It is recognized that VUR may be an intermittent phenomenon and that results may vary using the same technique on different occasions.

Direct radionuclide cystography (DRC) is performed with the child lying on top of the gamma camera following bladder catheterization and instillation of ^{99m}Tc-pertechnetate until the bladder is full. Images of the bladder and kidneys are acquired during micturition. Although sensitive for detecting reflux, the procedure provides no anatomical information about the urethra and is invasive. The technique delivers a significantly lower radiation absorbed dose than conventional MCUG, but increasing use of pulsed-sequence fluoroscopy (as described above) overcomes this difference and is likely to reduce demand for DRC in the future.

IMAGING PATHWAYS IN COMMON PRESENTATIONS OF UROLOGICAL DISORDERS

Antenatal hydronephrosis

The postnatal management of antenatal hydronephrosis is focused first on assessing whether the hydronephrosis is transient or represents ongoing pathology. Initial postnatal assessment should comprise ultrasound within the first 24 hours if antenatal hydronephrosis was significant, particularly in the presence of bilateral hydronephrosis and bladder distension in boys. The most important diagnosis to make at this stage is posterior urethral valves: early treatment is vital if renal function is to be preserved.

The crucial observation is of a thickened bladder wall, since a thickness of 4 mm or above is virtually diagnostic of posterior urethral valves in this context. However, even in the absence of this finding, bilateral hydronephrosis in the male neonate requires urgent MCUG to exclude valves. (Figure 49.8). This must be performed under intramuscular or intravenous gentamicin cover, as even an aseptic technique has the risk of inducing a bacteraemia, which can lead to overwhelming sepsis in the presence of an obstructed system. If posterior urethral valves are confirmed, then the bladder must be recatheterized immediately on completion of the study.

As mentioned previously, if the postnatal ultrasound scan at 24–48 hours appears normal, then this should be repeated at approximately one week to exclude hydronephrosis masked by relative dehydration. The subsequent follow-up of hydronephrosis depends on the diameter of the renal pelvis, and a variety of diagnostic pathways has been suggested. The principle of imaging here is to identify kidneys that are likely to deteriorate by distinguishing obstructive from non-obstructive hydronephrosis, enabling appropriate selection for surgical intervention. Another important discriminator is the presence of calyceal dilation, which should prompt further evaluation with MCUG, ^{99m}Tc-DMSA renography or ^{99m}Tc-MAG$_3$ renography, even in the absence of significant pelvic distension. The main trigger for acceleration of investigations is increasing hydronephrosis on consecutive ultrasound scans.

The definition of obstruction in asymptomatic infants is unclear and may be established only in retrospect on the

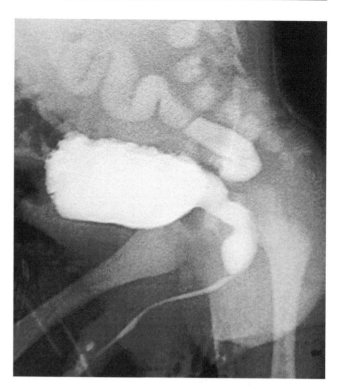

Figure 49.8 *Micturating cystourethrogram, showing a trabeculated bladder, dilated posterior urethra and valve. There is reflux into a dilated tortuous ureter.*

basis of a documented deterioration in renal function. A baseline ^{99m}Tc-MAG$_3$ renogram is, therefore, valuable at one to three months of age, with follow-up renography to assess any subsequent change in differential function and drainage. The timing of later imaging depends on renal function, shorter intervals being recommended for poorly functioning kidneys. Figures 49.9 and 49.10 show typical appearances in hydronephrosis compared with outflow obstruction at the level of the pelviureteric junction.

^{99m}Tc-DMSA imaging is of value when there is persistent hydroureteronephrosis or when the antenatal hydronephrosis is attributable to VUR.

Abdominal mass in the infant

The vast majority of abdominal masses presenting in the neonatal period are related to the urogenital system. Of these, the hydronephrotic kidney is the most common. The first investigation should be abdominal ultrasound; this will differentiate solid from cystic masses, will characterize the mass and, in most cases, will confirm the structure of origin. Occasionally, if the mass is very large, however, the degree of distortion of the abdominal and pelvic structures is such that the site of origin cannot be assessed confidently. Masses arising from the kidney usually can be recognized as such, as can bladder lesions. One pitfall is the misinterpretation of a cystic pelvic mass, e.g. an ovarian cyst, as the bladder.

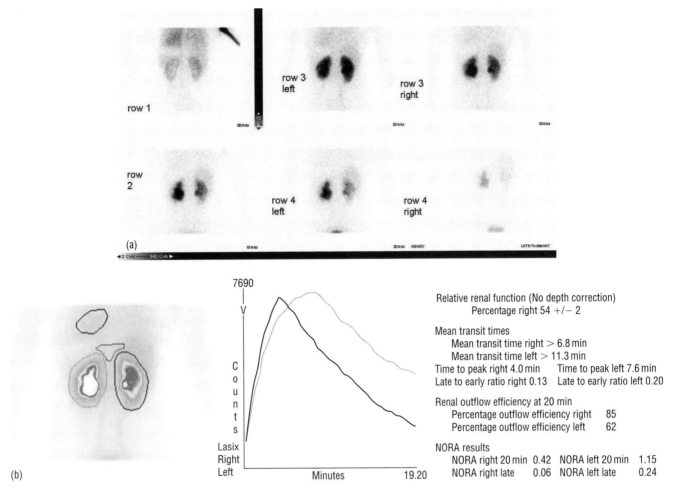

Figure 49.9   *Technetium-labelled trimercaptotriglycine (^{99m}Tc-MAG$_3$) renogram. (a) Composite posterior images showing left hydronephrosis. Initial hold-up in dilated left renal pelvis (0–20 minutes), with complete drainage at 60 minutes following diuretic challenge. (b) Time–activity curves: left hydronephrosis. See also Colour Plate 19.*

If hydronephrosis is identified, then the level of any obstruction can be suggested by the typical sonographic appearance of pelviureteric junction obstruction, with a convex renal pelvis and undetectable ureter, or hydroureteronephrosis with tapering ureter, as in vesicoureteric junction obstruction. Bilateral hydronephrosis with distended bladder suggests bladder outlet obstruction or gross reflux. Obstruction must be confirmed by dynamic imaging, most commonly ^{99m}Tc-MAG$_3$. MCUG will confirm or exclude reflux.

Renal tumours in the infant are likely to be mesoblastic nephromas or nephroblastomas. These present as solid lesions of heterogeneous echogenicity, which may contain areas of central low echogenicity representing tumour necrosis, and focal calcification. Occasionally, Wilms tumours are predominantly cystic.

Sonographic assessment should include midline encroachment, invasion of adjacent organs, lymphadenopathy, the presence of tumour thrombus in the renal vein or inferior vena cava and involvement of the contralateral kidney. Furtherstaging involves CT or MRI of the abdomen, together with chest CT. Current recommendations are that histology should be obtained by percutaneous biopsy under imaging guidance.

Renal cystic disease occasionally presents as an abdominal mass. Again, ultrasound generally will be diagnostic. Autosomal recessive polycystic disease manifests as bilateral enlarged kidneys containing multiple microcysts, which represent the dilated collecting tubules. A collecting system occasionally may be seen and certainly does not preclude the diagnosis. Moreover, this type of polycystic disease does not necessarily involve both kidneys uniformly, and areas of relatively normal renal parenchyma may be visible. Autosomal dominant polycystic disease may, on occasion, present in the infant; this can be surprisingly difficult to differentiate from autosomal recessive disease, as when evident at this early stage, the kidneys look large and echogenic and any visible cysts may be small.

Multicystic dysplastic kidneys generally are easier to diagnose, provided that the variably sized non-communicating cysts are not confused with a hydronephrotic kidney (Figure 49.11). ^{99m}Tc-DMSA imaging is of value in documenting the relative contribution of the dysplastic kidney to overall function.

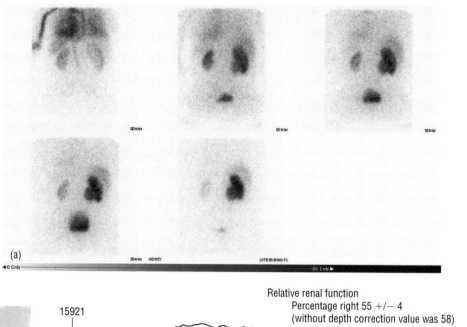

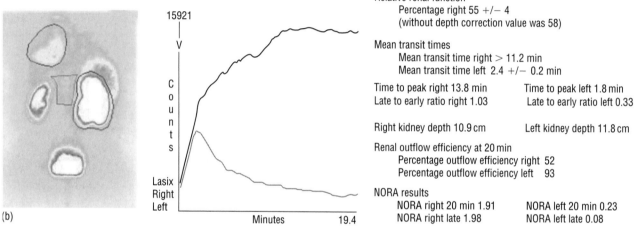

Relative renal function
Percentage right 55 +/− 4
(without depth correction value was 58)

Mean transit times
Mean transit time right > 11.2 min
Mean transit time left 2.4 +/− 0.2 min

Time to peak right 13.8 min   Time to peak left 1.8 min
Late to early ratio right 1.03   Late to early ratio left 0.33

Right kidney depth 10.9 cm   Left kidney depth 11.8 cm

Renal outflow efficiency at 20 min
Percentage outflow efficiency right 52
Percentage outflow efficiency left   93

NORA results
NORA right 20 min 1.91   NORA left 20 min 0.23
NORA right late 1.98   NORA left late 0.08

Figure 49.10 *Technetium-labelled trimercaptotriglycine (*^{99m}*Tc-MAG$_3$) renogram. (a) Composite posterior images, showing outflow obstruction at the right pelviureteric junction. Progressive hold-up in dilated right renal pelvis (0–20 minutes), with no drainage at 60 minutes despite diuretic challenge, change of posture and bladder emptying. (b) Time–activity curves: right pelviureteric junction obstruction. See also Colour Plate 20.*

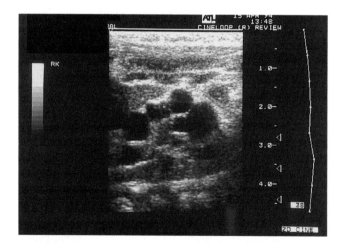

Figure 49.11 *Ultrasound of right kidney, showing multiple non-communicating cysts with some solid renal parenchyma interspersed. Appearances are typical of multicystic dysplastic kidney.*

Renal vein thrombosis can present with renal enlargement. The sonographic features are variable, but the kidney is generally echogenic in the acute stage, with loss of renal architecture. Colour Doppler fails to demonstrate flow in the intra-renal veins. Occasionally, renal vein thrombosis is secondary to adrenal haemorrhage, when the adrenal ultrasound will suggest the diagnosis.

Urinary tract infection

Considerable controversy still surrounds the topic of appropriate imaging and management of UTI. The fundamentals of management are to prevent or limit renal damage, and imaging is directed towards identifying any predisposing factors and documenting evidence of scarring. Most authorities are agreed that UTIs presenting in the first year of life deserve full investigation, regardless of the sex of the child. This would include ultrasound, ^{99m}Tc-DMSA and MCUG, with ^{99m}Tc-MAG$_3$ renography if obstruction is suspected. An ultrasound in UTI should look for the following: bladder-wall thickening (outlet obstruction or inflammation), echogenic debris in the urine (acute infection), ureterocele with or without a duplex collecting system, ectopic ureter, hydronephrosis (obstruction or reflux), urothelial thickening (acute infection or intermittent dilatation), cortical thinning, echogenic renal sinus with loss of corticomedullary differentiation (acute pyelonephritis), a focal area of abnormal echogenicity exerting mass effect (focal nephronia) and renal abscess.

Three particular conditions deserve special mention. In pyonephrosis, ultrasound may reveal a dilated collecting system containing multiple low-level echoes. This is a critical finding that requires immediate intervention in order to preserve renal function. In fungal infections, collections of hyphae and debris may form into balls, which can obstruct the pelvi-ureteric junction. These present as well-defined rounded foci within the pelvicalyceal system and may be associated with other sonographic evidence of *Candida*, such as renal enlargement and increased echogenicity.

Xanthogranulomatous pyelonephritis is an uncommon condition with extensive destruction of renal parenchyma, usually following incomplete treatment of UTI. Ultrasound reveals an enlarged echogenic kidney with normal renal architecture replaced by hypoechoic dilated and distorted calyces interspersed with echogenic debris and occasional calculi.

^{99m}Tc-DMSA imaging is the reference standard for renal scarring. Scarring distorts the integrity of the cortical margin, leading to an irregular outline and progressive loss of functioning renal tissue. Unilateral scarring may be associated with a reduction in the contribution of the affected kidney to divided function. Duplication may lead to loss of function in the upper moiety, usually secondary to obstruction, or may lead to scarring of the lower moiety secondary to vesicoureteric reflux. The relative contribution of each moiety to total renal function can be quantified. An example of renal scarring is shown in Figure 49.12.

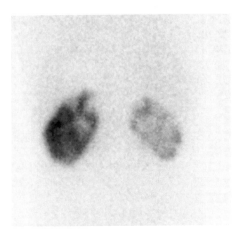

Figure 49.12 *Radio-labelled dimercaptosuccinic acid (^{99m}Tc-DMSA) study, showing bilateral renal scarring.*

The role of ^{99m}Tc-DMSA imaging in acute pyelonephritis is controversial. Acute infection leads to focal cortical ischaemia and altered tubular membrane transport, resulting in focal areas of reduced DMSA uptake. As ischaemia precedes tubular dysfunction, DMSA imaging may allow early diagnosis before significant tissue damage has occurred. Recognizing both the difficulty in distinguishing lower and upper urinary tract infection in young children and the potential sequelae of delayed diagnosis, ^{99m}Tc-DMSA scintigraphy has been advocated in the investigation of acute pyelonephritis. Conversely, it is accepted that acute parenchymal inflammatory change is usually transient and does not lead to irreversible renal scarring in the majority of cases. In the interests of minimizing exposure to ionizing radiation, most centres delay ^{99m}Tc-DMSA imaging until at least 12 weeks after infection. ^{99m}Tc-MAG$_3$ renography is useful to exclude outflow obstruction as a predisposing cause for infection, particularly in the context of renal duplication. Upper- and lower-moiety function can be quantified, and indirect cystography may show reflux.

Haematuria

There are five common causes of haematuria in childhood: UTI, calculi, trauma, tumour and renal vein thrombosis. The age of the child and the clinical presentation frequently differentiate between these, and imaging is used to confirm clinical suspicion. Ultrasound is likely to be the first investigation for all of these conditions.

Subsequent imaging in UTI, tumour imaging and the sonographic features of renal vein thrombosis were discussed earlier. Plain abdominal X-ray and IVU are obtained if stones are suspected, but these techniques may be supplanted by low-dose CT scanning in the future. The extent of investigation of haematuria in renal trauma should be guided by the mechanism of injury and the patient's condition. For microscopic haematuria, ultrasound is generally enough to exclude significant injury, provided that colour Doppler assessment of vascular integrity is included. In macroscopic haematuria, CT scanning frequently is indicated (Figure 49.13). It can be of benefit to the surgeon to obtain a plain abdominal X-ray immediately after contrast-enhanced CT to demonstrate the collecting systems in coronal plane. If vascular damage is suspected, then conventional angiography may be required, for both diagnostic and therapeutic purposes.

Hypertension

Renal pathology is the most common cause of hypertension in children over one year of age. The underlying pathology is usually scarring secondary to infection and/or reflux, but the differential includes renovascular disease and tumour. The first investigation is usually ultrasound to detect discrepancies in renal size, severe scarring, hydronephrosis and renal or adrenal tumours, followed by ^{99m}Tc-DMSA imaging.

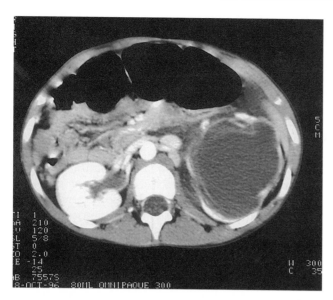

Figure 49.13 *Abdominal computed tomography scan, showing gross left hydronephrosis and perinephric haematoma. The patient presented with abdominal pain and haematuria after relatively minor trauma. Note the reversed position of the aorta and inferior vena cava, consistent with abdominal situs inversus.*

If the index of suspicion for renovascular disease is high, then Doppler ultrasound followed by ^{99m}Tc-MAG$_3$ renography before and after captopril administration are useful. In older children, the most common cause of renovascular disease is fibromuscular dysplasia, which is often bilateral and may affect branch arteries.

Renal perfusion is maintained through a stenosed vessel via the renin – angiotensin system. Administration of an angiotensin-converting enzyme inhibitor such as captopril leads to a fall in perfusion to the affected kidney. This delays the time to peak activity in the initial phase of the ^{99m}Tc-MAG$_3$ dynamic renogram and decreases the relative contribution of the affected kidney to total function. Captopril-induced segmental defects on ^{99m}Tc-DMSA imaging are particularly useful in detecting branch-artery renal artery stenosis (RAS), with a reported sensitivity of 59–73 per cent and specificity of 68–88 per cent for detecting renovascular disease. If pre- and post-captopril ^{99m}Tc-MAG$_3$ and ^{99m}Tc-DMSA imaging are normal, then the likelihood of renal hypertension is very low. The reference technique for renovascular hypertension remains selective angiography. The place of CT angiography, magnetic resonance angiography and colour Doppler ultrasound scanning as alternatives to invasive angiography in paediatric nephro-urology is under investigation.

Transplantation

Imaging plays a vital role in the prompt detection and diagnosis of complications following renal transplantation. The clinical presentation and timing after surgery may give clues as to the underlying cause and direct subsequent investigation.

Early complications occurring within days of surgery include acute tubular necrosis, hyperacute rejection and arterial or venous thrombosis. Over the next few months, rejection must be distinguished from ciclosporin toxicity. Late complications include infection, rejection, ciclosporin toxicity, outflow obstruction and recurrence of the original pathology. Accurate diagnosis is usually achieved by combining ultrasound with dynamic renography. The radiopharmaceutical of choice is usually ^{99m}Tc-DTPA, which allows imaging to be combined with venous sampling for accurate GFR measurement. The higher extraction efficiency of ^{99m}Tc-MAG$_3$ results in superior image quality, but experience in paediatric transplantation is more limited. As the two tracers are not interchangeable, consistent use of the same pharmaceuticals is essential for serial follow-up in an individual patient.

Infection is relatively common following transplantation, and a ^{99m}Tc-DMSA study three to four weeks postoperatively establishes a useful baseline for future comparison.

In acute tubular necrosis, the transplanted kidney is perfused but shows poor filtration and a prolonged transit time. Vascular occlusion, by comparison, leads to absent perfusion and no filtration. At a later stage, rejection typically is associated with both reduced blood flow and poor filtration, whereas perfusion generally is affected less severely in ciclosporin toxicity.

CONCLUSION

The major indications for renal tract imaging in childhood are infection and hydronephrosis. Although practice varies between centres, the importance of an integrated nuclear medicine and radiology approach is recognized. The development of consensus algorithms for paediatric renal investigation is essential in order to improve standards and ensure appropriate cost-efficient access to complex imaging.

FURTHER READING

Currarino G, Wood B, Majd M. Diagnostic procedures. In: Silverman F, Kuhn J (eds). *Caffey's Pediatric X-Ray Diagnosis: An Integrated Imaging Approach.* St Louis, MO: Mosby, 1993; pp. 1147–200.

European Association of Nuclear Medicine. EANM Guidelines on Pediatric Nuclear Medicine. www.eanm.org

Gordon I. Paediatric nephro-urology. In: Ell PJ, Gambhir SS (eds). *Nuclear Medicine in Clinical Diagnosis and Treatment.* London: Churchill Livingstone, 2004; pp. 1569–80.

50

Antenatal diagnosis of urinary tract anomalies

HK DHILLON

Learning objectives

- To understand the impact of prenatal ultrasound in identifying urinary tract anomalies.
- To be able to differentiate between prenatally diagnosed abnormalities that require investigation/intervention and those of no clinical significance.
- To understand the diagnostic pathways used in managing this new subpopulation.

INTRODUCTION

Maternal ultrasound has been incorporated into routine obstetric practice since the early to mid-1980s. In the UK, ultrasound scanning currently is carried out before 12 weeks' gestation, looking specifically for nuchal thickness as an indication of the risk of chromosomal abnormalities. This is followed by a detailed anomaly scan at approximately 20 weeks' gestation. Further scans are indicated if an abnormality is detected and for obstetric reasons.

This new population of children is unique, as they are healthy and outwardly normal at birth. They are thus not 'patients' in the conventional sense, and clinical signs and symptoms are present in fewer than ten per cent of these neonates. Optimal management is still evolving, and long-term studies will continue to elucidate the natural history of the various diagnostic groups. This will identify, prospectively, children whose prenatal abnormalities put them at risk of, for example, deterioration of renal function, urinary tract infections and pain. Such studies will also identify children with anomalies of no clinical importance. The lack of long-term outcomes has led to a tendency for excessive imaging, both pre- and postnatally. Prenatally detected anomalies generate considerable anxiety for the parents, and this is proportionate to the number of scans carried out. Greater emphasis needs to be placed on developing close links between obstetric/fetal medicine units and paediatric specialties in order to ensure that the parents are counselled appropriately.

INCIDENCE

The incidence of prenatally diagnosed uropathies reported from European centres averages around one in 500 pregnancies. Prenatal ultrasound identifies the whole spectrum of an abnormality, thereby necessarily including many children from the milder end of the spectrum who will never have a clinical problem.

Therefore, the challenge posed by maternal ultrasound is to differentiate between an abnormality of the urinary tract that is clinically important from one of no clinical significance. This distinction can be achieved only by recognizing that optimal management of this population is both prenatal and postnatal. Ideally, there should be joint clinics with obstetric colleagues in order to improve counselling for parents. Such collaboration also provides continuity of care. Even if there are

---

Box 50.1 Prenatal diagnosis: differential diagnosis of distended bladder

Urethral abnormality: posterior urethral valves, urethral atresia/hypoplasia, prune belly syndrome
Syringocele (often transient)
Vesicoureteric reflux
Urogenital sinus
Cloacal anomaly
Impacted ureterocele
Idiopathic

Box 50.2 Prenatal diagnosis: differential diagnosis of non-visualization of bladder

Renal agenesis/lower-tract agenesis
Bladder extrophy
Cloacal extrophy
Epispadias
Urogenital sinus anomaly
Cloacal anomaly
Bilateral single ectopic ureters

---

practical difficulties that prevent paediatric specialists from being involved prenatally, it is mandatory that the prenatal history is obtained before any investigations are planned.

Failure to obtain the precise details of the prenatal history is a major cause of confusion and excessive and inappropriate investigations. These neonates are referred to paediatric specialists solely because of the prenatal findings, which thus represent the only history available. It is unacceptable to investigate a healthy neonate on the basis of phrases such as 'prenatal right hydronephroses', which are non-specific and represent anomalies that range from life-threatening to clinically insignificant. Moreover, the prenatal milieu is a stable environment with the additional benefit of having the amniotic fluid acting as an ultrasound medium. The placenta maintains this *in utero* environment as well as full hydration of the fetus, which allows for more accurate assessment of the urinary tract.

Prenatal history should include the timing and findings of all scans, even if they were normal. As well as hydronephrosis being described as 'mild', 'moderate' or 'severe', precise measurements in the same transverse plane as is used postnatally should be included. The absence or presence of calyceal involvement should be noted. Visualizing the bladder, measuring the bladder-wall thickness and recording that it empties completely excludes bladder outflow obstruction and complex urological anomalies such as bladder extrophy and cloacal anomalies (Boxes 50.1 and 50.2). Documentation of the volume of amniotic fluid will identify a fetus with reduced liquor, which, if of renal origin, implies an infant who is likely to have compromised renal function.

Fetal intervention is indicated only where there is the possibility of a bladder outflow obstruction, which can have a poor prognosis in terms of compromised renal function. The published results of vesicoamniotic shunting relate to fetuses that already have a severe degree of renal impairment and have shown little benefit from this procedure. However, there is the possibility that early shunting may be of benefit when bilateral hydronephrosis and bladder distension are not accompanied by oligohydramnios and abnormal urine biochemistry. There is an urgent need to reappraise the indications for fetal intervention in those cases where there is a better prospect of improving the outcome.

All neonates with a prenatally detected anomaly will have a postnatal ultrasound between two and seven days of life. Unilateral abnormalities with an entirely normal contralateral kidney should not be imaged before 72 hours, as postnatal scans may appear to show an improvement in relation to the prenatal scans due to inadequate hydration. Further imaging should always be based on prenatal findings.

POSTNATAL EVOLUTION AND SEQUENTIAL IMAGING

The nature of the investigative sequence will depend upon the significance and severity of the prenatal findings. Several key indices will dictate postnatal action.

Clinically significant anomalies

These require either early admission or early outpatient investigation.

EARLY ADMISSION

All neonates with a prenatal history of an abnormal bladder (whether distended or absent) will require early admission, as the differential diagnoses include life-threatening and/or complex urological abnormalities. Fetuses with a urinary-tract abnormality associated with oligo- or anhydramnios have potentially abnormal renal function and also warrant early investigation for assessment of renal function. Bilateral abnormalities of the parenchyma such as echogenic kidneys or large kidneys, which may represent the spectrum of polycystic disease, also merit early admission for nephrological input. Similarly, a small proportion of severe bilateral hydronephrosis (>20 mm) or solitary kidneys with severe hydronephrosis may have overall reduced renal function and will require admission and even intervention.

EARLY INVESTIGATION

Some neonates will require more investigations than simple ultrasound follow-up in the first few months of life. A micturating cystourethrogram (MCUG) is indicated when certain criteria are fulfilled, as detailed in Box 50.3. The findings on MCUG dictate subsequent investigations. The finding of vesicoureteric reflux is followed by a dimercaptosuccinic acid (DMSA) scan. However, a normal MCUG raises the possibility of an 'obstruction' at the vesicoureteric junction, and mercaptoacetyltriglycerine (MAG_3) would be the radioisotope of choice.

Some neonates warrant a radioisotope study without a prior MCUG. These children are derived almost exclusively from the population with a potential pelviureteric junction 'obstruction'. All neonates who had a prenatal severe hydronephrosis (renal pelvis >20 mm) with dilated calyces warrant a MAG_3 study close to one month of age. The more severe the dilation, the greater the risk that the kidney may already have reduced function.

These investigations will define a number of different diagnostic groups, which will be examined individually below.

Clinically insignificant anomalies

There are a number of prenatal 'abnormalities' that have been found to have little clinical relevance. The most important of these is the detection of a unilateral dilation of less than 10 mm both pre- and postnatally with normal calyces and a normal contralateral kidney.

The main controversy surrounding the investigation of unilateral mild dilation is its possible association with reflux. Several publications justify routine cystography on the basis that unilateral mild dilation may be associated with severe reflux. This premise is correct only if the prenatal scans are ignored. All children with severe reflux would have had *in utero* findings that identified the need for a cystogram. However, postnatal scans may not visualize a dilated ureter if the child has just voided or is dehydrated. The term 'mild dilation' should be used only in reference to postnatal scans when the prenatal findings were similar.

A mild unilateral dilation of less than 10 mm pre- and postnatally may also be associated with reflux. Routine unselected cystography has identified that such children will have lesser degrees of reflux into a normally functioning kidney on a DMSA scan. This reflux will have resolved before two years of age (Godley et al. 2001). The majority (more than 75 per cent) of this population are male and historically did not present clinically.

SPECIFIC DIAGNOSES

Prenatally diagnosed hydronephrosis: ?pelviureteric junction obstruction

Approximately 50 per cent of all children with a prenatally diagnosed hydronephrosis will have an isolated upper-tract dilation that is labelled as a pelviureteric junction 'obstruction'. However, a significant proportion of this population are not obstructed and do not require a pyeloplasty. Controversy surrounds the ability of the furosemide (frusemide) renogram to define obstruction in view of drainage being unreliable and also dependent upon the state of hydration, bladder emptying, kidney function and severity of the hydronephrosis.

Conservative management for these infants is based on ignoring post-furosemide drainage and utilizing the uptake phase of the curve to assess the function of the hydronephrotic kidney. Surgery is indicated if the function decreases to below 40 per cent or if the child develops symptoms. Early studies used diethylenetriamine-pentacetic acid (DTPA), but this has been superseded by MAG_3.

A natural history study and a randomized clinical trial conducted at Great Ormond Street Hospital for Children found that ultrasound was the most useful imaging modality in differentiating children with a pelviureteric junction obstruction that justified pyeloplasty from hydronephrosis that remained stable or resolved spontaneously (Ransley et al. 1990; Dhillon 1998). The anteroposterior diameter of the renal pelvis in the transverse plane of the kidney proved to be the most useful predictor of outcome.

The potential of ultrasound to identify prospectively children with a true pelviureteric junction obstruction was tested by analysing 914 children with a prenatal hydronephrosis referred between 1980 and 2000. Pre- and postnatal ultrasound findings were correlated to eventual outcome. Bilateral dilation was included if both renal pelves were less than 15 mm. All kidneys with a hydronephrosis of more than 15 mm had a normal contralateral kidney. Three-quarters of these children have been followed for 10–18 years.

Children with a dilation of less than 20 mm represent more than 60 per cent of prenatally diagnosed hydronephrosis. Only seven per cent of this large group have justified pyeloplasty. Surgery was required when there was an intra-renal type of hydronephrosis, with a minimal extra renal component but severe calyceal clubbing. Pyeloplasty also was indicated in cases where the early postnatal scan showed an artificially 'improved' degree of dilation, which subsequently reverted to the prenatal dimensions of >20 mm with calyceal involvement. It is worth repeating that the label of 'mild' hydronephrosis should be applied only to a postnatal dilation when the *in utero* scans (including a late third trimester scan) record a similar or lesser degree of mild dilation. Therefore, children with a dilation of less than 20 mm pre- and postnatally and no calyceal involvement need only simple ultrasound follow-up. The presence of calyceal dilation will justify a radioisotope study.

Children with hydronephroses of more than 30 mm and with clubbed calyces are at high risk and have a greater than 75 per cent chance of subsequently requiring surgery. Early pyeloplasty is justified in this smaller population, as they would otherwise require frequent radioisotope imaging.

Children with a dilation of between 20 and 30 mm and dilated calyces require longer follow-up, in order to identify prospectively those patients who will benefit from pyeloplasty. Currently, equal numbers will demonstrate functional deterioration or spontaneous improvement or remain stable. The majority of the functional deterioration and spontaneous resolution occurs in the first three years. Initial management of this group therefore should be conservative. The smaller group of patients who remain stable at three years of age either can continue to be managed conservatively or can be offered pyeloplasty.

The management of this large population with a potential pelviureteric junction obstruction has been simplified greatly by using both pre- and postnatal ultrasound to determine the possibility of requiring surgery and tailoring the imaging and intervention appropriately.

Multicystic dysplastic kidney

The multicystic dysplastic kidney (MCDK) provides an excellent example of the impact of maternal ultrasound. Historically, such a kidney presented clinically as a palpable abdominal mass, but only 25 per cent of prenatally diagnosed multicystic kidneys are easily palpable. Clinically important MCDKs therefore will be easily palpable or have an abnormality of the contralateral kidney. Imaging requires no more than two ultrasounds in the first year and one radioisotope study (DMSA/MAG₃). MCUG is indicated in the presence of a contralateral or lower urinary tract anomaly pre- or postnatally. Ultrasound appearances and the radioisotope study are not reliable at assessing function, and a formal estimation of the glomerular filtration rate (GFR) is preferable. Children with normal GFR can be discharged with advice to have their blood pressure recorded at approximately yearly intervals, despite the reported risk of hypertension being very low (in the order of 0.01–0.1 per cent). The MCDK tends to involute spontaneously in the first few years of life, so there are very few indications for nephrectomy. An MCDK measuring more than 6 cm in length in the first three months of life is unlikely to involute; hence, nephrectomy is justifiable in cases where there is a large palpable MCDK or in the presence of an ipsilateral abnormality (ureterocele, distal reflux), which may predispose the infant to urinary tract infections. Prophylactic nephrectomy should not be advocated for the very low risk of hypertension or tumour (Thomas 2002).

Duplex kidneys

Children with duplex kidneys and with severe dilation of either moiety, especially if associated with a large ectopic ureterocoele, are at risk of sepsis. Current thinking is divided between early endoscopic puncture of the ureterocele and upper-pole nephrectomy. Successful endoscopic puncture of the ureterocele leads to decompression of the upper tract and ureter and avoids hemi-nephrectomy in 50 per cent of cases.

PRE- AND POSTNATAL PATHOLOGY

Prenatal history occasionally will document a course of events that are transient and result in radiological abnormalities of varying clinical significance.

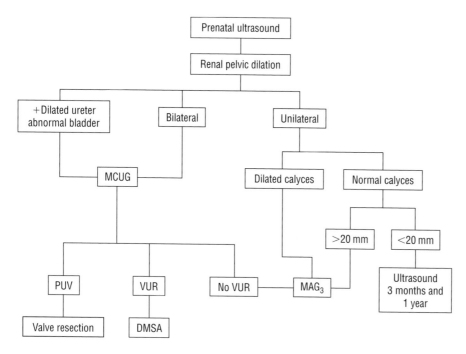

Figure 50.1 *Prenatally diagnosed hydronephrosis: diagnostic pathways.* DMSA, dimercaptosuccinic acid; MAG₃, mercaptoacetyltriglycine; MCUG, micturating cystourethrogram; PUV, posterior urethral valve; VUR, vesicoureteric reflux.

An excellent example of such an *in utero* event is a transient bladder outflow obstruction. The fetus will have bilateral hydronephrosis, dilated ureters and a distended bladder, with or without oligohydramnios. Before 28 weeks' gestation, the bladder will empty spontaneously, accompanied by an improvement in the upper-tract dilation and amniotic fluid volume. Postnatally, these babies are found to have reflux, dilated ureters, abnormal bladders or resolving hydronephroses. The most common cause of such a transient bladder outflow obstruction is a syringocele. Syringoceles arise from Cowper's glands in the anterior urethra of the male.

Cysts of the kidneys can involute *in utero* and result in abnormal radiology, which shows no evidence of the original anatomy. The MCDK may involute, so that it is not visualized by the third trimester. Historically, these children would have been labelled as having a solitary kidney. Cystic disease can also occur segmentally. Cysts in the upper or lower pole can involute, resulting in a globally smaller kidney, which represents the residual normal parenchyma. 'Segmental' cystic dysplasia may be the pathogenesis by which infants are born with small but otherwise 'normal' kidneys.

CONCLUSION

Fetal ultrasound is a window that allows observation of the evolution of urinary tract abnormalities. It has the potential to be a wonderful tool for reducing the morbidity from urinary tract pathology. However, it creates considerably anxiety and an imaging burden by also identifying abnormalities of no clinical significance. The great benefit to a relatively small percentage of children is therefore counterbalanced by the burden of unnecessary investigations performed without benefit on healthy infants without significant pathology. A suggested postnatal investigative pathway for antenatally diagnosed hydronephrosis based on current evidence is shown in Figure 50.1.

REFERENCES

Dhillon HK. Prenatally diagnosed hydronephrosis: the Great Ormond Street experience. *British Journal of Urology* 1998; **81** (Suppl 2): 39–44.

Godley ML, Desai D, Yeung CK, *et al*. The relationship between early renal status, and the resolution of vesico-ureteric reflux and bladder function at 16 months. *British Journal of Urology International* 2001; **87**: 475–62.

Ransley PG, Dhillon HK, Gordon I, *et al*. The postnatal management of hydronephrosis diagnosed by prenatal ultrasound. *Journal of Urology* 1990; **144**: 584–7.

Thomas DFM. Cystic renal disease. In: Thomas DFM, Rickwood AMK, Duffy PG (eds). *Essentials of Paediatric Urology*. London: Martin Dunitz, 2002; pp. 97–104.

FURTHER READING

Dhillon HK. Prenatal diagnosis. In: Thomas DFM, Rickwood AMK, Duffy PG (eds). *Essentials of Paediatric Urology*. London: Martin Dunitz, 2002; pp. 105–12.

Duffy PG. Posterior urethral valves and other urethral abnormalities. In: Thomas DFM, Rickwood AMK, Duffy PG (eds). *Essentials of Paediatric Urology*. London: Martin Dunitz, 2002; pp. 87–96.

Thomas DFM. Vesicoureteric reflux. In: Thomas DFM, Rickwood AMK, Duffy PG (eds). *Essentials of Paediatric Urology*. London: Martin Dunitz, 2002; pp. 45–55.

51

Renal function, renal failure and renal transplantation

RODNEY GILBERT AND AMIR AZMY

Learning objectives

- To understand the changes in renal function that occur in the neonate and infant.
- To understand the principles of measurement of glomerular filtration rate and the proper interpretation of plasma creatinine concentrations.
- To understand the most common causes of acute renal failure, especially the surgical aspects.
- To understand the principles of management of acute and chronic renal failure.
- To understand the principles of renal transplantation, rejection and immunosuppressive treatment.

FETAL AND NEONATAL RENAL FUNCTION

Fetal kidneys receive only two to four per cent of cardiac output, compared with 20 per cent in the adult. This low rate of renal blood flow is associated with high renal vascular resistance and a fairly constant glomerular filtration rate (GFR) in the fetus of about 1 mL/min/kg body weight. Fetal GFR is significantly reduced in about 70 per cent of complicated pregnancies. The principal function of the fetal kidneys is to maintain amniotic fluid volume. To this end, the fetus passes about 1000 mL of urine per day at term. Fetal kidneys contribute very little to homeostasis, which is achieved through the action of the maternal kidneys and the placenta, the latter receiving almost 50 per cent of the fetal cardiac output.

Glomerular filtration rate

This averages about $8\,mL/min/1.73\,m^2$ in babies born at 28 weeks' gestation and $20\,mL/min/1.73\,m^2$ at term. The healthy term infant copes well with this low level of renal function, partly because of the following:

- Breast milk provides a low solute load for the kidney to excrete.
- Only 25–35 per cent of absorbed amino acids are oxidized, and thus produce urea for the kidneys to excrete, with 65–75 per cent being incorporated into the body for growth.

Urea production can easily outstrip the ability of the immature kidneys to excrete it in a number of scenarios, including if the infant is rendered catabolic by infection, surgery or drugs, such as dexamethasone.

The low GFR in neonates and infants is an important consideration in prescribing drugs that are eliminated via the kidneys, e.g. gentamicin and vancomycin. Careful monitoring of plasma levels is required to prevent toxicity.

In preterm infants, nephrogenesis is not complete until 34 weeks after conception. GFR increases slowly until then, after which acceleration of GFR takes place, such that in term infants the GFR doubles by two weeks of age. The GFR does not reach adult values ($80–120 \, mL/min/1.73 \, m^2$) until the second year of life.

Creatinine

The cord-blood creatinine concentration largely reflects maternal renal function at the time of birth. Plasma creatinine then falls during the next three to four weeks to a level dependent on renal function. The average term infant has a plasma creatinine concentration of about $70 \, \mu mol/L$ at birth. This falls to $30–40 \, \mu mol/L$ by three weeks. Very low-birth-weight babies have an average plasma creatinine concentration of about $110 \, \mu mol/L$ on day one, falling to about $40 \, \mu mol/L$ at three weeks. It rises again after one year as muscle mass increases faster than GFR rather than proportional to GFR.

This maturation of renal function has important implications for babies with congenital renal abnormalities, such as renal dysplasia. Even those infants with apparently severe renal failure at birth may have sufficient improvement in renal function to require no dialysis for months or even years.

Sodium and electrolytes

In the adult, more than 99 per cent of filtered sodium is reabsorbed by the tubules. In contrast, the fetus tends to be in a volume-expanded state and renal sodium reabsorption is much lower. When volume-depleted, however, the fetus is able to conserve sodium, at least to some extent.

Fractional excretion of sodium, a measure of sodium loss (sodium clearance divided by creatinine clearance, FE_{Na}) is in the range of five to ten per cent in the fetus, whereas term babies adjust rapidly from a sodium-losing state to sodium conservation, with typical FE_{Na} values of one per cent within a day or two of birth.

Preterm infants have immature tubular function and remain in a sodium-wasting state. These infants will routinely require oral sodium supplements of $3–6 \, mmol/kg/day$, although the optimal time for starting these supplements is unresolved. Fetal urine is usually hypotonic with respect to plasma; typical osmolality is in the range $100–250 \, mosmol/kg$. The fetus can increase urine concentration but cannot concentrate urine to adult levels.

The plasma bicarbonate concentration is low in term infants ($18–22 \, mmol/L$) and even lower in very low-birth-weight babies ($14–18 \, mmol/L$) due to a decreased proximal

renal tubule threshold for bicarbonate. The excretion of an acid load is not impaired, and these physiologically acidaemic babies generally thrive.

Estimation of glomerular filtration rate

The composition of urine is determined almost exclusively by dietary intake of inorganic solutes and the rate of formation of end products of metabolism, such that all urinary components are a product of the balance between production and utilization of that component.

One way to measure the excretory efficiency of the kidneys is to calculate the apparent volume of plasma from which a substance is completely removed in a given time. This is the urinary clearance of a substance. It is usually expressed as millilitres per minute or litres per day.

$$C_x = (U_x \times V)/P_x \qquad (51.1)$$

U_x and P_x must be expressed in the same units. This may seem obvious, but many laboratories report plasma creatinine concentrations in micromoles per litre and urinary creatinine concentrations in millimoles per litre.

GFR is equal to urinary clearance of that substance, provided that:

- it is freely filtered at the glomerulus, such that the concentration in the plasma is equal to the concentration in the glomerular filtrate;
- it is neither secreted nor reabsorbed by the tubules;
- it is neither metabolized nor synthesized by the kidneys;
- it is not bound to plasma protein, or, if it is, free and bound portions can be measured separately.

GFR also can be measured by total plasma clearance of a substance that fulfils the above criteria and:

- is not excreted by any route other than in the urine;
- is neither synthesized nor catabolized in the body.

The fructose polysaccharide inulin meets these criteria. In this situation,

$$GFR = (U_{in} \times V)P_{in} \qquad (51.2)$$

For day-to-day estimation of renal function, the plasma creatinine concentration gives an adequate guide to renal function. The usefulness of plasma creatinine can be enhanced considerably by using the following formula:

$$GFR \cong (height \times 40)/plasma \; creatinine \qquad (51.3)$$

where GFR is measured in millilitres per minute per $1.73 \, m^2$ body surface area and height is measured in centimetres.

It must be emphasized that this method has many pitfalls and gives only a very rough guide to GFR, which can be grossly overestimated in children with low muscle bulk. Further errors occur because of increased tubular secretion of creatinine. Hyperfiltration by remaining nephrons within damaged kidneys also can lead to an underestimate of the extent of renal damage but frequently contributes to progressive renal impairment.

For situations in which a more accurate estimation of renal function is required, GFR should be measured by one of the following methods:

INULIN CLEARANCE

Inulin clearance remains the gold standard for measurement of GFR. Inulin clearance is now seldom measured except in research situations, because it is cumbersome to perform and laboratory measurement of inulin is difficult.

PLASMA DISAPPEARANCE METHOD

This is the most commonly used method for measurement of GFR in clinical practice. If a bolus of a substance that fulfils all six of the criteria given above is given intravenously, then there is a brief period of redistribution, following which the plasma concentration decays exponentially at a rate dependent on GFR. Total plasma clearance (C), which equals GFR, is given by:

$$C = D/A$$

where D is the dose of the administered substance and A is the area under the decay curve.

The curve can be defined adequately by taking several timed blood samples. The dose is simple to measure, but A cannot be measured accurately, as the curve extends to infinity. Equations have been derived to address this difficulty, but a detailed discussion is beyond the scope of this chapter. Commonly used markers include ^{51}Cr-edetate calcium sodium (EDTA) and ^{99}Tm-diethylenetriamine-pentacetic acid (DTPA).

RENAL FAILURE

Acute renal failure

Acute renal failure is the sudden loss of renal function, resulting in elevated plasma concentrations of nitrogenous waste products, with or without a change in urine volume. In the UK, acute renal failure in children usually occurs in one of two situations: haemolytic uraemic syndrome and so-called 'acute tubular necrosis', with varying combinations of shock, sepsis and intoxication.

Haemolytic uraemic syndrome in Europe is commonly caused by infection with *Escherichia coli* strain O157 H7-producing Shiga-like toxin; in Africa and the Indian subcontinent, it is usually caused by infection with *Shigella dysenteriae* type 1. The toxin-producing organisms colonize the bowel and release toxin, whose toxin A subunit is absorbed into the endothelial cell, inactivates the 28s ribosomal subunit and inhibits protein synthesis, causing cell damage and death. Thrombosis within the glomerular capillary tuft follows, resulting in impaired glomerular perfusion and the classic triad of renal failure, microangiopathic haemolytic anaemia and thrombocytopenia.

Treatment is supportive, as there is no effective specific therapy. Acute mortality is less than two per cent in the UK. The majority (about 80 per cent) of patients will recover normal renal function, although some will show late deterioration due to hyperfiltration of surviving nephrons.

Acute tubular necrosis is usually due, at least in part, to impaired renal perfusion. Changes on renal biopsy tend to be subtle. Typically, there is loss of the proximal renal tubule brush border and flattening of the epithelium. Occasional mitotic figures may be seen in renal tubular epithelial cells, as surviving cells spread out and divide to replace those lost. Functionally, there is loss of the normal polarity of epithelial cells.

In children, acute hypotension due to haemorrhage or severe dehydration secondary to diarrhoea rarely causes renal failure severe enough to require dialysis, unless complicated by sepsis, hypernatraemia or nephrotoxins. In the majority of cases, renal failure is due to a combination of two or more of the following: low blood pressure, renal vasospasm caused by inotropic agents such as adrenaline, poor cardiac output, sepsis and the administration of nephrotoxic drugs.

Renal failure is oliguric in approximately 30 per cent of cases and non-oliguric in 70 per cent. Oliguria is usually defined as a urine flow rate of less than 1 mL/kg/hour and anuria as less than 0.5 mL/kg/hour. There is evidence that in non-oliguric renal failure, the renal insult is less severe, the prognosis is better and the patients are much easier to manage.

Management of acute renal failure is supportive. Loop diuretics such as furosemide (frusemide) sometimes can 'convert' oliguric to non-oliguric renal failure, but they have no effect on GFR. 'Renal doses' of dopamine (2–5 µg/kg/min) have been advocated to improve renal perfusion, but well-conducted studies in adults have shown no benefit in survival, time spent on dialysis, time spent in intensive care or time spent in hospital.

Management consists of maintaining fluid and electrolyte balance and ensuring adequate nutrition. Prescription of standard maintenance fluids in oliguric patients will result in fluid overload and pulmonary oedema but may result in dehydration in polyuric patients. Patients initially may be hypovolaemic or volume-overloaded. Initial fluid therapy should be potassium-free until plasma potassium is known to be low or normal with a source of potassium loss. Calculation of fluid losses should include insensible losses, urine output and other losses, such as nasogastric drainage, surgical drainage, fluid lost through burns and diarrhoea. Typical electrolyte concentrations of various body fluids are shown in Table 51.1.

Patients with acute renal failure are generally in a catabolic state, at least initially. Animal studies and uncontrolled human data suggest that adequate nutrition can significantly

Table 51.1 *Typical electrolyte content of body fluids*

Fluid	Na (mmol/L)	K (mmol/L)	Cl (mmol/L)
Gastric	60–90	5–20	100–150
Pancreatic	120–140	5–15	40–80
Bile	120–140	5–15	80–120
Small bowel	100–140	5–15	90–130
Ileostomy	45–135	5–15	20–115
Diarrhoea	10–90	10–80	10–110

improve outcome in children with renal failure. Nutritional therapy has three main goals in these patients:

- To provide sufficient protein and calories to minimize catabolism, limiting the rise of the plasma urea concentration.
- To limit potassium and phosphate intake.
- To avoid excessive fluid volume intake.

The traditional recommendation is for an intake of 1.5 g of protein per kilogram of body weight and a calorie intake that is 20–30 per cent higher than for resting energy expenditure, but even at this level of intake, most patients will be in negative nitrogen balance. Wherever possible, enteral nutrition is preferred over parenteral nutrition, partly because of the benefit of even small amounts of luminal nutrition in maintaining gut integrity.

If fluid and electrolyte balance cannot be achieved by conservative means, then some form of renal replacement therapy (RRT) will be necessary. Other indications for RRT include hyperkalaemia, other electrolyte and acid–base disorders unresponsive to conservative management and severe azotaemia. It is not possible to give succinct guidance on when to initiate RRT; consultation with an experienced nephrologist or intensivist is essential.

There are several options in terms of RRT, including peritoneal dialysis, intermittent haemodialysis, continuous venovenous haemofiltration (CVVH) and continuous venovenous haemodiafiltration (CVVHD). The advantages and disadvantages of these methods are summarized in Table 51.2.

CVVH is usually the treatment of choice in the intensive care environment.

Chronic renal failure

Chronic renal failure is a progressive and irreversible loss of renal function.

CAUSES

The causes of chronic renal failure differ between populations, according to both genetic and environmental factors. Table 51.3 shows the frequency of various diagnostic categories causing end-stage renal failure in children under 15 years of age in the UK.

CONSERVATIVE MANAGEMENT

Management of chronic renal failure aims to:

- minimize the deterioration in renal function;
- correct metabolic abnormalities caused by inadequate renal function.

Progression of renal failure can be retarded in several ways:

- Therapy with corticosteroids and other immunosuppressive therapy, such as cyclophosphamide.
- Tight control of blood pressure, as renal disease is often associated with hypertension, which in turn can cause renal damage.
- Inhibition of the renin–angiotensin–aldosterone system with angiotensin-converting enzyme inhibitors, particularly if used together with angiotensin II receptor blockers. This exerts a renoprotective effect in patients with proteinuric renal disease.

The normal GFR beyond infancy is 80–120 mL/min/ 1.73 m^2. There is little metabolic effect until the GFR falls below 50–60 mL/min/1.73 m^2. As the GFR falls below this point, the following features may be seen in varying combinations:

Acidosis
The metabolic acidosis of chronic renal failure is mainly due to inadequate hydrogen ion secretion in the cortical collecting duct. Acidosis exacerbates renal osteodystrophy and contributes to anorexia and growth failure. Treatment is usually with oral sodium bicarbonate in a dose titrated to maintain normal plasma bicarbonate values. The typical dose is 1–2 mmoL/kg/day.

Anaemia
This is due mainly to a failure of erythropoietin secretion by the kidney. However, anorexia may contribute by rendering the patient deficient in iron, folate, vitamin B12 and other essential building blocks for erythropoiesis. Anaemia can cause impaired effort tolerance and contributes to anorexia and cardiac hypertrophy. Treatment is by adequate nutritional rehabilitation and injections of erythropoietin.

Anorexia and vomiting
Acidosis, anaemia and high plasma urea concentrations (above about 20 mmol/L) all contribute to the causes of anorexia and vomiting. Anorexia may exacerbate high plasma urea concentrations by rendering the patient catabolic. There is frequently abnormal gastric motility, including delayed gastric emptying and gastro-oesophageal reflux. Plasma concentrations of cholecystokinin are elevated and contribute to a sensation of satiety. Poor nutrition contributes to growth failure and increased mortality. Poor feeding in a child with a chronic illness often causes great anxiety in the parents. This can easily lead to food forcing and food refusal, which exacerbate the problem.

Table 51.2 *Advantages and disadvantages of various methods of renal replacement therapy*

Method	Staff	Equipment	Fluid and solute removal	Comment
Peritoneal dialysis	Little training	Simple, inexpensive; peritoneal catheters susceptible to blockage and leaks	Slow, unpredictable; may not be adequate in highly catabolic patients	No haemodynamic instability or disequilibrium syndrome; may not be possible after abdominal surgery
Intermittent haemodialysis	Highly trained	Complex, expensive; large-calibre venous catheter required	Rapid, intermittent, easily controlled; adequate solute clearance may require daily or twice-daily therapy	Tolerated poorly in seriously sick children; risk of disequilibrium syndrome
CVVH, CVVHD	Highly trained	Complex, expensive; large-calibre venous catheters required	Slow, continuous, easily controlled; adequate fluid and solute removal usually easy to achieve	Well-tolerated, even in haemo-dynamically unstable patients

CVVH, continuous venovenous haemofiltration; CVVHD, continuous venovenous haemodiafiltration.

Table 51.3 *Causes of chronic end-stage renal failure in the UK*

Category	%
Renal dysplasia	28
Obstructive uropathy	19
Glomerulonephritis	18
Reflux nephropathy	6
Tubulo-interstitial disease	7
Congenital nephrotic syndrome	8
Vascular disorders	4
Metabolic disease and drug toxicity	5
Polycystic kidney disease	3
Malignancy	2

Children, especially those under five years of age, with chronic renal failure frequently require enteral feeding via a gastrostomy or nasogastric tube to achieve adequate nutrition. About 20–25 per cent will benefit from a fundoplication as well. These procedures ideally should be done well before starting peritoneal dialysis. If the patient is already on peritoneal dialysis, then an open gastrostomy can be performed safely, but percutaneous gastrostomies frequently are complicated by peritonitis, especially with *Candida* spp.

Hyperparathyroid bone disease

A reduction in renal function leads to impaired ability of the kidneys to regulate the plasma inorganic phosphate concentration. Two things then happen:

- High plasma phosphate concentrations stimulate parathyroid hormone (PTH) secretion and cause a decrease in the plasma calcium concentration.
- Decreased 1-alpha-hydroxylation of vitamin D also contributes to hypocalcaemia, and any reduction in plasma calcium further provokes increased PTH secretion.

Normally, PTH acts on the kidneys to increase urinary phosphate excretion and 1-alpha-hydroxylation of vitamin D, leading to increased gastrointestinal calcium absorption. Both of these responses are attenuated in renal failure. The only remaining pathway to maintain the extracellular calcium concentration is via the action on PTH on bone, where it promotes osteoclastic activity and resorption of bone. This leads to restoration of the plasma calcium concentration but causes a further increase in the plasma phosphate concentration. This sets up a vicious cycle, as high plasma phosphate directly stimulates PTH secretion.

Treatment plans include the control of plasma phosphate concentration by limiting dietary phosphate intake, using phosphate binders such as calcium carbonate with meals to reduce phosphate absorption, and giving vitamin D analogues such as alfacalcidol or calcitriol to bypass the impaired 1-alpha-hydroxylation. Care needs to be exercised to prevent hypercalcaemia, particularly in the presence of hyperphosphataemia, as this can easily lead to metastatic calcification.

Hyperkalaemia

Hyperkalaemia is seldom a problem until renal failure is very far advanced. However, potassium-sparing diuretics such as spironolactone, angiotensin-converting enzyme inhibitors, angiotensin II receptor blockers and beta-blockers can cause hyperkalaemia in the presence of moderate renal failure, especially if used in combination.

Hypertension

The major cause of hypertension in chronic renal failure is salt and water overload. In some patients, such as those with severely scarred kidneys, polycystic kidney disease or haemolytic uraemic syndrome, overactivity of the renin–angiotensin system may play an important role. Treatment is usually with antihypertensive drugs, but occasionally bilateral native nephrectomy is required.

Growth failure

Some children grow poorly in spite of adequate nutrition and control of the metabolic and physiological complications of chronic renal failure. Recombinant human growth hormone has been shown to be safe to use in these children. At least in the short to medium term, this is effective in increasing growth velocity, provided that the other factors impacting on growth have been addressed, but the effect on final adult height is still a matter of investigation.

Psychosocial factors

Chronic renal failure is an incurable life-threatening condition. Therapy is very demanding on both the patient and their family. It is important to remember that the greatest burden of management is borne by the patient and their family. This imposes significant disruption of normal routines and causes a good deal of stress within the family, and psychological support and counselling are essential. Treatment regimens should be structured to maximize compliance and to minimize hospital admissions and interference with school attendance. Explanations of the disease, the treatment and the likely outcomes must be clear and often have to be repeated. As far as possible, normal discipline should be maintained. The emotional needs of unaffected siblings must also be considered.

Salt wasting

This is particularly a problem of conditions such as dysplasia (including posterior urethral valves), nephronophthisis and sickle cell-associated renal disease, rather than glomerulonephritis. It is partly a consequence of hyperfiltration by surviving nephrons. This results in an increase in glomerular filtrate in the proximal tubule. Sodium is required for growth, so affected children may fail to thrive in spite of adequate calorie intake. Treatment is with sodium supplements. Sometimes, it is necessary to increase the dose until either hypertension or hypernatraemia occurs, and then to reduce the dose by 10–20 per cent.

DIALYSIS

The indications for starting dialysis therapy in children are not agreed universally. It is not possible to define a specific level of plasma urea or creatinine at which dialysis should be initiated. Rather, a variety of clinical and biochemical factors need to be considered. Ideally, dialysis should be started early enough to avoid malnutrition and uraemic symptoms. Dialysis is usually required when the creatinine clearance (not the GFR) falls below 9–13 mL/min/1.73 m^2.

Peritoneal dialysis

Peritoneal dialysis is the usual first-choice option for dialysis in children. The advantages include the fact that dialysis takes place over 24 hours per day for chronic ambulatory peritoneal dialysis (CAPD) or about ten hours per day for automated peritoneal dialysis (APD). Thus, fluid and solute removal proceeds almost continuously, allowing far fewer dietary and fluid restrictions. The relative simplicity and safety of peritoneal dialysis allow it to be done at home in all but the most exceptional circumstances, allowing the child on peritoneal dialysis to attend school and engage in other childhood activities. The greatest drawback with peritoneal dialysis is the ever-present risk of infection. Recurrent peritonitis is the single biggest cause of technique failure in children.

Peritoneal access for chronic dialysis is achieved via a surgically placed Tenckhoff catheter, a soft catheter usually with two Dacron cuffs. The distal cuff is placed just outside the peritoneum, usually buried within the rectus muscle. The catheter is then brought out through the skin via a subcutaneous tunnel, with the proximal cuff within the tunnel a few centimetres from the exit site. The exit site should point laterally or downwards, but never upwards, to prevent the accumulation of water or debris. Catheters with upward-pointing exit sites have twice the infection rate of those with downward-pointing exits. A large number of modifications of the original design have been tried. 'Swan-neck' catheters with a U-bend between the two cuffs have been shown to be superior in terms of infection risk to straight catheters.

The tip of the catheter should be free within the pelvis. In our unit, laparoscopically assisted insertion of Tenckhoff catheters has proven very useful to ensure correct placement and freedom from entanglement with bowel loops or omentum. Trials comparing straight-tipped with curled catheters have not shown a definite advantage for either design. Some surgeons routinely perform an omentectomy at the time of catheter insertion, but others do not. Those outcome data that do exist do not show a clear benefit for either approach. The main complications of Tenckhoff catheters are infection (exit-site infection, tunnel infection, peritonitis), blockage (usually with omentum) and leaking.

Haemodialysis

Vascular access for haemodialysis is usually via a central venous catheter for the following reasons:

- The vessel size in small children makes the formation of a fistula technically difficult and any such fistula is highly likely to thrombose.
- Repeated needling of a fistula may cause psychological problems in young children.
- The waiting times for dialysis in the UK are much lower for children than for adults.

Native arteriovenous fistulae are usually reserved for adolescents who have become sensitized to large numbers of tissue antigens and therefore are likely to have a long wait for a donor organ.

The site of choice for a haemodialysis central venous catheter is the internal jugular vein. The subclavian vein should be avoided because it is more likely to develop stenosis, potentially making the later creation of an arteriovenous fistula impossible in that arm. The tip of the catheter should lie within the right atrium. This is because the high blood flow rates (typically eight to ten per cent of total blood volume per minute) required for haemodialysis are difficult to achieve if the catheter is in a vein. The most important complications of haemodialysis central venous catheters are infection and blockage.

Home haemodialysis is used increasingly in adults, as it is cost-effective and allows a more normal lifestyle in suitable patients. In children, haemodialysis usually is performed in hospital. This is because extracorporeal blood volume and blood flow rates are a much greater proportion of total blood volume in children, who therefore tend to be more haemodynamically unstable and require greater nursing supervision.

Haemodialysis requires three sessions per week of three to four hours per session. Thus, there is a large impact on lifestyle and quality of life. There are also relatively infrequent but abrupt fluid and electrolyte shifts that require much tighter regulation of fluid and electrolyte intake than is necessary with peritoneal dialysis. For these reasons, haemodialysis is usually reserved for patients in whom peritoneal dialysis is impractical or has failed.

PAEDIATRIC RENAL TRANSPLANTATION

The results of paediatric renal transplantation have improved considerably over the past two decades. Transplantation in children is now being considered as the best replacement therapy in children with end-stage renal disease (ESRD), due to improvement in children's survival, graft survival and quality of life. The establishment of specialized nephrology units dealing with children with ESRD has been supported and encouraged by advancement in immune suppression, improvement in surgical techniques of renal transplantation, urologist involvement in correction of underlying causes, and preparation of the abnormal bladder before receiving the transplanted ureter.

There is a great reluctance to recognize that renal transplantation in children is different from that in adults. In a study of 4329 transplants recorded between 1987 and 1996, obstructive uropathy, renal dysplasia and hypoplasia were the underlying cause in 32 per cent of cases, vesicoureteric reflux in 5.7 per cent and prune belly syndrome in 2.9 per cent (Benfield et al. 1999).

Pretransplantation evaluation

General evaluation is mandatory for each case. Every effort should be made to minimize the complications of renal insufficiency in order to improve the general health of the child before transplantation:

- Correction of anaemia using erythropoietin has reduced the need for packed red-cell transfusion and obviated the risk of transfusion-related infections.
- Correction of osteodystrophy with phosphate binders and activated vitamin D should be considered.
- Correction of growth retardation with aggressive calorie supplements. Some children may require nasogastric

tube feeding or gastrostomy feeding. Growth hormone should be given to children whose weight is under the fifth centile for age.

A pretransplantation urological evaluation is now considered of utmost importance, including the following:

- History of urological problems: voiding dysfunction, urinary tract infection, obstructive uropathy, vesicoureteric reflux, stones, previous surgery on the urinary tract.
- Presence of a scar from a previous operation, a stoma-diverted urinary tract or an abdominal catheter, e.g. gastrostomy tube may interfere with the site of transplantation. Urine culture, renal ultrasound, post-voiding bladder ultrasound to detect the amount of residual urine and a voiding cystourethrogram may be necessary to assess bladder capacity, the state of the bladder neck and the patency of the urethra. This may be coupled with urodynamics and cystourethroscopy. Patients with urinary tract diversion or a continent pouch may require retrograde studies, intravenous urogram and magnetic resonance imaging (MRI) urography to assess the suitability of the pouch for the transplanted ureter.
- Pretransplantation nephrectomy: bilateral nephrectomies may be considered before transplantation in cases of uncontrolled hypertension, persistent or recurrent renal infection, renal calculi (calcular pyonephrosis), severe proteinuria and acquired cystic renal disease with tumours. Bilateral nephrectomies may be performed at the time of renal transplantation.

Screening for suitability

When screening for donor suitability, the ABO group (the donor should be ABO-compatible with the recipient) and the human leucocyte antigen (HLA) system are the most important factors determining suitability. Over 50 per cent of transplanted kidneys have been from living donors, mostly family members; however, living unrelated donors should be considered.

There are a number of advantages of living related donor kidneys, including the following:

- Improved graft survival compared with cadaver donor kidneys.
- The waiting list for renal transplantation is increasing steadily, and the patient may wait for a long time for a cadaver kidney. Using a live related donor shortens the waiting time and the transplant can be planned accordingly.

There are, however, a number of risks with living related donors. Reported mortality in donors is 0.025 per cent. Mild and serious morbidity are reported to be 17 and 2.5 per cent, respectively.

Laparoscopic donor nephrectomy has reduced the morbidity, improved postoperative recovery and shortened the length of hospital stay.

Contraindications to transplantation

In very young children with ESRD, it is generally accepted that transplantation should be delayed because of the reported poor outcome in children under the age of two years. In patients under the age of one year at transplantation, graft and patient survival are poor, especially with cadaver kidney, and this has discouraged transplant surgeons to operate on this age group.

Immune suppression has discouraged transplantation in human immunodeficiency virus (HIV)-positive children who develop ESRD. A history of malignancy is an absolute contraindication, with the possible exception of Wilms tumour, when the patient may be transplanted after one year when the child is considered cured and free of the disease. Multiorgan disease, including in children with neurological impairment, is a relative contraindication, but cases should be discussed individually for suitability of possible transplantation. Down syndrome is not considered a contraindication.

Kidney preservation

The donor kidney is usually preserved by cold storage after flushing with ice-cold high-concentration potassium solution. Heparin 30 units/kg is injected intravenously before application of arterial clamps, followed by low-dose heparin 5–10 units/kg intravenously for three to five days postoperatively (one of the common complications in children is vascular thrombosis). It is important to minimize warm ischaemia time to preserve the renal vessels and the blood supply to the ureter.

Operative procedure of renal transplantation

The patient lies in a supine position. Under general anaesthesia, a central venous catheter for venous pressure monitoring and an arterial line for administration of fluids, drugs, transfusion and blood sampling are inserted. The skin of the abdomen and genital area is prepared with antiseptic solution, and a Foley catheter is inserted into the bladder.

An extraperitoneal approach is possible in children weighing more than 20 kg. The renal vascular anastomosis is determined after placing the kidney graft in the wound to assess the best position for the vascular anastomosis. The renal artery is usually anastomosed first; the left kidney is usually transplanted in the right iliac fossa.

In small children with a large transplanted kidney, a transperitoneal approach is appropriate. The renal artery is anastomosed to the lower aorta or common iliac artery and the renal vein to the interior vena cava or common iliac vein.

For ureteroneocystostomy, an extravesical technique is preferred rather than a transvesical technique, because less ureteric length is required and a separate cystostomy is not required.

Advantages of renal transplantation

Renal transplantation:

- avoids long periods of dialysis;
- reduces the need for vascular access;
- overcomes malnutrition;
- heals renal osteodystrophy;
- promotes linear growth;
- improves life expectancy and quality of life for all groups of patients, regardless of the cause of renal failure (Wolfe et al. 1999).

Outcome of renal transplants

Factors affecting the outcome of renal transplants include:

- cadaver versus live donor;
- age of the donor and the recipient;
- HLA matching;
- immunosuppression (post-ciclosporin);
- underlying disease;
- compliance.

Long-term outcome of allografts is improving steadily. A report from the European Dialysis Transplant Association paediatric registry indicated that 91 per cent of transplanted children were attending school (Donckerwolcke et al. 1980). Transplanted children and their families were found to return to their pre-illness psychological and social equilibrium within one year after transplantation when the transplant was successful (Fine et al. 1977).

Allograft survival at five years does not guarantee continued allograft function. It is estimated that live donor graft survival at five years ranges from 55 to 73 per cent. However, cadaver kidney graft survival ranges from 39 to 43 per cent.

In December 2001, 6101 patients were waiting for renal transplantation in the UK (Transplant Activity Report 2000). The waiting list tends to grow by about three per cent each year.

RECENT DEVELOPMENTS

- The outcome of renal transplantation has improved to more than 88 per cent for cadaver kidney and 95 per cent for live donor graft.
- Renal transplantation improves survival in all age groups.
- There is more use of live donor grafts.
- Laparoscopic nephrectomy minimizes morbidity in living related donors.

PROBLEMS TO BE RESOLVED

- Inadequate supply of donor organs.
- Side effects of treatment (immunosuppression, malignancy).

An abnormal lower urinary tract is not a contraindication to transplantation. In children with obstructive uropathy, corrective procedures could be performed and the bladder could be utilized without significant complication, even in some cases of defunctionalized bladder due to early diversion. If the bladder is not suitable, then an ileal conduit or a non-refluxing colon conduit could be utilized.

Detrusor instability and detrusor sphincter dyssynergia increase the risk of urinary tract infection, vesicoureteric reflux and failure of anti-reflux surgery. These children would require treatment with anticholinergic drugs, adequate bladder drainage or sometimes even auto-augmentation or ileocystoplasty in preparation for transplantation.

Complications of transplantation

Technical complications occur in 13 per cent of transplantation procedures (35 per cent resulting in graft loss). Urological complications occur in 5.6 per cent; these include urinary leakage, urethral anastomosis stenosis, ureteral necrosis and symptomatic vesicoureteric reflux (31 per cent resulting in graft loss).

Renal vascular complications occur in 5.5 per cent, of which 3.2 per cent are due to technical reasons (renal artery stenosis, renal artery thrombosis, renal vein thrombosis). Renal artery and vein thrombosis result in a high incidence of graft loss. Wound complications occur in 4.2 per cent (primary lymphocele, haemorrhage, infection).

Complications of treatment

Patients who have been immunosuppressed may develop malignancy: skin cancer, lymphoma, Kaposi sarcoma and proliferative disorders have been reported.

IMMUNOSUPPRESSION

There is no universally accepted regimen for either the prevention of rejection or for its treatment when present. Several anti-rejection drugs are in routine use and several others are being developed or are undergoing clinical trials. Most protocols include steroids, a calcineurin inhibitor (ciclosporin, tacrolimus) and an antiproliferative agent (azathioprine, mycophenolate). Other agents coming into use are monoclonal interleukin 2 (IL-2) receptor antibodies and sirolimus. Each class of agent blocks a different aspect of the immune response.

Steroids have major effects on T-cell function by decreasing T-cell receptor expression as well as reducing expression of cell-surface adhesion molecules. T-cell receptors enable T-lymphocytes to recognize foreign antigens presented by antigen-presenting cells. They also prevent mitogen- and antigen-induced T-cell proliferation and inhibit gene transcription and the secretion of various cytokines, including the cytokines interleukin 1 (IL-1), IL-2, interleukin 6 (IL-6) and tumour necrosis factor (TNF). They also decrease cytotoxic activity of natural killer (NK) cells and antigen-specific cytotoxic lymphocytes. Corticosteroids have many important

side effects, including obesity, impaired glucose tolerance, hypertension, myopathy and behavioural changes. The lowest dose compatible with the desired clinical outcome should always be used.

Ciclosporin and tacrolimus are structurally unrelated compounds that prevent the activation of calcineurin within the cytoplasm of T-cells. The net result is that these agents block the IL-2-dependent growth and differentiation of T-cells. While the introduction of ciclosporin in the early 1980s made a big difference to one-year graft survival, there has been no effect on ten-year graft survival. Both drugs have a narrow therapeutic index, and careful monitoring of blood levels is required. Major side effects include nephrotoxicity, hypertension, seizures and, in the case of ciclosporin, gum hyperplasia.

Azathioprine and mycophenolate mofetil act as inhibitors of purine synthesis and therefore prevent the lymphoid proliferation associated with rejection. Both may cause leucopenia and thrombocytopenia. Mycophenolate mofetil frequently causes gastrointestinal upsets.

Monoclonal IL-2 receptor antibodies have been introduced into clinical practice. They are used as induction agents, given early in the postoperative course. They are effective in reducing the incidence of acute rejection in the first 6–12 months, but they are not effective in reversing established rejection episodes.

Sirolimus inhibits calcium-independent and calcium-dependent transduction of signals delivered by IL-2, interleukin 4 (IL-4), interleukin 7 (IL-7) and interleukin 15 (IL-15), therefore exerting multiple effects on T-cell maturation. It acts synergistically with ciclosporin. *In vitro* studies suggest an antagonistic effect when used with tacrolimus, but *in vivo* studies have suggested a more than additive effect. Common side effects include thrombocytopenia, leucopenia and hyperlipidaemia.

A variety of anti-lymphocyte preparations is available. A murine monoclonal anti-CD3 antibody and a polyclonal anti-thymocyte globulin are used for induction therapy of highly sensitized individuals and for rescue therapy for steroid-resistant rejection. These drugs may result in chills, fever and arthralgia due to the large load of foreign protein. Thrombocytopenia and leucopenia are not uncommon. The incidence of post-transplant lymphoproliferative disease (PTLD), cytomegalovirus (CMV) infection and other opportunistic infections is increased with increasingly aggressive immunosuppression.

REJECTION

Hyperacute rejection occurs when the recipient has preformed alloantibodies induced by previous blood transfusions, pregnancy or organ transplants against the donor tissue antigens. These antibodies bind to endothelial cells, causing rapid and irreversible necrosis within minutes to hours after reperfusion of the graft. Graft nephrectomy is invariably required. Hyperacute rejection is very rare, as a direct cross-match between recipient serum and donor lymphocytes is performed routinely. Modern cross-matching techniques, such as flow cytometry, can detect minute amounts of preformed antibodies.

Despite modern immunosuppressive medication, acute rejection remains a significant problem. Although most problematic in the early post-transplant period, it can occur at any time. The classic presentation of acute rejection with fever, graft tenderness, oliguria and proteinuria are now not specific and have become infrequent with the use of modern immunosuppression. In practice, acute rejection is suspected when there is an abrupt increase in plasma creatinine concentration of ten per cent or more. A number of causes other than rejection can produce an abrupt decline in renal function. These include drug toxicity, especially with calcineurin inhibitors, volume depletion, acute tubular necrosis, urinary obstruction, lymphocoele, urine leak and recurrence of the primary disease.

Ultrasound imaging with calculation of the resistive index can exclude many of these causes and provide supportive evidence of rejection. Fine-needle aspiration cytology is used for confirmation by some centres, but core biopsy of the graft remains the gold standard for the diagnosis of acute rejection. Core biopsy is also the only reliable means of diagnosing recurrence of the primary disease and is important in the diagnosis of calcineurin inhibitor toxicity. Given the serious consequences of very heavy immunosuppression, biopsy before treatment seems justified.

Treatment of acute rejection is usually with high-dose steroids. In the first six months following transplantation, these are given intravenously. Commonly used regimens consist of methylprednisolone 10–15 mg/kg/day for three to five days. Increasing the dose of calcineurin inhibitor or switching from ciclosporin to tacrolimus or from azathioprine to mycophenolate may be necessary. Antibody therapy with the anti-CD3 antibody OKT3 or with anti-thymocyte globulin may reverse steroid-resistant rejection but carries a high price in terms of severe immunosuppression and the risk of both infections and later malignancy.

Chronic rejection is understood poorly. Clinically, it manifests as slowly progressive deterioration of renal function. About five per cent of grafts are lost per year through chronic rejection. Immune attack, drug toxicity, hypertension, hyperlipidaemia and other factors may contribute to renal damage.

OPPORTUNISTIC INFECTION

The renal transplant recipient may suffer from any or all of the infections to which the immunocompetent host is susceptible. Common infections frequently have more severe consequences unless they are treated early and aggressively. Several organisms cause few problems in immunocompetent hosts but are a major cause of morbidity and even mortality in transplant hosts.

Viruses
CMV disease typically occurs four to ten weeks after transplantation. The biggest risk factor is CMV positivity of the donor. It increases the risk of other infections such as *Pneumocystis carinii* pneumonia and can trigger acute rejection. Treatment is usually with ganciclovir intravenously for two to four weeks.

Epstein–Barr virus (EBV) infection may cause a mononucleosis syndrome. The most important complication is the development of PTLD (see below).

All transplant recipients should be screened for varicella antibodies and immunized preoperatively if antibodies are not detected. Cutaneous zoster is about ten times more common in transplant recipients than in the general population. Much more serious is the occurrence of chickenpox. This can be devastating in transplant patients. Complications include pneumonia, encephalitis, hepatitis, pancreatitis and disseminated intravascular coagulation. Patients who develop chickenpox should be treated with intravenous aciclovir 10 mg/kg every eight hours for seven to ten days.

Polyoma virus is usually acquired in childhood and remains latent in the kidney. Following transplant, reactivation may occur, causing interstitial nephritis, fibrosis and progressive deterioration of renal function. A reduction in immunosuppression may stabilize graft function.

Bacteria
Urinary tract infections, pneumonia and sepsis syndrome are the most common bacterial infections in transplant recipients. The spectrum of urinary tract organisms is similar to that in community-acquired infection, but infections are more likely to be hospital-acquired and drug-resistant. *Streptococcus pneumoniae, E. coli, Pseudomonas aeruginosa, Klebsiella pneumoniae* and *Staphylococcus aureus* are the most common causes of pneumonia and septicaemia.

Other organisms
P. carinii pneumonia is a frequent complication in severely immunosuppressed patients. Many centres use co-trimoxazole prophylaxis, but there is no agreement on either the necessity for this or the optimum duration of treatment. Diagnosis rests on the demonstration of the causal organism, usually on broncho-alveolar lavage. Treatment is with high-dose co-trimoxazole or pentamidine.

Infection with fungi such as *Aspergillus* spp., *Histoplasma capsulatum, Coccidiodes immitis* and *Cryptococcus neoformans* may occur in a variety of sites, including the lungs, brain and abdomen. The mortality from these infections is extremely high. Survival depends on early diagnosis, aggressive therapy and the ability to reduce immunosuppression.

MALIGNANCY

Cancer is ten times more common in children who have received a kidney transplant than in the general population. Twenty-five years after starting dialysis or having a transplant, about 17 per cent of patients will have developed cancer. The majority of malignancies occur more than ten years after transplantation. The most common form of cancer in transplant patients is non-melanoma skin cancer, which accounts for about 50 per cent of cases and is more than 200 times more common in renal transplant recipients than in the general population. Most cases of skin cancer in children who have received kidney transplants do not occur until adulthood.

The second most common malignancy is non-Hodgkin's lymphoma, including PTLD, which accounts for about 25 per cent of all cancers in these patients. PTLD is usually caused by a combination of immunosuppression and infection with EBV, although only a small proportion of patients who get EBV infection will get PTLD. Patients who get EBV infection after their transplant are more likely to get PTLD than those who have had EBV infection before the transplant. Gradual reduction of the immunosuppressive drug dosages can cure some cases of PTLD. In many cases, this can be done without losing the graft. The remaining cancers that occur in children who have had transplants can affect any part of the body.

Disease recurrence and *de novo* nephritis

Recurrence of the primary renal disease in the paediatric transplant recipient is uncommon. Perhaps the most important of these is focal segmental glomerulosclerosis (FSGS). At present, it is almost impossible to predict which patients will have a recurrence. Those with a rapid progression to ESRD, and those with the best HLA matching of the donor kidney (including living related transplant recipients), have the greatest risk of recurrence. Approximately 25 per cent of patients develop a recurrence in the first graft. Second grafts in patients who had a recurrence in the first graft have an 85 per cent recurrence risk. Recurrence in FSGS is typically early, with massive proteinuria developing within days of the transplant. Median graft survival in untreated patients is reduced to about five months. There is no universally accepted treatment, but intensive immunosuppression combined with plasmapheresis has been successful in several cases. The response is best in patients treated early.

Other diseases with a significant risk of recurrence include membranoproliferative glomerulonephritis and non-diarrhoea-associated haemolytic uraemic syndrome.

CLINICAL SCENARIOS

Case 1

A male infant was born at term to a healthy mother. Routine antenatal ultrasound scans had shown no abnormality. At one week of age, the child was noted to have deep rapid breathing. A blood test revealed metabolic acidosis, with a plasma creatinine of 250 µmol/L, sodium of 130 mmol/L and potassium of 4.0 mmol/L. An ultrasound scan showed normal-sized kidneys with no corticomedullary differentiation.

He was managed conservatively, with sodium bicarbonate and sodium chloride supplements. By six months of age, his plasma creatinine concentration was 60 mmol/L. He was feeding and thriving well.

Antenatal ultrasound at 20 weeks misses a significant number of urinary tract abnormalities. Dysplastic kidneys may be of normal size, and typically these are missed on antenatal ultrasound. Significant maturation of renal function may occur, even in infants with severe dysplasia.

Case 2

A 13-year-old girl received a renal transplant from a CMV-positive donor. Six weeks later, she developed abdominal pain and diarrhoea. Her plasma creatinine concentration rose from 65 µmol/L to 120 µmol/L. Her tacrolimus blood level was 11 µg/L. A renal biopsy showed no evidence of rejection. The CMV polymerase chain reaction (PCR) was strongly positive.

The tacrolimus dose was reduced to achieve a trough level of 6–7 µg/L and she was treated with intravenous ganciclovir for two weeks. The renal function returned to baseline levels, and the CMV PCR became negative.

Acute graft dysfunction has many causes, including infection obstruction, rejection and drug toxicity. Careful evaluation is necessary: increasing the anti-rejection therapy in this child because of an assumed diagnosis of rejection would have made the situation worse.

REFERENCES

Benfield MR, McDonald R, Sullivan EK, *et al.* The 1997 Annual Renal Transplantation in Children Report of the North American Pediatric Renal Transplantation Cooperative Study (NAPRTCS). *Pediatric Transplantation* 1999; **3**: 152–67.

Donckerwolcke RA, Chantler C, Broyer M, *et al.* Combined report on regular dialysis and transplantation of children in Europe, 1979. *Proceedings of the European Dialysis and Transplant Association* 1980; **17**: 87–115.

Fine RN, Edelbrock HH, Riddell H, *et al.* Renal transplantation in children. *Urology* 1977; **9**: 61–71.

Transplant Activity Report 2000. www.uktransplant.org.uk/b2dasp

Wolfe RA, Ashby VB, Milford EL, *et al.* Comparison of mortality of all patients on dialysis, patients on dialysis awaiting transplantation and recipients of a first cadaver transplant. *New England Journal of Medicine* 1999; **341**: 1725–30.

FURTHER READING

Hinman F, Jr. Renal construction: renal transplantation in children. In: Hinman F, Jr (ed.). *Atlas of Urologic Surgery*, 2nd edn. Philadelphia, PA: WB Saunders; pp. 962–3.

52

Urinary tract infection and vesicoureteric reflux

SRINIVASAN R BABU AND HENRIK A STEINBRECHER

Learning objectives

- To understand what a urinary tract infection is.
- To understand the natural history of urinary tract infection and vesicoureteric reflux.
- To understand how to investigate and manage a urinary tract infection.
- To understand the management options available in the treatment of vesicoureteric reflux.

INTRODUCTION

Despite the advances in antenatal diagnosis, urinary tract infection (UTI) still continues to be a common way in which a child with a urological abnormality presents. Approximately five per cent of girls and 1.5 per cent of boys develop symptoms of UTI during childhood. Compared with adults, children with UTI are more likely to have an underlying urinary tract abnormality and are more likely to suffer renal damage. Around 30–50 per cent of children investigated for UTI have an underlying (refluxing or obstructive) urinary pathology. The presentation is often atypical in children. The diagnosis and management of UTI in children needs a systematic approach, which, in essence centres on the prevention of the serious long-term consequences of UTI, such as renal scarring, hypertension and renal failure. Understanding the pathogenesis of UTI and the interplay between host and organism factors is of paramount importance in the investigation and management of these children.

PATHOGENESIS

The balance between host factors and bacterial factors plays a major role in development of UTI (Table 52.1). It is essential to understand this, as identifying the factor involved in the aetiopathogenesis could help in the management.

Host factors

The mechanical factors that interfere with rapid clearance of organism include any impediment to urine flow, such as obstruction, stasis or reflux. Dysfunctional voiding, constipation and periurethral bacterial colonization are well-established factors that increase the incidence of UTI. Koff's complex is a vicious cycle of UTI, vesicoureteric reflux (VUR) and dysfunctional voiding and needs to be interrupted to achieve resolution of recurrent UTIs. The higher incidence of UTIs in uncircumcised boys during the first few months of life has been attributed to foreskin and prepucial colonization.

Table 52.1 *Pathogenesis of urinary tract infection (UTI)*

Host factors	Organism factors
Urine stasis (obstruction, reflux)	Bacterial virulence
Dysfunctional voiding, constipation	Fimbriated strains (e.g. *E. coli*)
Urethral, perineal and prepucial colonization	
Native immunity, urinary IgA, breastfeeding	
P blood group phenotype (more prone to having a UTI)	

E. coli, *Escherichia coli*; IgA, immunoglobulin A.

Individuals with P blood group phenotype have been shown to have increased susceptibility to UTIs due to the P blood group antigen acting as a receptor for bacterial P-fimbriae. Native immunity, urinary immunoglobulin A (IgA) and breastfeeding may have an influence in reducing the incidence of UTI. The type and extent of faecal colonization have indirect consequences on periurethral and perineal colonization.

Organism factors

Escherichia coli is the causative organism in more than 80 per cent of cases. Receptors for P-fimbriae are present on urothelial cells and renal tubular cells. Bacterial virulence and the ability of fimbriated forms of *E. coli* to adhere to the urinary tract lining are important factors in determining the occurrence of a UTI. P-fimbriated *E. coli* are also more likely to induce febrile reactions, due to increased urinary interleukin 6 (IL-6) response.

CLINICAL PRESENTATION

It is essential to differentiate between upper UTI (pyelonephritis) and lower UTI (cystitis), as this aids in planning the extent of investigation. Therefore, the history-taking and examination should centre on these. Upper-tract symptoms often include fever, rigor, vomiting and being systemically unwell. Renal involvement should be suspected in the presence of a high-grade fever exceeding 38 °C and rigors during infancy. Isolated loin pain is suggestive of unilateral obstructive renal pathology.

Symptoms of lower-tract infection (cystitis) include frequency, dysuria, pain and secondary enuresis. Although older children sometimes report these classic symptoms, often the presentation is one of perineal irritation or stinging on voiding, which can present as crying episodes during voiding. In infancy, the symptoms are not typical and often the parents report cloudy foul-smelling urine, although this is not always indicative of a UTI. Children with lower UTI are generally

---

Box 52.1 History in a child presenting with urinary tract infection (UTI)

Upper UTI symptoms

High-grade fever (>38 °C)
Rigors
Vomiting
Malaise, systemically unwell
Central/loin pain

Lower UTI symptoms

Dysuria
Frequency, urgency, urge incontinence
Nocturia, enuresis
Suprapubic pain, perineal irritation
Epididymo-orchitis

History to look into underlying aetiological factors

Constipation (pain, stool consistency, stool frequency)
Bladder instability (frequency, urgency)
Dysfunctional voiding (holding, straining, Vincent's curtsey sign)
Toileting habits (position, wiping post-void)
Infrequent voiding
Drinking history (quantity, quality), bladder stimulants (caffeine, blackcurrant)
Bathing habits (bubble-baths, shampoo before bath)
Family/social history

---

systemically well and often do not require hospitalization. Haematuria can occur due to haemorrhagic cystitis or urethritis. In boys, UTI can present as epididymo-orchitis. Box 52.1 summarizes the detailed history required in a child presenting with UTI.

DIAGNOSIS

When considering referrals for a 'proven UTI', it is important to establish the nature of specimen collection and ascertain the details of the actual culture report. Immediate transport of a fresh sample is crucial for a reliable result. Methods used to prevent the growth of contaminants include immediate chilling to 4 °C and later transfer in a cooled container. The various collection methods, in the order of least to most reliable to diagnose UTI, include collection bags, urine pads, clean catch, catheter sample and suprapubic aspiration (Table 52.2).

In the emergency setting, four determinants in urine analysis can be supportive of UTI (Table 52.3): microscopy for white cells, microscopy for bacteria, urinary leucocyte esterase and urinary nitrite. A significant pyuria includes a white cell count over 5×10^6 in boys and over 40×10^6 in

Table 52.2 *Methods of urine collection*

Per-urethral	Bladder	From upper tract
Midstream or clean catch	Suprapubic aspiration	Ureteric/ nephrostomy
Perineal bag	Suprapubic catheter	
Urine pads		
Catheter		

Table 52.3 *Diagnosis of urinary tract infection based on urine analysis*

Urine microscopy	Urine dipstick
For white cells (pyuria)	Leucocyte esterase
For bacteria	Nitrite

Table 52.4 *Culture criteria for diagnosis of urinary tract infection*

Method of collection	Count (pure culture)	Probability (%)
Suprapubic aspiration	Gram-negative bacilli (any number)	>99
	Gram-positive cocci	>1000
Catheterization	>10^5	95
	10^4–10^5	Likely
	10^3–10^4	Suspicious
	<10^3	Unlikely
Clean catch	>10^5 (two specimens)	90
	>10^5 (one specimen)	>80
	10^4–10^5	Suspicious
	<10^4	Unlikely

girls. Microscopic identification of bacteria in urine is more sensitive in detecting UTI than pyuria.

Urine leucocyte esterase detects breakdown products of white cells and is negative in the absence of pyuria. The nitrite test measures dietary nitrates, which are reduced to nitrite by Gram-negative bacteria. However, this takes several hours of bacterial reduction and is, therefore, useful only on the first morning-voided specimen. Most Gram-positive bacteria do not reduce nitrates, thereby providing a false-negative response. A combination of urinary nitrites and leucocyte esterase provides a high sensitivity and specificity to diagnose UTI in the emergency setting.

The accepted definition for diagnosis of UTI is a pure growth of more than 10^5 organisms per millilitre on culture. When the results are equivocal (insignificant colony count, mixed growth, unconventional pathogens), one should first investigate the nature of collection, as this could be the result of bag specimens or urethral specimens when there is colonization (Table 52.4). Not infrequently do parents confess to having collected the urine from a potty. If there is an equivocal

result in the presence of strong clinical suspicion, then a suprapubic sample often helps, as any growth on suprapubic aspirate is considered significant. Suprapubic aspiration ideally is done under ultrasound guidance to ensure a full bladder and avoid damage to viscera or vessels.

FURTHER INVESTIGATIONS

The aims of radiological investigations in children with UTI are twofold: (i) to identify underlying anatomical or functional abnormality (e.g. obstruction, reflux), and (ii) to assess the extent of upper-tract pathology (function, scarring). Clinical variables, such as family history, presence of febrile UTI, recurrent UTIs, age and gender, historically are used to plan the extent of investigation, although they have poor correlation with the presence of an underlying abnormality. In 1991, the Royal College Paediatrics and Child Health guidelines recommended that:

- all children should have an ultrasound scan of the urinary tract, and an abdominal X-ray;
- all children under seven years of age should have a dimercaptosuccinic acid (DMSA) scan;
- all children under one year of age should have a micturating cystourethrogram (MCUG).

More recent studies have shown that DMSA scanning has a low yield of positive results if a child is over one year of age, and that there is no evidence of any impact on change in management in the age group of one to seven years. It has been recommended that DMSA scanning could be omitted in children over one year of age with a first simple UTI and not sufficiently ill to be admitted to hospital. This would result in a more simplified approach to investigation of children with UTI:

- In children up to one year of age: ultrasound, MCUG and DMSA scan.
- In children over one year of age: ultrasound only (DMSA scan only if systemically unwell).

The timing of the investigations after UTI is worth mentioning. An ultrasonogram is useful in acute scenarios to exclude obstructive lesions. An MCUG should be done after complete recovery of a UTI with prophylaxis. An early DMSA scan often gives false results due to pyelonephritis and is best delayed to two to three months after UTI to identify scarring. A local departmental policy often helps to prevent over or under-investigation of these children. Table 52.5 summarizes the guidelines at Southampton General Hospital, Southampton, UK, to investigate children with UTI.

TREATMENT

In an emergency situation, a positive urine analysis in the presence of clinical symptoms can be considered a valid reason

Table 52.5 *Investigation of a child with a urinary tract infection (UTI) at Southampton General Hospital, Southampton, UK*

Age under two years	USS: early to exclude obstructive lesion MCUG: timing depends on USS; early if obstructive uropathy suspected; if reflux suspected, wait until six months or/and free of infection DMSA scan: two to three months after UTI to detect scarring
Age two to five years	USS: early to exclude obstructive lesion DMSA scan: two to three months after UTI to detect scarring (Indirect cystogram if DMSA scan shows scarring or in presence of recurrent UTI or family history of reflux)
Age over five years	USS: pre- and post-micturition (DMSA scan only if pyelonephritis suspected)

DMSA, dimercaptosuccinic acid; MCUG, micturating cystourethrogram; USS, ultrasound scan.

to start antibiotic treatment. In any case, once diagnosed, a UTI should be treated promptly with antibiotics. The route of administration depends on the severity of infection and age. Intravenous antibiotics (aminoglycosides, co-amoxiclav, cephalosporin) are preferred in infants or older children with systemic symptoms and pyrexia. In cooperative older children with reliable parents, outpatient therapy with oral antibiotics is possible.

Systematic reviews have shown that a shorter course (two to four days) of oral antibiotics is as effective as 7–14 days of treatment in eradicating lower UTI in children. However, the duration of treatment for an upper UTI is still seven to ten days.

Following treatment of an acute UTI, the child should be maintained on prophylaxis until appropriate radiological evaluation is completed. Antibiotics commonly used for prophylaxis include trimethoprim, nitrofurantoin, amoxicillin and cefalexin.

It is essential to manage appropriately constipation and voiding dysfunction and also to address issues that promote colonization (toilet/bathing/drinking habits). Eating bio-yoghurts has been shown to be beneficial in altering gastrointestinal flora. Box 52.2 summarizes the aspects of medical management.

Treatment of asymptomatic bacteriuria is controversial. It is now recommended that school-age children with asymptomatic bacteriuria should not be treated with antibiotics, as they are not at increased risk of impaired renal growth or deterioration in renal function when untreated. The practice of taking urine samples regularly to check for bacteriuria in an asymptomatic child is usually completely unnecessary and can raise anxiety levels in parents dramatically.

Box 52.2 Medical management of urinary tract infection (UTI)

Appropriate treatment of acute UTI
Prompt investigation following UTI
Low-dose antibiotic prophylaxis
Explain rationale to parents (ensure compliance)
Management of other predisposing factors:
- reduce residual volume: regular, frequent, complete/double voiding;
- correction of constipation;
- drink at regular intervals, avoid irritants (caffeine, blackcurrant);
- discourage disinfectants, shampoos and surface-tension-lowering in bath;
- prevent local irritation (treat thread worms, avoid tight cloths);
- use of oral bio-yoghurts.

VESICOURETERIC REFLUX

Definition and description

VUR is the retrograde movement of urine from bladder into the ureter on either bladder filling or bladder voiding, or both. The prevalence of VUR in children is around one to two per cent. It can be an intermittent phenomenon. VUR is present in 30 per cent of children diagnosed with UTI. Understanding the natural history of VUR is very important in the management of these children.

Aetiology

PRIMARY VESICOURETERIC REFLUX

When there is no underlying pathology, the VUR is considered primary. The normal ureterovesical junction has a submucosal tunnel of at least four to five times the size of the ureter, thereby providing a flap-valve mechanism to prevent reflux of urine from bladder into the ureter. In primary VUR, the ureteric orifice is situated more laterally on the trigone, and is wider or larger than normal, and the submucosal tunnel is shorter, resulting in deficiency of the valve mechanism. Primary VUR has a strong family history reported in around 30 per cent of siblings and 50 per cent of offspring. The natural history of primary VUR is one of spontaneous resolution.

SECONDARY VESICOURETERIC REFLUX

Secondary VUR occurs when urine is stored in the bladder or is emptied from the bladder at an abnormally high pressure. The underlying pathology could be anatomical obstruction (posterior urethral valves, other urethral obstructions),

Table 52.6 *Aetiology of vesicoureteric reflux (VUR)*

Primary VUR	Laterally placed ureteric orifice Poor submucosal tunnel Familial
Secondary VUR	Obstructive (posterior urethral valves, urethral stricture, meatal stenosis) Neuropathic (myelomeningocele, spinal dysraphism, post-pelvic surgery) Dysfunctional (detrusor sphincter dyssynergia, urge syndrome, constipation)

neuropathic bladder dysfunction (spinal dysraphism, myelomeningocoele, neuropathy following pelvic operations) or non-neuropathic bladder dysfunction (detrusor-sphincter dyssynergia, detrusor instability). Table 52.6 summarizes the various causes of VUR in children.

Consequences of scarring and reflux nephropathy

VUR may be completely asymptomatic and non-consequential, with no long-term sequelae. However, in up to 25–40 per cent of children with VUR, renal scarring is already established at presentation. What decides whether scarring does or does not occur? The normal renal papillae have a conical shape, which protects against the intra-renal reflux. Abnormally flat 'compound' papillae occur mainly at the poles of kidney, making them prone to pyelonephritis and scarring. Previously, high-grade reflux in the neonatal period was though to produce scars by the 'water-hammer effect' (mechanical damage secondary to a high-pressure jet). However, current experimental and clinical evidence indicates that reflux of sterile urine under normal voiding pressure does not result in scarring. Focal renal scarring requires the combination of urinary infection and intra-renal reflux. In the absence of one of these, scarring does not occur.

Ransley's 'big-bang theory' suggests that renal scarring is maximal after the first episode of infection.

The development of renal scars is dependent on a balance between at least six different factors (Table 52.7). The risk of renal scarring is highest in the neonate, falling rapidly as age advances. Several factors contribute towards this. Immature neural control pathways and central coordination result in detrusor-sphincter dyssynergia and high-pressure voiding during infancy. Poor host immunity is one of the factors responsible for the high rate of scarring in neonates. In addition, symptoms of neonatal UTI are often vague and non-specific and treatment inadequate or delayed.

Release of enzymes and superoxide and oxygen radicals from neutrophils is responsible for the tubular damage and scarring after pyelonephritis. The resulting tubular dysfunction, especially if bilateral, results in reduced urinary concentrating ability. End-stage renal failure is reported in 10–15

Table 52.7 *Factors determining development of renal scarring*

Aggressive factors	Protective factors
Virulence of organism Intra-renal reflux	Host immunity Age (scarring reduces as age advances)
High urinary tract pressure	Prompt treatment

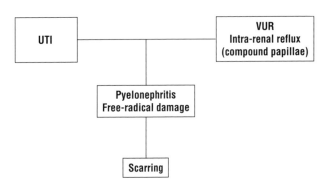

Figure 52.1 *Pathogenesis of reflux nephropathy. Focal scarring requires a combination of urine infection and intra-renal reflux. Medical management controls urinary tract infection (UTI) while surgery prevents vesicoureteric reflux (VUR).*

per cent of patients with reflux nephropathy. Figure 52.1 summarizes the pathogenesis of reflux nephropathy.

Hypertension secondary to scarring is a late phenomenon, usually occurring 15–18 years later. The incidence is ten per cent with unilateral scarring and 20 per cent with bilateral scarring. The aetiology of hypertension is understood poorly. Although scarring is invariably present in patients who develop hypertension, studies have shown that there is no correlation between the incidence of hypertension and the extent of scarring. The renin–angiotensin system is likely to be involved in the development of hypertension. Studies have suggested that genetic makeup (DD genotype) could be a common factor responsible for increased susceptibility to scarring and increased angiotensin II levels.

Presentation

Symptomatic UTI is the most common mode of presentation with VUR. An increasingly common presentation is antenatally detected hydronephrosis, of which VUR accounts for 15–20 per cent. Studies have shown that VUR presents in different ways in males and females. In boys, the reflux usually is high-grade and presents early, and anatomical factors play an important role. In girls, often the reflux is low-grade and presents late, and dysfunctional factors play a major role.

VUR may be identified during investigation of wetting in girls. Presentation for the first time with renal failure and hypertension in adolescence is becoming very rare. Box 52.3 summarizes the different types of presentation of VUR.

Box 52.3 Different types of presentation of vesicoureteric reflux

Urinary tract infection
Hydronephrosis (antenatal/postnatal)
Wetting, bladder dysfunction
Reflux nephropathy (scarring/small kidney on routine ultrasound)
Hypertension, renal failure

Further investigation

SUSPECTED VESICOURETERIC REFLUX

Ultrasound is the initial investigation performed in a child presenting with UTI or antenatal hydronephrosis. However, ultrasound has a very poor pick-up rate for reflux or scars, one study reporting normal ultrasound in up to 74 per cent of patients. MCUG is the definite way to prove or disprove VUR; however, this is an invasive procedure with associated morbidity. It is generally performed after six months of age, unless an obstructive uropathy, especially in a male infant (in the form of posterior urethral valve), needs to be excluded. The reasons for this 'late' investigation are as follows: if the VUR is clinically thought to be primary, then management is conservative initially with prophylactic antibiotics, so an early MCUG does not change treatment. Early MCUGs have been associated with episodes of severe sepsis in neonates and young infants, making it a considerably risky investigation.

ESTABLISHED VESICOURETERIC REFLUX

A DMSA scan helps to identify scars and assess renal function but has no way of identifying persistent reflux. An indirect cystogram is less invasive than an MCUG and has the advantage of emitting less radiation in a cooperative potty-trained child. It is, however, not accurate in identifying low grades of reflux, although it could be argued that low-grade reflux is clinically insignificant in the majority of cases. An MCUG is the gold-standard investigation for identifying reflux, although because of the intermittent nature of VUR, it is not 100 per cent effective at proving its resolution. MCUG is the only test that provides accurate grading. It also gives anatomical details and excludes underlying lesions that could cause secondary VUR. The grading devised by the International Reflux Study Committee (1981) is used widely (Table 52.8).

Medical management

The principles of management of primary VUR have evolved with understanding of the natural history of the disease, especially after the Birmingham Reflux Study (1987) and the International Reflux Study in Children (1992). These studies

Table 52.8 *Grading of vesicoureteral reflux*

Grade	Features
I	Reflux into **ureter only**; no dilation
II	Reflux into **ureter, pelvis, calyces**; **no dilation**
III	**Mild** or moderate **dilation** and/ or tortuosity of ureter; mild or moderate dilation of renal pelvis; slight blunting of fornices
IV	**Moderate dilation** and/or tortuosity of ureter and moderate dilation of pelvis and calyces; **obliteration of angle of fornices**; papillary impressions maintained in majority of calyces
V	**Gross dilation and tortuosity** of ureter; gross dilation of pelvis and calyces; **loss of papillary impressions** in majority of calyces

Essential features are in **bold**.

comparing medically and surgically managed groups reported that there was no significant difference between the groups with respect to incidence of breakthrough UTIs, renal function, renal growth and progression of old scars or new scar formation. This has led to widespread use of conservative management of VUR, the rationale being as follows:

- In the absence of UTI, isolated low-pressure VUR does not lead to scar formation.
- Uncomplicated primary reflux resolves spontaneously.

Figure 52.2 summarizes the practical approach to management of VUR. The principles of medical management include effective treatment of the acute episode of UTI and prevention of further infection and scarring. Once an acute episode of UTI has been treated, it is essential to complete investigations to exclude anatomical causes of secondary VUR. A large proportion of children, even after a normal DMSA scan and MCUG, have significant factors, such as constipation, dysfunctional voiding and bladder instability, all preventing resolution of VUR. These factors need to be treated aggressively with laxatives, bladder-training programmes or anticholinergics, as required. Regular follow-up, parental commitment and patient compliance are essential for success of medical treatment.

Prognosis and follow-up

Several studies have reported the resolution rate of VUR treated conservatively. Among the predictive factors, neither sex nor laterality (unilateral versus bilateral) could help in predicting resolution; grade was the best predictive parameter. In broad terms, the resolution rate can be summarized as follows: grade I, 80 per cent; grade II, 60 per cent; grade III, 40 per cent; and grades IV and above, ten per cent. The duration to resolution since diagnosis has been reported as follows: grade I, 2.5 years; grade II, five years; and grades III and IV, eight years. The frequency of renal scarring is proportional to

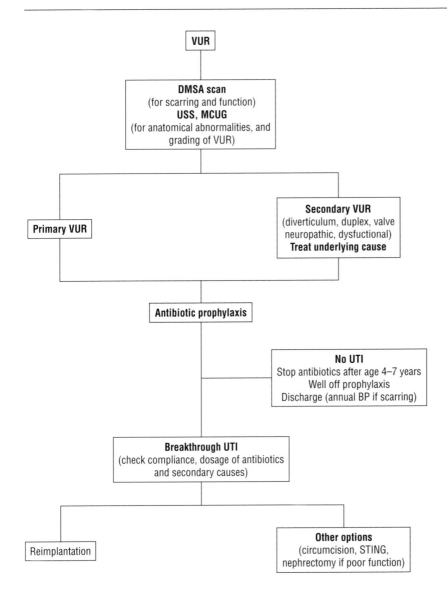

Figure 52.2   *Management of vesicoureteric reflux (VUR).*

BP, blood pressure; DMSA, dimercaptosuccinic acid; MCUG, micturating cystourethrogram; STING, subureteric Teflon™ injection; USS, ultrasound scan; UTI, urinary tract infection.

the number of episodes of pyelonephritis and the severity of reflux. The risk factors for new scarring are younger age group, high-grade reflux and previous scarring. The reported scarring rate with different grades is as follows: grade I, ten per cent; grade II, 17 per cent; and grades III and above, 60 per cent.

How long should the antibiotic prophylaxis be continued? Studies have shown that the mean age of resolution of low-grade reflux is around 4.6 years and the risk of developing new scars falls to zero after the age of four years. However, caution should be exercised in children with high-grade reflux, bilateral reflux and existing scars. Should one ensure that VUR has resolved completely before stopping prophylaxis? Opinion differs on the need for a repeat cystogram to identify reflux resolution before stopping prophylaxis. Some studies have recommended two negative indirect cystograms a year apart before stopping prophylaxis. In the authors' opinion, if medical treatment is successful, then antibiotic

prophylaxis can be stopped between the age of four and seven years without any repeat cystogram.

Surgical management

Both primary and secondary VUR are managed conservatively initially. However, the presence of anatomical factors such as a para-ureteric diverticulum or reflux into a duplex system make spontaneous resolution less likely. In these children, surgical treatment may be considered sooner. Refluxing obstructed mega-ureters are always managed surgically. Controversy exists between different countries regarding the management of bilateral grade IV reflux, grade V reflux and reflux in the presence of multiple scarring. In the UK, the general policy is to reserve re-implantation only for breakthrough infections and worsening function. The different surgical options for primary VUR are discussed below.

Management of VUR secondary to lower-tract obstruction is discussed in Chapters 55, 58 and 59.

CIRCUMCISION

Prepucial colonization has been described as a cause of UTI, and it is claimed that neonatal circumcision reduces the incidence of UTIs. Routine neonatal circumcision is not practised in UK and the same applies for boys with VUR. However, in the presence of recurrent *Proteus* spp. infection, or demonstrable phimosis with pooling of urine under the prepuce, circumcision can be considered as a first option.

SUBURETERIC TEFLON™ INJECTION

Originally developed in 1980, subureteric Teflon™ (polytetra-fluoroethylene) injection (STING technique) has achieved a success rate of over 75 per cent with one to two injections in experienced hands. The principle involves increasing the submucosal tunnel length via cystoscopic subureteric injection of a bulking agent. Migration of Teflon to lymph nodes, lungs and brain has been reported in animals. The other substances that have been developed for the same purpose include gluteraldehyde cross-linked bovine collagen, polydimethylsiloxane (Macroplastique™), dextranomer in sodium hyaluronan solution (Deflux™) and autologous chondrocytes. Although the technique is simple and repeatable, the success rate for correction of high-grade VUR is lower than with re-implantation. As a result of this, a greater number of investigations (invasive and non-invasive) may have to be repeated to decide whether the reflux has been treated adequately.

URETERIC RE-IMPLANTATION

There are a number of different techniques of re-implanting the ureter surgically. All aim to lengthen the submucosal tunnel, which the ureter takes as it enters the bladder. The aim is to achieve a tunnel length-to-ureteric diameter ratio of five to one or more. This is more difficult in mega-ureters, which require additional ureteric reduction or plication manoeuvres.

Cohen technique

The most favoured operation for VUR is the cross-trigonal ureteric advancement described by Cohen. This has the benefits of being easy to learn and a success rate of 95–100 per cent. It has a low incidence of postoperative obstruction and is useful for both normal-sized ureters and mega-ureters. Its drawback includes the transposition of the ureteric orifice across to the other side of the bladder, making any future endoscopic manipulation almost impossible. It involves opening the bladder, with a greater incidence of postoperative haematuria and bladder spasm than in other techniques.

Politano–Leadbetter technique

In this operation, instead of advancing the ureter across to the other side, the ureteric hiatus is lateralized. The ureter is dissected intravesically from the surrounding detrusor and

mobilized. A new hiatus is created superolaterally by passing a right-angled clamp behind the bladder. The ureter is then passed through the new hiatus and the submucosal tunnel. The added benefit is that the ureteric orifice remains on its original side. It has a slightly lower success rate than the Cohen technique, due partly to the reduced availability of increasing the submucosal tunnel length if using just one side of the bladder wall. It also results more commonly in post-re-implantation obstruction due to an increased angulation of the ureter as it leaves the bladder muscle. This is often overcome by adding a psoas hitch to the ureter, thereby straightening out the angle.

Lich–Gregoir technique

The Lich–Gregoir technique has become more popular, especially for unilateral re-implantation, as it has reduced haematuria (because the bladder is not opened), causes less postoperative discomfort and reduces length of hospital stay. It also has the benefit of keeping the ureteric orifice in its natural side for potential endoscopic manipulation at a later date if necessary. This technique can be combined with a psoas hitch and ureteric tapering in patients with gross ureteric dilation to achieve an adequate ureter-to-tunnel ratio. It is preferable to avoid bilateral extravesical re-implantation, as this has been associated with a greater incidence of bladder dysfunction postoperatively.

Laparoscopic re-implantation

Laparoscopic extravesical re-implantation has been performed successfully in animals and in patients, with improved cosmesis and shortened hospital stay. Both the transperitoneal extravesical laparoscopic technique to carry out a Lich–Gregoir procedure and the transvesical method to perform a Cohen procedure have been performed safely. Laparoscopic re-implantation is, however, still in its infancy, and technical refinements and greater series are required to establish whether there are real benefits over the standard open re-implantation.

TRANSURETERO-URETEROSTOMY

This is a useful option following a failed re-implantation or in the presence of gross mega-ureter and a small bladder. One ureter is re-implanted with psoas hitch, while the contralateral ureter is anastomosed to the re-implanted ureter above the level of bladder. It is often the primary operation in gross reflux in infants due to a secondary bladder problem. In this way, a 'defunctioned' ureter can remain *in situ* until a definitive bladder procedure is carried out, e.g. augmentation using the ureter or Mitrofanoff bladder tube using the ureter.

HEMI-NEPHRECTOMY/COMMON CHANNEL RE-IMPLANTATION

In children with a duplex system and reflux into a classically non-functioning lower pole, a lower hemi-nephrectomy is a useful therapeutic option. If both poles of the kidney are functioning and reflux persists with intercurrent infections, then a common channel re-implantation is performed. In this technique, both ureters are mobilized *en bloc* with their covering sheath, advanced intravesically and re-implanted. It is possible to perform a common channel Lich–Gregoir extravesical re-implant. The STING procedure has also been used, but with a lower success rate than in a single-ureteric STING.

NEPHRECTOMY

Ultimately, nephrectomy is still a valid option in children with unilateral VUR, recurrent infection and a poorly functioning kidney (function on DMSA scan less than ten per cent). The refluxing ureter is ideally excised completely to prevent stump reflux. More and more commonly, this is carried out laparoscopically, using either a transperitoneal approach, allowing easy dissection to the entrance of the ureter at the bladder wall, or an extraperitoneal approach.

PROGNOSIS AND SCREENING

After the first episode of UTI, there is a 50 per cent chance of re-infection within a year. Between 15 and 30 per cent have a scar at the time of diagnosis; of those who do not have a scar, 5–15 per cent develop new scars. The worst prognostic group includes children with recurrent UTIs, high-grade reflux and scarring at first presentation. Prompt investigation and management of the UTI help to prevent further renal damage. The incidence of hypertension is variable; presentation is late, with no correlation with extent of scarring. Hence, all children with recurrent UTI, VUR and any degree of scarring should undergo an annual check of blood pressure for life.

The screening of siblings and offspring is controversial. Since the natural history of VUR is one of spontaneous resolution, it can be argued that screening is of little use in asymptomatic older siblings. Ultrasonogram provides the first non-invasive step, although it has very poor sensitivity and specificity for diagnosing reflux. It may, however, pick up scarring in established cases. DMSA scanning and MCUG are too invasive to be used as screening modalities unless there are real suspicions of VUR in a sibling. Indirect cystogram is less invasive but difficult in younger children and can still miss low-grade reflux. Direct radionuclide cystography has been recommended as a screening method for younger siblings, especially in children under one year of age, in view of its lower radiation dose compared with MCUG.

CLINICAL SCENARIO

A ten-year-old girl, who was initially managed medically for grade III VUR (on MCUG), was referred to a urologist because she developed two episodes of UTI and abdominal pain after discontinuing prophylaxis. A DMSA scan revealed unscarred kidneys with normal function. A repeat MCUG confirmed persistent right-sided grade III reflux, and she was recommenced on prophylaxis. Since she had features of urgency and frequency, she was treated with anticholinergics to control her bladder instability. After a year, her symptoms of bladder instability improved, there were no further UTIs, and her medications were stopped. While off prophylaxis, she developed three further UTIs. An urodynamics examination revealed normal compliance with no instability. Prophylaxis was restarted, and she was advised to try bio-yoghurts and avoid the use of shampoo/bubble-bath. At the age of 12 years, she had one further UTI. There was some evidence of upper-pole scarring on the right kidney on a repeat ultrasonogram. In view of this, it was decided to treat her surgically; an extravesical ureteric re-implantation of the right ureter was performed. The postoperative period was uneventful, and prophylaxis was stopped after six weeks. Repeat ultrasound revealed no hydronephrosis and no further MCU was performed. At one-year follow-up, she remained free of UTIs without prophylaxis and was discharged.

REFERENCES

Birmingham Reflux Study Group. Prospective trial of operative versus non-operative treatment of severe vesico-ureteric reflux in children: five years' observation. *British Medical Journal* 1987; **295**: 237–41.

International Reflux Study in Children. Five-year study of medical or surgical treatment in children with severe reflux: radiological renal findings. *Pediatric Nephrology* 1992; **6**: 223–30.

International Reflux Study Committee. Medical versus surgical treatment of primary vesico-ureteric reflux: a prospective international reflux study in children. *Journal of Urology* 1981; **125**: 272–83.

FURTHER READING

Deshpande PV, Verrier-Jones K. An audit of RCP guidelines on DMSA scanning after urinary tract infection. *Archives of Disease in Childhood* 2001; **84**: 324–7.

Michael M, Hodson EM, Craig JC, Martin S, Moyer VA. Short compared with standard duration of antibiotic treatment for urinary tract infection: a systematic review of randomised controlled trials. *Archives of Disease in Childhood* 2002; **87**: 118–23.

Shortliffe LMD, Shinghal R, Seto EH. Pediatric urinary tract infections. In: Gearhart JP, Rink RC, Mouriquand PDE (eds). *Pediatric Urology*. Philadelphia, PA: WB Saunders, 2001; pp. 237–58.

Thomas DFM. Vesicoureteric reflux. In: Thomas DFM, Rickwood AMK, Duffy PG (eds). *Essentials of Paediatric Urology*. London: Martin Dunitz, 2002; pp. 45–55.

Working Group of the Research Unit Royal College of Physicians. Guidelines for the management of acute urinary tract infection in childhood. *Journal of the Royal College of Physicians of London* 1991; **25**: 36–42.

53

Upper urinary tract duplication

PETER CUCKOW

Learning objectives

- To understand the embryology of upper-tract duplication anomalies.
- To recognize the difference between pathological and benign variants.
- To be able to investigate the variants appropriately.
- To learn both surgical and conservative management of upper-tract duplication anomalies.

INTRODUCTION

Duplication of the upper urinary tract is the most common urinary tract anomaly, occurring in approximately one in 125 individuals at post-mortem. There is a female preponderance (70 per cent) and a familial tendency (11 per cent of first-degree relatives also have a duplication), and in 20 per cent of patients it is bilateral. Duplex kidneys have two separate poles or moieties (upper and lower), each with a separate collecting system. The ureters from these either enter the lower urinary tract separately in a complete duplex (40 per cent of cases) or join above the bladder and drain via a common orifice in an incomplete duplex (60 per cent of cases). The position of the ureteric orifice on the trigone may be called ectopic, when it is away from the expected ureteric position (either lateral or medial to it).

Duplex kidneys may not cause clinical problems for the patient; indeed, the majority may be completely benign. Ureteric problems of vesicoureteric reflux, abnormal drainage (ectopic ureter) and cystic swelling of the lower end (ureterocele), however, do cause significant complications and often require surgical management (see below). With increasing antenatal diagnosis, the difficulty is to separate patients who require intervention from those who need only to be observed or even discharged without follow-up.

BASIC SCIENCE

The embryological theory of Mackie and Stevens helps to explain the formation of duplex systems. Normal kidney induction occurs when the ureteric bud grows into the metanephric blastema to form the collecting system and renal parenchyma, respectively. The normal origin of the ureteric bud on the mesonephric (or Wolffian) duct ensures that when the latter is absorbed into the developing bladder wall, the ureteric orifice ends up in the correct or orthotopic position on the lateral corner of the trigone (Figure 53.1).

Duplex kidneys arise in two situations (Figure 53.2). The ureteric bud may bifurcate before entering the blastema cells, inducing two separate collecting systems with a common origin on the mesonephric duct and, thus, a single

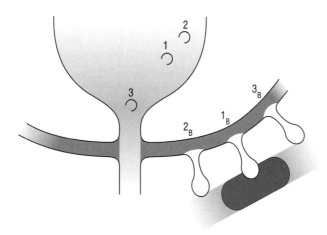

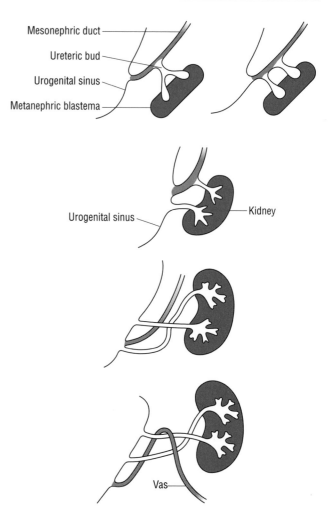

Figure 53.1 *Embryological theory of Mackie and Stevens. The normal ureteric bud (1_B) develops as an outgrowth of the mesonephric duct and meets the metanephric blastema cells. This induces a normal kidney whose ureteric orifice is normally located on the trigone of the developed bladder (1_O). A more distally sited ureteric bud (2_B) does not meet normal metanephric blastema cells, so an abnormal or dysplastic kidney may result. Additionally, its orifice (2_O) is incorporated earlier into the bladder and is sited more laterally on the trigone, where it is prone to reflux due to a short intramural tunnel. More proximal location of the ureteric bud (3_B) also leads to dysplastic kidney formation by a similar mechanism. The orifice, however, is incorporated later into the developing bladder and is medial to the 'normal' position (3_O). It may be associated with mesonephric (Wolffian) duct remnants.*

Figure 53.2 *Embryogenesis of ureteric duplication. Division of the ureteric bud results in partial duplication, with two separate collecting systems and a single ureteric orifice. Two separate ureteric buds result in two separate collecting systems, each with its own orifice. The first orifice to enter the developing bladder from the lower pole migrates further across the trigone and ends above and lateral to the upper-pole ureter that arrives later, thus resulting in the apparent reversal of orifice position and the crossing of ureters, otherwise known as the Weigert–Meyer law.*

ureteric orifice (bifid system). Alternatively, two separate ureteric buds may arise, leading to two separately drained moieties, each with its own orifice. If the origin of the ureteric bud is such that it does not enter the middle of the blastema cells, then an abnormal renal moiety results. Thus, ureteric buds arising significantly away from the normal origin on the Wolffian duct may induce abnormal or dysplastic renal moieties.

When the distal Wolffian duct is absorbed into the bladder to form the trigone, the ureteric orifices migrate superolaterally. Orifices located nearer to the bladder on the duct (as in the case of lower-pole ureters) arrive earlier and migrate further. The resulting orifice is located lateral to the 'normal' position, i.e. it is laterally ectopic. A short intramural tunnel results, and incompetence of the valvular anti-reflux mechanism is more likely. Lower-pole ureters are located lateral to upper-pole ureters in complete duplex systems, are prone to vesicoureteric reflux, and may be associated with significant renal dysplasia. Upper-pole ureters arrive at the bladder later and migrate less across the trigone, so their position is medial to the 'normal'. Their course through the bladder wall is longer, and so reflux is unlikely; however, if they fail to separate from the Wolffian duct, they will drain into its derivatives – the vasa, seminal vesicles, upper urethra and veru montanum in males and the urethra, vestibule and vagina in females. These ectopic

ureters are associated with more severe dysplasia. In females, this will result in dribbling incontinence due to drainage below the continence mechanism. In males, all drainage sites are above the striated urethral sphincter, so incontinence is not a feature. Crossing of the lower and upper pole ureters in complete duplex systems is referred to as the 'Weigert–Meyer rule'.

Ureteroceles are cystic swellings of the distal ureter. The embryological origin is unclear, although various mechanisms have been proposed, including lower ureteric obstruction due to a persistent membrane and delayed canalization of the distal ureter. Ectopic ureteroceles are usually associated with dysplastic upper-pole moieties and can obstruct the bladder

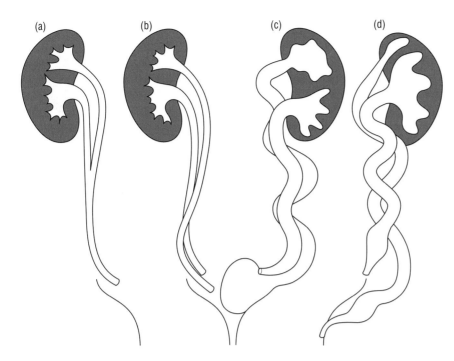

Figure 53.3 *Range of duplex anomalies:*
(a) Partial duplication with single orifice.
(b) Complete uncomplicated duplex.
(c) Dysplastic upper-pole ureter associated
with ureterocele and dilated lower-pole system.
(d) Ectopic upper-pole ureter and laterally
ectopic (refluxing) lower-pole ureter, with
bipolar dysplasia.

outlet, thereby impacting potentially on all renal moieties. Orthotopic ureteroceles are in the 'normal' position on the trigone and are associated more often with a single system than with duplication. The kidney is more normal in its function (according to Mackie and Stevens' theory).

Figure 53.3 shows the range of duplex abnormalities that may be found in children.

DIAGNOSIS

The increasing efficacy of antenatal diagnosis is bringing to our attention more patients with asymptomatic duplications. Diagnosis may be non-specific and, as with other uropathies, based on the finding of renal dilation. More specific features of duplication at the kidney level include separate collecting systems (of which one or both may be significantly dilated) and a larger than expected renal length. Dilated ureters can be seen, and at the bladder level ureteroceles can be identified within the lumen (see Case 1 below).

If suspected prenatally, then the patient is started on prophylactic antibiotics and investigated after birth to reveal the specific features of the duplication. Apart from a repeat ultrasound, a micturating cystogram is important to confirm a ureterocele and, in particular, its position relative to the bladder neck, where it may obstruct the outlet. Vesicoureteric reflux, which may also occur into contralateral single system ureters in 20 per cent of cases, can be characterized according to the degree of dilation and graded in the standard way. The majority of reflux is into lower-pole systems, where calyces are fewer compared with in single systems and point downwards and laterally – the so-called 'drooping flower appearance'. After three months, a mercaptoacetyltriglycine (MAG_3) renogram is used to define the functional component of each moiety and to decide the form of surgical management, if required (see below).

As was the case before the advent of antenatal ultrasound, patients may also present clinically; the most common way is with urinary tract infection. In infants, the symptoms vary from acute life-threatening sepsis to a more chronic failure to thrive. Infection is related to reflux, stasis in the upper urinary tract and poor bladder emptying. Occasionally, in infant girls the ureterocele may prolapse through the urethra and present as a mass in the perineum. Other clinical signs include palpable abdominal masses (ureters and bladders).

Whether the patient presents antenatally or clinically, radiological investigation will reveal the features of the ureteric duplication, which are usually reflux, ureterocele or ectopic ureter, or any combination of these. Management priorities are to prevent infection, to treat obstruction and to preserve renal parenchyma.

DUPLEX REFLUX

Reflux is more common in duplication than in single systems and is found in 70 per cent of patients who present with infection. Although reflux affects the lower-pole moiety most commonly (90 per cent), nine per cent affects both poles (both ureters laterally ectopic or bifid ureter with laterally ectopic orifice); in one per cent of patients, reflux may be into the upper pole alone (ruptured ureterocele or urethral ectopic ureter that refluxes during voiding). In addition, 20 per cent of contralateral single-system ureters also reflux.

The grade of reflux on cystogram tends to be higher with duplication than that seen in the population with single-system reflux. Also, there are more likely to be associated renal parenchymal abnormalities on functional imaging, whose presence in non-infected antenatal cases confirms their dysplastic aetiology. Nonetheless, conservative management with antibiotics and observation (see Chapter 52) is appropriate, as spontaneous resolution may occur – although the rate is lower (at 3.5 years: 85 per cent grades I and II, 35 per cent grade III). Reflux will not resolve in grades IV and V, or when both moieties are involved, but antibiotics are effective at preventing infection and thus deferring surgery until the child is older.

Indications for surgical intervention are severe reflux, severe renal damage, failure of antibiotic prophylaxis, failure of resolution, and as part of an operation for another duplex problem. Poorly functioning moieties are probably best treated by lower-pole hemi-nephrectomy or total nephrectomy if upper-pole function is also poor. As duplex ureters run in a common sheath and share a blood supply near the bladder, a small stump is left in order to avoid injuring the upper-pole ureter, and only rarely may this have to be removed at a later date due to complications. When good function dictates an anti-reflux operation, then the subureteric Teflon™ injection (STING) procedure is available, but with a higher failure rate than in single systems (34 per cent). Open re-implantation is usually performed of both ureters, which are dissected together and re-implanted within their common sheath by a Cohen or Leadbetter technique. Recurrence of reflux is less than five per cent, and ureteric tapering is rarely indicated, as with the most dilated systems excision is indicated due to their poor function (see Case 3 below).

URETEROCELE

The overall incidence of ureterocele is about one in 4000 people. Ureteroceles usually are associated with a dilated upper-pole moiety and ureter on ultrasound. Reflux is demonstrated in as many as 50 per cent of lower-pole ureters and 30 per cent of contralateral single ureters. A micturating cystogram can reveal weakness in the posterior trigone, whose wall may be deficient behind the ureterocele and bulge outwards on voiding. The most important function of the cystogram, however, is to confirm or rule out outlet obstruction by the ureterocele at the bladder neck.

Non-operative management of ureteroceles may be indicated in antenatally diagnosed, uncomplicated cases. However, most will come to surgery. Endoscopic puncture has gained favour in recent years as the simplest and least invasive way to decompress a ureterocele. It is particularly indicated to acutely decompress an infected upper moiety (after adequate resuscitation of the patient) or to relieve bladder outlet obstruction. Care must be taken to choose the right puncture site: too low and within the bladder neck, and the orifice will be held closed; too high, and reflux may be produced into the upper-pole ureter. In practice, it may be difficult to orient a large ureterocele endoscopically, and the technical difficulty of this procedure should not be underestimated. Although good results are reported, failure of decompression, continued bladder outlet obstruction by the ureterocele wall, infection and reflux are all indications for a more invasive approach in around 50 per cent of ectopic ureteroceles. In intravesical ureteroceles, puncture appears to be much more successful. However, the often excellent or normal function of the (mostly single-system) kidney and a relative lack of complications make any intervention in these patients questionable.

Upper-pole hemi-nephro-ureterectomy has been the preferred treatment for duplex ureteroceles and is vindicated by the severe dysplasia and secondary abnormalities found in excised moieties. It is the most effective way to decompress a ureterocele and, as a primary procedure, will avoid the complication of reflux. The kidney is approached through a flank incision, and its upper pole and pedicle are exposed. The upper-pole vessels are identified and divided, and the moiety is removed with diathermy. To help this, its ureter may first be identified below the main renal pedicle and separated from the lower-pole ureter. It can then be divided and its proximal end brought behind the vessels and retracted above them. This manoeuvre helps in the identification of the extent of the upper pole and aids in its separation from the lower pole. The author keeps a rim of capsule attached to the lower moiety and uses this to close the raw area with absorbable monofilament sutures to further secure haemostasis. The distal ureter is then separated carefully from the lower pole ureter and divided as low down as possible, leaving a distal stump. The need for further surgery may be as low as ten per cent and depends largely on the surgeon's approach to lower-pole reflux, which may follow ureterocele decompression and loss of support for the distal lower-pole ureter. Obstruction of the bladder outlet by the ureterocele remnant and bladder neck insufficiency are the major indications for a secondary bladder-level procedure.

If functional imaging suggests good upper-pole function (which is rare in duplex ureterocele), then ureterocele excision and bipolar re-implantation may be indicated. More commonly, bladder-level procedures are carried out following failure of puncture or upper-pole hemi-nephrectomy. Thus, in the vast majority, difficult and damaging bladder surgery may be avoided or at least postponed until later in childhood. Total excision of the ureterocele may extend down into the proximal urethra, and a lack of any residual obstructing tissue should be confirmed by passing a large catheter antegradely. Any deficiency of the bladder neck or trigone can be repaired at the same time (see Cases 1 and 2 on p. 467).

ECTOPIC URETER

Ectopic ureter is found in one in 2000 people, of whom 80 per cent are female. Eighty per cent of cases involve the upper pole of a duplex kidney, ten per cent are bilateral, and a contralateral duplex system is found in 40 per cent. In the past, the majority of these patients presented with complications, either early with urinary infection and abdominal mass (from huge dilated ureters) or in older girls with urinary incontinence. Increasing numbers of infants are now presenting antenatally with dilated ureters. Single ectopic ureter is strongly associated with other major anomalies, such as tracheo-oesophageal fistula, myelomeningocele and diaphragmatic hernia, and 50 per cent are found as a result of working up these patients.

In females, ectopic drainage sites include the urethra beyond the bladder neck (35 per cent), the vestibule (34 per cent), the vagina (25 per cent) and the uterus (five per cent). These are all below the level of continence, and hence the classic presentation of a little girl with dribbling incontinence but an otherwise normal voiding pattern. These girls have never been dry and often present with long stories of failed continence management. In boys, the ectopic drainage sites are the posterior urethra (47 per cent), the seminal vesicles (33 per cent), the prostatic utricle (ten per cent), the ejaculatory duct (five per cent) and the vas deferens (five per cent). As all these are above the striated sphincter, incontinence is not a problem, and these boys present with unusual infections and sepsis.

Confirming the diagnosis of ectopic ureter as a source of wetting may be difficult and requires persistence. Although dilated lower ureters can be traced through the pelvis, the upper-pole moiety and its proximal ureter may be small and difficult to detect on ultrasound. Frequent lack of function renders most invisible on intravenous urogram (IVU), although the so-called 'drooping flower appearance' of the lower-moiety calyces alludes to the presence of an upper pole. A micturating cystourethrogram (MCUG) can demonstrate reflux into urethrally ectopic ureters whose orifices are open and reflux during voiding. Functional imaging identifies small upper-pole defects alluding to an occult moiety, helping in the planning of surgery. Magnetic resonance imaging (MRI) may also identify dilated non-functioning systems.

Diagnosis should be based on a clear suspicion from the clinical history and a careful clinical examination of the female perineum, for a visible source of the wetting should always be performed. Cystoscopy helps to clarify the anatomy of the ureteric orifices, and longitudinal ridge in the anterior vaginal wall may represent an underlying ureter. It is important to characterize both sides due to the high incidence of bilaterality, as the obvious duplex may not be the source of the problem. Various dye tests have been devised to help confirm the diagnosis of ectopic ureter and identify the orifice position, but in practice these are messy and unreliable. Even with exhaustive investigations, the ectopic orifice remains unfound in 30 per cent of cases.

As upper-pole function is usually very poor, the most common surgical approach to duplex ectopic ureter is upper-pole hemi-nephro-ureterectomy. The results in curing incontinence are dramatic and make this one of the most satisfying operations in paediatric urology. In up to ten per cent of cases, complications from the stump may require its later excision. If the upper-pole function is worth preserving, then a common sheath re-implantation of the ureters is indicated.

RARER DUPLICATION PROBLEMS

Pelviureteric junction obstruction can also be seen in the context of ureteric duplication, where it usually affects the lower-pole ureter. It can be managed in a similar way to single systems. Reflux of urine between ureters in partial duplication rarely may cause loin pain in later life. This is otherwise known as 'yo-yo reflux' and can be demonstrated on isotope renography. The solution is either to carry out separate re-implantation of the ureters or to join them higher up, depending on the anatomy.

CLINICAL SCENARIOS

Case 1

Screening ultrasound revealed a dilated right kidney in a 19-week-old fetus. Further ultrasound at 24 weeks revealed a duplex kidney, with dilation of both poles and a ureterocele in the bladder. Postnatal investigation of a healthy baby girl confirmed the diagnosis of duplex right kidney with gross dilation of the upper pole and a large ectopic ureterocele encroaching on the bladder neck. Cystography confirmed the ureterocele, which everted on further bladder filling, and also ipsilateral lower-pole reflux, with a drooping flower appearance to the lower pole. Functional imaging confirmed a non-functioning lower pole, so a right upper-pole hemi-nephrectomy was performed.

Case 2

A nine-year-old boy presented with a history of recurrent urinary tract infections and haematuria. IVU at his local hospital showed a duplex left kidney. A cystogram was performed, which demonstrated reflux into the lower pole. Poor function was confirmed on a MAG$_3$ renogram. He was treated by lower-pole hemi-nephrectomy.

Case 3

A six-year-old girl presented with a history of dribbling incontinence and never being dry, in spite of a normal micturition pattern. Review of her ultrasound suggested a small occult upper pole of the right kidney, and this was seen as a defect on a DMSA scan. Careful examination showed a persistent dampness of the perineum. At cystoscopy, an ectopic ureteric orifice was found and cannulated. After right upper-pole hemi-nephrectomy, she was completely dry.

FURTHER READING

Cuckow PM. The management of ureteric duplication in children. *European Urology Update Series* 1998; **7**.
Walsh PC, Retik AB, Stamey TA (eds). *Campbell's Urology*, 6th edn. Philadelphia, PA: WB Saunders, 1992.

54

Upper urinary tract obstruction

PETER CUCKOW AND DIVYESH DESAI

Learning objectives

- To understand the different types of upper urinary tract obstruction and their pathophysiology.
- To differentiate antenatally diagnosed patients who can be followed conservatively from those who need surgical intervention.
- To be familiar with the available investigative modalities and their interpretation.
- To learn the surgical and conservative management of upper urinary tract obstruction.

INTRODUCTION

Obstruction of the upper urinary tract may be due to congenital anomalies of the ureter at the level of the pelviureteric junction (PUJ) or the vesicoureteric junction (VUJ). Nowadays, most of these cases present with antenatal ultrasound. These two diagnoses contribute to the majority of cases of upper urinary tract obstruction; therefore, discussion of them will be the main focus of this chapter. In addition, in children, there are a few acquired conditions that may cause obstruction of the ureter, either by intraluminal blockage (stones, papillary necrosis) or extraluminal compression (retroperitoneal tumour, intra-abdominal mass). Ureteric strictures in children are unheard of without a history of surgical intervention.

BASIC SCIENCE

When a kidney is acutely and completely obstructed, such as by a calculus or acute PUJ obstruction, there is a rapid sequence of events. Initially, filtration continues, and although there may be some reabsorption of urine from the renal pelvis, the pressure within the renal capsule rises, causing a reduced blood flow. Nephron loss follows – about 50 per cent loss by six days, and total loss after six weeks. Complete obstruction, therefore, ultimately is associated with complete loss of the kidney, a process that is accelerated greatly by the coincidence of urinary infection. The majority of so-called 'obstructions' are associated with some renal function and cannot by definition be complete, so some surgeons prefer to use the term 'urine-flow impairment'. Exactly what is meant by the term 'obstruction' has caused much debate, but perhaps the most useful definition is 'any restriction to urine flow, which if left untreated will cause progressive renal deterioration' (Koff and Campbell 1994).

Hydronephrosis is a term commonly used to describe dilation of the renal pelvis. The term hydroureteronephrosis is used when the ureter is also involved. Although dilation is almost always present with obstruction, the latter is not the only cause of dilation. Hydronephrosis could be due to renal dysplasia, as in an ectopic kidney. Hydroureteronephrosis could be due to vesicoureteric reflux, for example. Neither term should ever be used synonymously with obstruction. A series of investigations therefore is required to determine whether the hydronephrotic kidney is compromised and fits within our definition. It is often necessary to repeat these investigations at intervals in order to determine whether any changes have taken place and to decide whether surgical intervention is required.

DIAGNOSTIC TESTS

Antenatal and postnatal ultrasound

Ultrasound is the first investigation for imaging upper tract obstruction. It is the only modality currently available to diagnose dilation of the urinary tract antenatally. It is good at identifying the severity of dilation (determined classically by measuring the anteroposterior (AP) diameter of the renal pelvis). This provides a number used to monitor progress throughout the pregnancy and beyond. Severity is generally greater when the dilation is seen early compared with that appearing later after a normal initial scan. In addition to the AP diameter, ultrasound gives some information about the anatomy of the renal calyces, whose dilation may be related to the severity of 'obstruction' and the likely outcome (vide infra) and also about the level of dilation. If the ureter is seen, then the diagnostic focus shifts to the VUJ and the need for a postnatal cystogram to rule out vesicoureteric reflux arises. The level of renal function cannot be determined on antenatal ultrasound, but a helpful positive feature is a good thickness of renal parenchyma with a 'normal' echo pattern. In bilateral cases, bladder cycling with normal volumes of liquor is also reassuring. Conversely, a bright parenchyma may indicate renal dysplasia, and a low volume or lack of liquor is almost always a bad sign. Postnatally, ultrasound provides similar information, although good images are generally easier to acquire. If the first postnatal scan is performed less than five days after birth, however, the relatively dehydrated state of the infant during this time may lead to an underestimate of the severity of dilation and a false sense of security. For this reason, all babies with antenatal dilation should have a repeat scan at six weeks, regardless of the result of the first postnatal scan.

Doppler tracings of the renal vessels can be used to derive the resistive index. This is a measure of renal blood flow, which theoretically may be reduced when intracapsular, and thus parenchymal pressure is increased by rises in pressure in the pelvis of an obstructed kidney. This measurement has not been found to be useful in children and generally is not used.

Micturating cystourethrography

This is indicated postnatally in patients in whom ureteric dilation has been seen and in bilateral cases where there is a need to exclude reflux and (in boys) lower tract obstruction. It is probably not necessary to perform it routinely in patients with dilated renal pelvis alone and certainly not in those presenting later and without an antenatal history.

^{99}Tc-Mercaptoacetyltriglycine diuretic renography

Together with ultrasound, ^{99}Tc-mercaptoacetyltriglycine (MAG3) diuretic renography has become the mainstay of diagnosis in upper tract obstruction. MAG3 is filtered only partially by the glomerulus but obtains high levels in the renal filtrate by an active filtration mechanism in the proximal convoluted tubule. The physiological maturation of renal and specifically proximal tubular function in the early postnatal period limits the usefulness of early scans, which may have a high background activity, but these can nonetheless be used to assess renal function in selected cases. The first MAG3 scan therefore is usually delayed until around three months, when good images may be obtained.

MAG3 is administered by a rapid intravenous bolus with the patient already positioned on the scinti-scanner to allow immediate acquisition of data. Regions of interest are drawn around each kidney for analysis in order to isolate renal activity, and corrections are made to allow for general background activity. The rate of uptake of the renal parenchyma is measured during the second minute and is used to provide a differential function for the two kidneys, which is derived from the gradient of the upslope of the renogram curve and expressed for each kidney as a percentage of the total. After this, the tracer enters the renal collecting system and transits through the pelvis and ureter to the bladder, which results in a drop in activity over the kidney. This information is expressed both as a series of images and as a curve of renal activity against time, as shown in Figure 54.1a. When tracer is held up in the renal collecting system, this fall in activity is delayed or lost, raising the possibility of an obstruction (Figure 54.1b). If the renal collecting system is dilated, however, then the radioactive tracer will drain slowly due to dilution in the renal pelvic urine, and a large volume of urine is required to wash it out. For this reason, a weight-related dose of furosemide (frusemide) is administered, classically after 20 minutes, to produce diuresis and refine the drainage curve. The response to diuretic may be that the activity decreases (drainage occurs; Figure 54.1c) but no response suggests continued hold-up or obstruction (Figure 54.1d). At the end of the study, the patient is taken from the scanner (where he or she has lain supine throughout), held upright to change the posture, and allowed to micturate. Further images are acquired subsequently to assess longer-term drainage.

It is important to recognize two things about the interpretation of MAG3 renograms. First, true obstruction will result in a compromise of renal function and a falling differential function in unilateral cases. Second, drainage curves are affected both by the degree of hydration (and urine flow) of the patient and by the volume of the collecting system, which may vary

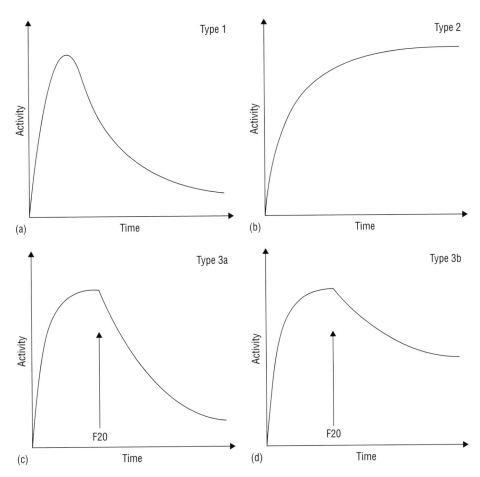

Figure 54.1 *Renogram curves. (a) Normal renogram with a steep peak of activity followed by a rapid fall as the tracer is washed out of the renal pelvis. (b) Obstructed: the activity continues to rise and there is no fall on administration of diuretic, showing that all tracer is held up in the collecting system and fails to drain. (c) Non-obstructed: tracer is washed out with diuretic and activity falls, showing drainage. (d) Equivocal: there is little response to furosemide (frusemide), but a fall in activity suggests that some slow drainage is occurring.*

considerably in children. For these reasons, paediatric urologists focus more on differential function and its changes over several scans than on drainage curves in their decision-making process.

Contrast radiology

Intravenous urography is no longer part of the routine assessment of hydronephrosis. However, occasionally it can provide useful anatomical information in difficult and older patients. Other contrast studies of the collecting system require a general anaesthetic to be performed. Retrograde pyelography at cystoscopy has been routine for some surgeons before proceeding to pyeloplasty and gives a better definition of ureteric anatomy. Antegrade pyelography via a puncture of the renal collecting system is more invasive but is used in difficult cases to define anatomy and give an impression of flow through the PUJ. Whitaker (1973) tried to refine the antegrade study by measuring the pressure gradient along the ureter when saline is infused into the renal pelvis at a constant rate. Unfortunately, in children the numbers obtained do not correlate well with obstruction defined by other means, so the Whitaker test is used rarely.

PELVIURETERIC JUNCTION OBSTRUCTION

Urine flow impairment at the PUJ is the most common form of upper tract obstruction. It is found equally in males and females and is twice as likely to affect the left kidney. The aetiology of the obstruction is variable, but recognizable anatomical variants include a narrow segment of ureter at the level of and below the PUJ (intrinsic stenosis), ureteric folds in the proximal ureter, and crossing accessory vessels to the lower pole of the kidney, causing kinking of the proximal ureter. There is also an important rare association of PUJ obstruction and vesicoureteric reflux, in which folding of the upper ureter or a narrow segment may prevent drainage of the refluxed urine and be an additional cause of renal compromise. This is a potential catch to the unwary surgeon, but the situation can be clarified by performing renography with the bladder on catheter drainage or with retrograde or antegrade contrast studies. Less commonly, an upper tract obstruction may be associated with a retrocaval ureter, in which the ureter of the right kidney winds around the back of the vena cava and gives a characteristic 'fish-hook' appearance on intravenous urography (IVU). PUJ-type obstructions are also recognized in the lower poles of duplex kidneys and in horseshoe kidneys.

With the advent of antenatal screening ultrasound, there was a five-fold increase in the number of patients presenting for evaluation. The size of this problem is considerable, as upper tract dilation is now found in nearly one in 300 pregnancies, and over 40 per cent of these are labelled PUJ after initial postnatal evaluation. The advantage of antenatal diagnosis may be in the early expeditious treatment of cases, reducing morbidity, complications and improving outcomes. A concern, however, is that this diagnosis not only causes a great deal of anxiety for parents but also may lead to many patients being over-treated. The current incidence of pyeloplasty (the most common operation for PUJ obstruction) in children is around one in 1500, reflecting a more conservative modern approach.

Over the past two decades, experience and several prospective studies of observation versus conservative treatment have provided clarification and enabled both more accurate prenatal counselling and better selection of patients for intervention postnatally. The challenge to the surgeon is to identify patients who will most benefit from an operation and to separate them from those who are unlikely to need this intervention and can be discharged from follow-up. In this respect, comparing measured parameters with long-term outcomes has enabled triggers for surgical intervention to be developed.

The degree of renal pelvic dilation on antenatal and postnatal ultrasound scans can be related to the likely need for surgery. Kidneys are at high risk of deterioration if severe dilation is present early in the pregnancy (<20 weeks) or if there are large increases in dilatation prenatally. Postnatally, renal pelvic AP diameter on the first (fully hydrated) scan can predict the likelihood of intervention for poor or deteriorating function. All patients with dilation over 50 mm will come to surgery, which often is simply to excise a non-functioning kidney. With dilation over 40 mm, 80 per cent will need an operation; with dilation over 30 mm, 55 per cent will need surgery; with dilation over 20 mm, 20 per cent will need an operation; and if the AP pelvic diameter is below 20 mm, then only one to three per cent are operated on. Most surgeons agree that patients with a hydrated AP diameter of less than 15 mm can be discharged with no follow-up. Gross calyceal dilation also alludes to more severe renal compromise and a greater likelihood of deterioration. It is a qualitative measure that dictates pyeloplasty even if the more quantitative AP diameter is lower. On follow-up, an increasing AP diameter may be an indication for surgery in itself but usually determines the need for a new renogram to be performed.

The MAG3 renogram provides an accurate differential function, and follow-up studies in unilateral cases have also enabled risks of intervention to be determined. If the initial function is over 40 per cent, then only 17 per cent come to surgery on follow-up; a similar number (20 per cent) come to surgery if the initial differential is above 30 per cent. Below 30 per cent, two-thirds of patients will need an operation for deterioration of function. If the function is very low on the initial scan (less than ten per cent), then there has been no benefit from short-term drainage via a nephrostomy; these patients do not recover their function and nephrectomy is indicated. A catch is that hyper-function (i.e. differential function significantly above 50 per cent on the affected side) is not an infrequent finding in a unilateral case with significant dilation and may indicate a kidney responding to stress. Around half of these kidneys may deteriorate and come to surgery when followed up.

After ultrasound scanning at six days and six weeks and MAG3 renography at three months, follow-up scans and their frequency for conservatively managed patients will depend largely on the initial findings. In general, ultrasound scans are performed at three-monthly intervals, and a MAG3 is repeated at six months and one year. If dilation is stable, then the frequency of scans is reduced after the first year and MAG3 renography is reserved as a second-line investigation, to be triggered by changes in ultrasound appearance (increased dilation). Prophylactic antibiotics are administered routinely to all patients from birth, but once the diagnosis of PUJ obstruction is made and other anomalies excluded, antibiotics may be stopped.

Conservative follow-up reveals that many patients with initial severe dilation and decreased function return to more normal parameters without any intervention. Indeed, of all those patients presenting with antenatal dilation, 75 per cent will not need surgery. This is probably a very significant contributor to the excellent results of pyeloplasty in historical series, when the majority of patients were operated on but would have done well without surgery. The indications for continuation of conservative management are the opposite of the indications for surgery, i.e. lack of symptoms, stable or decreasing dilation, and stable or improving function.

Bilateral cases present a more difficult situation, as the differential function on MAG3 scanning is unable to provide a comparison to normal. Decision-making therefore is often on the basis of ultrasound appearance, and the threshold to operate is lower. The more severely affected kidney on MAG3 scanning is usually operated first, although bilateral synchronous pyeloplasties are also performed.

Apart from antenatal diagnosis, PUJ obstruction may present with clinical signs and complications in later childhood. These include severe sepsis due to an obstructed infected kidney (which may be a bag of pus), intermittent abdominal pain (which may or may not be related to the ipsilateral loin), an incidental finding of a mass or a dilated kidney on an ultrasound scan performed for another reason, or rarely haematuria. The presence of a clinical scenario such as urinary tract infection makes decision-making much easier and will tip the balance towards surgical intervention in any patient on conservative follow-up.

Table 54.1 *Summary of indications for pyeloplasty*

Modality	Criteria
Antenatal ultrasound	Severe early dilation
	Rapidly increasing and gross dilation
Postnatal ultrasound	AP diameter >30 mm
	AP diameter >20 mm and calyceal dilation
MAG3 scan	Initial function <30%
	Deteriorating function on follow-up
Symptoms	Loin pain
	UTI or other symptoms

AP, anteroposterior; MAG3, ^{99}Tc-mercaptoacetyltriglycine; UTI, urinary tract infection.

A classic mode of presentation of PUJ obstruction in an older child (usually over four years of age) is with intermittent abdominal pain. This may be severe and associated with vomiting, loin pain and tenderness and tends to be self-limiting. Alternatively symptoms can be rather vague in nature, and so there is often a prolonged history of non-specific and uninvestigated symptoms. In most cases, evaluation with abdominal ultrasound identifies hydronephrosis limited to the kidney and confirms the diagnosis, although renography may be normal. It is logistically difficult to scan patients during their episodes (i.e. when dilation is likely to be more severe), and in those with only mild dilation on routine scans it may take some time to evaluate their symptoms and come to a conclusion. The indication for surgery is pain, and post-operative evaluation of this is the outcome measure. At operation, crossing vessels are often found, in which case the anastomosis is made anterior to them.

A summary of the indications for pyeloplasty is shown in Table 54.1.

The definitive surgery for PUJ obstruction in children is pyeloplasty. Although several techniques have been described, the Anderson-Hynes dismembered pyeloplasty is the standard approach. This is usually performed through an antero-lateral loin muscle-cutting incision, although the author has found the muscle-splitting incision applicable in all age groups. The lumbotomy incision is also described, but this provides more limited access to the kidney and it is not possible to make the anastomosis anterior to crossing vessels. Some surgeons are advancing a laparoscopic approach and this may become the standard, especially with the advent of robotic instrumentation for suturing. The principle of Anderson-Hynes remains the same for all routes, however; it is illustrated in Figure 54.2.

Occasionally, when a patient presents acutely with a dilated kidney and especially when there is suspicion of infection, temporary drainage of the upper tract with a per-cutaneously placed pigtail nephrostomy is indicated. This allows the clinical emergency to settle and the definitive pyeloplasty to be performed on a routine list once the infection has settled. If function is likely to be poor, then a MAG3 scan can be performed to determine whether nephrectomy is indicated instead. Various percutaneous techniques are

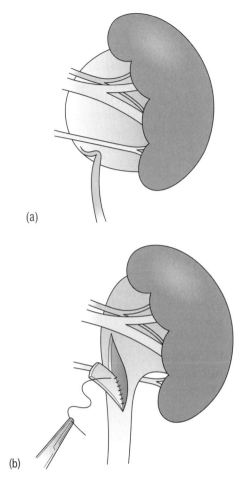

(a)

(b)

Figure 54.2 *Anderson-Hynes pyeloplasty. (a) Appearances at operation: a dilated renal pelvis with a tortuous or stenotic pelviureteric junction (PUJ) and/or crossing lower-pole vessels. The PUJ is excised with a variable amount of renal pelvis to reduce its volume. A wide spatulated anastomosis is made between the renal pelvis and normal calibre ureter (b).*

described for dilation and incision of the PUJ, followed by a period of intraluminal stenting. These have not found an application in children due to high complication rates and poor results. Stents are used routinely following pyeloplasty by many surgeons. A JJ stent needs to be removed under a further general anaesthetic, so a nephrostomy stent (an external draining tube continuous with an indwelling JJ stent) is popular. This allows a period of external drainage in addition to stenting the anastomosis and can simply be pulled out without anaesthetic after a few days. A drain external to the anastomosis is rarely used, and the author reserves this (as well as internal stenting) for difficult cases. In the majority of patients, careful anastomosis with fine absorbable sutures and a temporary urethral catheter (for 24–48 hours) are sufficient.

The results of pyeloplasty are very good, with a reported success rate of over 96 per cent and a low complication rate. Postoperative pain and fever may indicate an anastomotic leak and/or a failure of drainage through the neo-PUJ. This is confirmed on ultrasound and is treated with a percutaneous nephrostomy and/or a period of JJ stenting. Some patients may require a revision following this complication.

Follow-up surveillance is with ultrasound and MAG3 scanning; initially, these are performed after three months. It is important to realize that a very dilated kidney will continue to look dilated on ultrasound and may never return to normal. Providing that this is not severe and it is stable on at least two follow-up scans, the patient can be discharged. The MAG3 scan is mainly to assess function following the surgery, similar to the preoperative evaluation, although an improvement in the drainage curve is often seen due to a reduction in volume of the renal pelvis. If the patient has been operated on following a drop in the kidney's function, then it will remain stable or improve in almost all of them. It is not necessary to perform more than one follow-up MAG3 scan if function is satisfactory and the ultrasound appearance is stable. Further studies may be indicated by increased dilation on ultrasound follow-up.

'OBSTRUCTED' MEGAURETER (VESICOURETERIC JUNCTION OBSTRUCTION)

The next most common site of upper tract obstruction is at the VUJ. Research into the diameter of ureters in children has confirmed that the normal ureter never exceeds 6 mm and can rarely be seen on ultrasound in the absence of pathology. Megaureter (literally meaning 'big ureter') is a term referring to ureters that can be seen along their length, which may be due to a variety of causes. These causes may be primary, i.e. due to an intrinsic pathology of the VUJ, or secondary to another external influence such as lower tract obstruction or a neuropathic high-pressure bladder. A cystogram helps to divide them further into refluxing and non-refluxing types. Although the majority of 'obstructed' primary megaureters do not reflux, a caveat is that it is possible for reflux and obstruction to coexist, but this is relatively rare.

Primary non-refluxing megaureter accounts for 12 per cent of antenatally diagnosed uropathies (which today is the most common mode of presentation), is more common in males than females, and has a left-sided predisposition. Various theories have been put forward to explain the urine flow impairment at the VUJ, including an aganglionic segment of distal ureter (akin to Hirschsprung's disease of the bowel). Histology confirms the presence of ganglion cells, however, but has identified features including a narrow distal segment with deficient muscle fibres and increased collagen and an area of muscular hypertrophy in the dilated ureter immediately above. Similar to the findings with PUJ obstruction, follow-up of antenatally diagnosed asymptomatic cases shows a tendency for spontaneous improvement postnatally, justifying an initially conservative approach.

The antenatal features of VUJ obstruction are a dilated renal pelvis, which is continuous with a dilated ureter to the level of the bladder. This may be difficult to identify initially in the fetus, but it becomes clearer with repeated scans or on postnatal evaluation. Postnatal ultrasound is followed immediately by a micturating cystourethrogram to rule out reflux into the dilated system (and lower tract obstruction if the dilation is bilateral). A thorough general examination is performed to rule out causes of secondary megaureter, such as neuropathic bladder and prune-belly syndrome. MAG3 renography and repeated ultrasound scans are performed at about three months, unless the dilation is severe and earlier intervention seems necessary. This is true particularly in bilateral cases, where earlier functional assessment is important to plan management.

Of the antenatally diagnosed cases, 35 per cent will resolve on conservative follow-up (prophylactic antibiotics and surveillance) and 50 per cent will remain stable in terms of their function and dilatation. One in six (15 per cent) patients will require intervention because of poor function, deterioration or complication (mainly infection). Conservative follow-up is based on regular ultrasounds and a repeat MAG3 at one year of age, or sooner if there is increasing dilation or infection.

Reimplanting a large dilated ureter into a relatively small infant bladder may have severe long-term consequences for its development and function, and it has been a relief that this surgery is no longer thought to be necessary in the majority of patients. Where surgery is indicated, if the initial function is poor (less than ten per cent) and there is a normal contralateral kidney, then the best treatment is nephro-ureterectomy performed open or laparoscopically. This leaves the normal bladder and kidney undisturbed. If the function is better or in a bilateral case, then reimplantation surgery may be delayed by the placement of a ureteric JJ stent. This has to be inserted via an open operation in babies; the stent is placed with one limb up each ureter. After three to six months, the stent is removed and follow-up imaging is performed. This shows improvement in at least 50 per cent of cases, and so more invasive surgery can be avoided. In the remainder, the period of stenting has delayed reconstructive surgery until the second year of life and has also decompressed the ureter for a period, reducing the risks and difficulties of reimplantation. Megaureters are reimplanted using a Leadbetter–Politano technique, as shown in Figure 54.3. Their diameter is reduced using a Starr plication and the bladder is fixed using a psoas hitch to secure the submucosal tunnel. A period of postoperative stenting is usually required. Follow-up is with repeat ultrasound and functional imaging. In total, one in 12 (seven per cent) patients from the antenatal group will require this definitive operation.

Patients who present clinically may do so with severe sepsis and require drainage with a percutaneous nephrostomy to resolve the acute situation and allow a full assessment to be carried out. These are most likely to come to surgical management, and many will come to nephro-ureterectomy due to poor function. If function is worth preserving, then a period of stenting is probably not indicated, so one should proceed to definitive reconstruction.

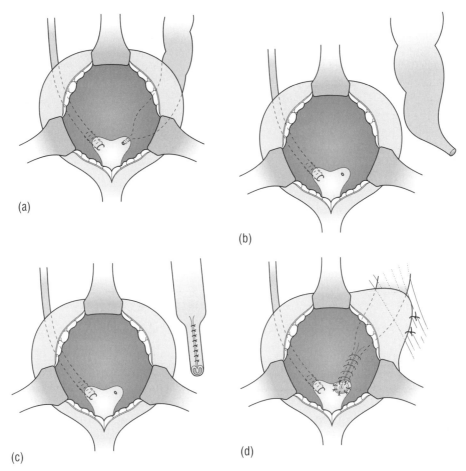

Figure 54.3 *Reimplantation of megaureter. (a) The bladder is opened to reveal the ureteric orifice, which is dissected through its hiatus and detached from the bladder wall (b). The distal segment is removed, and a Starr plication of the lower 2 cm is performed to narrow this distal segment (c). The ureter is brought through the bladder wall and tunnelled down to the original orifice position submucosally (d). The bladder wall is fixed with a psoas hitch of prolene sutures to secure the tunnel.*

OTHER CAUSES OF UPPER TRACT OBSTRUCTION

The next largest group of patients with upper tract obstruction are those presenting with intraluminal obstruction from renal and ureteric calculi. The diagnosis and management of these is covered elsewhere in this book. Large retroperitoneal tumours are relatively rare in children but cause extraluminal compression of the ureter(s) and can present with upper tract obstruction. This is often asymptomatic and identified on cross-sectional imaging of the tumour, unless bilateral obstruction leads to renal failure or there is super-added sepsis. Although nephrostomy drainage is often used to relieve the obstruction acutely, endoscopic retrograde insertion of JJ stents is also effective and has the added advantage of avoiding external drainage. Although there are risks associated with general anaesthesia in these often severely ill patients, the retrograde approach avoids needling the kidney, which is hazardous in patients with abnormal clotting. Chemotherapy is usually effective at reducing the size of these tumours and thereby resolving the obstruction, and the stents are usually only temporary.

CLINICAL SCENARIOS

Case 1

A baby boy presented following an antenatal diagnosis of right hydronephrosis. Postnatal ultrasound showed significant hydronephrosis, which increased over a year with calyceal dilation (Figure 54.4a). Over this period, the initially good differential function of 48 per cent deteriorated to 39 per cent, and a pyeloplasty was performed (Figure 54.4b).

Case 2

Following an antenatal diagnosis of unilateral hydronephrosis, postnatal evaluation of a baby girl revealed significant (35 mm) renal pelvic dilation with calyceal involvement (Figure 54.5a). A MAG3 scan showed reduced function (35 per cent of the differential) and drainage from the right kidney (Figure 54.5b). Pyeloplasty was performed. Follow-up imaging three months later demonstrated an improvement in the ultrasound

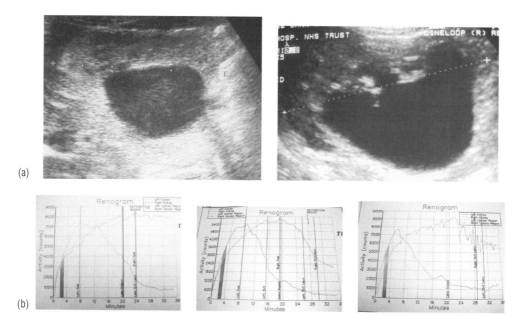

Figure 54.4   *(a) Increasing dilation on ultrasound. (b) Decreasing function and continued poor drainage, leading to a decision to operate.*

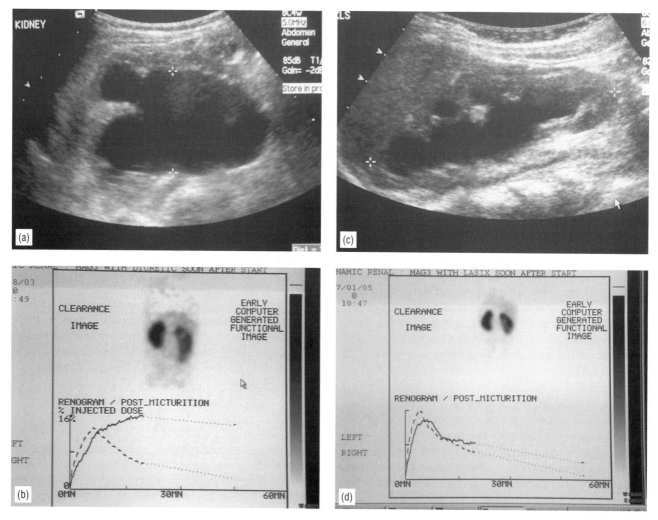

Figure 54.5   *Massive dilation on ultrasound (a) and reduced function at 35 per cent and poor function on MAG3 (b). Significant improvement in all modalities following pyeloplasty (c, d).*

appearance (Figure 54.5c) and in both the nephrogram and differential function on MAG3 scanning (39 per cent).

Case 3

A patient with antenatally diagnosed hydronephrosis was found to have good function at postnatal imaging. The dilation at one year was significantly less with no surgical intervention (Figure 54.6).

Case 4

Evaluation of a boy with antenatally diagnosed hydroureteronephrosis showed a dilated kidney and ureter to the level of the bladder (Figure 54.7a). Follow-up imaging at six months suggested persistence of the dilation, with a massive megaureter behind the bladder (Figure 54.7b). The child remained well on

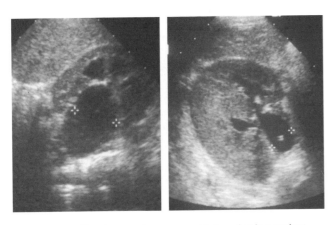

Figure 54.6 *Spontaneous improvement in imaging in a patient with initially normal function and dilation. Appearance at six weeks and one year.*

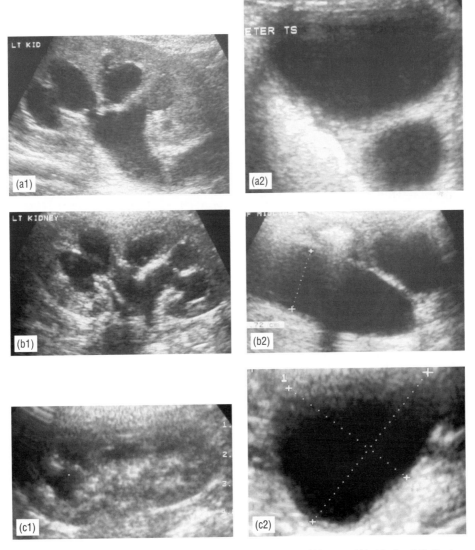

Figure 54.7 *Spontaneous improvement in ultrasound appearance of a megaureter at kidney and bladder level. Patient was studied at (a) six weeks, (b) six months and (c) 18 months.*

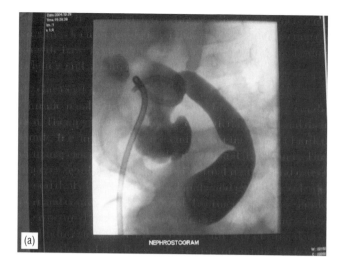

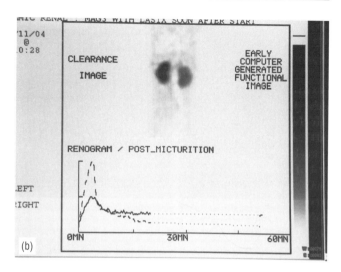

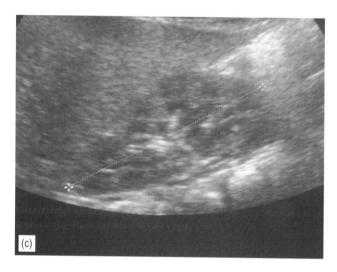

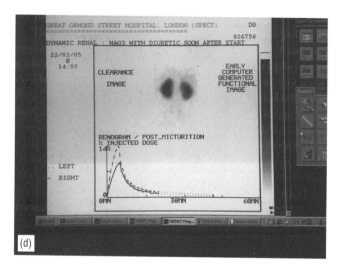

Figure 54.8 *Megaureters complicated by infection and treated with nephrostomy drainage (a). Ultrasound after tapered ureteric reimplantation (c) and improvement in function (b, d).*

prophylactic antibiotics. Repeat imaging at 18 months showed a great improvement in the ultrasound appearance, with continued good function.

Case 5

A six-month old baby presented following an admission via casualty with a high fever and urinary tract infection. Acute investigation revealed a severely dilated right collecting system and ureter. Initial treatment was with percutaneous nephrostomy (Figure 54.8) and intravenous antibiotics. A MAG3 functional scan was performed with nephrostomy drainage with a differential function of 30 per cent. Six weeks later, a tapered ureteric reimplantation with psoas hitch was performed. Follow-up ultrasound showed significant reduction of the hydronephrosis and MAG3 scanning showed an improvement of function to 39 per cent and good drainage.

REFERENCES

Koff SA, Campbell. The nonoperative management of unilateral neonatal hydronephrosis: natural history of poorly functioning kidneys. *Journal of Urology* 1994; **152**: 593–5.

Whitaker RH. Methods of assessing obstruction in dilated ureters. *British Journal of Urology* 1973; **45**: 15.

FURTHER READING

Nguyen HT, Kogan BA. Upper urinary tract obstruction: experimental and clinical aspects. *British Journal of Urology* 1998; **81** (suppl 2): 13–21.

55

Lower urinary tract obstruction

SN CENK BÜYÜKÜNAL

Learning objectives

- To understand the types and mechanisms of urethral pathology.
- To understand the pre- and postnatal presenting symptoms, clinical findings and specific complications.
- To know about the diagnostic imaging characteristics of valves and other lower urinary tract obstructions.
- To have a working knowledge of the surgical treatment modalities and long-term complications and their evaluations.

INTRODUCTION

Obstruction of the lower urinary tract is essentially a disease of the male, due to lesions such as posterior and anterior urethral valves, polyps, strictures, syringoceles and meatal stenosis.

Both in males and in females, the effects of lower urinary tract obstruction may be far-reaching, involving the bladder with abnormal bladder function, vesicoureteric junction obstruction, hydroureteronephrosis, dysplasia and even, in severe cases, renal failure. These factors must be considered when lower urinary tract obstruction is suspected and diagnosed. They are most common and relevant in the situation of posterior urethral valves.

Lesions causing urethral obstruction are less common in females than males. The main reasons for urethral obstruction in females are ureteroceles, cloacal abnormalities, bladder outlet obstruction due to severe hydrocolpos and imperforate hymen, and female hypospadias.

Prolapsed ectopic ureteroceles can present as an intralabial smooth, round, oedematous mass (Figure 55.1) and may create obstructive symptoms. Ultrasonography and intravenous urogram may be helpful in making the diagnosis. Transurethral incision may relieve the obstructive symptoms.

Sarcoma botryoides or rhabdomyosarcoma of the vagina and/or bladder appears as a lobulated mass protruding from the introitus. A blood-spotting red mass should alert the physician. Some of these lesions may cause obstructive urinary symptoms (Figure 55.2). Biopsy is necessary for exact diagnosis.

A low simple imperforate hymen may give rise to urinary obstructive symptoms (Figure 55.3). A bulging intralabial centrally located mass is a very pathognomonic sign. This may create severe hydrocolpos in a neonate due to maternal oestrogen stimulation. A simple incision and drainage is the treatment of choice.

MEATAL STENOSIS

This is a relatively common and usually acquired abnormality in the distal part of the male urethra, as a result of either circumcision or hypospadias repair. Irritation of the meatus

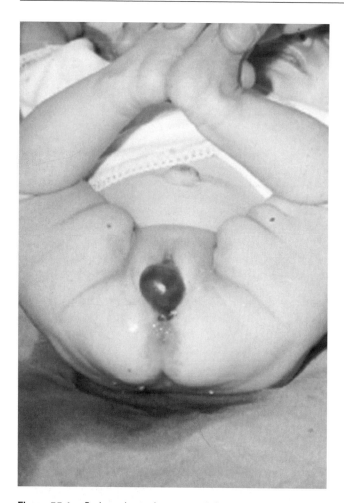

Figure 55.1   *Prolapsed ectopic ureterocele in an 11-month-old girl.*

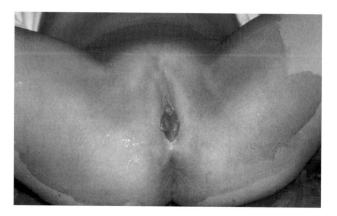

Figure 55.2   *Sarcoma botryoides (rhabdomyosarcoma) protruding from the vagina in a three-year-old female with obstructing urinary symptoms.*

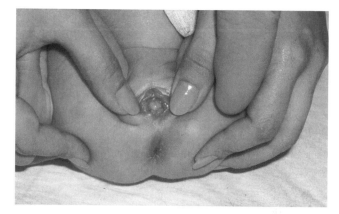

Figure 55.3   *Imperforate hymen. Note the bulging hymen in a neonate in the midline location.*

bloody spotting, intermittent dysuria or enuretic episodes may be seen.

Care should be taken not to overdiagnose this clinical entity, based on the visual and anatomical appearances of the meatus. Despite its 'pinpoint' appearance, the external meatus may enhance normal urination with its elasticity. Calibration of the meatus and observation of the urinary stream are usually enough for diagnosis. Thickening of the bladder wall and pathological changes in uroflowmetry can be detected in severe cases. However, these diagnostic tools have no advantage over obvious physical visual examination.

Treatment consists of an anterior meatotomy. To prevent future re-stricture formation, we always prefer to use three to four 7/0 absorbable sutures (Vicryl™ or polydioxanone suture). Lubricant creams are used routinely to prevent re-adhesions.

In one study, 190 neonates without any co-existing urological pathologies, were circumcised. Fusidic acid ophthalmic ointment was applied to the meatus for ten days. In our retrospective study, we found no evidence of meatal stricture formation.

URETHRAL POLYPS

Urethral polyps are usually benign single congenital lesions. They are usually located in the posterior urethra. Polyps are seen in males and usually originate from the verumontanum. Polyps may have a 1–3 cm long pedicle. The outer surface is covered by a transitional urinary epithelium. Abnormal protrusion of the urethral wall and histopathological changes due to maternally induced oestrogens are the only well-known aetiological factors.

Intermittent urinary obstruction, dysuria, haematuria, urgency, incomplete emptying, diminution in the calibre of the urinary stream and intermittent incontinence are the most prominent presenting symptoms. Polyps are not very frequent, and there are not enough data about their incidence. In the study of Gleason and Kramer (1994), most children

of a neonate after neonatal circumcision may lead eventually to a stricture formation. For this reason, neonatal circumcision has always been blamed as an aetiological factor in the formation of meatal stenosis.

The presenting symptom is almost always a very narrow and upwardly deflected urinary stream. In older children,

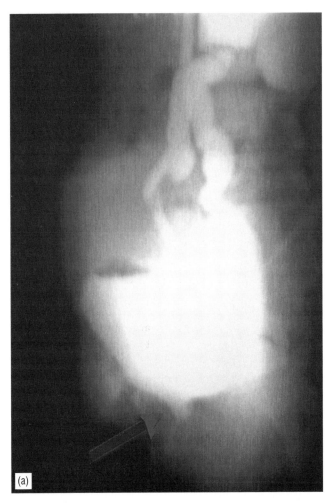
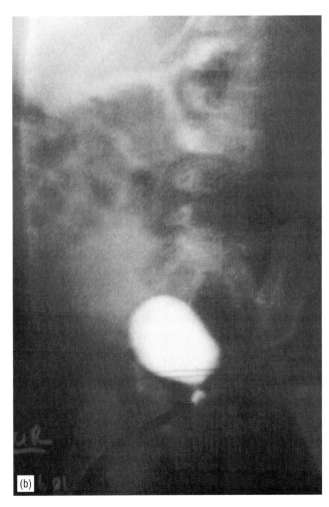

Figure 55.4 *(a) Minor syringocele in a one-month-old boy. Note the filling defect and enlarged posterior urethra in voiding cystourethrography. (b) An obstructive syringocele with severe bilateral reflux and dilation of the upper tract.*

with urethral polyps were eight to nine years of age at presentation. A difference in their voiding patterns due to obstruction in the lower urinary tract was the most frequent symptom.

A filling defect in the urethra detected by a meticulously performed voiding cystourethrography (VCUG) is the most important diagnostic sign. Some polyps may protrude up to the bladder neck with their long pedicles; these may be detected by bladder ultrasonography.

Cystoscopy is necessary for confirmation of diagnosis and treatment. Transurethral excision can be performed easily. Risk of recurrence is small if the base is excised sufficiently.

CYSTIC COWPER'S GLAND DUCTS OR SYRINGOCELES

The bulbourethral (Cowper) glands are paired and situated in each side of the bulbar urethra and corpus spongiosum. The main Cowper's glands are drained via two ducts, canalized directly to the bulbous urethra through the corpus spongiosum. These ducts are fenestrated to the urethra by tiny openings. Cystic dilations may occur due to obstructions in these tiny orifices. The cystic dilations and diverticular formation of Cowper's glands were named 'Cowper's gland syringoceles' by Maizels *et al.* (1983).

The cysts may stay as non-symptomatic microscopic findings or become gross submucosal cysts. They may have thin walls and sometimes rupture spontaneously, with the remnants of the cyst wall protruding into the urethra. A group of syringoceles may open into the urethra by a spatulous ostium; these are classified as perforated syringoceles.

Syringoceles can remain silent and without clinical problems in infants and young children. Ruptured syringoceles cause urethral infections, haematuria, spotting at the meatus, dysuria and dribbling. Non-perforated syringoceles may produce obstructive problems and voiding difficulties.

Most of these abnormalities are diagnosed incidentally on VCUG undertaken for various reasons, including haematuria, infection and obstructive problems (Figure 55.4). Care should be taken during VCUG not to perforate the thin wall of the cyst with catheterization. On cystoscopic examination, these lesions may appear as cystic lesions with thin walls.

Most children remain asymptomatic and do not require any treatment. In symptomatic cases, transurethral marsupialization of the cyst is necessary.

Seven syringocele cases were treated in our unit during one study. The mean age was 40.5 months (range 1–150 months). Recurrent urinary tract infection and obstructive voiding symptoms were the most frequent findings. High-grade vesicoureteric reflux (VUR) was detected in five patients. Two of the seven patients had prenatal hydronephrosis. Cystoscopy and unroofing was the treatment of choice in all of our patients. Two required additional anti-reflux procedures. All patients were free of symptoms in the average two-year follow-up.

ANTERIOR URETHRAL VALVES

Anterior urethral valves seem to occur almost seven to ten times less frequently than posterior urethral valves. They are membranous tissues, filamentous cusps or iris-like diaphragm-type lesions. Most are located in the bulbous urethra (40 per cent), penoscrotal junction (30 per cent) and penile urethra (30 per cent). An associated diverticulum may be seen in some cases.

Several embryological theories have been presented for the occurrence of anterior urethral valves, including:

- failure of the recanalization process between the proximal and distal parts of the urethra, resulting in a valve-like tissue remnant;
- a disorganization process during the creation of a duplicated urethra;
- congenital cystic dilation of a periurethral gland, resulting in a flap-like valve.

Most children are diagnosed during early infancy. The most important and frequent presenting symptoms are difficulty in voiding, dribbling incontinence and recurrent urinary tract infection. 'Ballooning' in the urethra during urination is the pathognomonic finding of a distally located valve. In our experience, a long penile tissue with defective corpus spongiosum and difficulty in voiding during the first weeks of life seems to be the most frequent finding (Figure 55.5).

VCUG is the gold-standard investigation for detection of anterior urethral valves. A linear defect along the ventral side of the urethra and an immediate change in the diameter of the urethra are the most demonstrative radiological findings. In addition, VUR can be detected in almost one-third of cases. A visible urethral diverticula can be seen in about a third of cases. Upper-tract dilation can be detected by ultrasonography in nearly half of these patients.

Cystoscopy is essential for diagnosis and treatment. Fulguration of the valves is possible. However, insufficient corpus spongiosum tissue is a real risk factor for postoperative subcutaneous extravasations and urethrocutaneous fistulae formations. For this reason, patients with diverticular

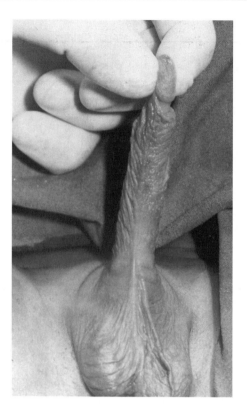

Figure 55.5 *Long loose penis in a 1.5-year-old male with anterior urethral valve. Note the defective spongios tissue. In cystoscopic examination, a valve was located in the proximal portion of the anterior urethra.*

formation and a defective corpus spongiosum may benefit from open surgery. In our experience, open surgery seems safer than endoscopic treatment.

URETHRAL STRICTURES

A number of conditions or events can cause urethral strictures, which are then responsible for lower-urinary tract infections:

- *Congenital strictures:* these are extremely rare. It is estimated that 14 per cent of all paediatric urethral strictures are of congenital origin.
- *Infectious strictures:* these are due mainly to indwelling catheters used during the postoperative period following any surgery.
- *Traumatic strictures:* these may be iatrogenic or non-iatrogenic in their origin. Diagnostic or therapeutic endoscopic procedures, traumatic catheterizations and post-surgical strictures due to hypospadias surgery are the most frequent causes of iatrogenic strictures. Traumatic injuries due to road-traffic accidents are the most frequent cause of non-iatrogenic injuries.

The clinical evaluation and treatment of these problems are beyond the limits of this chapter and will be discussed elsewhere.

POSTERIOR URETHRAL VALVES

Introduction

Posterior urethral valves (PUVs) are the most common cause of bladder outlet obstruction in boys. The incidence varies between one in 4000 to one in 25 000 live male births. A dilated posterior urethra, thickening of the bladder neck and hypertrophy of the detrusor muscle, hydroureteronephrosis, diverticular formation, poor renal growth, and sometimes urinoma formation or urinary ascites are typical pathological findings. Poor urinary stream, inadequate emptying of the bladder, VUR and, occasionally, renal failure are the pathophysiological results of these conditions.

Relevant basic science

According to the literature, there have been several reports on twin and non-twin siblings. For this reason, a polygenetic mode of inheritance has been reported by various authors.

The existence of other coexistent anomalies has been investigated by various studies. Undescended testis seems to be the only significant coexisting pathology. Its reported coincidence is 12–17 per cent.

In 1919, Young and colleagues mentioned three different types of valvular obstruction of the posterior urethra:

- *Type I valve:* a bicuspid-type malformation between the urethral floor, the lateral sides of the verumontanum and the anterior part of the urethra.
- *Type II valve:* located between the verumontanum and the bladder neck.
- *Type III valve:* circular non-oblique valve located distal to the verumontanum. These valves are seldom encountered. They are circular soft mucosal pathologies (Stephens *et al.* 1996).

Type I valves are the most common. During micturition, the valves fill with urinary flow and act like sails catching the wind.

There has been much debate regarding the existence of type II valves. Essentially their existence is questionable, and practically they do not exist as real obstructive structures. They may be seen as longitudinal folds in the posterior urethra.

In 1983, Stephens presented his theory on embryogenesis of posterior urethral valves. According to this theory, lateral folds in the posterior urethra, called plicae colliculi, located in the lateral edges of the verumontanum are responsible for the formation of posterior urethral valves. Their overdevelopment and anterior fusion seemed to be responsible in forming PUVs (Stephens *et al.* 1996).

In 1974, Hendren used the term 'mini-valves' for obstructive lesions graded between normal plicae colliculi and real type I valves.

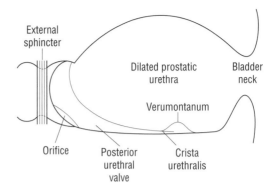

Figure 55.6 *Sagittal diagram of a posterior (type I) urethral valve.*

Dewan *et al.* in Australia reported interesting observations on PUV. They investigated uninstrumented infants with possible signs and symptoms of PUV. According to their observations, a PUV usually appeared as a single obstructive membrane, with a small hole in the mid-posterior portion (Figure 55.6). Due to these impressions, they called this entity 'congenital obstructing posterior urethral membrane' (COPUM). According to their experience, repeated catheterizations and cystoscopic examinations were responsible for the creation of a bigger passage in the obstructing membrane, as in type I valves.

General features and investigations

Since PUV is responsible for the deterioration of both kidneys and renal insufficiency, it is mandatory to diagnose this pathology as early as possible. Over the past two decades, many efforts have been made in the early antenatal diagnosis, follow-up and evaluation of PUV.

The main fetal sonographic findings are dilation of the fetal urinary bladder, proximal urethral dilation and thickening of the urinary bladder wall. Ureteral dilation and caliectasis may coexist. However, these are inconsistent findings in fetuses with PUV. Cystic formation and increased echogenicity may be reliable predictors of ultrasonographic investigations, although these findings were not very specific or sensitive.

Since karyotype abnormalities and other coexisting malformations are observed in 15–40 per cent of cases with obstructive uropathies, karyotype analysis and a meticulous scanning for other possible disorders are mandatory.

There is no general agreement about a sensitive technique for the assessment of risk of pulmonary hypoplasia. However, renal development and function can be estimated by use of the following investigations:

- *Investigation of fetal urine osmolality and electrolyte levels:* various authors have mentioned the importance of these parameters. Fetal urine sodium >100 mmol/L, chloride >90 mmol/L and osmolality >210 mosmol mean insufficient tubular reabsorption capacity and irreversible kidney damage. However, according to Wilkins *et al.* (1987), these measurements were not very sensitive in predicting renal outcome.

- *Investigating separate functions:* Nicolini *et al.* (1991, 1992) suggested sampling from both kidneys. According to their findings, this might provide better data for long-term prognostic studies.
- *Urinary microproteins:* according to various investigators, fetal urinary beta-2-microglobulin may be useful for evaluation of fetal renal function. Higher levels of beta-2-microglobulin have been found to be specific and sensitive for the prediction of renal insufficiency.
- *Amino acid measurements:* In the mid 1990s, the importance of the measurement of alanine/valine and valine/threonine ratios by using magnetic resonance spectroscopy was highlighted. By using this method, it was possible to predict the degree of kidney function as 'normal', 'compromised' or 'failure'.
- *Amniotic volume:* oligohydramnios is another predictive sign in the presence of high-grade severe obstructive uropathy.

Postnatal evaluation

Intrauterine growth retardation, failure to thrive, poor feeding, fever and vomiting due to severe urinary infection and sepsis are the most frequent early presenting symptoms in the neonatal period.

On physical examination, a palpable mass due to a distended bladder, or palpable masses due to hydronephrotic kidneys, can be detected easily. Abdominal distension due to urinary ascites is seldom seen. Straining during voiding and cessation in the urinary stream are typical findings in boys with PUV. However, many infants with PUV urinate normally. In severely obstructed cases, severe attacks of urosepsis and signs of renal insufficiency can be detected in the early period. Episodes of chronic and recurrent urinary infections and voiding problems, such as frequency, dribbling and incontinence, are presenting symptoms in older children. Children presenting in later periods generally have better renal function than neonates.

Diagnostic tools

VCUG remains the gold-standard investigation in the diagnosis of PUV. However, the general condition of many tiny neonates may not permit an early investigation to be performed. The radiological evaluation of the posterior urethra is extremely important. If the baby does not urinate, then help should be given by the Credé manoeuvre.

Type I valves are seen as linear oblique flaps across the urethra. These valves extend from the verumontanum to the distal anterior urethral wall. Type III valves are more

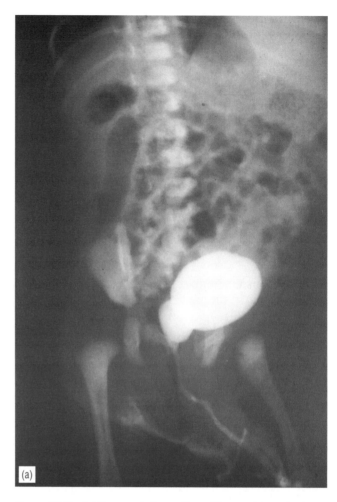

Figure 55.7 *(a) Huge posterior urethra with posterior urethral valve (PUV).*

perpendicular to the long urethral axis. The posterior urethra is less dilated in these patients.

The following findings are typical ultrasonographic and VCUG findings in the diagnosis of PUV:

- dilated posterior urethra (sometimes even larger than the bladder), prominent verumontanum and crista, thickness of the bladder neck, thick and trabeculated bladder wall, diverticular formation in bladder wall, bulging of the posterior urethra over the bulbous urethra and collapsed anterior urethra (Figure 55.7);
- VUR detected in up to 50 per cent of cases;
- true bladder volume may be surprisingly smaller than the expected bladder volume.

Radionuclide renal scans are very important for the assessment of kidney function. According to various investigators, mercaptoacetyltriglycine (MAG$_3$) is the most sensitive radiopharmaceutical agent as far as the assessment of kidney functions is concerned. Most clinicians prefer to perform nuclear studies at the end of the first month of life. However, these studies can be informative even two weeks after birth. In our hands, dimercaptosuccinic acid (DMSA) scanning static

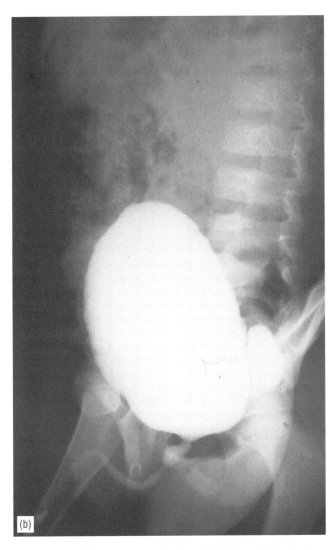

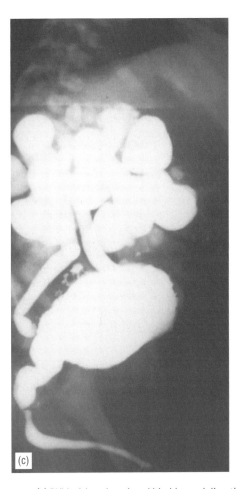

Figure 55.7 *(c) PUV with trabeculated bladder and diverticular formation plus bilateral gross vesicoureteric reflux.*

Figure 55.7 *(b) Type I PUV with enlarged bladder and diverticula formation.*

images can be as informative as MAG$_3$ studies for the early evaluation of kidney function.

Serum analysis is not very sensitive in reflecting kidney function in the first days of the life, because the effects of the maternal kidneys are still evident during the first 48 hours. After the initial period, serum creatinine levels, blood urea nitrogen and serum and urinary electrolytes should be monitored at routine intervals. Urine culture studies must be followed up carefully.

Management

PRENATAL PERIOD

If the karyotype is completely normal and there are no other life-threatening abnormalities, then the following may be potential sequelae:

- a fetus whose obstruction is severe enough to cause deterioration of pulmonary development;
- a fetus at risk of poor development of both kidneys;
- a fetus without any irreversible kidney damage and that may be a candidate for fetal intervention.

A number of antenatal options for treating a fetus with severe PUV are being developed:

- *Vesicoamniotic shunt:* currently, the most popular method seems to be the placement of a double pigtail vesicoamniotic catheter. However, complication rates are still high. Occlusion or migration of the catheter and preterm labour are the most frequent complications of this procedure.
- *Fetoscopic surgery:* the risks and high complication rates of open fetal procedures have popularized fetoscopic and minimally invasive procedures. Fulguration of the PUV of a fetus by fetal endoscopic approach using laser technology, and insertion of shunts using minimally invasive techniques, can be used in limited hands, although long-term follow-up is still being debated and assessed.

For the prenatal period, case selection seems to be the most important issue. We think that shunting procedures should be limited to fetuses with normal renal function and oligohydramnios before 24 weeks' gestation. For greater experience

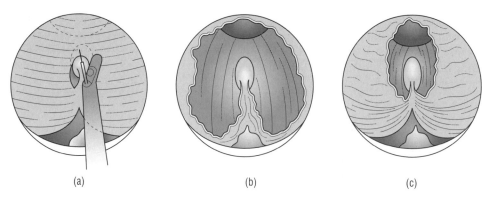

(a)   (b)   (c)

Figure 55.8   *(a) Fulgration of posterior urethral valve by using Bugbee electrode. (b,c) Relief of obstruction.*

in larger clinical series, progress in fetoscopic minimally invasive procedures, development in diagnostic methods for the prediction of fetal renal functions and improvement in fetal selection criteria are necessary.

INITIAL POSTNATAL EVALUATION AND TREATMENT STRATEGIES

In babies with antenatal diagnosis, antibiotic prophylaxis is initiated and VCUG is planned. In this period, serum electrolyte and creatinine levels, urinalysis and acid–base balance are investigated, and medical supportive treatment is planned if necessary. If the diagnosis is clear, the general condition of the baby is stabilized and there are no infectious problems, then endoscopic treatment is planned.

The following are the most popular methods for the treatment of PUV in neonates:

- endoscopic resection of valves;
- fulguration of valves by using Bugbee electrode during cystoscopic examination (Figure 55.8);
- rupture of valves by using Fogarty balloon catheter (Figure 55.9) or a Whittaker hook;
- in babies with a small penis and urethra, an antegrade suprapubic approach for endoscopic fulguration method can be performed successfully.

Care should be given to prevent any bleeding problems and to prevent possible injury to the urethra. A urethral catheter is left *in situ* for two days.

A control cystourethrogram is planned for three months after the valve ablation. This is necessary for the evaluation of post-instrumentation strictures, evaluation of valve remnants that give rise to urinary obstruction, and reassessment of the existence of VUR.

If there is no possibility of performing any type of valve ablation, or if there is functional impairment or ongoing severe urinary infections and upper tract dilations, then a cutaneous vesicostomy seems to be the easiest procedure with the lowest complication rates. The vesicostomy, which is concealed by a nappy, requires no further treatment or stoma bag. A special type of pyelostomy – the Sober-type ureterostomy – can be performed in selected cases.

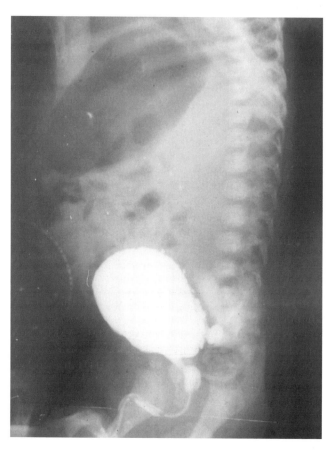

Figure 55.9   *Rupturing of posterior urethral valve (PUV) by using a Fogarty-like catheter. Note the contrast-filled elliptic balloon inserted in the anterior urethra, with the aim of mechanical destruction of the PUV.*

In our practice, prophylactic circumcision should be done routinely during valve ablation, although other centres do not include this as part of their routine. Trimethoprim 1–2 mg/kg/day is recommended routinely, especially during the first year of life.

During the first five-year follow-up period, if there is no evidence of VUR, the child is monitored annually and there is no need for specific prophylaxis. In about half of the cases, VUR disappears after the fulguration of PUV. If there is persistence of VUR and/or existence of tortuous and thick ureters, then prophylactic antibiotic therapy should be continued for a couple more years.

If there is persisting high-grade VUR and ipsilateral renal dysplasia, then a prophylactic pop-off mechanism probably exists. In this situation, it would be wise to keep this system for protection of the non-refluxing contralateral kidney. In the presence of recurrent urinary tract infections and attacks of hypertension, this refluxing system should be removed surgically.

Outcome

Urodynamics as a new diagnostic tool in paediatric urological practice has given us a new perspective and different vision into the evaluation of dysfunctional problems with PUV bladders (Lal et al. 1999). Problems such as hypocompliance, decreased bladder capacity and detrusor instability may give rise to clinical symptoms such as incontinence and renal impairment (Emir et al. 2002).

During the past two decades, developments in paediatric bladder augmentation techniques has helped tremendously to solve these problems.

Since 15–20 per cent of these boys may require renal transplantation and dialysis programmes, all patients should be followed up with measurement of blood pressure, investigation of plasma creatinine levels, urinary ultrasonography and urodynamics on an annual or at least biannual basis until adulthood.

CLINICAL SCENARIOS

Case 1

Antenatal scan at 23 weeks' gestation showed a grossly distended bladder in a male fetus with bilateral hydroureteronephrosis and oligohydramnios. No other coexistent abnormality or genetic disorders were detected. In follow-up, the degree of dilation persisted and oligohydramnios worsened. A percutaneous vesicoamniotic shunt replacement was performed without any complication. The postnatal period was uneventful. The baby was put on a prophylaxis programme. VCUG revealed a dilated posterior urethra and bilateral grade IV VUR. Valve fulguration by using a Bugbee electrode was performed in the second week of life. The baby now voids spontaneously and remains on a prophylaxis programme.

Case 2

An 11-year-old male was admitted to the clinic with daytime incontinence and attacks of severe recurrent urinary tract infections. He had a history of PUV and valve fulguration when he was one year old. He was followed up by routine controls. He had bilateral gross reflux and a non-compliant bladder, with a bladder volume of 65 mL. His creatinine level

was 0.90. Acid–base balance and electrolyte levels were within normal limits. It was decided to augment his bladder. An ileocystoplasty was performed. His gross reflux disappeared without any anti-reflux procedure. He had some difficulties due to pain during urethral catheterizations. For this reason, a continent appendicovesicostomy, using the Mitrofanoff principle was supplemented 1.5 years after the operation. He is now free of incontinence, recurrent urinary infections and reflux.

REFERENCES

Emir H, Eroglu E, Tekant G, et al. Urodynamic findings of posterior urethral valve patients. European Journal of Pediatric Surgery 2002; **12**: 38–41.

Gleason PE., Kramer SA. Genitourinary polyps in children. Urology 1994; **144**: 106–9.

Lal R, Bhatnagar V, Mitra DK. Long-term prognosis of renal functions in boys treated for posterior urethral valves. European Journal of Pediatric Surgery 1999; **9**: 307–11.

Maizels M, Stephens FD, King LR, Firlit CF. Cowper's syringocele: a classification of dilatations of Cowper's gland duct based upon clinical characteristics of 8 boys. Journal of Urology 1983; **129**: 111–14.

Nicolini U, Tannirandron Y, Vaughan J, et al. Further predictors of renal dysplasia in fetal obstructive uropathy: bladder pressure and biochemistry of fresh urine. Prenatal Diagnosis 1991; **11**: 159–66.

Nicolini U, Fisk NM, Rodeck C. Fetal urine biochemistry: an index of renal maturation and dysfunction. British Journal of Obstetrics and Gynaecology 1992; **99**: 46–50.

Stephens FD, Smith ED, Hutson JM. Congenital intrinsic lesions of the posterior urethra. In: Stephens FD, Smith ED, Hutson JM (eds). Congenital Anomalies of the Urinary and Genital Tracts. Oxford: ISIS Medical Media, 1996; pp. 91–116.

Wilkins IA, Chitkara U, Lynch L, et al. The nonpredictive value of fetal urinary electrolytes: preliminary report of outcomes and correlations with pathologic diagnosis. American Journal of Obstetrics and Gynecology 1987; **157**: 694–8.

Young HH, Frontz WA, Baldwin JC. Congenital obstruction of the posterior urethra. Journal of Urology 1919; **3**: 289.

FURTHER READING

Dewan PA. Congenital posterior urethral obstruction: the historical perspective. Pediatric Surgery International 1997; **12**: 86–94.

Glassberg KI, Horowitz M. Urethral valve and other anomalies of the male urethra. In: Belman B, King LR, Kramer SA (eds). Clinical Pediatric Urology. London: Martin Dunitz, 2002; pp. 900–945.

Holmdahl G, Sillén U, Hanson E, Hermansson G, Hjälmås K. Bladder dysfunction in boys with posterior urethral valves before and after puberty. Journal of Urology 1996; **155**: 694–8.

Mouriquand PDE, Thomas DFM. Posterior urethral valves and other congenital anomalies of the urethra. In: Thomas DFM (ed.). Urological Diseases in the Fetus and Infant-Diagnosis and Management. Oxford: Butterworth-Heinemann, 1997; pp. 195–208.

Smith GH, Canning DA, Schulman SL, Snyder HM, Duckett JW. The long-term outcome of posterior urethral valves treated with primary valve ablation and observation. Journal of Urology 1996; **155**: 1730–34.

Urolithiasis

W vAN'T HOFF AND PG DUFFY

Learning objectives

- To understand the aetiology of calculi.
- To plan relevant investigations for surgery.
- To coordinate metabolic assessment.
- To understand modern treatment modalities.
- To choose appropriate surgical treatment.

AETIOLOGY

Urolithiasis in childhood differs considerably from that in adults. It is much rarer (with a prevalence of between 0.1 and 0.9 cases per 1000 hospital admissions) in developed countries than in less developed countries. In children, the presentation is often less specific, the aetiology different and the management more complicated compared with that in adults. Interestingly, children presenting with renal stones tend to have a lower than average weight and height, suggesting either that they occur in chronically sick children or that they lead to poor growth, perhaps associated with chronic infection, vomiting or pain (Coward *et al.* 2003). Some children, especially those who are born prematurely and/or have profound immobility, are at higher risk of stones. The aetiology of paediatric urolithiasis is changing (Figure 56.1). Whereas the frequency of a metabolic abnormality was only 16 per cent in a series of 120 paediatric cases reported from the UK in 1977, current data from the same institution suggest a frequency of 44 per cent (Coward *et al.* 2003). Furthermore, urolithiasis is becoming more common in all age groups, and the age of first stone formation is falling, especially in women (Robertson *et al.* 1999). Twenty per cent of people who develop a renal stone do so before the age of 20 years. In adults, stones now occur almost as commonly in women as in men. However, in children, boys are still affected twice as frequently as girls, and at a younger age (Coward *et al.* 2003). Urea-splitting organisms, typically *Proteus mirabilis* (colonizing the foreskin) but also commonly *Escherichia coli* and other Gram-negative organisms, convert urea to ammonium, increasing urinary pH and favouring supersaturation of triple phosphate. Most infective stones occur in children with otherwise normal urological tracts, but there is an increased incidence in children with augmented bladders or obstructive lesions and in the presence of foreign bodies.

PRESENTATION

Modes of presentation are listed in Box 56.1. The most common presentation is with urinary tract infection (UTI), which often is persistent or recurrent. Such children may have

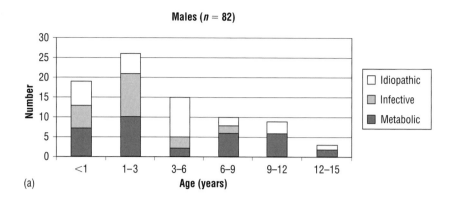

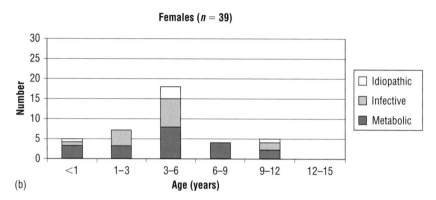

Figure 56.1 *Age at presentation, sex distribution and aetiological type of paediatric stones presenting to Great Ormond Street Hospital and the Middlesex Hospital in the period 1997–2001. (From Coward et al. 2003.)*

Box 56.1 Modes of presentation

Urinary tract infection/pain
Haematuria: microscopic/macroscopic
Failure to thrive
Chronic renal failure
Acute renal failure
Bilateral obstruction/obstruction solitary kidney
Mass: xanthogranulomatous pyelonephritis

---

infective (triple phosphate) stones, but approximately 50 per cent children with metabolic stones also present with UTI. A significant number (15 per cent) of children with stones are diagnosed incidentally during imaging for other symptoms, e.g. recurrent abdominal pain or backache. However, pain may not be perceived by the parents or carers in up to half of young children with stones. Ex-premature children are at much higher risk of stone formation. Fairly large stone bulk in one or both kidneys may cause no obvious symptoms, apart from failure to thrive. Rarely, obstruction causing acute renal failure may be due to a stone at the pelviureteric junction or in the ureter, and in such cases there may be no proximal ureteric dilation. Xanthogranulomatous pyelonephritis – chronic inflammation in a large kidney associated with calculi – presents as a large renal mass, which may resemble Wilms tumour, in a child with systemic symptoms, e.g. weight loss and anaemia.

Predisposing urological abnormalities may occur in approximately 20–30 per cent of children with urinary calculi. Stones associated with primary pelviureteric junction (PUJ) obstruction are uncommon and characteristically small and multiple. In most renal calculi, dilation of the pelvis is due to an obstructive stone at the PUJ, with or without infection. Stones may occur within mega-ureters or in a ureterocele. The presence or absence of vesicoureteric reflux can be assessed after complete stone clearance; the need to treat surgically is unusual. Intestinal segments for bladder reconstruction are accompanied by a significant risk (30–40 per cent) of stones.

INVESTIGATIONS

X-ray abdomen.

A plain abdominal X-ray is required for any child who has macroscopic haematuria or a proteus UTI, especially in a boy. This investigation may not demonstrate radiolucent calculi, and in the younger age group the renal area is often obscured by bowel gas.

Ultrasound

Stones in the kidney, lower ureter and bladder may be demonstrated by ultrasound scanning by the presence of a so-called 'acoustic shadow', which distinguishes calculi from other echogenic lesions within the renal collecting system. The most common echogenic lesions without significant shadow are blood clot and fungal balls. Ultrasound is excellent at demonstrating radiolucent calculi. It is not particularly good at showing stones in the middle and upper thirds of the ureter in the absence of dilation. Ultrasound may show stones in the kidneys, but it is inaccurate in describing the number and exact position within the pelvicalyceal system.

Intravenous urogram/dimercaptosuccinic acid scanning

This excellent combined study can be performed simultaneously using a single intravenous cannula. Intravenous urogram outlines accurately the collecting system and ureter and is extremely important to show the exact site of stones and the anatomy of the pelvicalyceal system. This is the premier study for planning the percutaneous approach to extract calculi. It is also important in outlining the pelviureteric system and to determine whether stone fragments will drain adequately after extracorporeal shockwave lithotripsy (ESWL). Dimercaptosuccinic acid (DMSA) scanning, which can be performed as a separate study, is important in order to reveal kidney function and also, as a baseline, to note whether damage occurs to the kidney during treatment with percutaneous nephrolithotomy (PCNL) or ESWL.

Spiral computed tomography, unenhanced

This can be used if there is a potential adverse risk to contrast media. It demonstrates very accurately the presence of stones and differentiates between stones in the collecting system and in the parenchyma. Unenhanced spiral computed tomography (CT) can be used in difficult cases, such as when the kidney is ectopic or the position of the kidney is distorted by a grossly abnormal spine in a patient with spina bifida. However, the radiation supplied by this is three times greater than that with IVP.

Micturating cystourethrogram

The ultrasound test will demonstrate the presence or absence of a thick-walled bladder and complete or incomplete bladder emptying. Therefore, the micturating cystourethrogram (MCUG) is not used routinely as an initial investigation in patients with stone disease. If, however, there is an abnormality of the bladder, MCUG may be required to exclude missed posterior urethral valves. Vesicoureteric reflux is not an abnormality that requires early assessment.

METABOLIC ASSESSMENT

Every child with urolithiasis should undergo a metabolic evaluation (Coward *et al.* 2003). The likelihood of finding an abnormality varies according to the population of children studied, with low figures (five per cent) in poorly developed countries and high rates (50 per cent) in more affluent developed areas. Biochemical evaluation is also important, because metabolic abnormalities are associated with an increased number of stones, with bilateral stone disease and with recurrent stone disease (Coward *et al.* 2003). The evaluation can be delayed until stones are cleared. Indeed, some transient metabolic abnormalities (e.g. hypercalciuria) can resolve when the child is stone-free. It is important to try and send any stone fragment removed or passed for detailed analysis, as this may reveal an underlying metabolic abnormality (e.g. cystine in cystinuria, 2,8-dihydroxyadenine in adenine phosphoribosyl transferase (APRT) deficiency). Identifying a specific metabolic stone may save the child from undergoing needless investigations. Triple phosphate stones are commonly seen after urinary infection, but this should not prevent a full metabolic evaluation, since occasionally such stones can occur in underlying metabolic disorders (Coward *et al.* 2003).

Metabolic evaluation is based on a routine set of plasma biochemical tests, including bicarbonate, calcium, phosphate, magnesium and urate, and analysis of the urine. Collection of 24-hour urine samples is not feasible in very young children (generally under three to four years); in this age group, random spot samples are all that can be tested. Normal ranges for urinary solute excretion in random samples in children are available, although there is some variation, dependent on the sample group, timing of urines, relationship to diet or feeds, etc. (see below). Catheterization is inappropriate, other than in exceptional cases. The key urinary solutes to determine are calcium, oxalate, cystine and urate. Abnormal urinary pH may indicate renal tubular acidosis, which is very uncommon. Measurement of urinary citrate may be helpful, and abnormalities in any of the above should be confirmed on several samples, preferably with a 24-hour collection. Further metabolic investigation may then be necessary, e.g. liver biopsy in hyperoxaluria and plasma and urine clearance studies in purine disorders.

Hypercalciuria is the most common metabolic abnormality and is found in about one-third of all children with stones. Urinary calcium excretion changes considerably during the day and is best assessed by a second morning sample (generally the lowest value). Repeated measurements and, where feasible, a 24-hour collection are necessary in abnormal cases. Most hypercalciuria occurs in the absence of other renal problems, but rarely it is a feature of a tubulopathy, e.g. distal renal tubular acidosis, hypomagnesaemia-hypercalciuria syndrome, Bartter syndrome or Dent's disease. In children, hypercalciuria is only rarely associated with hypercalcaemia. Most cases can be managed with dietary advice, such as increased fluids and low salt intake. Only a few patients need drug therapy (thiazide diuretics), as the risk of recurrent stones is low (less than five per cent in series from developed countries).

Two genetic (autosomal recessive) disorders – cystinuria and primary hyperoxaluria – each account for approximately ten per cent of paediatric stone cases. In cystinuria, there is defective urinary and intestinal uptake of dibasic amino acids, of which cystine is the most important, as it is poorly soluble and readily forms crystals in urine. Half of all cystinuric cases present in childhood, and bladder stones appear to be particularly common. The diagnosis can be made easily by testing the urine for excess cystine (screening by nitroprusside test, confirmation by ion-exchange chromatography). Aggressive management with a strict high fluid intake, urinary alkalinization and, occasionally, chelating therapy is necessary, as this is a lifelong disorder with a significant risk of renal damage and, occasionally, chronic renal failure.

Primary hyperoxaluria (PH) refers to a group of disorders characterized by defects in liver enzymes: alanine-glyoxalate transferase (AGT) in PH1 or glycerate reductase (GR) in PH2. Presentation varies between severe chronic renal failure in early infancy through recurrent stone episodes or nephrocalcinosis to an incidental finding. This illustrates the importance of environmental triggers (e.g. episodes of dehydration or sepsis) in urolithiasis. Hyperoxaluria also may be secondary to defective intestinal calcium absorption (e.g. in malabsorption states or after gut resection), can occur during parenteral nutrition, especially in premature infants, and can result from prolonged antibiotic use (e.g. in cystic fibrosis). Primary hyperoxaluria is diagnosed by measurement of urinary oxalate, but the result should be related to age-specific reference data, as there is a considerable change in excretion over the first few years of life. Initial measurements can be made in spot urine samples, and the result is factored by urine creatinine. Abnormal results should be confirmed by 24-hour urine collection, and other metabolites (glycolate, glycerate) should also be determined. A liver biopsy may be necessary to confirm a defect in AGT or GR activity. Treatment is with a high fluid intake and citrate therapy; patients with PH1 may respond to pharmacological doses of pyridoxine, a cofactor for AGT. Patients with primary hyperoxaluria are at especial risk if they have sustained renal damage, in which case they are not only unable to metabolize oxalate but also unable to excrete it via the only route of elimination (the kidney). As the glomerular filtration rate (GFR) falls, plasma oxalate rises, ultimately causing systemic oxalosis. Dialysis does not adequately clear oxalate, and isolated kidney transplantation has a poorer outcome than in other causes of renal failure, because the systemic oxalate burden is excreted and damages the kidney transplant. Most European authorities recommend combined liver–kidney transplantation for PH patients in renal failure. The urological imperative in PH is, therefore, to clear stones quickly to minimize renal damage.

Uric acid stones are rare in developed countries but common in developing countries, where hyperuricosuria is more prevalent. Uric acid stones tend to occur in the lower urinary tract and are often associated with UTI. Purine stones can occur in the rare metabolic disorders of APRT deficiency (leads to increased conversion of adenine to 2,8-dihydroxyadenine (2,8-DHA), which is much less soluble) and xanthinuria (deficiency of xanthine oxidase (XO), in which excess urinary xanthine causes stone formation). Purine stones are radiolucent

but are identifiable on ultrasound. Patients suspected of having these disorders require specialized metabolic review.

MODERN INSTRUMENTATION

Extracorporeal shockwave lithotripsy

ESWL (Figure 56.2) was introduced in the 1980s. It consists of generating a shockwave, which is transmitted through a fluid medium and focused on to the stone within the kidney. The shock wave can be generated by a high-tension electric spark plug, multiple vibrating piezoelectric crystals or electromagnetic plates. There are different types of lithotripters using these various energy sources. The original shockwave machine – the Dornier – utilized the electric spark plug; it produces a high-energy shockwave that can disintegrate the stone into large pieces. The shockwave generated by piezoelectric crystals tends to be of lesser energy, produces smaller fragments, and is less painful for the patient, but it takes a longer time to disintegrate the stone and may require multiple sessions. These machines visualize the stone using fluoroscopy or ultrasound. In children under the age of six or seven years, sedation or general anaesthetic is required for pain relief and to ensure that the child stays in the same position. It is usual to use this treatment modality for kidney stones measuring less than 2 cm. It is important to ensure that the collecting system is normal and that the fragments may drain satisfactorily from the pelvis into the collecting system and bladder.

If stones in the mid- and lower ureter can be visualized by ultrasound or fluoroscopy, then they may be treated with ESWL. They are usually smaller than 1.5 cm if in the ureter.

In the early series of the use of ESWL in adults, it was noted that the kidney parenchyma may be temporarily traumatized by the passage of the shockwave through the kidney on to the stone. Haematuria is well-recognized, and there is a

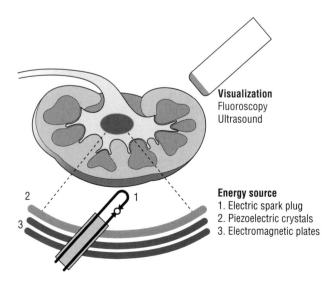

Figure 56.2 *Extracorporeal shockwave lithotripsy.*

temporary elevation of renal tubular enzymes. CT scans before and three months after treatment reveal in the adult population that serious renal damage is unlikely. It has not been demonstrated clearly that ESWL does not damage the growing kidney. Disadvantages of ESWL include the need for sedation or multiple general anaesthetics if the stone is slow to disintegrate. Care must be taken to ensure that there is adequate cover with intravenous antibiotics and hydration to prevent sepsis and the possibility of Steinstrasse obstruction due to multiple fragments usually collecting at the lower end of the ureter. JJ stents have been described as a necessity to prevent possible fragment obstruction, but this remains a controversial issue and is not used in all cases of children treated with ESWL. In younger children and babies, it may be necessary to place a foam block over the lower lung area to prevent damage by passage of the shockwave through the tissues.

Percutaneous nephrolithotomy

PCNL (Figure 56.3) was first described in the late 1970s. It is utilized for large stones in the pelvis of the kidney and for staghorn calculi. The approach is to insert a catheter retrogradely up the ureter. This allows retrograde insertion of contrast and clear outline of the calyces. A tract is formed using a needle and graded metal telescopic dilators, usually through a lower-pole calyx into the collecting system. A firm plastic Amplatz sheath is then passed over the dilators to keep the tract open from the skin to the kidney. The stone can be visualized with a telescope and may be removed simply by lifting it out through the Amplatz sheath, or it may be disintegrated using ultrasound, lithoclast or laser probes. The stones are broken down by the ultrasound probe using a form of energy that depends on the mechanical oscillation of the probe tip. The lithoclast disintegrates by using the principle of vibration created in a manner similar to that of a pneumatic drill. Laser energy is delivered through a very thin flexible quartz cable and affects the stone by causing tissue vaporization and the production of thermal energy.

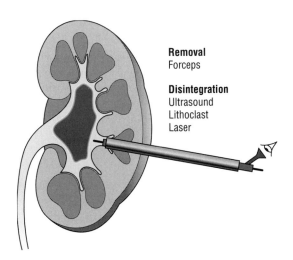

Removal
Forceps

Disintegration
Ultrasound
Lithoclast
Laser

Figure 56.3 *Percutaneous nephrolithotomy.*

The technique of PCNL has been used mainly in adults because of the large probes and tracts required to gain access to the kidney. There is increasing use of this technique in younger children, and tracts of 24F are very suitable for removing relatively large calculi. Mini tracts of 11–13Fr have been developed and a small endoscope can be passed through this with delivery of the laser fibre. This is used in special cases but is not of great use if the stone is relatively large, because of the inability to quickly remove the fragments through a small tract.

It is possible to gain access to the bladder percutaneously with the suprapubic approach, and fragments can be easily removed or disintegrated. In boys, if the stones are large it is not feasible to enter the bladder through the small urethra.

Ureteroscopy

Many ureteroscopes have been developed with very fine tips (4.2F). With these instruments, access can be gained to the ureter, and a stone may be removed with a metal basket or disintegrated with a laser fibre.

Laparoscopy

This technique has entered into the armamentarium of the paediatric surgeon and urologist. It has been used – although not frequently – to remove a large stone from an extra-renal pelvis or a large stone from a ureter.

TREATMENT

See Figure 56.4.

Obstruction

A stone blocking a pelviureteric junction or, more commonly a ureter in association with sepsis may destroy kidney function. The child should be treated with intravenous fluids and antibiotics. If there is no obvious improvement over the first 24–48 hours, then drainage of the system is mandatory. This is usually carried out with percutaneous insertion of a pigtail catheter. Renal function may be impaired acutely if there is bilateral blockage or unilateral blockage in a solitary kidney. Early relief of obstruction is mandatory. It is important to note that a peculiarity of obstruction in the child or infant is that he or she may become dehydrated, and dilation above the obstruction is not seen on ultrasound scan.

Open surgery

In the past, treatment of calculi in children was mainly with the traditional open approach (Figure 56.5). Open surgery is now reserved for children with large complex calculi and

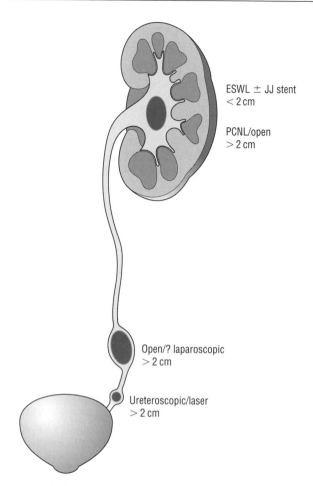

Figure 56.4 *Summary of treatment of upper urinary tract calculi. ESWL, extracorporeal shockwave lithotripsy; PCNL, percutaneous nephrolithotomy.*

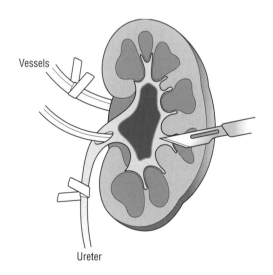

Figure 56.5 *Open surgery for treatment of upper urinary tract calculi.*

large ureteric stones. The open approach provides a very effective method of removing a large single stone from the pelvis of the kidney or systematic removal of the staghorn calculus, during which cooling of the kidney with vascular

control is necessary (Gough and Bailie 2000). The kidney may be X-rayed on the table to aid in removal of calculi in the more inaccessible calyces. This technique provides an excellent method of obtaining complete clearance of the kidney. If some small fragments remain, these can be treated with ESWL at a later date.

Extracorporeal shockwave lithotripsy

ESWL is now used more often in children, particularly with calculi under 2 cm in diameter. The disadvantages of ESWL are that the child may require sedation or, more usually, general anaesthetic, and several treatments may be required. In children with large stones, care must be taken to assess for obstruction due to fragments at the early period after treatment. In children under two years of age, it has been reported that large stones respond extremely well to ESWL (Lottmann *et al.* 2001). ESWL has a specific place in the treatment of stone fragments after PCNL or open surgery. Consideration should be given to different types of lithotripter, which utilize different energy sources and produce different fragment sizes. ESWL has been utilized to disintegrate calculi in the lower ureter.

Percutaneous nephrolithotomy

PCNL is reserved for large stones and staghorn calculi (Mor *et al.* 1997). More than one tract may be necessary to enter the kidney to gain access to calyceal fragments. Moderate-sized stones can simply be lifted out with graspers or disintegrated using probes, as described previously. The ultrasound probe produces very small fragments and sucks out the debris at the same time. The lithoclast produces larger fragments but is an extremely simple and reliable probe. The advantage of the laser is its very small size, which allows the operator to form an extremely small tract to gain access to the stone. Fragment removal may be a problem, and time must be spent in producing suitably small fragments within the pelvicalyceal system that will drain spontaneously.

The complications of PCNL are sepsis and blood loss. The patient must receive intravenous antibiotics, and blood must be available during the procedure. The kidney itself may bleed or a specific intra-renal vessel may be damaged. During disintegration of a large stone, the pelvicalyceal system may be penetrated and fluid irrigation may be lost into the retroperitoneal space, causing postoperative paralytic ileus or electrolyte imbalance due to reabsorption of fluid. The kidney may be damaged due to the tract piercing the parenchyma.

Ureteroscopy: ureteric calculi

Ureteric stones under 0.5 cm in diameter will pass spontaneously. As the stone increases in size, the rate of passage decreases. It is usually considered that a stone measuring 1.5–2 cm requires surgical attention. This stone may be within a ureterocoele; therefore, simply endoscopically incising the ureterocoele and lifting out the calculus may be all that is required. If the stone is in a mega-ureter, then access to the ureter can be obtained using a ureteroscope; disintegration is carried out with a laser probe. Fragments may be allowed to pass spontaneously or may be removed individually using a fine grasper or a wire basket. The ureteroscope is an extremely thin instrument and complications may include perforation of the ureter and damage to the ureteric wall with the laser probe.

Cystoscopy: bladder calculi

Stones in the bladder can be disintegrated with an endoscope passed per urethra and a laser fibre or litholast probe. Larger stones may be approached suprapubically and disintegrated with a laser fibre or an ultrasound probe. Extremely large stones should require open suprapubic removal.

SUMMARY

Paediatric renal calculi are rare in children and babies. They occur more commonly in boys than girls. Metabolic abnormalities have been detected in 44 per cent. All children with calculi should undergo a metabolic screen. The most common metabolic abnormality is hypercalciuria. The most common presentation is UTI. Modalities of surgical treatment include open surgery, ESWL and endoscopy, which can be percutaneous, ureteroscopic, cystoscopic or laparoscopic. In a unit managing paediatric patients with calculi, stone clearance was obtained with ESWL in 95 per cent, with PCNL in 89 per cent and with combined PCNL and ESWL in 100 per cent (Choong *et al.* 2000).

REFERENCES

Choong S, Whitfield H, Duffy P, *et al.* The management of paediatric urolithiasis. *British Journal of Urology International* 2000; **86**: 857–60.

Coward RJM, Peters CJ, Duffy PG, *et al.* Epidemiology of paediatric renal stone disease in the UK. *Archives of Disease in Childhood* 2003; **88**: 962–5.

Gough DC, Bailie CT. Paediatric anatrophic nephrolithotomy: stone clearance at what price? *British Journal of Urology International* 2000; **85**: 874–8.

Lottmann HB, Traxer O, Archambaud F, Mercier-Pageyral B. Monotherapy extracorporeal shock wave lithotripsy for the treatment of staghorn calculi in children. *Journal of Urology* 2001; **165**: 2324–7.

Mor Y, Elmasru, Kellett MJ, *et al.* The role of percutaneous nephrolithotomy in the management of paediatric renal calculi. *Journal of Urology* 1997; **158**: 1319–21.

Robertson WG, Longhorn SE, Whitfield HN, *et al.* The changing pattern of the age at onset of urinary stone disease in the UK. In: Borghi I, Meschi T, Briganti A, Schiani T, Novarini A (eds). *Kidney Stones.* Corenza: Editoriale Bios, 1999; pp. 165–8.

FURTHER READING

Barratt TM, Duffy PG. Nephrocalcinosis and urolithiasis. In: Barratt TM, Aer ED, Harmon WE (eds). *Pediatric Nephrology*, 4th edn. Baltimore, MD: Lippincott Williams & Wilkins, 1999.

William G, Van't Hoff WG. Renal and urinary tract stone disease in children. In: Davison AM, Cameron S, Grunfeld J-P, *et al.* (eds). *Oxford Textbook of Clinical Nephrology*, 3rd edn. Oxford: Oxford University Press, 2005; pp. 1281–91.

57

Bladder exstrophy and epispadias complex

LSL McCARTHY AND DUNCAN WILCOX

Learning objectives

- To understand the embryology of normal and abnormal bladder development.
- To understand the anatomical variations of bladder exstrophy and epispadias complex.
- To understand the antenatal and perinatal management of bladder exstrophy and epispadias complex.
- To understand the postnatal treatment plan and variation of bladder exstrophy and epispadias complex.
- To appreciate the long-term outcomes and complications of bladder exstrophy and epispadias complex.

INTRODUCTION

The bladder exstrophy–epispadias complex forms a spectrum of rare defects that extend from simple glanular epispadias to complex cloacal exstrophy.

DEFINITIONS

Male epispadias (Figure 57.1) is a deformity in which the urethra opens on the dorsum of the penis instead of at its tip (one in 100 000 live births). There is associated dorsal chordee. In *female epispadias* (Figure 57.2), the urethral opening extends to the clitoris, which is bifid (one in 400 000 live births). In both male and female epispadias, the urinary sphincters may be incomplete, with separation of the symphysis pubis, leading to incontinence.

Bladder exstrophy (Figure 57.3) means literally the eversion or turning inside-out of the bladder. The bladder is open anteriorly and the urethral plate and ureteric orifices are exposed, with splaying of the pubic bones and separation of the rectus muscles (one in 30 000 live births; three males to one female). Fifty per cent of patients born with bladder exstrophy have this classic type.

Cloacal exstrophy (Figure 57.4) has two laterally placed exstrophic bladders that are separated by a bar of intestinal tissue. Each hemi-bladder may have a ureteric orifice. From the intestinal plate, orifices lead to the terminal ileum. Appendices (often two) and a distal (hindgut) bowel orifice with an imperforate anus invariably are present (one in 200 000 live births; equal incidence in males and females).

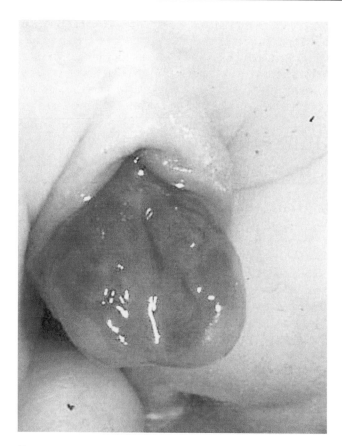

Figure 57.1   *Male epispadias.*

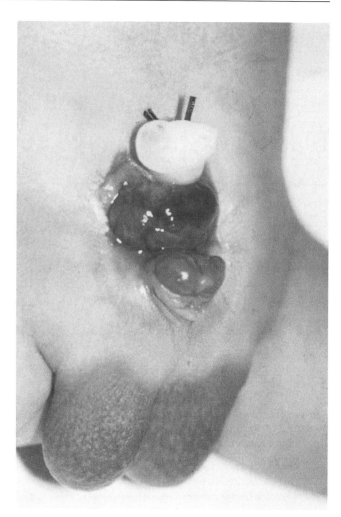

Figure 57.3   *Bladder exstrophy.*

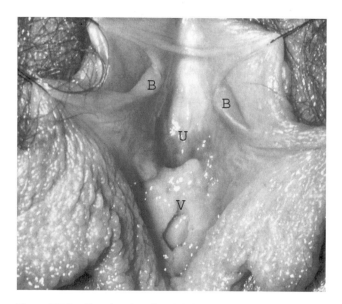

Figure 57.2   *Female epispadias. B, bifid clitoris; U, urethra; V, vagina.*

Rare exstrophy variants include *pubovesical cleft*, which describes a complete opening of the urethra to the bladder neck, but with an intact bladder, and *superior vesical fistula*, in which the muscular and skeletal defects are identical to those in classic bladder exstrophy, but the membrane has ruptured only in the cranial portion, giving the appearance of a congenital vesicostomy.

EMBRYOLOGY

By day 14 post-conception, the human embryo consists of two layers: the epiblast and the hypoblast. (Previously, these were termed ectoderm and endoderm.) On day 15, the primitive streak appears on the dorsum. It is at this point that the fundamental axes of the body are established: cranial/caudal, left/right, ventral/dorsal. The definitive endoderm and intra-embryonic mesoderm form by gastrulation through the primitive streak (Figure 57.5). Thus, the epiblast gives rise to the ectoderm, mesoderm and endoderm. During the third week, two depressions appear in the ectoderm, which fuse tightly with the endoderm, preventing ingrowth of the mesoderm; these are the buccopharyngeal membrane and the cloacal membrane. The allantois is a diverticulum of the endoderm

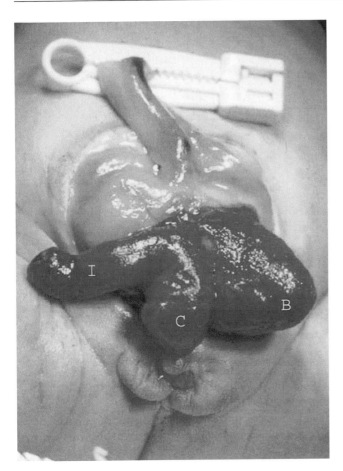

Figure 57.4 *Cloacal exstrophy, B, left hemi-bladder; I, ileum (prolapsed); C, colon (prolapsed). The right hemi-bladder is obscured by the prolapsed small and large bowel.*

that extends into the body stalk. Embryonic folding occurs during the fourth week, converting the flat trilaminar germ disc into a three-dimensional structure. This occurs because of rapid growth of the embryonic disc compared with the yolk sac. The endoderm at the lateral edge of the embryonic disc is attached to the yolk sac, so the expanding disc bulges into a convex shape. As a result of this folding, the cephalic, lateral and caudal folds meet in the midline. The endoderm now forms cranial and caudal blind-ending tubes (foregut and hindgut, respectively), with the future midgut between them, widely connected to the yolk sac. The foregut ends in the buccopharyngeal membrane and the hindgut at the cloacal membrane, both of which have moved on to the ventral surface of the embryo, as has the body stalk (Figure 57.6).

The ectoderm that was immediately caudal to the cloacal membrane in the bilaminar disc has now been rotated to lie adjacent to the body stalk, cranial to the cloacal membrane. The ingressing mesoderm that separates this ectoderm from the underlying endoderm has its origin as the mesoderm that migrated around the cloacal membrane at the end of week three and will form the anterior abdominal and bladder wall. This mesoderm forms a particular bulge in murine development that Kluth has described as the glandular hillock. Rathke's

folds in the lateral wall of the cloaca fuse with the Tourneux fold growing down cranially to produce the urorectal septum, which separates the cloaca into an anterior urogenital sinus and a posterior hindgut. Eventually, the bilaminar buccopharyngeal membrane and the cloacal membrane, which are not supported by mesoderm, break down.

Embryology of bladder exstrophy

If the origin of the mesoderm that forms the infra-umbilical anterior abdominal wall is examined, then it can be seen that this mesoderm has had to migrate around the cloacal membrane during gastrulation to reach its correct site (Figure 57.5). There are a number of hypotheses regarding the abnormal formation of this area. If this migration is primarily inhibited (Kluth's hypothesis), or if the fusion of ectoderm and endoderm at the cloacal membrane extends too far caudally in the bilaminar disc, secondarily preventing mesodermal ingrowth (hence, Muecke's hypothesis with regard to the cloacal membrane forming a wedge preventing mesodermal ingrowth), then it actually amounts to the same thing. A third possibility is that the mesoderm does migrate into this region but then undergoes inappropriate apoptosis (programmed cell death), leading to its loss. Where the endoderm and ectoderm are unsupported by mesoderm, then this membrane will break down, leading to exposure of the bladder and classic bladder exstrophy (Figure 57.6).

Embryology of cloacal exstrophy

If failure of mesodermal ingrowth from the anterior abdominal wall is also associated with a failure of the urorectal septum to form and divide the cloaca, then cloacal exstrophy will occur (Figure 57.7, p. 504). Posteriorly in the developing cloaca, the endoderm that normally would form the hindgut is placed centrally, with the endoderm that will form the bladder being placed laterally. This is the pattern described for cloacal exstrophy. If the tail gut has failed to regress, then this could be the origin of what is described as the hypoplastic 'hindgut'; it is always associated with an imperforate anus, as there was never any possibility of this tube opening anywhere but into the cloaca. Profound hypoplasia of the hindgut could also explain why the ileum empties straight on to the central intestinal mucosal bar in patients with cloacal exstrophy.

ANATOMICAL DEFECTS

Skeletal defects in classic bladder exstrophy include externally rotated posterior components of the pelvis and 30 per cent shortened and externally rotated pubic rami (Figure 57.8, p. 505). The pelvic floor is deficient. The abdominal wall has a triangular defect bounded by the recti laterally and an intrasymphyseal band (distorted urogenital membrane)

Normal gastrulation

Bladder exstrophy embryology

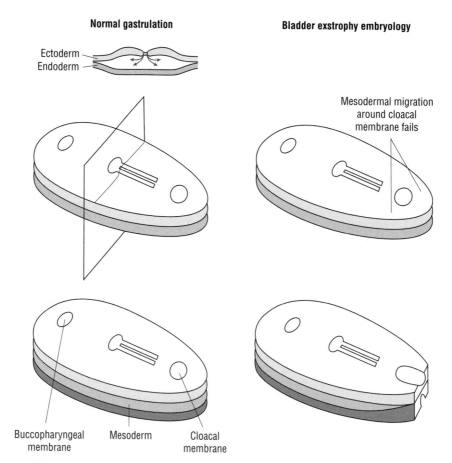

Figure 57.5 *Gastrulation. Epiblast cells detach from the epiblast layer and replace cells in the hypoblast, giving rise to the ectoderm (light grey) and endoderm (dark grey). Further migration of ectodermal cells occurs through the primitive streak producing the mesoderm. Two areas of ectoderm and endoderm remain stuck together: the buccopharyngeal membrane and the cloacal membrane. Mesoderm has to migrate around the cloacal membrane to reach the caudal end of the embryo. Failure of the mesoderm to migrate into this area will lead to a defect of the lower-abdominal wall and ventral bladder wall: bladder exstrophy and its variants.*

inferiorly. The exstrophic bladder fills this. The umbilicus is at the apex of this defect and may be associated with an umbilical hernia or a minor degree of exomphalos in cloacal exstrophy. Inguinal herniae occur in 80 per cent of boys with bladder exstrophy and ten per cent of girls. In boys, the penis appears short because of the widely split pubic bones and a 50 per cent deficit of anterior corporal tissue. In girls, the vagina is short, with a stenotic opening. The clitoris may be bifid; the fallopian tubes and ovaries, however, tend to be normal in classic bladder exstrophy. In cloacal exstrophy, in the male there may be bifid or absent phalli and in the female there may be two vaginas with separated uterine horns.

Cloacal exstrophy frequently is associated with spinal dysraphism and may be associated with short bowel syndrome.

INHERITANCE

Most cases are sporadic, although familial cases have been reported, with a sibling risk of one in 100. The future risk to

exstrophy patients of having an exstrophy child has been reported as one in 70.

ANTENATAL DIAGNOSIS AND MANAGEMENT

Diagnosis

Antenatal ultrasonography may reveal an absent bladder, abnormally positioned anterior-superior male genitalia of diminutive size, with a low insertion for the umbilical cord, widening of the pubic rami and a lower abdominal mass (Figure 57.9, p. 505). Amniotic fluid is normal. This is detectable from 16 weeks' gestation onwards. Differential diagnosis of an absent bladder includes the following:

- fetus has voided to completion
- bilateral renal agenesis
- technical failure of the ultrasound (obese patient, prone fetus)

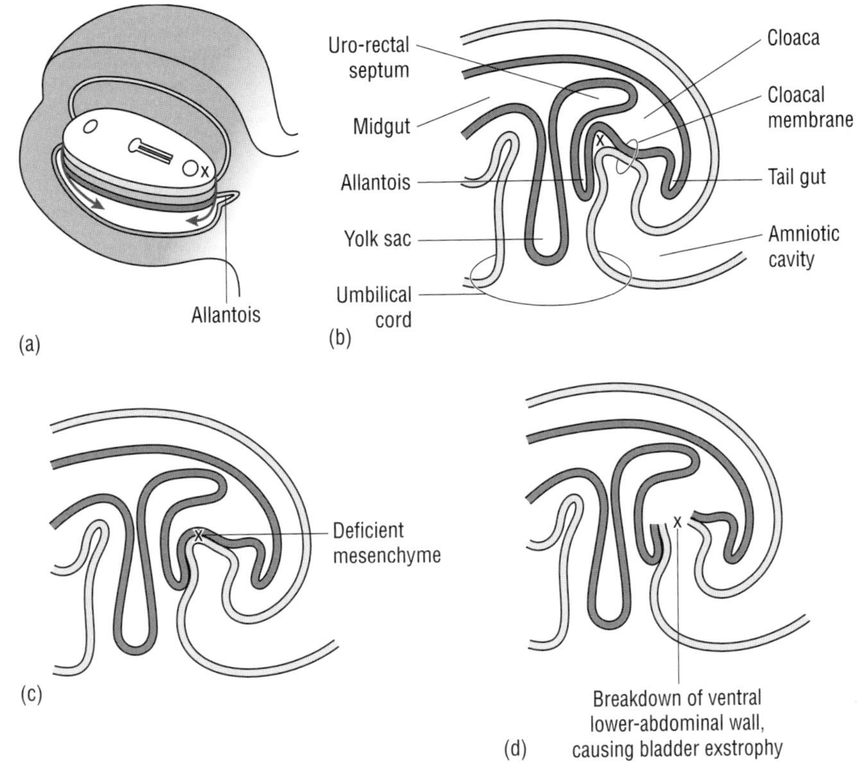

Figure 57.6   *Three-dimensional body folding. In the third week of life, rapid growth of the embryonic disc compared with the yolk causes three-dimensional folding of the embryo. (a) The arrows highlight the movements of the head fold and tail folds. (The embryo also rotates, but for simplicity the axis of the embryo is constant in these diagrams.) (b) The body stalk has been formed and contains two endodermal diverticulae: the yolk sac and the allantois. The endodermally lined hindgut connects to the cloaca, from which leads the tail gut (which is normally resorbed) and the allantois. The X shows the ventral position of the caudal end of the embryonic disc after three-dimensional body folding has occurred. (c) In bladder exstrophy, the mesoderm is deficient at the caudal end of the embryo and so is absent at the position marked by the X. (d) In the absence of the supporting mesoderm, the ectoderm and endoderm break down, resulting in a defect extending from the penis to the base of the umbilicus. In classic bladder exstrophy, the cloaca is still separated into the urogenital sinus and the rectum by the growth of the urorectal septum and Rathke's folds (not illustrated).*

- infantile polycystic disease
- severe intrauterine growth retardation.

Pregnancy management

Bladder exstrophy is normally an isolated abnormality. However, fetal echocardiography to exclude cardiac defects and karyotyping to determine fetal sex have been recommended. Twenty-five per cent of bladder exstrophy fetuses were aborted electively in a malformations surveillance programme at Brigham and Women's Hospital.

Delivery

There is no evidence of benefit from caesarean section. Once delivered, the open bladder plate should be protected from dehydration by covering with sterile cling film. Resuscitation is rarely required. The baby should be referred to a tertiary centre for early bladder closure.

POSTNATAL MANAGEMENT

Initial investigations should include imaging of the upper renal tract, pelvic radiography, routine preoperative bloods and karyotyping.

SURGERY

The aims of surgery for bladder exstrophy are:

- anatomical closure of the bladder and abdominal wall;
- preservation of renal function, with urinary continence;
- external genitalia that are functionally and cosmetically acceptable.

Classically, a three-stage reconstruction is performed (described below), although single-stage reconstructions are practised in some centres and Kelly and Eraklis (1971)

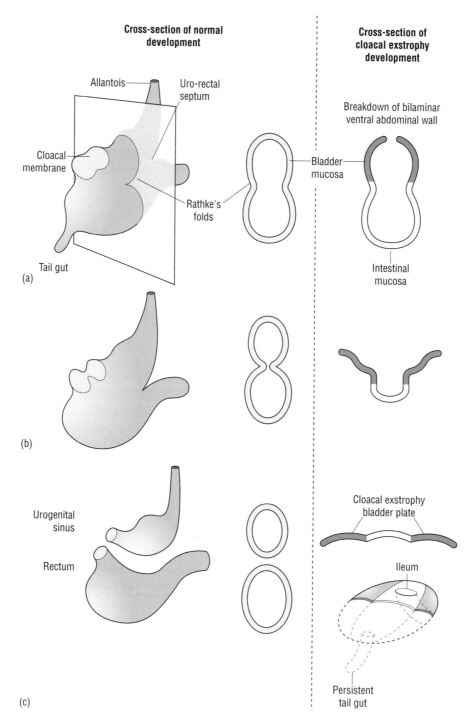

Figure 57.7 *Embryology of cloacal exstrophy. The embryo is rotated 180 degrees compared with that in Figure 57.6 and is lying supine in this figure. Only the endoderm is shown for clarity. (a) The cloaca has not yet been divided by the growth of Rathke's folds and the urorectal septum. If the cloaca is cut in the plane illustrated, then the cross-sections for normal development and cloacal exstrophy are illustrated. Grey shading indicates the bladder mucosa in the cloacal exstrophy cross-section. (b) The cloaca is nearly divided into the anterior urogenital sinus and the posterior rectum. (c) The urogenital sinus and the rectum are now separated, and the tail gut has regressed in normal development. In cloacal exstrophy, the bladder mucosa has formed two lateral plates, separated by a central band of intestinal mucosa, which normally would line the rectum. The ileum drains into the superior part of this and the tail gut may fail to regress, giving rise to a vestigial piece of large bowel that does not drain to any anus.*

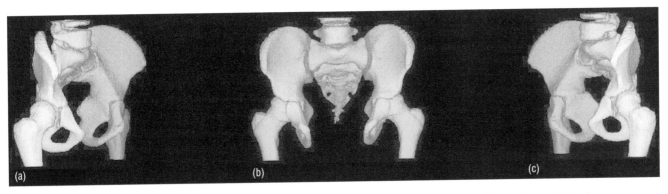

Figure 57.8 *Three-dimensional reconstruction of the pelvis in bladder exstrophy: (a) right oblique view; (b) anterior-posterior view; (c) left oblique view.*

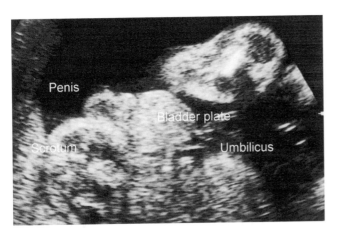

Figure 57.9 *Antenatal diagnosis of bladder exstrophy.*

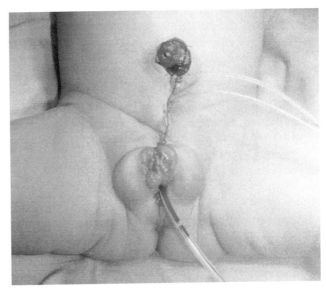

Figure 57.10 *Baby after bladder closure. There is a bladder catheter, and passing through the superior suture line two ureteric stents.*

described a staged procedure using a more radical soft-tissue dissection.

Closure of bladder, posterior urethra and abdominal wall with or without pelvic osteotomy

The aim of this procedure is to close the bladder and abdominal wall, converting bladder exstrophy into complete epispadias with incontinence. The bladder is separated from the skin by incising along the mucocutaneous junction, leaving the urethral plate. The rectus fascia is dissected off the bladder, the umbilical vessels are ligated, and the dome of the bladder is freed from the peritoneum. Ureteric stents and a catheter are placed, and the bladder and posterior urethra are closed. The pubic bones are approximated. This may require a pelvic osteotomy, with concomitant use of an external fixator (see below). The abdominal wall defect is then closed. Plaster-of-Paris splints can be applied to keep the legs together, reducing the risk of wound dehiscence.

Postoperatively, the plaster-of-Paris splint is kept on for two to six weeks. Urine drainage and ureteric stents are kept for two to four weeks (Figure 57.10). Antibiotic prophylaxis is given to cover this period. Following removal of the ureteric

catheters, an ultrasound is performed to look for upper tract dilation.

Both wound dehiscence and bladder prolapse may require reclosure. Multiple attempts at closure are associated with reduced bladder size and a worse final outcome. Urological complications include reflux, vesicoureteric junction obstruction (transiently following closure) and urinary tract infection, which may be fungal.

Following this procedure, all boys and the vast majority of girls will be incontinent, with no dry interval. A further bladder-neck procedure will be required, but by producing a degree of bladder outlet resistance by performing the epispadias correction first, bladder growth is increased. Bladder growth can be assessed by three-monthly cystoscopy and cystometrograms. Provided that the bladder is growing adequately, then epispadias repair and bladder-neck reconstruction can follow. If the bladder is not growing, then augmentation cystoplasty should be considered.

Epispadias repair at six months to one year: Cantwell–Ransley repair

The aims of this are to:

- produce a functional and cosmetically acceptable penis by correction of chordee, urethral reconstruction, penile skin closure and reconstruction of the glans;
- increase bladder outflow resistance to promote bladder growth.

The urethral plate is mobilized on its mesentery remaining attached at the glans. The neurovascular bundles are identified and preserved, and the corpora cavernosa are separated. Chordee is corrected by rotating the corpora in front of the tubularized urethra. The urethral plate is tubularized over an 8F catheter and then the corpora cavernosa are closed dorsally over the neo-urethra, which now lies ventrally. Glans wings are then closed dorsally over the neo-urethra.

Complications of this procedure include bladder spasm, fistula (4–19 per cent), stenosis (eight per cent) and superficial wound dehiscence (eight per cent).

Gerharz et al. (1999), in a study of boys following epispadias repair, showed that the neo-urethra was a good channel in 77 of 93 (83 per cent) by cystoscopy and catheterization. On standing, 87 (93 per cent) of patients had a downward-angled penis; the remaining patients needed further penile surgery (five with exstrophy, one with epispadias). The appearance of the penis was acceptable, and 10 of the 12 patients who were over 16 years of age had engaged in satisfactory intercourse and reported their penis to be acceptable, both functionally and cosmetically.

Bladder neck reconstruction at three to five years

Several operations are described in the literature, but one of the most commonly used is the Young-Dees–Leadbetter procedure. The aim is to produce a continent bladder neck that does not leak but that will allow micturition. Through a Pfannenstiel incision, the bladder is exposed and opened by a vertical incision. The ureters are mobilized (if low, they may have to be moved cephalad) and re-implanted using the Cohen cross-trigonal technique. A line of mucosa extending cranially from the posterior urethra is tubularized over a catheter, and the bladder is closed.

Postoperatively the bladder is drained by a suprapubic catheter for three weeks. Then the bladder is 'cycled' by clamping and releasing the suprapubic tube. When a suitable period of dryness is achieved, it is removed.

The success of Young-Dees bladder-neck repair varies from 25 to 80 per cent. The most important factor in achievement of continence is bladder volume before bladder-neck reconstruction. The main complications following bladder-neck reconstruction are failure of the procedure to produce continence and impairment of bladder function. Failure to achieve continence (which Gearhart defines as dry intervals of less than

three hours) can be treated in some cases by bladder-neck injections of collagen or Macroplastique™ to increase the outflow resistance. Multiple injections may be necessary. However, persistent wetness may require urinary diversion or bladder augmentation, or may be an indication for closing the bladder neck completely. However, there is an impact on bladder function following injections: Diamond et al. (1999) report that although bladder capacity increased, the presence of a normally compliant and stable bladder fell from 80 per cent preoperatively to 50 per cent postoperatively.

LONG-TERM OUTCOMES OF BLADDER EXSTROPHY RECONSTRUCTION

This can be divided into outcomes for urinary continence, renal function, fertility and psychosocial function.

Urinary continence following current reconstructive practice

Confusion exists in the literature regarding the outcomes of bladder exstrophy treatment, because of the interchangeable use of 'dryness' and 'continence of urine' used by some authors. 'Continence of urine' should mean that the bladder (or suitable storage organ) fills without leaking, with an adequate capacity, which can then be emptied voluntarily at an appropriate time and place. This system should preferably be of low pressure, in order to avoid damage to the upper renal tracts. Dryness, however, simply means that there is no leakage of urine. Chan et al. (2001) reported a series of 62 patients who had staged bladder exstrophy repair at the Johns Hopkins Hospital, Baltimore, USA: 74 per cent were continent (dry intervals of more than three hours), with no need for augmentation or catheterization; 16 per cent were socially continent, with occasional accidents; and ten per cent were wet. Only two patients in the series had required bladder augmentation. These exceptional results are, however, not reported universally. Bolduc et al. (2002) has described the experience of the Hospital for Sick Children, Toronto, Canada: 57 patients (49 bladder exstrophy, eight cloacal exstrophy) were operated on over 13 years from 1988. Thirty per cent needed bladder reclosure. Subsequently, 77 per cent required a continent urinary diversion by Mitrofanoff or Monti procedure, 66 per cent bladder augmentation and 47 per cent required bladder neck closure after unsuccessful bladder neck reconstruction. Those who had a bladder-neck closure were dry. Eighty-two per cent of those with a reconstructed bladder neck were dry, 12 per cent had acceptable results and five per cent were wet.

Urinary continence following previous reconstructive practice

Woodhouse (2001) has described poor outcomes in adulthood following childhood exstrophy surgery. This, however, reflects the outcome of surgical techniques from 20 years ago. Some of these patients have continent urinary diversion such as ureterosigmoidostomies and are content with this, even in the face of development of malignancy. Poor outcomes may follow an initially successful reconstruction that has then deteriorated or a failed initial reconstruction.

If spontaneous voiding is achieved, then the bladder neck repair and urethra can often remain intact. However, in patients who have to catheterize the bladder to drain it, the urethra can become progressively traumatized, strictured and, ultimately, obstructed. Failure of outlet resistance may occur rarely but is much more likely to be due to a change to a less structured lifestyle in the teenage years, with less regular drinking and voiding patterns. This is best treated by use of a Mitrofanoff continent catheterizable stoma.

Woodhouse has described primary bladder failure developing in the late teenage years in patients who appeared to have normal bladders at puberty. It is thought to occur because of chronic voiding against a fixed resistance, necessitating high-pressure detrusor contractions. The detrusor muscle eventually decompensates and fails. This has occurred in 23 per cent of patients. Chronic retention is treated by catheterization. Instability with poor compliance is treated by bladder augmentation. In extreme cases, ureterosigmoidostomy is considered.

Secondary bladder failure may be due to stone formation (risk 6–23 per cent). Carcinoma occurs in the exstrophic bladder, with a risk of four per cent at 30 years' follow-up, although so far all of these cases have been in diverted bladders.

Failed exstrophy reconstruction will occur even in the best series. Repeated attempts at reconstruction are associated with worsening of the final outcome. Eventually, some sort of diversion is required, such as closure of the bladder neck with Mitrofanoff formation or ureterosigmoidostomy.

Anterior abdominal-wall defects, with lateral displacement of the rectus muscles and pubic symphysis diastasis, are present in many exstrophy adults who did not have closure of the pelvic ring. This leaves a triangular defect closed by scar tissue, with pubic hair displaced inferiorly and laterally. This is cosmetically unsatisfactory but rarely leads to hernia formation. Male patients often complain that during intercourse, lack of support for the penis means that it is pushed back into the pelvis. The anterior abdominal wall can be reconstructed using mesh to reinforce the rectus fascia and provide support for the anterior abdominal wall and penis.

Upper tracts and renal function

In long-term follow-up studies, both Woodhouse and the Hospital for Sick Children in Toronto reported a 25 per cent rate of renal scarring. In the Toronto study, this damage occurred irrespective of whether the bladder neck was reconstructed or closed and of whether the bladder was augmented. It was, however, associated with recurrent urinary tract infections.

Sexual function and fertility

Woodhouse has reported that sexual function and libido in exstrophy patients are normal. The majority (87 per cent) of men are capable of having erections and achieving orgasm. However, ejaculation is not normal in the majority of exstrophy men, bladder neck closure being associated with retrograde ejaculation. Some exstrophy men are reported to have oligospermia. Epididymitis occurs in 33 per cent of cases and, when refractory, has necessitated vasectomy and orchidectomy. Only five per cent of exstrophy men have fathered children.

In female exstrophy patients, Woodhouse has reported that vaginoplasty is often necessary before sexual intercourse can take place. Forty-five women with exstrophy have borne 49 children according to the world literature. Half of exstrophy females will experience uterine prolapse associated with pregnancy. This is extremely difficult to treat. Pelvic osteotomy during initial reconstruction in childhood may reduce the risk of this severe complication and may prove to be a good indication for this procedure.

Psychosocial function

Stein *et al.* (1996) have reported that the educational achievements, occupation and social development of exstrophy patients are normal.

OTHER CONSIDERATIONS

Pelvic osteotomy

Pelvic osteotomy may be needed for primary closure and should be performed if dehiscence occurs (Figure 57.11). It may well reduce the risk of development of the devastating complication of severe uterine prolapse in females.

Gender assignment

Reassignment of gender in exstrophy patients is limited to male cloacal exstrophy patients with inadequate tissue for phallic reconstruction. Gender dysphoria has occurred in patients in whom testicular tissue was left, whereas orchidectomy in the first months of life has been associated with a better outcome.

Urinary diversion: ureterosigmoidostomy

This requires normal anal continence and is associated with serious complications, including pyelonephritis, hyperkalaemic acidosis, rectal incontinence, ureteral obstruction and delayed development of malignancy. It does, however, provide an alternative strategy for management of the exstrophic bladder that is too small for primary closure, and it provides a good alternative for patients who have had failed bladder reconstructions. At Mainz University School of

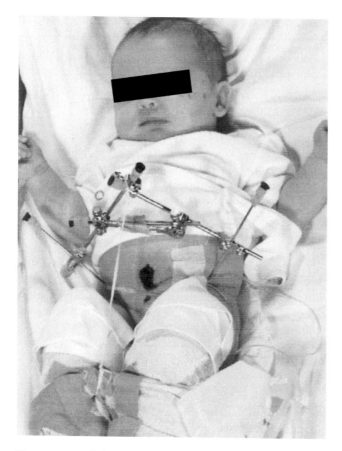

Figure 57.11 *Baby who required pelvic osteotomies. An external fixator is present to allow healing of the osteotomies.*

Medicine, Mainz, Germany, urinary diversion ('Mainz pouch') is performed primarily. In follow-up studies over more than 20 years, this has been associated with 95 per cent stability of the upper urinary tract. Neoplasia is reported by Woodhouse to occur in 22 per cent, but only 11 per cent have invasive carcinoma.

Single-stage reconstruction

Grady and Mitchell (1999) have described a single-stage reconstruction of bladder and cloacal exstrophy in 24 patients. This procedure is a combination of all three separate stages into a single procedure, but without ureteric reimplantation. Mitchell reports an 80 per cent continence rate (volitional voiding with dry intervals of at least two hours). Two boys have required bladder neck reconstruction subsequently, one of whom has also had bladder augmentation with fashioning of a Mitrofanoff stoma. Renal ultrasound is normal in 66 per cent of patients, although 66 per cent of the series did have vesicoureteric reflux.

The Kelly procedure involves complete disassembly of the epispadiac phallus. The posterior urethra is reconstructed along with reconstruction of the posterior urethral sphincter. The penis is then reconstructed, with the urethra placed ventrally, often in a hypospadiac position. The hypospadias is

reconstructed at a later date. For this technique to become popular, it has to be demonstrated that the long-term outcomes include a bladder that is stable and compliant, that the upper tracts are not damaged, and that ultimately urinary continence is improved.

Caione *et al.* (2000) have described extending the penile disassembly technique to include identification of the perineal striated muscle complex and appropriate periurethral reconstruction in primary exstrophy-epispadias reconstruction. Follow-up revealed good cosmesis in 12 of 13 patients, no severe hydronephrosis, and no renal function deterioration. Forty-six per cent had experienced pyelonephritis. Bladder capacity was 35–80 mL in exstrophy patients and 65–120 mL in epispadias patients. Twenty-three per cent were continent, 54 per cent had cyclic voiding patterns with 30–90-minute dry intervals only, and 23 per cent were incontinent?

CONCLUSION

The bladder exstrophy–epispadias complex forms a spectrum of rare malformations. Complete reconstruction in infancy should be the aim. The difficulty of achieving this aim, and the high risk of compromising final outcome if primary reconstruction fails, has led to the concentration of experience in management of this condition into two national centres in the UK.

CLINICAL SCENARIO

A young mother who is 20 weeks' pregnant is referred to you. The anomaly scan suggests a male fetus with bladder exstrophy. What is the management?

Confirming the diagnosis

The following features are seen antenatally:

- Absent bladder: checked with the presence of the umbilical vessels; as the bladder fills and empties over a 30-minute period, it is necessary to scan over this period
- bulging mass above the phallus
- low-set umbilicus
- abnormal short phallus
- rarely, separated pubic bones can be identified
- normal hydramnios.

Counselling

WHAT OPERATIONS NEED TO BE DONE?

- Usually, the bladder is closed at birth, and within the first year of life the penis is repaired. Then, within the first three years, a continence procedure is performed.

- In more than half of boys, a bladder augmentation and Mitrofanoff stoma are required after a continence procedure.

WHAT IS THE OUTCOME?

- *Urinary incontinence*: approximately 25 per cent of boys are dry and void. The vast majority of the remaining boys are dry but they will require lifelong catheterization.
- *Renal outcome*: it is very unusual for children with bladder exstrophy to have renal impairment.
- *Sexual outcome*: in adult males born with bladder exstrophy, erections sufficient for intercourse are normal. Ejaculation, however, is often retrograde and can be slow. Some men are fertile, but this may require assistance.

What are the options now?

- Continue as normal with pregnancy: a normal delivery is recommended following by early referral to an exstrophy unit.
- Termination of pregnancy due to the long-term problems that this child may have.
- Fetal intervention: currently, there is no clinical experience with fetal intervention.

REFERENCES

Bolduc S, Capolicchio G, Upadhyay J, *et al.* The fate of the upper urinary tract in exstrophy. *Journal of Urology* 2002; **168**: 2579–82.

Caione P, Capozza N, Lais A, Matarazzo E. Periurethral muscle complex reassembly for exstrophy-epispadias repair. *Journal of Urology* 2000; **164**: 2062–6.

Chan DY, Jeffs RD, Gearhart JP. Determinants of continence in the bladder exstrophy population: predictors of success? *Urology* 2001; **57**: 774–7.

Diamond DA, Bauer SB, Dinlenc C, *et al.* Normal urodynamics in patients with bladder exstrophy: are they achievable. *Journal of Urology* 1999; **162**: 841.

Gerharz EW, Riedmiller H, Woodhouse CR. Strategies for reconstruction after unsuccessful or unsatisfactory primary treatment of patients with bladder exstrophy or incontinent epispadias. *Journal of Urology* 1999; **162**: 1706–7.

Grady RW, Mitchell ME. Complete primary repair of exstrophy. *Journal of Urology* 1999; **162**: 1415–20.

Kelly JH, Eraklis AJ. A procedure for lengthening the phallus in boys with exstrophy of the bladder. *Journal of Pediatric Surgery* 1971; **6**: 645.

Stein R, Hohenfellner K, Fisch M, *et al.* Social integration, sexual behaviour and fertility in patients with bladder exstrophy: a long-term follow-up. *European Journal of Pediatrics* 1996; **155**: 678–83.

Woodhouse CRJ. The genitalia in exstrophy and epispadias. In: Gearhart JP, Rink RC, Mouriquand PDE (eds). *Pediatric Urology*. Philadelphia, PA: WB Saunders, 2001.

FURTHER READING

Embryology

Muecke EC. The role of the cloacal membrane in exstrophy: the first successful experimental study. *Journal of Urology* 1964; **92**: 659.

Antenatal diagnosis and management

Wilcox DT, Chitty LS. Non-visualisations of the fetal bladder: aetiology and management. *Prenatal Diagnosis* 2001; **21**: 977–83.

Management

Gearhart JP. Exstrophy, epispadias, and other bladder abnormalities. In: Walsh PC, Retik AB, Vaughan ED, Wein AJ (eds). *Campbell's Urology*. Philadelphia, PA: WB Saunders, 2000; pp. 1939–90.

58

Continence and the wet child

JC DJURHUUS, S RITTIG AND TM JØRGENSEN

Learning objectives

- To be able to discriminate between different types of wetness in children.
- To acquire knowledge about the pathophysiology of different types of childhood incontinence.
- To establish adequate diagnostic planning for wet children.
- To establish a pathophysiology-based differentiated treatment strategy for the wet child.

INTRODUCTION

The most frequent urological symptom in children is wetness. Between five and ten per cent of seven-year-olds wet their beds, and up to three per cent of children of the same age have day-time wetting. In addition, up to one-third of seven-year-olds have frequent voiding and urges to void. Voiding complaints *per se* are far less frequent. Only one per cent of seven-year-olds complain of voiding symptoms such as dysuria and interrupted stream. Over the past two or three decades, it has become increasingly obvious that an indiscriminate approach to the wet child is far from satisfactory. A detailed diagnostic approach predominantly using non-invasive diagnostic measures should lead to a far more focused treatment strategy and a better outcome, although the level of evidence for this focused strategy is still less than impressive.

BASIC SCIENCE

Lower urinary tract function is characterized by its complexity. Many mechanisms are understood incompletely, and basic knowledge about normality still contains significant shortcomings. During fetal life, there is a gradual transition of the cysto-urethral organ complex function from conduct towards reservoir. Animal studies have shown that in mid-pregnancy, the urine is transported in an almost peristaltic fashion through the bladder and urethra. Later, at the transition from the mid-third to the last third of pregnancy, the bladder acts increasingly as a reservoir, with intermittent emptying.

Full neurogenic control of lower urinary tract function is achieved at about four years of age. The neurological maturation is marked by a loss of the bladder-cooling reflex, a loss that is linked to a full outgrowth of the C-fibre component of the bladder nerves.

Bladder capacity continues to increase with age. Before birth, the frequency of bladder emptying is approximately once an hour. In the first year of life, the interval increases to every second hour. At the age of seven years, the frequency of voiding has decreased to three to seven per day. This frequency is maintained into adulthood.

There are several means of defining bladder capacity, including cystometric capacity and largest voided volume during daytime giving rise to equations describing the development of bladder capacity. One of the simpler equations based on largest void on a frequency volume chart is that bladder capacity increases with (age $\times$ 30) + 30 mL.

Bladder capacity is, however, not a fixed entity. There are several components describing what should be meant by a comprehensive description of functional bladder capacity. The average bladder capacity is the average of the voidings during daytime, except for the morning voiding. The maximal bladder capacity is usually equal to the morning voiding, frequently being the largest voiding, except in children with incontinence or monosymptomatic bedwetting. It can also be elucidated by maximal withholding or at cystometry.

CONTINENCE MECHANISM

Continence is ascribed to urethral and extra-urethral mechanisms. The urethral sphincter mechanisms consist of the predominantly sympathetically innervated internal sphincter at the bladder neck and the external striated sphincter a little distal to the middle of the urethra in females and below the prostate in males. The internal sphincter mechanism is quite well defined in boys, but in girls it consists only of some smaller muscle bundles scattered around the bladder neck. The structure is gaining increasing interest, with alpha-receptor-blocking agents for voiding dysfunctions now being used in children, especially boys.

The striated sphincter is situated predominantly in the front of the urethra, with muscle bundles becoming thinner posteriorly. It consists of up to 85 per cent slow-twitch fibres, which makes it well suited for being a significant continence mechanism. The high content of slow-twitch fibres causes muscle contraction to be very different from that of the surrounding musculature of the pelvic floor. The pelvic floor's much more substantial component of fast-twitch fibres makes this musculature well suited for supporting additional resistance during coughing and squeezing. The striated sphincter has its own special innervation. Neurotracing studies have shown that the sphincter control centre is the Onuf's nucleus, a collection of nerve cells in the medulla at the level of S2–3 and containing a very high concentration of serotonin and noradrenaline receptors. The therapeutic implications of the receptor content of the control centre for the sphincter are far from understood, but they may represent possible future targets for pharmacological intervention.

The reservoir function of the bladder is also far from understood in detail. During accumulation of urine, the bladder is not inactive. Chaotic micromotions have been indicated. However, the predominant function is a state of accommodation; probably, sympathetic beta-stimulation ameliorates urine accommodation. The bladder has a paradoxical response to filling. The higher the filling rate, the more it can accommodate. This is probably why the bladder capacity during fast-fill cystometry can be compared only with maximal bladder capacity during diuresis.

The initiation of voiding consists of a sudden decrease in urethral pressure caused by a relaxation in the sphincters, leading to introduction of urine into the proximal part of urethra, stimulation of the nociceptive system, transmission of signals to the medulla, and nervous stimulation of a bladder contraction followed by introduction of urine beyond the sphincter mechanism. In spite of being so complex, this voiding reflex can actually be initiated by stimulation of the pelvic nerve. There are strong indications as to an involvement of nitric oxide (NO) in the sudden relaxation of the urethra. The detrusor contraction is mainly a matter of muscarinic receptor stimulation, especially receptor subgroups II and III.

ASSESSMENT OF LOWER URINARY TRACT FUNCTION

A thorough history-taking with equal focus on the physical and intellectual status is important. Physical examination includes inspection of the lower back and the genitals, reflexes, observation of voiding and urine flow, ultrasound residual volume assessment and urine culture and dipstick analysis for infection and diabetes (Figure 58.1). A very important tool in the diagnostic assessment is a voiding diary (frequency–volume chart). Voiding diaries should be inviting and entertaining, making the child active and motivated in the further workout of the lower urinary tract problem.

Sufficient information is obtained from three days of voiding diaries. If the child is a night-time wetter, then the voiding diary should be supplemented for one week with night-time pad-wearing and subsequent weighing, which, together with the morning void, gives the night-time urine output.

The voiding diary provides voiding frequencies, average voided volume, maximum voided volume, the distribution of urine production and fluid intake over 24 hours and therefore offers a sound platform for deciding on relevant treatment strategy.

The diagnosis of constipation is also of paramount importance. Completely accurate diagnostic tools for this are still not established. One has to rely on history regarding bowel habits, description of stools, defecation pain, abdominal pain and rectal digital examination, optionally supplemented by a plain X-ray or ultrasound. Quite often, the consequence is a trial-and-error treatment strategy with laxatives. Anorectal neurophysiology and transport function may have to be evaluated, together with colonic transit time measurements, using the elimination time of radio-opaque fragments on X-ray or of isotopes by gamma-camera examination.

Urodynamic investigation

In patients without neurogenic lower urinary tract symptoms or physical signs related to neurogenic disorders, a urodynamic investigation is not first choice. It is generally agreed that this should be reserved for cases in which long-term antibiotics, bladder rehabilitation, biofeedback and pharmacological treatment have failed.

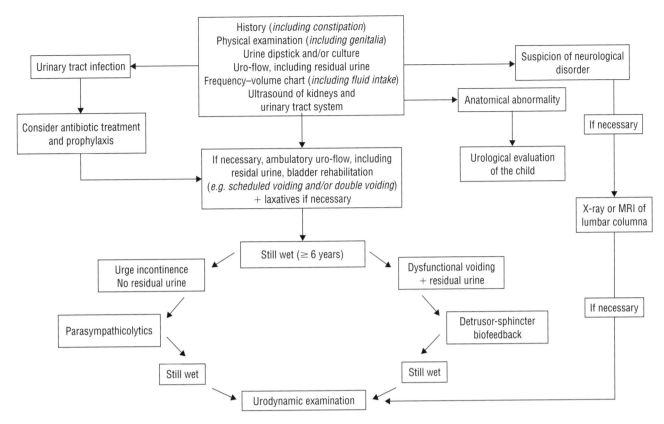

Figure 58.1 *Algorithm outlining a diagnostic strategy for the evaluation of the wet child.*
MRI, magnetic resonance imaging

The technical approach for urodynamic investigations is still a matter of fierce dispute. Some centres use transurethral catheterisation for cystometry and/or pressure-flow measurements, whereas others use a double-lumen small-size suprapubic catheter inserted either under general anaesthesia or, in older children, under local anaesthesia. The advantage of using a suprapubic catheter is that the examination is experienced by the child as minimally invasive, thereby permitting prolonged measurements and repeated measurements with the child's cooperation and confidence. Extended natural fill investigations, a further type of urodynamic technique, give rise to better correlation between symptoms and the urodynamic findings. Another advantage is that this category of measurement allows for voiding monitoring and reservoir function monitoring not only during the day but also during the night, which is of paramount importance for understanding individual symptoms both day and night.

Although it is invasive, suprapubic access still implies a very low complication rate. In fact, it seems to be lower than transurethral access in terms of the development of concomitant infection.

The disadvantages of using natural fill and a suprapubic catheter with extended measurements are that most monitoring equipment do not allow for an online analysis, measurements are complicated and demand extended experience, and the analysis is extremely time-consuming and has to be tailored to each patient.

Imaging

Ultrasound is the initial imaging modality. It comprises examination for congenital malformations of the kidneys and upper urinary tract and especially for detection of post-void residuals. Although abnormalities detected by way of ultrasound in incontinent children without infection and infection history are rare, the investigation is still recommended in most children.

Radiological investigation, sometimes in combination with urodynamics as video-urodynamics, has had widespread use. As well as detecting malformations and vesicoureteral reflux (p. 453), the combination of imaging and urodynamics adds valuable information, especially with regard to the circumstances under which reflux occurs. However, the increasing awareness of the risk of using X-rays in children has, in many centres, reduced the use of the investigation to selected complicated cases.

VOIDING SYNDROMES

There is increasing awareness of the fact that lower urinary tract symptoms in children should be regarded with a differentiated approach concerning both the aetiology and the treatment of the conditions. This includes a firm distinction between daytime and night-time wetness and between bladder reservoir problems and voiding problems. In the following sections, we describe the different syndromes, their prevalences and diagnoses, and how they should be treated.

The term 'nocturnal enuresis' (NE) should, according to the International Children's Continence Society (ICCS) standardization, be limited to conditions in which the wetness occurs during the night while the child is asleep and when no daytime symptoms are present. It is the most frequent symptom in children after asthma, with a prevalence of five to ten per cent at the age of seven years and of 0.5–1 per cent in adulthood. There are different opinions about when monosymptomatic bedwetters pass the physiological threshold. Most consider wetness beyond the age of five to be pathological, but in practice monosymptomatic bedwetting should be regarded as a disease only when the child and parents consider it so. In many countries, treatment is not considered before the age of six or seven years.

For centuries, it has been known that monosymptomatic nocturnal enuresis (MNE) has a strong hereditary component. During the past decade, several genetic aspects have been established in terms of loci on different chromosomes. These loci seem to be related specifically to MNE, and both MNE and day- and night-time incontinence have showed positive linkage. The role of genetics is still an open question, and specific gene and gene products have not been found.

The severity of NE has an impact on the here-and-now situation of the child and his or her parents. However, it also influences the prognosis of becoming spontaneously dry. The more severe the NE, the more unlikely is the probability of spontaneous resolution to becoming dry. This is in tandem with the fact that NE in adolescents usually is very severe.

MNE is a heterogeneous condition that presents in different forms, but all forms have in common a mismatch between the bladder capacity and the urine production at night (Figure 58.2).

Night–time polyuria

The most frequent MNE form (approximately two-thirds) is characterized by normal bladder function, including a normal bladder capacity both day and night, but an abnormally large urine production at night, exceeding the bladder capacity. More than a decade ago, it was substantiated that this type of MNE is associated with, or has its background from, a lack of a circadian rhythm of antidiuretic hormone (ADH). This lack of circadian rhythm, displayed as the same plasma concentration of ADH over 24 hours, is probably a sign of a delay in maturation. Children who become dry are either enhanced by treatment or spontaneously develop a normal circadian rhythm of urine production.

TREATMENT

When night-time polyuria has been confirmed by way of voiding diaries with pad weighing, night-time antidiuresis treatment should be initiated. The child should be treated with desmopressin, starting at a low dose and then titrating towards full dryness or maximal dose. Treatment should be continued for three months, followed by a non-treatment period. Treatment should be restarted immediately if wetness recurs. Drug treatment can be continued for years, and in a few patients it is a lifelong treatment. There is no tachyphylaxis and the risk of complications is minimal. However, instruction against polydipsia should be enforced. If breakthrough of wetness occurs during treatment, a diagnosis should be pursued meticulously, focusing especially on possible infection or diabetes mellitus.

Treatment with desmopressin is symptomatic at first. The antidiuresis restores the balance between urine output and the bladder capacity. The long-term effects and cure rate are not established. There are some indications as to a curative effect, but this has not been proven.

CLINICAL SCENARIO

A seven-year-old boy presented with nocturnal enuresis three to five nights per week. These symptoms had persisted since infancy (=primary NE). The boy had no other urological complaints, in particular no daytime urgency or incontinence

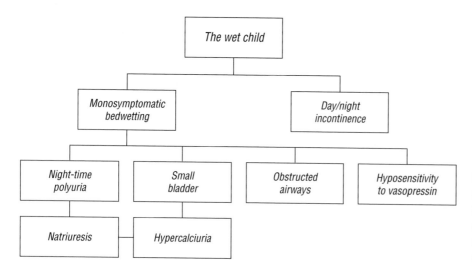

Figure 58.2 *Differentiation between day and night incontinence and monosymptomatic bedwetting in the wet child. The current concept of subgrouping monosymptomatic nocturnal enuresis is outlined.*

(=MNE). Urinalysis was normal, as was physical examination. A frequency–volume chart showed a normal daytime functional bladder capacity (largest void) of 290 mL. Pad-weighing and morning urine volume measurements showed a large nocturnal urine production of 378 mL on wet nights. Treatment with oral desmopressin 0.20 mg at bedtime resulted in complete relief of symptoms. The boy's family was instructed to continue treatment in three-month intervals interrupted by treatment-free breaks of a few days to check whether spontaneous cure had occurred.

'Small' bladder capacity

Another frequent cause of MNE is small bladder capacity syndrome. The child has a normal circadian rhythm of urine production but has a reduced bladder capacity during the night. In most cases, the functional bladder capacity is also reduced during the day. There is an increased frequency of voiding during the day, close to or beyond the upper limit of normal (seven per day), accompanied by a bladder capacity below 70 per cent of what should be expected for age. This is usually the most severe form of enuresis, often with more than one episode each night. Often, it is unclear whether the decreased bladder capacity is related to overactivity of the bladder. This could be proven urodynamically by way of night-time bladder pressure monitoring or indirectly as the result of anticholinergic treatment.

TREATMENT

The treatment of choice in this type of enuresis is alarm-clock treatment. For many years, it was a mystery as to how this treatment actually worked, i.e. was it a modulation of the arousal mechanism leading to nocturnal bladder control or a change in urine output? Recent research has shown that small bladder enuresis dryness is achieved by way of a significant increase in the night-time bladder capacity, whereas nocturnal urine output is unchanged, thereby establishing a balance between urine production and bladder capacity.

There are several different types of alarm-clock treatment devices, but they all have in common a moisture sensor that triggers an alarm, ideally waking the child. Frequently, however, the child does not wake; therefore, one of the parents must be nearby so that they can wake up the child. This treatment modality demands much professional support, not only for the child but also for the family. Therefore, it is of paramount importance that frequent contact between the nurse monitoring the treatment and the child and his or her parents is established. Normally, the treatment should continue for eight weeks.

The outcome of treatment presents conflicting results in the literature. In its early days, miraculous treatment responses were reported, but with the increasing demands required of the scientific quality of reports on treatment, the long-term outcome has decreased to approximately 34 per cent permanent dryness in later years.

Other types

Nasal adenoid vegetations lead to obstructed airways and some degree of hypoxia. Together with the mechanical efforts of respiration and its impact on atrial stretching, this results in an increased production of atrial natriuretic peptide, causing nocturnal natriuresis and polyuria. Ablation of the adenoid vegetations is the treatment of choice. The scientific documentation of the condition and the results of its treatment is less than satisfactory.

There is an increasing awareness of the importance of nocturnal solute excretion in MNE. Natriuresis in connection with obstructive upper airways has been mentioned. This is, however, not the only entity associated with natriuresis. A certain number of polyuric patients without other symptoms have polyuria predominantly with an increased solute excretion. The major cause is probably large sodium excretion, but hyperabsorptive hypercalciuria also has been implicated.

Drugs modulating sodium excretion, such as non-steroidal anti-inflammatory drugs (NSAIDs), have been reported to be effective. They are, however, probably not suitable for long-term medical treatment, not least because of the ensuing changes of the vascular resistance in the kidneys. Antidepressants also have been shown to have a significant impact on nocturnal polyuria, with pronounced modulation of solute excretion. The potential significant cardiac side effects of these drugs, especially when taken in overdose, make them recommendable only in special cases.

Dietary modulation of calcium intake has been advocated in hypercalciuria patients. Some effect has been reported in a few studies, but it is still an open question as to how frequent the hypercalciuria actually is and how effective the treatment might be.

CLINICAL SCENARIO

An eight-year-old girl had day- and night-time incontinence since infancy. There was no history of urinary tract infection or constipation. She had two to three small incontinence episodes every day, often associated with urge and squatting, and she wet her bed every night. A frequency–volume chart revealed 9–11 micturitions per day (normal three to seven per day) and a clearly reduced functional bladder capacity (140 mL). Urinalysis and physical examination were normal. The child was given voiding instructions by the family doctor, but with unsatisfactory response. After referral to a paediatric urologist, the evaluation was supplemented by a rectal examination (normal) and ultrasound investigation of the urinary tract. Ultrasound was normal, except for a thick bladder wall. A uroflowmetry showed a tower-shaped curve with a maximum flow rate of about 20 mL; no residual urine was found. Intensive bladder rehabilitation with scheduled voiding supervised by a urotherapist did not resolve the symptoms fully. Anticholinergic therapy with oxybutynine 5 mg twice daily, however, cured the daytime symptoms. As the night-time wetting continued, nocturnal urine production was determined by pad-weighing and was found to be within the normal range. Eight weeks of alarm-clock treatment cured the night-time wetting.

Dysfunctional voiders

Voiding dysfunction in children is rather rare. Approximately one per cent of seven-year-olds will have voiding patterns clearly deviating from normal. The predominant pattern is that of staccato voiding, which consists of frequent interruptions of detrusor-initiated voiding. The staccato voiding has many terms, including 'non-neurogenic detrusor sphincter dyssynergia' and 'overactive urethra', but most authors adhere to the descriptive term 'staccato voiding'. Symptoms are those of the frequency/urgency syndrome.

Sometimes, urgency incontinence is caused by secondary detrusor overactivity or a significant residual urine caused by an underactive detrusor. More seldom, a plateau flow pattern is encountered, consistent with an infravesical obstruction.

It is generally agreed that a consistent pattern of three characteristic flows measured consecutively are prerequisites for the diagnosis. The aetiology of staccato voiding has not been elucidated fully. The most simple theory is that it can be a long-time effect caused by the voiding pains following a urinary tract infection, in which the child learns to protect the urethra from the full urine stream by contracting the sphincter and continues to do so after the urethral pain has disappeared. However, it may also be caused by long-term overtraining of the pelvic floor and the urethral sphincter during the holding situation in a child with an overactive bladder. It is also hypothesized that it is a sign of a delayed maturation of the interaction between the detrusor and the pelvic floor or an increased nociceptive receptor response in the proximal part of urethra.

TREATMENT

Primarily, an obstruction should be treated. Previously and even today, different pharmacological modalities have been tried in the management of dyscoordinated voiding. Initially, tranquillizers or parasympatholytics were used; later, alpha-blocking agents were used. In our opinion, the primary treatment of choice is biofeedback. This may be preceded by behavioural treatment, in order to correct improper toilet habits. Biofeedback treatment is very effective, both short- and long-term. Biofeedback is a visualization of a biological event to the patient by way of electronic equipment. The visualization apparatus consists of perianally placed surface electrodes with a ground electrode on the thigh combined with an electromyography amplifier for visualization of the pelvic floor activity. A urotherapist repeatedly instructs the child in maximal contraction and maximal relaxation of the pelvic floor. This is followed by repetitive voidings visualized on the screen and by using a loudspeaker assisted by instructions from the urotherapist. The session takes one full day, with the child on increased fluid intake, followed by another session one week later and another approximately one month later. Children are usually very responsive to this type of treatment

from the age of six years and onwards, but frequently a brush-up session is necessary. The endpoint of the treatment is obvious: normalization of the urine flow, leading to symptom-free voiding.

In a few cases, and almost exclusively in boys, voiding may look to be obstructed. It is plateau-shaped and very often may be due to congenital obstruction in the urethra. Such a flow configuration is usually accompanied by frequency/urge syndrome and, sometimes, pain. Urethrography will show a narrowing in the bulbar urethra (strictures, congenital posterior urethral valves, Cobb's collar, Morman's ring). The diagnosis can be confirmed and the condition treated during urethroscopy.

Vaginal urine retention

In a substantial number of girls, the hymen is funnel-shaped or the labia is partly fused. During voiding, part of the stream enters the vagina (vaginal reflux), and the urine dribbles after the patient has left the toilet. Some girls, especially if they are obese, tend to sit on the toilet with their thighs close together; consequently, some urine enters the vagina during micturition.

Symptoms are diagnostic with dribbling just after leaving the toilet. The treatment is simple in most cases: the child changes to a backward-facing position on the toilet, placing one leg on each side of the toilet, so that she is forced to spread her legs widely.

Anatomical abnormalities

In a few girls, examination of the genitalia shows an epispadia (p. 497), or a history of normal voiding and constant dribbling will raise suspicion of ectopic ureter to be corrected by surgery.

Overactive bladder

Two to three per cent of seven-year-olds have incontinence with concomitant signs of an overactive bladder, and up to one-third of seven-year-olds have some urgency, with increased voiding frequency. There is often posturing to avoid wetting (especially in older children), by crouching down during an urge, and the heel of the foot being pressed on to the perineum until the urge has resolved (Vincent's curtsey). This syndrome has undergone a conceptual change over the past decade. Previously, there was a clear-cut urodynamic definition of the overactive bladder, with detrusor contractions during filling initially with a contraction amplitude of more than $15\,cmH_2O$. Now it is simply any contractions. The same symptoms without contractions on the cystometry were known as 'sensory urge'.

Realizing that a solitary urodynamic diagnosis probably is insufficient, the International Continence Society today prefers the term 'overactive bladder', in which the symptom is due to bladder and/or urethral dysfunction. Detailed urodynamic investigations have shown that there are different patterns

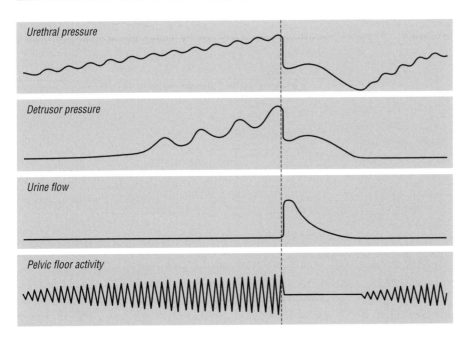

Figure 58.3 *Schematic drawing of type I overactive bladder, in which the bladder pressure is consistently increasing towards a certain level, where the patient has to relax the pelvic floor and overactive voiding takes place.*

behind the symptomatic overactive bladder. Figures 58.3 and 58.4 show schematic representations of the two types. Type I consists of a build-up of bladder contractions with increasing amplitudes, counteracted by pelvic floor contractions until the point at which the child has to give in and relaxes the pelvic floor, frequently before reaching the toilet. After initiation of micturition, the bladder pressure suddenly decreases and normal bladder pressures are achieved during the rest of the voiding.

Type II is caused primarily by abnormal function of the urethra. For decades, it has been known that the urethra has spontaneous activity of smooth-muscle origin. This spontaneous activity in the urethra has been interpreted, wrongly, as urethral instability. It is, however, a complex type of spontaneous activity in the musculature, present both in the urethra and in the anal canal (Figure 58.4).

This spontaneous urethral activity does not appear to have any relation to the first type, but it is sudden and an abrupt decrease in urethral pressure leading to the introduction of urine into the urethra. This activates a detrusor contraction unless the pelvic floor activity is activated immediately after the introduction of urine. In the case of any delay in pelvic floor reaction, a detrusor contraction develops and leakage may occur. This type of overactive bladder will be depicted only if bladder pressure is seen as a single contraction of the bladder without the build-up of preleakage bladder contractions. One could consider this type of overactivity as a premature micturition reflex, since the manifestations and the sequences in biological events are quite similar to those of normal micturition.

TREATMENT

Treatment of overactive bladder is elimination of constipation and any urinary tract infections present followed by behavioural treatment. This modality will cure at least 50 per cent of affected children. The cornerstone in behavioural treatment is first to establish the child's awareness about his or her particular voiding habits. Different referral centres have different strategies. Most include a correction of fluid intake and abolishment of caffeine-containing beverages, including tea, coffee and cola, as well as other stimulant drinks, such as concentrated blackcurrant. Most centres also include an initial increase in the number of voidings followed by a gradual decrease to normality. If inappropriate postures are part of the child's voiding habits, then they should be corrected. It is of paramount importance that health workers are educated appropriately before they become urotherapists. Special education of nurses should include achievement of a profound knowledge of physiology and pathophysiology of the lower urinary tract. These qualified instructions can be conveyed to the child in frequent and repeated sessions, starting with very frequent voidings followed by gradual postponement.

If the above treatment for a couple of months does not abolish the symptoms, then pharmacotherapy with antimuscarinics should be tried. There are few such drugs with substantiated effects in children, and some of them do have significant side effects, especially in children with symptoms of attention-deficit hyperactivity disorder (ADHD). The later-developed antimuscarinics seem to have less influence on cognitive function and therefore are tolerated better.

Drug titration until dryness is achieved, or until significant side effects become limiting, is recommended, with a treatment period of at least eight weeks. Children will usually tolerate larger dosages of antimuscarinics than are tolerated by adults.

Lazy bladder syndrome

The aetiology of lazy bladder syndrome is multifactorial. Filthy school toilets and urethral pain during voiding or

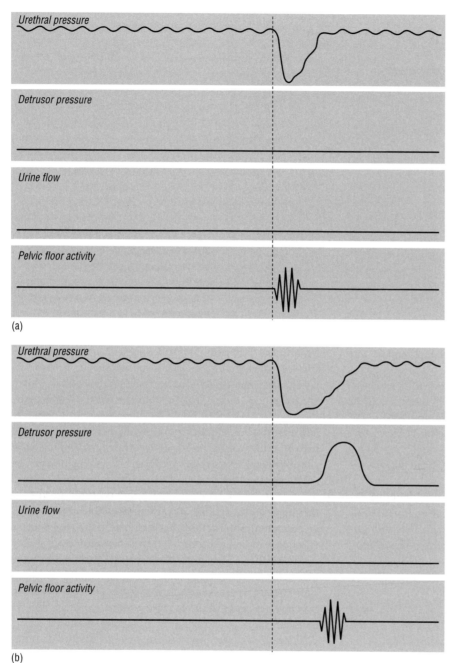

(a)

(b)

Figure 58.4 *Urethral origin of 'overactive' bladder: (a) Sudden relaxation of the urethra leads to an immediate reaction from the pelvic floor counteracting a detrusor contraction. Previously, this was called 'sensory urge'. (b) Urethral pressure drop followed by a delayed pelvic floor contraction. The delay causes the development of a detrusor contraction.*

following urinary tract infection will, in some children, lead to infrequent voiding. In some children, the syndrome has a previous infravesical obstruction as background. These children characteristically void only twice every 24 hours, or less, but voiding frequency can simulate normality if the bladder emptying is poor. The condition is often associated with constipation and recurrent urinary tract infection.

A diagnostic clue is that the patient does not empty their bladder after waking up in the morning, despite having been dry during the night.

In order to establish the correct diagnosis, it is often necessary to perform a urodynamic examination and to exclude underlying neuropathy (p. 521). Cystometry will show large bladder capacity, most often a weak detrusor, a negative

bethanechol test and no signs of obstruction on the pressure flow examination.

TREATMENT

Treatment consists of bladder rehabilitation, frequently timed voidings and double voidings at least twice a day. Sometimes, clean intermittent catheterization is necessary for a shorter or longer period.

Giggle incontinence

Intense giggling, typically during prepuberty, has for a long time been known in some individuals to be followed by

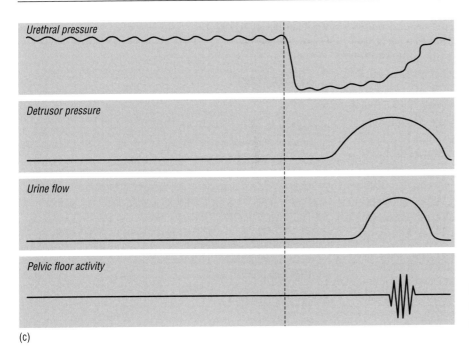

Figure 58.4 *(c) Urethral relaxation with a very delayed pelvic floor contraction, which leads to detrusor contraction and leakage.*

(c)

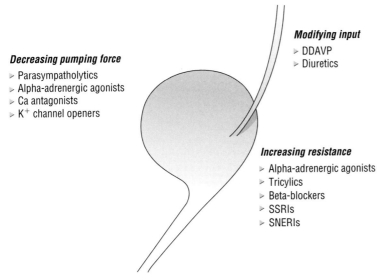

Decreasing pumping force

➢ Parasympatholytics
➢ Alpha-adrenergic agonists
➢ Ca antagonists
➢ K⁺ channel openers

Modifying input

➢ DDAVP
➢ Diuretics

Increasing resistance

➢ Alpha-adrenergic agonists
➢ Tricylics
➢ Beta-blockers
➢ SSRIs
➢ SNERIs

Figure 58.5 *Principles for treatment of lower urinary tract symptoms in children. Only with parasympatholytics and desmopressin (DDAVP) treatment has effect been proven to a scientifically satisfactory level. The other modalities are either experimental or theoretical suggestions for future treatment.*

SNERIs, specific noradrenaline reuptake inhibitors; SSRIs, selective serotonin reuptake inhibitors.

partial or often complete emptying of the bladder. The aetiology is more or less unknown. Physical and urodynamic examination are most often normal. It has been postulated that giggling triggers, via central nervous system centres, a reflex relaxation of the urethral sphincter, which reflexly starts a bladder contraction.

TREATMENT

The syndrome is very often highly disturbing for the affected child, and it is of little comfort to the child to be told that the condition generally improves in the course of time. Many different treatment modalities have been tried, but none have been tested adequately and most are ineffective: sympathomimetic agents, phenylphenidate and imipramine, and biofeedback training for better pelvic floor control and for control of the sphincter, are some of the choices.

CONCLUSION

Apart from the polyuric type of MNE, most manifestations of wetness and voiding dysfunction in children should be treated with elimination of constipation and changed habits, even in a rather intensive form as dedicated programmes, camps or schools. Only when these actions have failed should drug treatment be instigated. Figure 58.5 outlines the principles of drug action in these children.

CLINICAL SCENARIO

A nine-year-old girl had daytime incontinence and faecal soiling since the age of four years. She also had a history of at least four lower urinary tract infections during the past eight months and a history indicative of constipation. She had several incontinence episodes during the day, often without a sensation of urge. The frequency–volume chart revealed only three micturitions per day, with large volumes often exceeding 500 mL. Physical examination revealed palpable abdominal masses. There was faecal impaction on a rectal examination and normal ultrasound of the urinary tract, except for a large residual urine of 120 mL. Uroflowmetry showed a fractionated curve (staccato pattern) indicative of bladder–sphincter dyscoordination. Long-term antibiotic prophylaxis was instituted, together with laxatives. Furthermore, thorough voiding instructions were given by the urotherapist, who also instructed in scheduled voidings every three to four hours and triple voiding twice daily to improve bladder emptying. As the staccato voiding continued, two biofeedback training sessions were performed. After five months, the daytime incontinence, constipation and faecal soiling were resolved, and uroflowmetry and bladder emptying improved.

FURTHER READING

Djurhuus JC, Rittig S. Nocturnal enuresis. *Current Opinion in Urology* 2002; **12**: 317–20.

Hoebeke PB, Vande Walle J. The pharmacology of paediatric incontinence. *British Journal of Urology International* 2000; **86**: 581–9.

Nijman RJM. Classification and treatment of functional incontinence in children. *British Journal of Urology International* 2000; **85** (suppl. 3): 37–42.

Nijman R, Butler R, Van Gool J, Bowers W, Hjaelmaas K. Conservative management of urinary incontinence in childhood. In: Abrams P, Cardosa L, Khoury S, Wein A (eds). *Incontinence*, 2nd edn. Plymouth: Plymbridge Distributors, 2002; pp. 515–51.

Norgaard JP, van Gool JD, Hjalmaas K, Djurhuus JC, Hellstrom AL. Standardization and definitions in lower urinary tract dysfunction in children. International Children's Continence Society. *British Journal of Urology* 1998; **81** (suppl. 3): 1–16.

The neuropathic bladder

THOMAS BOEMERS

Learning objectives

- To understand the basic neuroanatomy and neurophysiology of normal lower urinary tract function.
- To understand the clinical implications of neuropathic bladder–sphincter dysfunction.
- To understand the diagnostic work-up of neuropathic bladder–sphincter dysfunction.
- To understand the conservative management of neuropathic bladder–sphincter dysfunction.
- To understand the basic principles of operative management of neuropathic bladder–sphincter dysfunction.
- To be able to set up a preliminary management plan for a newborn with myelomeningocele with respect to neuropathic bladder–sphincter dysfunction.

INTRODUCTION

The lower urinary tract is composed of the bladder, the bladder neck, the urethra and the urethral sphincter, which is part of the perineal and pelvic floor musculature. The main function of the lower urinary tract consists of storage and timely evacuation of urine, while preserving renal function. This is achieved by two functional units: the bladder (detrusor muscle), which serves as a reservoir, and the outlet (bladder neck, posterior urethra and external urethral sphincter), which controls evacuation. These subunits are innervated by the peripheral nerve supply to the genitourinary tract, which is under control of the central nervous system. In children, coordinated function generally requires normal maturation of the nervous system as well as normal anatomy. Disruption of the anatomy of the lower urinary tract, disintegration of the nervous system and dyscoordination of sequential functional steps result in lower urinary tract dysfunction, with secondary problems such as urinary incontinence, obstructive uropathy, urinary tract infection (UTIs, vesicoureteral reflux (VUR) and renal damage. The morbidity of neuropathic lower urinary tract dysfunction is immense and usually necessitates lifelong medical treatment and surveillance.

Congenital and acquired lesions of the nervous system responsible for the innervation of the lower urinary tract generally will lead to dysfunction of the urinary bladder and urethral sphincter mechanism. Therefore, the term 'neuropathic bladder' is a misnomer, because it draws attention to only one part of the lower urinary tract, the bladder. Generally speaking, the term should be 'neuropathic bladder–sphincter dysfunction' (NBSD). However, for the ease of communication in this text, the term 'neuropathic bladder' always refers to both units of the lower urinary tract, the bladder and urethral sphincter.

RELEVANT BASIC SCIENCE

Innervation of the lower urinary tract

PERIPHERAL INNERVATION

Peripheral innervation is achieved by three different nerve groups:

- sacral parasympathetic nerves (pelvic splanchnic nerves)
- thoracolumbar sympathetic nerves (hypogastric nerves)
- sacral somatic nerves.

These nerves transmit efferent (centrifugal) and afferent (centripetal) innervation to the genitourinary tract and pelvic floor muscles.

Parasympathetic nerves

The efferent sacral parasympathetic nerves to the lower urinary tract are carried within the pelvic splanchnic nerves. They provide the major autonomic motor innervation to the bladder (detrusor muscle). The pelvic splanchnic nerves are formed by coalescence of the sacral ventral roots S2, S3 and S4. The nerve fibres are both preganglionic and postganglionic. Acetylcholine is the primary neurotransmitter; therefore, detrusor contraction can be elicited by administration of acetylcholine to these nerves, and they can be blocked by anticholinergic drugs, one of the main medical treatment modalities in the management of NBSD.

Sympathetic nerves

The sympathetic fibres originate in the T10–L2 spinal cord segments and emerge in the ventral nerve roots. The nerve fibres synapse in the paravertebral ganglia of the lumbar sympathetic chain and branch out to form the superior hypogastric plexus (anterior to the aorta), which bifurcates into the left and right hypogastric nerves. Ultimately, they intermingle with pelvic parasympathetic nerves to form the pelvic plexus. The hypogastric nerves mainly convey efferent sympathetic innervation to the muscles of the bladder base, bladder neck and proximal urethra. The main postganglionic neurotransmitter is noradrenaline; therefore, the nerves are termed 'adrenergic'. Sympathetic innervation elicits inhibition of detrusor muscle, excitation of the bladder base and urethra, and closure of the bladder neck and posterior urethra.

Pelvic plexus (hypogastric plexus)

Parasympathetic fibres from the pelvic plexus innervate the pelvic organs and corpora cavernosa of the penis and clitoris (cavernous nerves). The pelvic plexus lies deep within the pelvis, with the main part located laterally to the bladder base and adjacent to the rectum in men and upper vagina and uterus in women.

Somatic pelvic nerves

The somatic nerves to the pelvic floor muscles are typical motor neurons. The cell bodies originate in Onuf's nucleus in the anterior horn of the S2–S4 segments and form the pudendal nerve. The pudendal nerve carries the somatic innervation to the perineal and pelvic floor muscles, including the external striated urethral sphincter.

CENTRAL NERVOUS CONTROL

Unlike other visceral functions, which are purely involuntary, lower urinary tract function is under voluntary control. However, micturition depends on a learning process and maturation of the nervous system, which takes place during childhood. The neural control of lower urinary tract function occurs at different levels within the central nervous system. The main influence of the cerebral cortex on the lower urinary tract is central inhibition of the micturition reflex. It allows voiding to be deferred if the circumstances are not appropriate. However, induction of voiding at will is also possible. Through the cerebral cortex, micturition can also be influenced by psychological, behavioural and social aspects. The thalamus, hypothalamus and limbic system act as a relay station for sensory axons and organize the autonomic nervous system involved in micturition. The basal ganglia and cerebellum have an inhibitory effect and suppress spontaneous reflex contractions of the detrusor. The pontine-sacral pathways connect the pontine micturition centre to the sacral micturition centre and are important for activating the micturition reflex. The sacral micturition centre is located in the spinal cord segments S2–S4, which equate to the vertebral levels T11–L1. The micturition reflex consists of a series of events that ultimately result in coordinated relaxation of the striated urethral sphincter, opening of the bladder neck, and contraction of the detrusor muscle, leading to complete elimination of urine.

Function of the lower urinary tract

Lower urinary tract function consists of storage and regular expulsion of urine. These functions are under control of the peripheral and central nervous system and are accomplished by interaction of the vesicourethral unit with the striated external sphincter and pelvic floor muscles.

STORAGE PHASE

Under physiological conditions, the bladder fills slowly and the bladder wall is continuously stretched, thereby accommodating large volumes of urine without a significant rise in intravesical pressure. This property, mainly referred to as 'bladder compliance', is dependent largely on intrinsic bladder-wall tension and elasticity. A normal bladder compliance with low pressures throughout the filling phase is essential for protecting the kidneys and preserving renal function. Continence during storage is achieved by the fact that urethral closing pressure remains greater than intravesical pressure. During bladder filling, stretch receptors within the bladder wall are increasingly activated, causing a steady rise of activity in the afferent pelvic nerves. The afferent pelvic nerves are under constant inhibitory control, which ensures that activation of efferent fibres is reached only at a critical level (micturition threshold). Failure of the inhibitory mechanism, as in many cases of NBSD, may lead to high intravesical pressure and unphysiological detrusor overactivity during the storage phase.

VOIDING PHASE

The micturition reflex is initiated by relaxation of the urethral sphincter. This fall in urethral pressure is followed by contraction of the detrusor muscle; simultaneously, the bladder neck and posterior urethra open. A prerequisite for a normal voiding reflex to occur is an intact neural pathway between the pontine and sacral micturition centres. Lesions below the sacral micturition centre create an areflexic decentralized bladder, commonly classified as a 'lower motor-neuron lesion'. A lesion above the sacral micturition centre causes hyperreflexia (spasticity) of the bladder, classified as an 'upper motor-neuron lesion', with uncoordinated micturition (detrusor-sphincter dyssynergia). Mixed lesions are classified as 'intermediate bladder'. Normal voiding is influenced greatly by central nervous control, allowing voluntary facilitation or inhibition.

LOWER URINARY TRACT FUNCTION IN CHILDREN

It is assumed that micturition in children under the age of three years occurs purely on a reflex basis, without central neural control. However, recent studies have challenged this concept and suggest that development of voluntary control is probably only a modulation of pre-existing and already well-formed reflex pathways.

Nonetheless, development of continence and voluntary voiding in children is a multifactorial process that mainly involves maturation of the nervous system and learning. As the child gets older, he or she becomes aware of bladder fullness and is able to postpone micturition by external sphincter contraction rather than central inhibition. This process usually evolves during the second year of life. With gradual maturation, continence and voluntary voiding occurs around three years of age. At this stage, the child learns to defer micturition by central inhibition and does not solely use external

sphincter contraction. In children with neuropathic bladder, this process does not take place.

GENERAL FEATURES

Classification and terminology of neuropathic bladder

NBSD can be classified on a neurotopographical basis according to whether the lesion is located above or below the sacral micturition centre, i.e. as an upper motor-neuron lesion or a lower motor-neuron lesion. If the lesion is complete, then the type of bladder-sphincter dysfunction is predictable. However, if the lesion is incomplete or located at various levels, then many diverse patterns can result, i.e. mixed upper- and lower motor-neuron lesions. In contrast to spinal-cord trauma, in which lesions are usually complete and located at a distinct anatomical level, congenital lesions of the spinal cord (e.g. myelomeningocele, MMC) often demonstrate mixed patterns. Therefore, a neuroanatomical classification in the paediatric population is highly complex and demanding, since most cases of NBSD are due to MMC and other forms of neurospinal dysraphism. However, clinically, classification of lower urinary tract dysfunction is essential for a specific therapeutic approach. Complex neuroanatomical descriptions do not serve this purpose, and with the evolution of urodynamic testing, a clinically oriented classification has evolved, based on specific urodynamic findings.

The two main functions of the lower urinary tract, namely storage and timely evacuation of urine, depend on the interaction of the bladder with the urethral sphincter. The urodynamic classification system therefore describes these two units in terms of function and coordination. Function may be normal, overactive or underactive, and interaction between bladder and sphincter is either coordinated (synergic) or uncoordinated (dyssynergic). The resulting patterns of bladder-sphincter dysfunction are depicted in Figure 59.1, and the percentages of the different patterns are given in Figure 59.2.

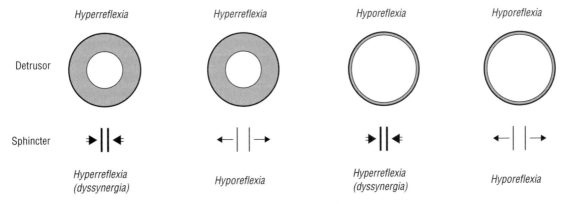

Figure 59.1 *Urodynamic classification of neuropathic bladder-sphincter dysfunction.*

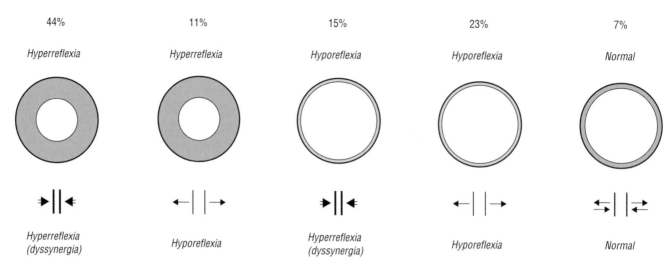

Figure 59.2   *Percentages of urodynamic patterns found in children with neurospinal dysraphism.*

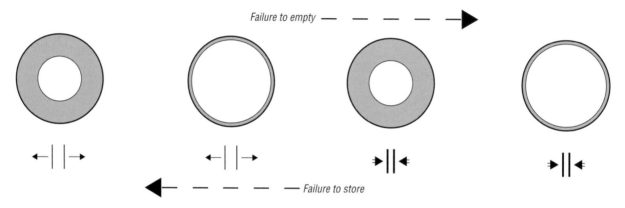

Figure 59.3   *The two main clinical problems in children with neuropathic bladder-sphincter dysfunction.*

The different types of NBSD will lead to two main clinical problems: failure to store and failure to empty (Figure 59.3).

Even though these pattern are not always as obvious and clear, they can be used clinically as guidelines for therapy, and they have prognostic implications as well. According to the definition by the International Continence Society (ICS), overactivity or underactivity of detrusor function should be termed 'hyperreflexia', 'hyporeflexia' or 'areflexia', respectively, in cases of neuropathy. In addition to the specific pattern, two other urodynamic findings are of clinical significance and prognostic importance: bladder compliance (elasticity of the bladder wall) and the leak-point pressure (intravesical pressure at which urethral leakage occurs). Low bladder compliance, especially when seen early in the filling phase, as well as a leak-point pressure above 40 cmH$_2$O have a bad prognosis in terms of renal function. Children with low bladder compliance or high leak-point pressure have a high risk of renal deterioration. Often, a high leak-point pressure and a low bladder compliance coincide, and there are data to suggest that non-compliant bladders are acquired because of high outlet resistance. However, high intravesical pressures during filling and leakage are also seen with pure detrusor-sphincter dyssynergia in the

absence of poor bladder compliance, and this is also a risk factor for renal deterioration. It must be remembered that when evaluating NBSD, one should not only look at the urodynamic parameters but also include clinical and radiographic findings in order to reach an overall conclusive diagnosis of a specific type of NBSD.

Aetiology of neuropathic bladder in children

Causes for neuropathic bladder can be classified into congenital and acquired lesions. Congenital structural disorders of the spinal cord account for more than 90 per cent of cases of neuropathic bladder in children.

MYELOMENINGOCELE

MMC results from failure of tubularization and closure of parts of the vertebral column and spinal cord, resulting in a dysraphic lesion with a more or less marked neurological defect (Figure 59.4). With an incidence of one to two per 1000 newborns, MMC is a common and serious birth defect. MMC is a spectrum that, in the majority of cases, involves the lumbar

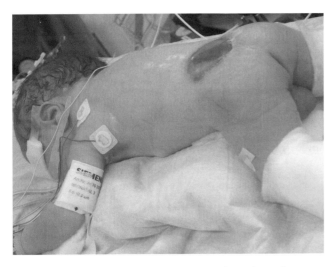

Figure 59.4 *Newborn with lumbosacral myelomeningocele.*

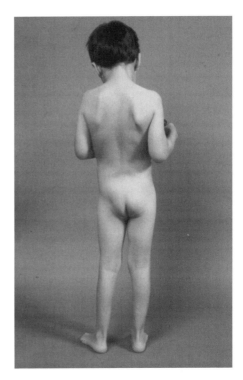

Figure 59.5 *Boy with occult neuropathic bladder-sphincter dysfunction due to sacral agenesis.*

and sacral vertebral column and the corresponding spinal cord segments. The thoracic and cervical vertebral column and corresponding spinal cord segments may also be affected, especially with very large defects. The neurological lesion in MMC is variable and not predictable as in patients with traumatic lesions of the spinal cord. Most children demonstrate incomplete lesions with sensory or motor sparing, and classification of the neurological deficit in relationship to the sacral micturition centre into upper- or lower motor-neuron lesion often is not possible. Neurological involvement of bladder and bowel function is seen in 95 per cent of affected children. Almost all children with MMC also have the Arnold–Chiari malformation, which causes hydrocephalus. Mental impairment to a more or less severe degree also accompanies MMC. The neurological deficit has a negative impact on mobility in children with MMC. The degree of paralysis of the lower extremities depends largely on the level of the cord lesion, but generally most children with MMC will become wheelchair-dependent throughout childhood and adolescence. Furthermore, children with MMC have spinal deformities with marked kyphoscoliosis. It is necessary when treating NBSD in children with MMC to take into consideration all secondary problems associated with this condition, as these problems may have a direct impact on urological management.

OTHER FORMS OF CONGENITAL NEUROSPINAL LESION

Other forms of congenital neurospinal lesion are often referred to as occult spinal dysraphism. However, if one is alert to these lesions, then usually they can be detected by routine clinical examination. Occult spinal dysraphism includes lipomyelomeningocoele, lumbosacral lipoma, tight filum terminale, dorsal dermal sinus and spina bifida occulta. Often, these conditions are referred to as primary tethered spinal cord syndrome. In tethered spinal cord syndrome, it is suggested that the lesion imposes traction on the filum terminale and sacral nerve roots, leading to a progressive neurological

deficit with growth of the child. In general, these lesions are not associated with hydrocephalus, and affected children demonstrate only isolated NBSD and anorectal dysfunction, with constipation and faecal incontinence. Most children are ambulatory and do not have the profound mental and neurological problems seen in children with MMC.

SACRAL AGENESIS

Sacral agenesis is a congenital anomaly of the sacral spine that forms the central component of a spectrum of anomalies comprising the caudal regression syndrome. Sacral agenesis encompasses complete absence of the sacrum (total sacral agenesis) to minor defects of distal sacral vertebral segments (partial sacral agenesis). Patients with sacral agenesis demonstrate a variety of neurological problems. The severity of the problems seems to be proportional to the degree of the sacral defect. Sacral agenesis is missed frequently, since the defect produces little external deformity (Figure 59.5). Even with marked defects, there is often no sensory deficit, and impaired motor function is often limited to the muscles of the pelvic floor and perineum. Frequently, urinary and faecal incontinence is the only clinical sign in patients with isolated sacral agenesis. Faecal incontinence and constipation resulting from neuropathic anorectal dysfunction are also found in children with sacral agenesis, and associated sacral agenesis is found in at least 25 per cent of children with anorectal malformations. The most common clinical findings in sacral agenesis are urological complications secondary to NBSD.

TRAUMATIC INJURIES OF THE SPINAL CORD

Traumatic spinal cord injury is rare in children, and there is no difference compared with spine injury in adults. Following injury, a period of 'spinal shock' with areflexia of the bladder may ensue, due to oedema of the neural tissue, which may last for a few weeks. In some patients, voiding eventually returns to normal. In others, however, lower tract dysfunction may be permanent. Most traumatic injuries involving the spinal cord produce an upper motor-neuron lesion with detrusor overactivity and detrusor-sphincter dyssynergia. Management of NBSD is the same as in congenital spinal cord lesions.

IATROGENIC LESIONS

Pelvic surgery can damage the nerve supply to the genitourinary tract and pelvic floor muscles and, consequently, cause NBSD, a fact well known to adult urologists, gynaecologists and colorectal surgeons. Anatomical studies have demonstrated that damage to the pelvic splanchnic nerves and pelvic nerve plexus can occur during dissection of the distal rectum and surgical procedures at the level of the rectovesical and recto-uterine pouch. Iatrogenic nerve damage affects the peripheral nervous system, which results in a lower motor-neuron-type lesion, with areflexia or hyporeflexia of the bladder.

Iatrogenic neural injury may occur during paediatric surgery for anorectal malformations, persistent cloaca, urogenital sinus, bilateral ureteric re-implants with extravesical mobilization, sacrococcygeal teratoma and Hirschsprung's disease.

OTHER CAUSES

Other causes of NBSD include cerebral palsy, head injury, meningitis, encephalitis, Guillain–Barré syndrome, transverse myelitis and tumours of the nervous system.

Clinical implications of neuropathic bladder–sphincter dysfunction

The morbidity of neuropathic lower urinary tract dysfunction is immense and necessitates lifelong medical treatment and surveillance. The main problems seen in patients with NBSD are:

- urinary incontinence
- loss of renal function
- recurrent UTI.

Since these problems are related directly to the type of NBSD, proper treatment depends on assessing lower tract function by clinical urodynamic testing in combination with other examinations, such as ultrasound, voiding cystourethrography and renal scintigraphy.

INCONTINENCE

One of the major problems seen in children with NBSD is urinary incontinence. At least 90 per cent of children with MMC are incontinent without any medical or surgical treatment. In young children, urinary incontinence is acceptable and can be managed with nappies/pads. However, in school-age children and adolescents, persistent incontinence imposes a social handicap and limits quality of life significantly. Management of children with NBSD should include a clear concept for treating urinary incontinence.

Generally, urinary incontinence can be classified into three main categories:

- reflex incontinence due to detrusor overactivity (hyperreflexia) with bladder pressures rising above the urethral closing pressure;
- stress incontinence due to low outlet resistance, seen with denervation of the urethral sphincter muscle or neuropathic incompetence of the bladder neck. In these patients, an intravesical pressure rise, e.g. with coughing or straining, will lead to leakage;
- overflow incontinence, which occurs in patients with denervation of the bladder or a fixed high urethral outlet resistance. The bladder never empties completely, and constant dribbling of urine with a palpable bladder is seen.

URINARY TRACT INFECTIONS

Recurrent UTIs are common in children with NBSD. However, UTIs are easily overlooked in children with NBSD, because obvious signs and symptoms such as dysuria and frequency are often absent in this patient group. Generally, UTIs are caused by incomplete emptying of the bladder with significant residuals, e.g. in detrusor-sphincter dyssynergia or acontractile detrusor with high outflow resistance. Residual urine will become contaminated with bacteria, and the step from contamination to infection is just a matter of time. Recurrent UTIs cause chronic inflammation of the bladder, with consecutive structural changes of the bladder wall, such as fibrosis and collagen deposition. This will cause further deterioration of bladder-wall compliance. Recurrent UTIs often cause pyelonephritis, especially in the presence of high-grade VUR, leading to renal scarring, functional impairment and hypertension.

RENAL FUNCTIONAL LOSS

Renal deterioration in children with NBSD is a serious complication that, at worst, results in renal insufficiency. In about 15 per cent of children born with MMC, renal impairment is present at birth. Generally, in most children with NBSD, this is caused by high intravesical pressures resulting from low bladder compliance or functional outflow obstruction, as in detrusor-sphincter dyssynergia and detrusor hyperreflexia. High intravesical pressures will lead to secondary VUR and obstruction at the vesicoureteral junction due to hypertrophy of the bladder wall. Since maturation of the renal parenchyma is not fully present at birth, the kidneys are especially vulnerable during the first two years of life. Therefore, in young children, high-pressure reflux, obstructive uropathy and pyelonephritis, or at its worst a combination of all three, may cause severe renal damage, with scarring of the renal parenchyma. The main goal of any form of treatment of NBSD should aim to preserve renal function.

INVESTIGATIONS

History and physical examination

The diagnosis is clear in 90 per cent of children with NBSD, especially those with MMC. However, a small number of children may have an occult neuropathic disorder. In order to treat these children properly and to avoid a therapeutic delay, it is crucial to make the correct diagnosis early. History-taking and physical examination aim to obtain information that suggests a neuropathic cause of voiding dysfunction. It is important to substantiate whether any of the child's family members are afflicted with neurospinal dysraphism. Moreover, it is essential to verify whether the child has a congenital anomaly that concurs with neurospinal dysraphism or structural genitourinary anomalies, e.g. anorectal malformation or persistent cloaca. Information should be gained on pregnancy and delivery and possible trauma to the nervous system. Important signs and symptoms that may suggest a neuropathic aetiology are constant dribbling or leakage of urine, loss of urine on exertion, interrupted stream, straining, urinary retention and recurrent UTIs.

Neuro–urological evaluation

Neuro-urological evaluation assesses the integrity of the nervous system involved in lower genitourinary function. This can be accomplished by clinical neurological examination and urodynamic testing (neuro-urological examination).

A good estimate of the integrity of the nervous system involved in lower tract function can be gained through clinical examination (Table 59.1). Testing of genital and perineal sensation will give information on the integrity of afferent innervation of the S2–S5 spinal cord segments. Evaluation of the patellar (L2–L4) and Achilles (L5–S2) deep tendon reflexes provides an indication of segmental spinal cord function. Hypoactivity suggests a lower motor-neuron lesion, whereas hyperactivity generally indicates an upper motor-neuron lesion. A positive Babinski sign implies an upper motor-neuron lesion. The bulbocavernosus reflex (BCR) consists of contraction of the bulbocavernosus muscle after stimulation of the penile glans or clitoris and is mediated by the pudendal nerve; as such, it represents a local spinal cord reflex (S2–S4). The reflex is absent in all patients with a complete lower motor-neuron lesion but can be elicited in people with incomplete lesions and is present in 90 per cent of patients with an upper motor-neuron lesion. Therefore, absence of the BCR is indicative of a lower motor-neuron lesion, but presence of the reflex does not rule out neuropathy. Tonic activity of the external anal sphincter at rest depends on the integrity of the spinal

Table 59.1 *Physical examination of the child with neurospinal dysraphism*

Inspect the spine	Scoliosis or kyphosis
	Cutaneous back lesions
	Pelvic obliquity
	Deviation of natal cleft
	Short natal cleft ('flat bottom')
Inspect lower extremities	Muscle atrophy (calves)
	Foot deformity
	Asymmetry of feet
	Cutaneous lesions (pressure sores)
Neurological examination	Elicit leg reflexes
	Babinski sign
	Cremaster reflex
	Bulbocavernosus reflex
	Anocutaneous reflex
	Test perineal and perianal sensation
	Check general coordination
	Observe gait
Genital examination	Inspect penis and meatus
	Inspect introitus in girls
Anorectal examination	Check position of anus
	Check anal sphincter tone

cord segments S2–S4. Good sphincter tone rules out a complete lower motor-neuron lesion, and volitional contraction and relaxation of the external anal sphincter (EAS) suggests intact control by supraspinal centres. Reflex contraction of the EAS after pinprick of the mucocutaneous anal junction constitutes the anocutaneous reflex (ACR). The reflex activity of the ACR is similar to that of the BCR. Contraction of the external anal sphincter with coughing or abdominal straining is also a low spinal reflex and seems to have the same clinical implications as the BCR. Testing of perineal sensation can also give information on the neurological status. Absence of perineal sensation is a good indicator of neuropathy and virtually always coincides with NBSD. However, the presence of perineal sensation does not rule out neuropathy. The Credé reflex can be elicited in patients with neuropathic bladder dysfunction by tapping the suprapubic abdominal wall, which then leads to an involuntary bladder contraction, followed by leakage or voiding. Patients with a positive Credé reflex generally have an upper motor-neuron lesion, i.e. a lesion located above the sacral micturition centre.

Laboratory investigations

Laboratory investigations include urine analysis and repeated urine cultures. Otherwise, serum analysis of creatinine, electrolytes and urea-nitrogen should be checked yearly.

Imaging

All children with voiding dysfunction should receive a screening ultrasound study of the urinary tract in order to detect upper-tract dilation, which suggests either VUR or obstruction. Ultrasound can demonstrate structural anomalies of the urinary tract and allows measurement of kidney size, bladder-wall thickness and post-voiding residual urine. Children who demonstrate anomalies on ultrasound should undergo a voiding cystourethrogram (VCUG) in order to differentiate between reflux and obstruction and to determine lower-tract anatomy. Any child who is suspected of having NBSD should have a plain X-ray study of the lumbosacral spine. In infants, screening for intraspinal pathology is possible by spinal ultrasound. In older patients, magnetic resonance imaging (MRI) is the best method for demonstrating intraspinal pathology, especially in occult spinal dysraphism. Children with VUR, obstructive uropathy and renal anomalies are generally submitted to renography (mercaptoacetyltriglycine (MAG$_3$), dimercaptosuccinic acid (DMSA) scanning) in order to obtain information on split renal function, scarring and upper tract drainage.

Urodynamics

Urodynamic testing consists of assessing bladder and urethral sphincter function. Individual studies such as recording of the intravesical pressure during bladder filling and voiding (leakage) are often combined with other studies performed simultaneously, e.g. measurement of the urinary flow rate and sphincter electromyography (EMG). In children with NBSD, urodynamic testing should be combined with simultaneous cystography, which is referred to as video-urodynamics. This allows us to correlate the occurrence of VUR or urethral leakage with intravesical pressure and EMG activity. Differentiation between high- and low-pressure reflux may be important in the management and prediction of renal deterioration. The information gained by urodynamics helps in establishing a clinical urodynamic diagnosis on which therapy can be based, e.g. detrusor–sphincter dyssynergia or bladder compliance. Specific urodynamic parameters, especially the leak-point pressure, i.e. the pressure at which urethral leakage occurs, have a predictive value with respect to renal deterioration. Pressures above 40 cmH$_2$O coincide with a high rate of nephropathy. As the type of NBSD can change with time, regular assessment of lower urinary tract function should be done, usually on a yearly basis. Nowadays, proper management of NBSD without regular urodynamic testing is outdated.

MANAGEMENT

Management of children with NBSD is variable and based on individual findings. Besides treating the urinary tract, other aspects have to be addressed, especially in children with MMC, such as gender, mental abilities of the child, motor skills and ambulation. In particular, wheelchair-bound girls will not be able to perform clean intermittent self-catheterization (CISC) easily. In addition, an important consideration is

age, since infants and very young children are hardly ever treated surgically. Sometimes, socioeconomic considerations and cultural aspects may play a role in choosing a specific treatment plan.

Preservation of renal function is the main goal in treating NBSD.

All therapeutic considerations, in particular with operative treatment of urinary incontinence, have to be judged with respect to the possible negative impact on the upper urinary tract. Other treatment objectives are achievement of continence for urine and prevention of recurrent UTIs. Management must be adapted to the type of dysfunction and, in general, conservative treatment should be considered before choosing a surgical option. However, medical and surgical treatments often are used in combination. When planning treatment, the child's ability to become independent has to be considered, especially their ability to perform CISC. Ideally, the child should be dry before reaching school age; however, this goal has to be adapted to the overall status of the child's mental and physical abilities. Also, parental compliance and competence with respect to the different treatment modalities chosen for their child have to be considered. Treatment of NBSD, whether conservative or surgical, remains an individual decision for each child, and no standard approach can be applied, except in newborns and young infants, who should always be treated by prophylactic antibiotics and clean intermittent catheterization (CIC) until the child has been assessed fully, including urodynamics.

Conservative management

PHARMACOLOGICAL TREATMENT

Antibiotic therapy

One of the mainstays in preventing recurrent UTIs is the administration of prophylactic antibiotics. Especially in infants, it is important to prevent pyelonephritis, as the renal parenchyma is highly susceptible to infection. Moreover, reducing the number of episodes of cystitis will reduce the probability of structural changes of the bladder wall leading to a low compliant bladder with high intravesical pressures. Antibiotic prophylaxis is generally achieved with trimethoprim or nitrofurantoin (2 mg/kg/day). Prompt antibiotic treatment of acute pyelonephritis is mandatory in order to prevent renal damage. In general, treatment should be done using broad-spectrum penicillins or cephalosporins given intravenously in young children. In older children, oral antibiotics can be given.

Anticholinergic therapy

Relaxation of detrusor smooth muscle by anticholinergic therapy is a good treatment option for detrusor hyperreflexia and low bladder compliance. In non-compliant bladders, however, treatment is not as consistent as in hyperreflexia, since bladder-wall stiffness is also due to intrinsic bladder-wall fibrosis. These drugs, e.g. oxybutynin chloride, tolterodine and hyoscamine, increase bladder capacity and lower intravesical pressure.

Generally, they should be used in conjunction with CIC. Side effects are frequent but not severe. Usually, children complain of dizziness, a dry mouth and hot flushes. Previously, oxybutynin has also been administered intravesically through the catheter after having performed CIC. Side effects are much less with this method, and the effect on the detrusor muscle is more effective.

Alpha-blockade

Alpha-adrenergic-blockers, such as phenoxybenzamine and alfuzosin, have been administered to treat outflow obstruction. Results are inconsistent, and CIC seems to be a much better treatment option. These drugs have carcinogenic potential and cannot be recommended for use in children.

Alpha-adrenergic drugs

Alpha-adrenergic drugs, such as ephedrine, increase the tone of the bladder neck, but not sufficiently enough to produce continence.

CLEAN INTERMITTENT (SELF-) CATHETERIZATION

Complete bladder emptying at low intravesical pressures is important for preventing recurrent UTIs. With introduction of the concept of clean intermittent catheterization in 1972 by Lapides, other forms of bladder evacuation such as the Credé manoeuvre, manual expression of the bladder and long-term placement of indwelling catheters have become almost obsolete. Numerous studies have shown an improvement in continence, renal function and infection rate with the use of CIC. The aim of CIC is to provide periodic complete bladder emptying. Success depends highly on parental and patient compliance. With CIC, stable upper tracts are achieved in about 80 per cent of children; however, continence rates lie around 30 per cent. It cannot be emphasized enough that a successful CIC programme depends highly on compliance and motivation of the carers and the child. Nowadays, there is general agreement that CIC should be initiated in the newborn or young infant and should be combined with antibiotic prophylaxis and in selected cases (low bladder compliance, detrusor–sphincter dyssynergia) with anticholinergic drugs.

Treatment of vesicoureteral reflux

VUR is common with NBSD. It may be present at birth or develop later in life. In general, VUR is secondary to NBSD, especially in patients with high leak-point pressures, low compliant bladders, detrusor sphincter dyssynergia (DSD) and detrusor hyperreflexia. It is unclear whether sterile reflux may cause renal damage, but urinary infections in the presence of high-grade reflux can cause rapid and profound renal deterioration (Figure 59.6). Therefore, all children with NBSD and VUR should be kept on antibiotic prophylaxis until at least two years of age. After this time, maturation of the kidneys has taken place and renal damage is less likely to occur. However, in children with severe NBSD, it is generally accepted to continue prophylactic antibiotics for longer. Moreover,

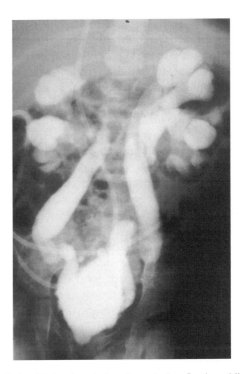

Figure 59.6 *Bilateral grade 5 vesicoureteric reflux in a child with myelomeningocele with low bladder compliance and high leak-point pressure.*

VUR should be treated by lowering bladder pressures with anticholinergic medication and CIC. Many reports in the literature have demonstrated resolution of VUR after proper treatment of bladder dysfunction with CIC and anticholinergic medication. In a very selected group of patients who do not respond to conservative treatment, ureteral re-implantation may be an option. However, the failure rate of ureteral re-implants in children with NBSD is significant, and in some cases re-implantation may cause severe secondary ureterovesical obstruction with an even greater risk of upper tract deterioration. Therefore, in patients with high-pressure reflux not amenable to conservative treatment, bladder augmentation with continent urinary diversion should be done. Surgical conversion of a high-pressure bladder into a low-pressure reservoir often will lead to resolution of reflux without ureteral reimplantation. In very severe cases of unmanageable VUR in children too young to undergo continent urinary diversion, cutaneous vesicostomy or urethral dilation may be a treatment option. Recently, treatment of VUR by endoscopic subureteral injection of bulking agents has shown fairly good results, even in patients with NBSD.

Treatment of urinary incontinence

The main principle of conservative treatment for urinary incontinence is regular bladder evacuation in order to prevent overflow incontinence and treatment of reflex incontinence due to uninhibited detrusor contractions, as well as creation of an adequately large bladder capacity to allow storage of urine at low pressures. Conservative management of urinary incontinence is achieved with CIC. In children with high intravesical bladder pressure, low compliant bladders and small functional bladder capacity, administration of anticholinergic medication (e.g. oxybutynin) either orally or intravesically can be helpful. Reliable continence rates with conservative treatment are low and do not exceed 20 per cent in the majority of cases. However, in some children, incontinence can be minimized to a socially acceptable degree. Nevertheless, for some children, wearing pads or appliances is still an acceptable solution. Good results for treating detrusor hyperreflexia have been reported with injection of botulinum toxin type A into the bladder wall. However, this method is still under investigation, and experience, especially in children, is limited. As for operative management of incontinence, the potentially negative effect on the upper urinary tract has to be kept in mind at any time. Regular assessment of renal function and serial ultrasound of the upper urinary tract as well as regular, usually yearly, urodynamic studies are part of every treatment plan. Management should be done in relation to bladder and urethral sphincter dysfunction.

Operative management

Because of the limitations of conservative management for NBSD, especially with respect to continence rates, surgical treatment frequently is necessary in children with NBSD. There is general agreement that major surgery for NBSD should not be performed in infants and toddlers. Usually, surgical treatment is performed in children over six years of age. Three main surgical procedures are performed in NBSD: temporary decompression of the urinary tract, bladder augmentation and procedures to increase outflow resistance. The latter are often combined with a continent, catheterizable stoma to facilitate CIC.

TEMPORARY DECOMPRESSION OF THE URINARY TRACT

Cutaneous vesicostomy

In failure of CIC in infants in the presence of severe VUR, obstructive uropathy or recurrent episodes of pyelonephritis or severe renal impairment, a cutaneous vesicostomy can be a good alternative. If placed correctly, the vesicostomy acts as a pop-off valve, lowering intravesical pressure, while allowing some storage function of the bladder to take place. Since infants will wear nappies anyway, it is an ideal technique for children under 18 months of age. Long-term vesicostomy can be performed in severely disabled children who cannot perform CIC and are therefore not candidates for continent diversion procedures.

Urethral dilation

Lower tract decompression in infants, usually girls, can be performed by rigorous urethral dilation. This technique is an alternative to cutaneous vesicostomy. It seems to have almost the same effect as a vesicostomy. However, it is argued that in children with high outflow resistance and the ability of achieving continence with CIC alone, the otherwise sufficient continence mechanism is altered permanently, necessitating an additional surgical procedure later in life. Often, urethral dilation has to be repeated. This technique can also be used for long-term decompression in severely disabled children.

Sphincterotomy

External sphincterotomy or bladder-neck incisions are more or less outdated in the era of CIC.

INCREASING BLADDER CAPACITY

Augmentation cystoplasty is one of the mainstays in the treatment of children with NBSD. The indication for augmentation is a small functional bladder capacity due to low compliance of the bladder wall or detrusor hyperreflexia. The goal of bladder augmentation is to create an acontractile large-capacity reservoir that enables storage of urine at low pressure. Augmentation traditionally is carried out with isolated bowel segments, either ileum or sigmoid. The choice of bowel segment remains controversial, and no stringent recommendation can be given. It is important to detubularize the bowel segments and to split the native bladder wide open into two halves, thereby preventing autonomic contractions of either bowel segment or remaining bladder. Enough bowel must be used to create a sufficiently large reservoir; usually, the segment length is 20–30 cm. The isolated bowel segment is reconfigured in a U-shape fashion and stitched between the two bladder halves. The bladder has to be split all the way down to the trigone; some surgeons fix the two bladder halves to the left and right psoas muscle to prevent the remaining bladder from contracting. In some cases, with extremely fibrotic and thick-walled bladders, it is better to resect the bladder down to the trigone and perform a substitution cystoplasty rather than a bladder augmentation. Because of the possible negative metabolic effects of intestinal segments incorporated into the urinary tract, such as hyperchloraemic acidosis, and the possibility of malignant transformation of the bowel mucosa, other ways of augmentation have been tried. Some surgeons perform auto-augmentation, which consists of subtotal resection of the detrusor muscle, leaving only the bladder mucosa in place. The success rates are variable and not good enough to recommend this method uniformly. Recently, some authors have reported success with auto-augmentation combined with only a demucosalized seromuscular bowel segment (sigmoid) on to the remaining bladder mucosa. Success rates seem to be reasonable enough to continue investigating this method.

As well as the typical surgical complications of abdominal surgery, bladder augmentation has specific problems and complications. Metabolic complications may be reabsorption of chloride, with consecutive hyperchloraemic acidosis, electrolyte imbalance, reabsorption of urea and ammonia and problems with bone materialization. Acidotic patients have to be treated with sodium bicarbonate. Another problem is mucus production, making regular bladder irrigations necessary. Stone formation is frequent. Overdistension of the bladder, especially if the bladder is not emptied thoroughly by the child or the parents, may lead to bladder perforation, with peritonitis, septicaemia and shock, and is potentially life-threatening. Bacteriuria is a common finding in children with intestinal bladder augmentation. Generally, antibiotic treatment is necessary only in symptomatic cases. In children who have undergone augmentation with intestinal segments, yearly cystoscopies are recommended in order to detect malignant transformation of the intestinal mucosa, starting eight years postoperatively. However, there are no valid data available regarding the possibility and incidence of the formation of adenocarcinoma in bladder augmentations.

CONTINENT CATHETERIZABLE STOMAS

Following bladder augmentation, CIC is usually mandatory in order to empty the bladder at regular intervals. Although some children are able to perform urethral CIC, many will benefit from the creation of a continent catheterizable stoma. The most common stoma used is a continent appendicovesicostomy, which was described by Mitrofanoff in 1980 and thus is often referred to as a 'Mitrofanoff stoma'. If the appendix has been removed, other intestinal segments can be surgically shaped into a 'neo-appendix', e.g. tubularized small bowel, as in the Monti procedure.

INCREASING OUTLET RESISTANCE

There are many surgical methods of increasing outlet resistance, but there is no uniformly accepted method. In some children, continence can be achieved with bladder augmentation and CIC alone. However, a significant number will still need some surgery of the bladder outlet in order to become dry.

Bladder neck procedures

Many different methods of bladder neck reconstruction or lengthening and narrowing of the posterior urethra have been devised. The most common is the Young-Dees–Leadbetter procedure, which consists of lengthening of the posterior urethra and adding full-thickness bladder-wall support to the bladder neck region. Other procedures include the Kropp procedure and the Pippi Salle procedure, among many others. All procedures incorporate the following principles: urethral lengthening, reconfiguration of the bladder neck and, sometimes, creation of a flap-valve mechanism. With these procedures, continence is achieved more by compression and controlled urethral obstruction or by a valve mechanism, rather than functional closing mechanisms. Continence rates with these procedures are estimated to be about 60–80 per cent.

Bladder neck closure

A straightforward method with almost 100 per cent success rates is complete bladder neck closure in combination with a continent catheterizable stoma. A disadvantage is that once the bladder neck is closed, access to the bladder in an emergency, such as overdistension, can be difficult and there is no pop-off mechanism left.

Colpo-wrap

The Colpo-wrap is a method devised by the author of this chapter to increase outflow resistance in girls with NBSD. The anterior vaginal wall on both sides of the urethra is pulled upwards and wrapped around the bladder neck and urethra, thereby adding extrinsic urethral compression and support. The advantages of this procedure are that it is very simple and it leaves the possibility of performing urethral CIC undisturbed.

Sling operations

Sling procedures consist of external compression of the urethra and bladder neck by pulling either a fascial sling (rectus fascia) or Gore-Tex® sling around the urethra in a hammock-like fashion. This supports and compresses the urethra and bladder neck, increasing the leak point pressure, while a pop-off mechanism remains. Success rates of 70 per cent are similar to those seen in bladder neck procedures.

Artificial urinary sphincter

The artificial urinary sphincter is a mechanical-hydraulic device consisting of a cuff placed around the urethra or bladder neck, a balloon pressure reservoir and a pump control. Implantation of this device is reasonable in only a very select group of children with NBSD, mostly children with at least a marginal ability to void spontaneously. Generally, these patients have normal or near-normal detrusor function with outlet failure only. Continence rates are similar to those reached by other procedures. However, only a small number of children are able to void spontaneously with this system. The revision and complication rates in most series reach 60 per cent.

CLINICAL SCENARIOS

Case 1

A newborn with MMC (Figure 59.4) underwent closure of the defect. Postoperatively, the child had a palpable bladder and leaked urine constantly. On renal ultrasound, moderate bilateral dilation of the upper tracts was seen. Clinically, the child had 'spinal shock', with bladder denervation, overflow incontinence and high outlet resistance. After drainage of the bladder for two weeks with an indwelling catheter, the upper tracts looked normal. The catheter was removed and the child was put on CIC and prophylactic antibiotics. Regular ultrasound of the urinary tract was performed on a monthly basis in the first three months and video-urodynamics planned at age three months.

Case 2

A five-year-old boy is seen with primary 'enuresis' and 'encopresis' in the outpatients' clinic. His mother reports constant dribbling of urine, which increases on exertion. Furthermore, the boy has severe constipation, with soiling. A thorough examination shows a short natal cleft and hypoplastic gluteal muscles (Figure 59.5). Genital sensation is normal. A plain radiograph of the lower spine demonstrates partial sacral agenesis. The cause for urinary incontinence and constipation is neuropathic in origin.

Case 3

A ten-month-old girl with MMC who was lost to follow-up was seen with massive bilateral upper tract dilation on ultrasound. Video-urodynamics showed a low compliant bladder with a leak-point pressure above 40 cmH$_2$O. There was bilateral grade 5 VUR (Figure 59.6). She had experienced three episodes of pyelonephritis and chronic UTI with *Pseudomonas*. There was mild elevation of serum creatinine, and renal DMSA scanning demonstrated bilateral scarring. The parents did not follow the CIC programme and stopped giving prophylactic antibiotics a few weeks after the child was dismissed following neonatal back closure. Because of upper tract deterioration, the child received a cutaneous vesicostomy. Following vesicostomy, upper tract dilation normalized and chronic UTI resolved.

FURTHER READING

Bauer SB, Hallett M, Khoshbin S, *et al*. Predictive value of urodynamic evaluation in newborns with myelodysplasia. *Journal of the American Medical Association* 1984; **252**: 650–52.

Boemers TM. Urinary incontinence and vesicourethral dysfunction in pediatric surgical conditions. *Seminars in Pediatric Surgery* 2002; **11**: 91–9.

Lowe JB, Furness PD, III, Barqawi AZ, Koyle MA. Surgical treatment of the neuropathic bladder. *Seminars in Pediatric Surgery* 2002; **11**: 120–27.

McGuire EJ, Woodside JR, Borden TA, Weiss RM. Prognostic value of urodynamic testing in myelodysplastic patients. *Journal of Urology* 1981; **126**: 205–9.

Rickwood AMK. Assessment and conservative management of the neuropathic bladder. *Seminars in Pediatric Surgery* 2002; **11**: 108–19.

60

The prepuce, hypospadias and other congenital anomalies of the penis

PIETER VERLEYEN AND GUY BOGAERT

Learning objectives

- To understand the embryological base of congenital anomalies of the penis.
- To know the clinical relevant subclassification and respective management of the congenital anomalies of hypospadias and urethral duplication.
- To know the difference between pathologic phimosis and the normal foreskin.
- To understand the management of phimosis.
- To remember the important points of technique in penile surgery.

DEVELOPMENT OF THE PENIS, URETHRA AND PREPUCE

At six weeks, the genital tubercle appears between the cloaca and the umbilical cord (Figure 60.1). The descending urorectal septum then divides the cloaca into the urogenital sinus and the anal canal. The urogenital sinus develops into a short tubular pelvic part (future site of prostate) and a flattened phallic part (distal portion of urethra).

In the second month, the genetic information of the Y-chromosome influences the undifferentiated gonad to develop into a testis. The testis produces testosterone and Müllerian inhibiting factor, which influences further male differentiation. The genital (phallic) tubercle grows over the urogenital membrane by proliferation of mesoderm and forms the coronal sulcus of the glans. The urethral plate forms on the caudal surface of the phallic tubercle as a strip of endodermal cells. It deepens progressively, and on either side urethral folds

rise as a mesenchymal proliferation. The endodermal urethral plate invades the mesenchyme and forms the urethral groove, which loses the overlying ectoderm.

The urethral folds fuse to form the penile urethra, with the distal urethra being the last to close. The mesenchyme in the urethral folds forms the corpus spongiosum.

The glanular urethra is formed by a plug of ectoderm coming from the tip of the glans going to the mesenchyme as an ectodermal intrusion. The ventral segment of this invading ectoderm comes to lie dorsal to the distal extremity of the advancing urethral plate. When both structures make contact, the intervening double wall breaks down and the new ectodermal lumen comes in continuity with the proximal endodermal urethra. Thus, the distal and dorsal walls of the fossa navicularis are ectodermal stratified epithelium, while most of the urethra is endodermal stratified epithelium.

At eight weeks, prepucial folds appear in the coronal sulcus. The base of the fold is the glanular lamella, an actively proliferating layer. It rolls the prepucial folds progressively

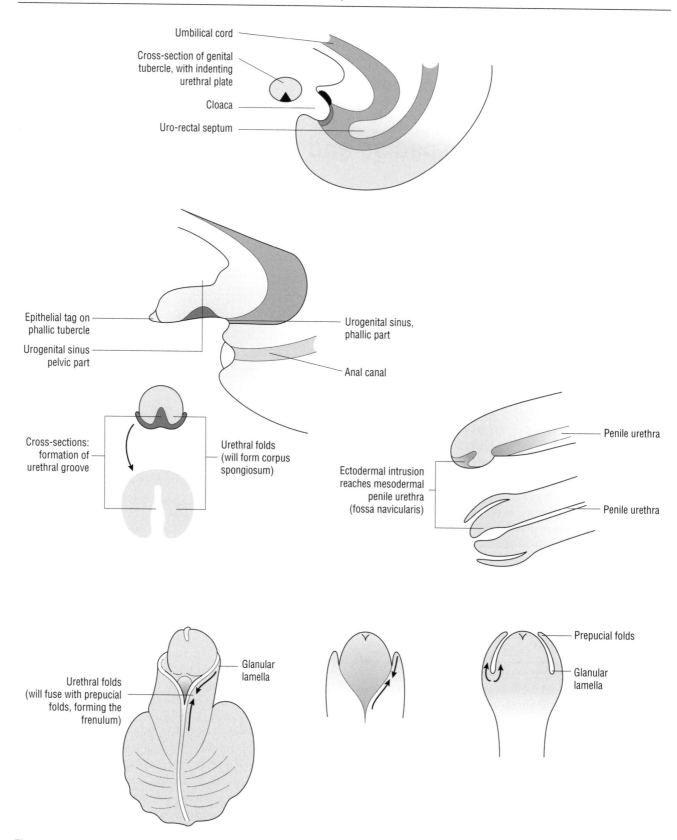

Figure 60.1   *Development of the penis, urethra and prepuce.*

over the base of the glans. The glanular lamella is continuous with the urethral folds on the ventrum. As these folds join at the base of the glans, the lamellar margins fuse with the prepucial folds, forming the frenulum. At 12 weeks, the distal urethra has formed and the prepucial fold covers the entire glans.

The glanular lamella forms a single epithelial layer between the prepuce and the glans, which only later degenerates into two layers. This process of separation between glans and prepuce starts distally and continues after birth. For this reason, the prepuce is still attached to the glans at birth.

CLINICAL PROBLEMS: PHIMOSIS, PARAPHIMOSIS AND BALANOPREPUCIAL ADHESIONS

Definitions

- *Phimosis* is a pathological narrowing of the opening of the prepuce, preventing it from being drawn back over the glans penis.
- *Phimosis* can be a result of chronic inflammation or scarring (as in balanitis xerotica obliterans or after forcible premature retraction).
- *Paraphimosis* is a painful constriction of the glans penis by the retracted foreskin. Prolonged retraction leads to lymphatic obstruction, which causes lymphoedema distally and constriction of the glans.

Natural history

In the newborn, the foreskin is still adherent to the glans. In 50 per cent, it cannot be retracted far enough to visualize the meatus. At six months of life, 20 per cent will have a retractable foreskin; by five years, more than 90 per cent will have a retractable foreskin. At the age of 20 years, the prevalence of phimosis is one per cent.

In ten per cent, the penis will be 'naturally circumcised', having the appearance of a circumcised penis without circumcision (congenital short foreskin).

Genital hygiene in small boys does not require retraction of the foreskin. Painful retraction can lead to bleeding, scarring, pathological phimosis and psychological trauma for the child and his parents.

Normal elasticity of the prepuce only comes with puberty, under the influence of endogenous testosterone and the first sexual activity, such as masturbation.

Non-operative management

Narrow foreskin or balanoprepucial adhesions can be treated with a topical corticoid cream (e.g. 0.05 per cent betamethasone) for six weeks. This makes the prepuce retractable in more than 70 per cent of children and is cost-effective. There are few side effects. It gives moisture and elasticity to the skin and makes retraction possible without trauma and scarring. It is probable that there is some local effect on maturation of the foreskin (Figure 60.2).

In case of paraphimosis, manual compression of the oedematous glans penis is necessary before reduction. In severe cases, a surgical release of the constricted foreskin is needed (dorsal slit). This can be performed under topical or local anaesthesia.

Retraction of the foreskin in order to dilate the narrow ring of the foreskin must not be carried out, because of the risk of microtrauma, balanitis and subsequent scarring.

Operative management

CIRCUMCISION

Circumcision is the most common operation performed in the USA, although the American Academy of Pediatrics and the UK Royal College of Obstetrics and Gynaecology have stated that 'there is no absolute medical indication for circumcision

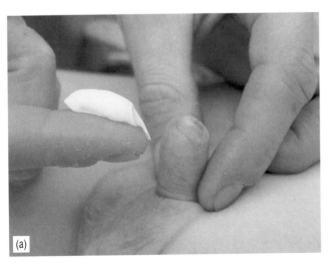
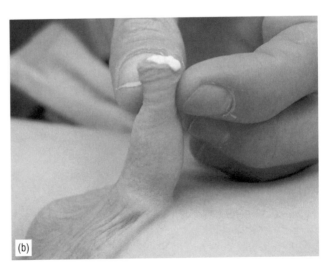

Figure 60.2 *Non-operative management of phimosis: application of a topical corticoid cream for six weeks.*

in the neonatal period'. The goal of circumcision is to remove an adequate amount of shaft skin with inner-prepucial skin to obtain an adequate cosmetic result and prevent future phimosis or paraphimosis.

Mostly, circumcision will be performed for emotional, cultural or religious reasons. Possible advantages of circumcision remain very controversial: circumcision may eliminate the risk of penile and cervical cancer and may decrease transmission of sexually transmitted diseases. Other studies, however, have shown the opposite. It seems that uncircumcised males are more susceptible to genital ulcer diseases, while circumcised men are more prone to urethritis, which is more common in developed nations. Recently, there has been growing interest in the psychosexual impact of this intervention. There are controversial arguments, such as the suggestion that the section of nerve endings and loss of redundant foreskin could have a negative effect on sexual satisfaction for men and women. Others have found that circumcised men have oral sex more often with their partners, probably due to hygiene issues. Recent studies have shown that circumcision without anaesthesia, even in newborns, who apparently cannot remember the event itself, is a very painful event. This may have an indirect influence on pain sensation later in life.

Absolute medical indication for circumcision is pathological phimosis due to balanitis xerotica obliterans.

Relative indications are:

- recurrent balanoposthitis;
- high risk of urinary tract infection (UTI) in boys with congenital urogenital malformation, e.g. high-grade vesicoureteral reflux. The incidence of UTI can be reduced ten-fold if the neonate is circumcised.

Contraindications for circumcision are penile anomalies such as hypospadias, epispadias and megalourethra, in which the foreskin can be useful in surgical reconstruction.

Techniques of circumcision

Without removal of skin:

- *Dorsal slit:* incision of the dorsal foreskin, exposing the glans. The cosmetic result is not satisfactory, and therefore this technique should be reserved for acute paraphimosis that cannot be reduced manually.
- *Other plasties of the foreskin:* different techniques have been described, using the principles of a Y–V or a Z-plasty. The disadvantage is that the foreskin should be retracted frequently after operation in order to prevent scarring. This can be a painful experience for the child, and when retraction is traumatic it can cause additional scarring, with re-stenosis.

With skin removal:

- *Shield technique, and its modifications* (Mogen, Gomco and Plastibell clamp): first the adhesions between the foreskin and glans are freed. A protective shield is brought over the glans and the excess foreskin is excised at a demarcation-line on the shield. Haemostasis is performed by manual compression (Mogen) or by pressure between the ring and the clamp (Gomco). In the Plastibell technique, the foreskin necroses off (within three to seven days) by placing a tight absorbable suture across the excess foreskin (Figure 60.3).
- *Freehand surgical excision:* a first circular incision is made in the inner prepuce, just proximal to the coronal groove. A second incision is made on the outer foreskin. The prepucial skin between both incisions is then excised. The wound is primarily closed with small absorbable sutures (Figure 60.4).

Important points of technique

If electrocautery is used, then bipolar coagulation is recommended, because of the risk of thrombosis of the underlying blood supply and necrosis of the glans penis or urethra with unipolar coagulation.

It is important to keep all shaft skin, and remove only the non-elastic or scarred foreskin, so that the penis will not be buried in the prepubic fat during erection. For good cosmetic results, the distal incision should be just 1–2 mm under the sulcus coronarius of the glans (Figure 60.4).

Most complications can be avoided by paying careful attention to complete separation of the glans from the inner prepuce, symmetrical removal of the inner and outer prepucial skin collar and good haemostasis.

For postoperative comfort, it is recommended to place a penile block with a long-acting local anaesthetic, such as bupivacaine.

Outcome and complications

Complications occur in 0.2–10 per cent of cases. Acute complications include the following:

- Bleeding: this is the most common complication. Control by direct compression (rarely, suture placement or bipolar coagulation is necessary).
- Infections usually are self-limiting and treated with local dressing changes. Serious necrotizing soft-tissue infections are very rare.
- If excess foreskin is resected, then this can be treated by local wound care with a barrier cream, with the penile skin being allowed to heal by secondary intention.

Non-acute complications include the following:

- Meatal stenosis can be a result of meatitis and meatal ulcers when the meatus is no longer protected by foreskin. It is probably a result of ammonia irritation, bacteria and rubbing in a urine-soaked nappy. If the urinary stream is deviated by more than 30 degrees upwards, then a meatotomy is indicated. Meatal stenosis can also occur due to excessive diathermy of bleeding points, especially at the frenular area.
- Skin issues include inadequate or asymmetric skin removal, excessive removal, skin bridges (adhesion of cut foreskin edge to the glans), inclusion cysts (when an

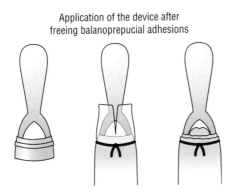

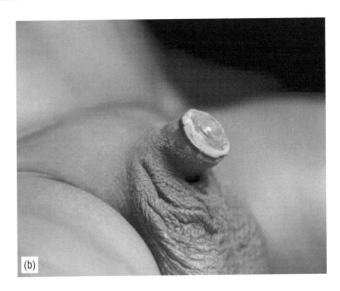

Figure 60.3 *Plastibell technique of circumcision.*

island of skin is left underneath the new foreskin) and penile curvature (skin tethering secondary to scar tissue if the operation was performed during acute inflammation).

- Urethral fistula may result due to aggressive removal of the foreskin with entrapment of the urethra and ischaemia from a crush injury or from monopolar coagulation.

RESTORING FORESKIN

Although there are no scientific data on the importance of the foreskin for sexual experience, some circumcised men claim that their sexual problems are due to their lack of foreskin. It has therefore been a challenge to attempt to restore foreskin.

Most of the devices tried have been used to stretch the foreskin and to try to recover the glans, but they are not effective.

Surgical techniques have been developed. However, the most important problem is that penile shaft skin is hairless and almost none of the other body skin can be used as a flap or graft. Most recent techniques use split-thickness skin grafting to restore the length of the foreskin.

HYPOSPADIAS

Definition and embryology

Hypospadias is a congenital disorder of the penis resulting in an incomplete development of the anterior urethra, corpus spongiosum and prepuce. At 12 weeks, incomplete development of the penile or glanular urethra (with failure of the urethral plate to close) does not allow the prepucial folds to fuse ventrally. Consequently, the ventral foreskin is absent, and there is excessive foreskin on the dorsal surface (hooded foreskin).

The meatus is ectopic and positioned ventrally and more proximal. The glans is open ventrally. A blind pit is found at the site of the normal meatus, a remnant of the normal ectodermal intrusion (fossa navicularis). Fifty per cent of patients will have anterior hypospadias with the meatus on the glans or subcoronal; 20 per cent have the meatus on the shaft of the penis; and 30 per cent have the meatus between perineum and the penoscrotal junction (Figure 60.5). The corpus spongiosum surrounding the distal urethra is developed incompletely, typically causing chordae on both sides of the distal urethra and meatus and resulting in ventral curvature. The frenulum and the arteria frenularis are absent.

The urinary stream may be deflected in a downward fashion, and infertility may be a problem because of difficulty in semen delivery.

Incidence and associated abnormalities

Hypospadias occurs in one in 300 male births. There is a 14 per cent incidence in male siblings and an eight per cent incidence in offspring. Inguinal hernias or undescended testes are found in nine per cent of hypospadias patients. Müllerian remnants or a utricle are present in a high number of patients with severe hypospadias. Other urinary tract anomalies are infrequent because of the earlier development of the kidneys, ureter and bladder. Only when hypospadias is associated with other organ-system anomalies (e.g. cardiac murmur, imperforate anus, pyloric stenosis) is renal and bladder imaging with abdominal ultrasound required. In severe hypospadias with undescended testes, emergency intersex evaluation should be done, with karyotyping and further endocrinological workup. The child should not be registered as male or female until the definitive sex of rearing has been decided upon, as it can be very difficult in some countries, including the UK, to change the sex of a child once registered.

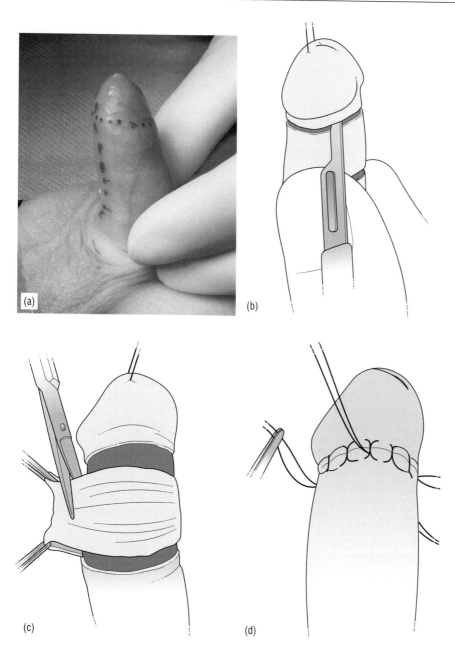

Figure 60.4   *Circumcision. (a) Incision on the outer foreskin. (b) Incision on the inner foreskin. (c) Excision of the prepuce. (d) Suturing of the foreskin with small absorbable sutures.*

Operative management

Surgical reconstruction of hypospadias is recommended because of functional, psychological and cosmetic aspects. Surgical techniques should restore the three main functions of the penis: a tube to be able to void straight, the possibility of sexual intercourse and as part of the reproduction organs. Reconstruction ideally should be completed before the age of 2.5 years. There is minimal scarring tissue and the penile skin will continue to grow with the child. At this age, toilet-training starts. If it is carried out before 2.5 years, the child probably will not remember the operation. A first operation can be done at the age of 10–12 months. Sometimes, a second operation is needed, which should be performed six months later. The

necessity of a second operation varies in the literature, from two to 20 per cent. This may be influenced by the severity of hypospadias and the technique used.

HISTORY

Historically, three periods in hypospadias surgery can be recognized. In the nineteenth century, Thiersch and Duplay described a technique in which the urethral plate was tubularized. In the twentieth century, multistage operations were popular, often using inadequate tissues such as scrotal hairy skin, leading to strictures, stones and infection.

Since the 1980s, modern principles have been standardized and offer better anatomical and functional results. The use of

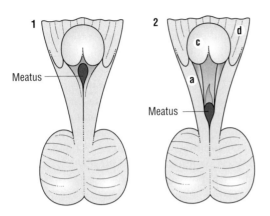
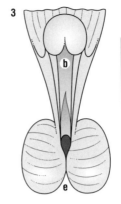

(1) Anterior (distal) hypospadias
(2) Midshat hypospadias
(3) Proximal hypospadias

(a) Diverging corpus spongiosum and chordae
(b) Urethral plate
(c) Blind fossa navicularis
(d) Excess dorsal foreskin
(e) Bifid scrotum

Figure 60.5   *Degree of hypospadias.*

the urethral plate as an anatomical entity and the use of pedicled non-hairy skin flaps or mucosal grafts (buccal, inner prepucial, bladder) have allowed single-stage repair in almost all cases.

Of the more than 300 described techniques, about 100 are still used. The choice of technique depends on the position of the meatus, the degree of chordae and the experience of the surgeon.

STAGES OF REPAIR AND DIFFERENT TECHNIQUES

Hypospadias repair can be described in three steps:

- Correction of chordae and penile curvature.
- Urethroplasty of absent urethra.
- Reconstruction of a normal ventral radius: glans, corpus spongiosum and skin.

Correction of chordae

The chordae derive from tethering of the hypoplastic ventral skin to the underlying structures, tethering of the urethral plate on the ventral surface of the corpus cavernosum, and the atretic distal corpus spongiosum, which diverges laterally from the ectopic meatus to the glans.

Chordae are corrected by degloving of the penile skin, careful dissection of the urethral plate and dissection of the lateral corpus spongiosum and the wings of the glans. Only in rare cases (five per cent) is a plicature of the dorsal corpora cavernosa necessary.

Urethroplasty

In the case of a wide urethral plate, it can simply be tubularized to form a new urethra (Thiersch–Duplay technique) (Figure 60.6).

If the urethral plate is narrow, an on-lay urethroplasty can be performed. A rectangular flap is used as an on-lay to close the urethral plate. A flap of ventral shaft skin can be rotated into the defect (perimeatal-based flap; also called the 'flip-flap procedure', Mathieu 1932) (Figure 60.7). A pedicled dorsal preputial flap (on-lay island flap, Elder 1987) or a free graft can also be used. As a free graft, buccal mucosa, or alternatively bladder mucosa, is preferred. In 1994, Snodgrass described a

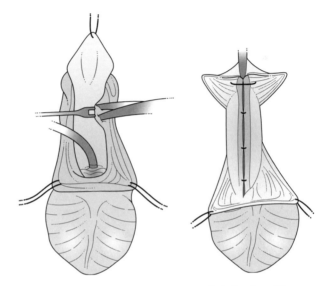

Figure 60.6   *Thiersch–Duplay techique: tubularization of the urethral plate.*

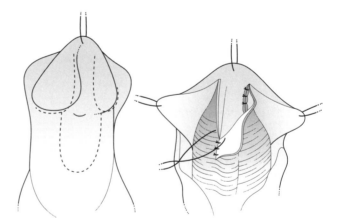

Figure 60.7   *Mathieu 'flip-flap' repair, using a perimeatal-based flap.*

technique in which the urethral plate is incised longitudinally to allow ventral closure of the plate (tubularized incised plate (TIP) urethroplasty) (Figure 60.8). In the gap where the incision was made, the urethral mucosa regenerates. This gap can alternatively be laid in with a buccal mucosa flap. Nowadays, TIP urethroplasty is the most commonly used technique for proximal and distal hypospadias repair because it is simple and has cosmetically very well-accepted results; the complication rate remains below ten per cent.

In the situation of significant ventral curvature and a very short urethral plate, the urethral plate can not be used as it is. In this case, a tubularized flap of the redundant dorsal foreskin can substitute the urethra. This is called the tubed prepucial island flap (Wacksman 1986). A long defect can thus be reconstructed. However, due to the circular anastomosis, stricture formation is more frequent with this technique.

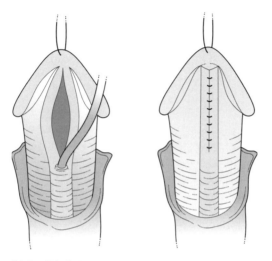

Figure 60.8   *Tubularized incised plate urethroplasty (after Snodgrass): longitudinal incision of the urethral plate and tubularization.*

In severe cases of proximal hypospadias with chordae and poor prepucial skin, a planned two-stage procedure is still an acceptable option (Durham-Smith, Bracka: Smith 1981; Bracka 1995). The first stage involves correction of the chordae, opening of the glans and placement of an on-lay free graft (buccal). This is followed by the second stage six months later of tubularization and reconstruction of penile skin.

Occasionally, a combination of primary tubularization of the proximal urethra and a distal free graft followed by distal tubularization six months later is possible.

For distal hypospadias, frequently the meatal advancement and glanuloplasty incorporated (MAGPI) procedure is used (Duckett 1981) (Figure 60.9). The septum between the meatus and the glanular ectodermal sinus is divided longitudinally and sutured transversally. This causes deepening of the glanular groove. The ventral lip of the urethra is subsequently lifted towards the meatus. The lateral wings of the glans are then brought together ventrally and sutured over the meatus. This procedure is in fact only a glanuloplasty, giving the impression of a meatal advancement. The technique is quite simple to perform, but meatal regression can be a problem later on. Different variations have been described, using the mucosa of the glanular groove. The glans approximation procedure (GAP) (Zaontz 1989) is possible in the case of a wide glanular groove.

Table 60.1 lists the different techniques in relation to the severity of hypospadias.

Reconstruction of the ventral radius

A new meatus is constructed at the blind-ending ectodermal pit where the normal meatus is expected (meatoplasty).

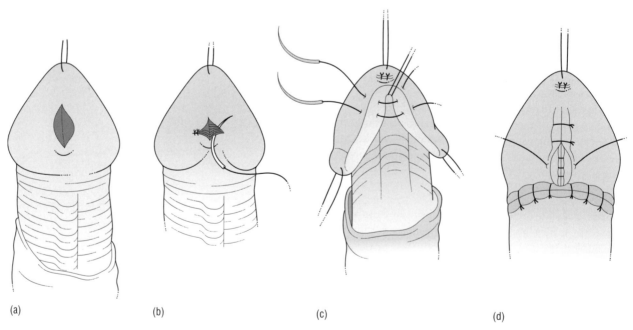

(a)   (b)   (c)   (d)

Figure 60.9   *Meatal advancement and glanuloplasty incorporated (MAGPI) procedure. (a) Longitudinal incision of the septum and between the blind fossa navicularis and the meatus. (b) Transversal suturing (creates deepening of the glanular groove). (c) Dissection of the glanular wings and lifting up of the meatus, to (d) allow vertical closure of the glans.*

The ventral glans is reconstructed by folding the two glanular wings over the new urethra (glanuloplasty). When possible, the spongiosa pillars are brought together over the new urethra (spongioplasty). The neo-urethra can be covered using subcutaneous tissue or a tunica vaginalis flap to protect the anastomotic sutures and make the anastomosis watertight. The last step is to bring excess dorsal penile skin to the ventral side of the penis in order to restore a normal ventral skin length. The dorsal foreskin is split longitudinally, either vertically (Byers flap) (Figure 60.10) or following venous drainage (Van Der Meulen flap). Both flaps are sutured together ventrally, forming a raphe and creating a penis with a circumcised aspect.

Important points of technique

- Microsurgery is performed using magnification glasses (at least 2.5 ×) and fine microsurgical instruments and sutures.
- Injection of a one in 100 000 adrenaline solution (mostly in combination with a local anaesthetic) can help with dissection and provide haemostasis. Alternatively, a small

Table 60.1 *Use of different techniques in relation to the severity of hypospadias*

Severity of hypospadias	Technique used
Distal hypospadias	MAGPI (for short urethral defects) Flip-flap procedure GAP
Mid-shaft hypospadias	Flip-flap procedure On-lay island flap TIP
Proximal hypospadias	On-lay island flap Tubed prepucial island flap TIP Planned two-stage procedure

GAP, glans approximation procedure; MAGPI, meatal advancement and glanuloplasty incorporated; TIP, tubularized incised plate.

penile tourniquet (without using adrenaline) can be used for 10–15 minutes during glanular dissection and suturing.

- Moderate use of only bipolar coagulation.
- Watertight anastomoses with running sutures of polyglycolic acid 6/0 to 8/0.
- Good antiseptic preparation and prophylactic antibiotics.
- Experienced surgeon.
- Right choice of technique.
- Avoid circular anastomoses. If unavoidable, use spatulated or oblique anastomosis.
- Use well-vascularized and hairless tissues (flaps rather than grafts).
- Cover the reconstructed urethra:
  - avoid anastomotic sutures of different layers on the same line;
  - approximate the diverted corpus spongiosum and eventually use tunica vaginalis flaps to cover the urethral anastomosis.

Complications of hypospadias repair

Complications are quite common. The next surgical correction should be delayed six months after the initial operation to allow total recovery of all tissues.

- *Fistula* can occur because of three problems: meatal strictures, infected haematomas and necrotic patches of the used tissue. A second corrective operation is not always needed. In the case of a persistent fistula, narrowing of the newly formed urethra must be ruled out before resection of the fistula. During the second operation, the fistula can be excised and sutured at its base. Drainage is not needed in most cases; if needed, however, it can be performed in a day-case setting.
- *Urethral stenosis* occurs mainly after a circular anastomosis, which is avoided in modern techniques. It can also be a result of insufficient ingrowth of a free graft or a result of the new tube suture line being advanced too

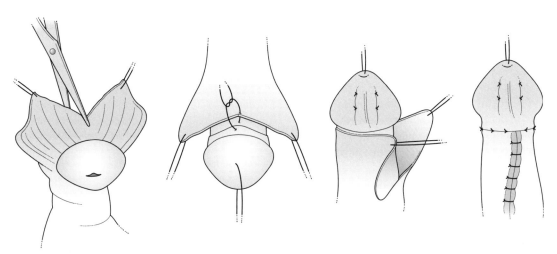

Figure 60.10 *Lengthening of the ventral shaft skin with Byers flaps. The excess dorsal foreskin is incised and brought ventrally.*

distally and creating a narrow meatal ring. A new urethroplasty frequently is needed.

- *Urethrocele:* the neo-urethra can dilate as a result of distal stenosis. The excess urethral tissue should be excised and the stenosis corrected.
- *Balanitis xerotica obliterans* is a rare problem resulting from chronic inflammation and fibrosis of the glans and meatus. Early topical steroids are applied. Rarely, a meatoplasty is needed.
- *Meatal regression or glanular dehiscence* can be a result of inadequate mobilization of the glanular wings. A flip-flap repair can give good results in some cases.
- *Other complications:* when bladder mucosa is used as a free graft, mucosal ectropion and pseudo-polyps can occur. After resection, recurrence and meatal stenosis are common. Hairy (scrotal) flaps should not be used, as this can lead to infection, urethral stones and stenosis. A new urethroplasty is required and the scrotal skin should be replaced by buccal mucosa. Persistent chordae must be corrected by excising the chordae or dorsal plication (shortening of the penis).

'Cripple hypospadias' is a term that was once used after several failed surgeries for hypospadias repair with persistent chordae, fistulas, excessive scarring and asymmetrical skin. The term should be avoided as it is disrespectful towards the patient. In some patients, total reconstruction of the penis is needed. However, the urethral plate sometimes can be spared. Buccal mucosa and tunica vaginalis flaps can be very helpful in these reconstructions.

OTHER CONGENITAL ANOMALIES OF THE PENIS

Urethral duplication

Urethral duplication is a rare congenital anomaly. It is defined as the presence of two urethral channels, which can be totally separate or linked, blind-ending or patent. Sometimes, two meati are found. The urethra can split in two and then reunite (spindle urethra). If one urethra does not pass a normal sphincter, then urinary leakage can be the presenting symptom. Urethral duplication can be a component of partial or complete caudal duplication, with duplication of the phallus or bladder and frequently anomalies in other organ systems. It can be a result of defective canalization of the urethral plate, or when the invading mesenchyme pinches off part of the urethra to form two, or secondary to abnormal downgrowth of the urorectal septum.

If clinical suspicion for urethral duplication exists, then an antegrade and retrograde voiding cystourethrogram should be performed. Urethrocystoscopy with simultaneous catheterization of the second channel can be useful. Treatment is necessary in case of problems such as infertility, infection, incontinence and deviation during erection. The accessory urethra can be excised, endoscopically incised or fulgurated (the latter not being the primary treatment of choice because of the risk of postoperative curvature).

Duplication of the penis

The duplication can be total or partial, in a sagittal or horizontal plane, and with or without urethral duplication. It is often associated with imperforate anus and other regional abnormalities. The penis and scrotum may be transposed (no switch of scrotal swelling below the genital tubercle), requiring cosmetic surgery to correct the penoscrotal transposition. If the corpus spongiosum is absent, then the spongious urethra can be enlarged, resulting in a megalourethra and leading to infections and stone formation, occasionally requiring surgical correction by complete urethral replacement or urethral duplication.

Penile agenesis

Abnormal differentiation of the genital tubercle in the sixth week can lead to penile agenesis. Frequently, other anomalies are associated, which are often incompatible with life. In 25 per cent, it is an isolated phenomenon. The scrotum is normal and the urethra opens into the anterior perineum or rectum or is formed inadequately.

Microphallus

Penile development can be retarded because of inadequate androgen priming. Alternatively, the penis may develop abnormally in a normal endocrine environment. It is then often associated with other anomalies, such as accessory penis, buried penis, cryptorchidism and anomalies of other organs.

It is important in these situations to consider sex of rearing and to fully involve genetic, endocrine and paediatric specialists in the treatment plan. Very rarely is a genetic male brought up as a phenotypic female.

REFERENCES

Bracka A. Hypospadias repair: the two stage alternative. *British Journal of Urology* 1995; **76**: 31.

Duckett JW. MAGPI (meatoplasty and glanuloplasty): a procedure for subcoronal hypospadias. *Urologic Clinics of North America* 1981; **8**: 513.

Elder JS, Duckett JW, Snyder HM. Onlay island flap in the repair of mid and distal hypospadias without chordee. *Journal of Urology* 1987; **138**: 376.

Mathieu P. Traitement en un temps de l'hypospade balanique et juxta-balanique. *Journale de Chirugie* (*Paris*) 1932; **39**: 481.

Smith ED. Durham-Smith repair of hypospadias. *Urologic Clinics of North America* 1981; **8**: 451.

Snodgrass W. Tubularized, incised plate urethroplasty for distal hypospadias. *Journal of Urology* 1994; **151**: 464.

Wacksman J. Use of the Hodgson XX (modified Asopa) procedure to correct hypospadias with chordee: surgical technique and results. *Journal of Urology* 1986; **136**: 1264.

Zaontz MR. The GAP (glans approximation procedure) for glanular/coronal hypospadias. *Journal of Urology* 1989; **141**: 359.

FURTHER READING

Circumcision. *British Journal of Urology* 1999; **83** (suppl. 1): 1–113.

Berdeu D, Sauze L, Ha-Vinh P, Blum-Boisgard C. Cost-effectiveness analysis of treatments for phimosis: a comparison of surgical and medicinal approaches and their economic effect. *British Journal of Urology* 2001; **87**: 239–44.

Bogaert G. Urethral duplication and other urethral anomalies. In: Gearhart JP, Rink RC, Mouriquand PDE (eds). *Pediatric Urology*. Philadelphia, PA: WB Saunders, 2001; pp. 607–19.

Hinman F, Jr. Penis and male urethra. In: *Atlas of Urosurgical Anatomy*. Philadelphia, PA: WB Saunders, 1993; pp. 418–29.

King LR. Hypospadias. In: King LR (ed.). *Urologic Surgery in Infants and Children*. Philadelphia, PA: WB Saunders, 1998; pp. 194–208.

61

Ambiguous genitalia and intersex

IEUAN HUGHES AND PADRAIG MALONE

Learning objectives

- To understand the terminology used in intersex conditions.
- To understand the process of sex determination in embryogenesis.
- To be able to categorize intersex conditions.
- To be able to develop a management plan for children with intersex.

INTRODUCTION

Sex determination followed by sex differentiation is an orderly sequence of events coordinated in a time- and threshold-dependent manner via a network involving numerous genes and hormones, particularly sex steroids. Understanding this process is a prerequisite to the investigation of a newborn infant with ambiguous genitalia. Indeed, much of the current knowledge about the genetic control of sex determination has been gleaned from studying individuals with syndromes of sex reversal, such as complete XY gonadal dysgenesis and the XX male. Similarly, the study of individuals with defects in steroid biosynthesis or action has provided information about novel pathways of steroid production and the mode of action of hormones at target sites.

Sex assignment as either male or female is instantaneous at birth for the vast majority of infants. If this is not possible because of ambiguity of the external genitalia, then it is essential that the neonatologist, paediatric endocrinologist and paediatric surgeon/urologist work in a coordinated manner

to support the family during a difficult early phase in management. Further confusion can be created by injudicious use of terminology and inappropriate guesswork as to the sex of the infant. Time is of the essence in reaching a decision on sex assignment, but this should not be at the expense of an adequate investigative protocol undertaken in specialized centres (Ogilvy-Stuart and Brain 2004).

TERMINOLOGY

The subject of intersex is confusing enough without adding to the problem by the use of terminology such as 'pseudo'. The terms 'female pseudo-hermaphroditism' and 'male pseudo-hermaphroditism' traditionally have been used for masculinization of an XX individual and undermasculinization of an XY individual, respectively, but they should not be used nowadays. The term 'hermaphroditism' should be reserved for describing ambiguous genitalia in an individual in whom both testicular and ovarian (containing follicles) tissue is present.

Such a description can be applied only when there is histological confirmation of the nature of the gonads. Geneticists use the term 'sex reversal' prefaced by 'XY' or 'XX'. In its complete form, there is no ambiguity of the external genitalia, such as in complete androgen-insensitivity syndrome. The partial form of sex reversal typically is associated with ambiguous genitalia, such as that seen in congenital adrenal hyperplasia. Such descriptive terms maintain an orderly approach to the assessment of newborn intersex. The pragmatic model used in this chapter is the masculinized female (previously, female pseudo-hermaphroditism) and the undermasculinized male (previously, male pseudo-hermaphroditism).

The assignment of sex at birth is a physical attribute coupled inextricably with issues of gender. It is not the brief of this chapter to relate the subject of intersex to postnatal psychosexual development, but it is important to note that the following definitions are germane to understanding the management of ambiguous genitalia:

- *Gender (sex) assignment*: the decisive allocation of male or female at birth.
- *Gender identity*: the sense of self as being male or female.
- *Gender role*: denotes aspects of behaviour and preferences.
- *Sexual orientation*: target of sexual arousal.
- *Gender attribution*: assignation of a person as male or female.
- *Gender dysphoria*: a transsexual state.

Transsexualism is not considered in the context of intersex, as individuals with gender dysphoria usually are not born with ambiguous genitalia. However, it is possible that intersex individuals in later life may not be satisfied with their sex assignment and may wish to have further surgery, as appropriate. There are examples of this occurring with severely masculinized females with congenital adrenal hyperplasia (CAH) who have been assigned quite late as females only to wish for sex assignment to male when older. This kind of experience makes it essential that all professionals working in the field of intersex pool their knowledge of longer-term outcome data.

EMBRYOLOGY

The embryology of the gonads and reproductive tract is reviewed in standard texts, and in this chapter only a few key processes are highlighted (Grumbach *et al.* 2003).

The urogenital ridge region, genetically coded for by a number of genes, is the site of development of not only the kidneys and gonads but also the adrenal glands. When the gene *WT1* is disrupted, there is absence of both kidney and gonad development. When the gene *SF1* is disrupted, the adrenal glands and gonads are absent. Gene-inactivating mutations cause syndromes such as Denys–Drash and Frasier syndromes (*WT1*) and XY sex reversal with adrenal failure (*SF1*).

The mesonephros is key to the development of the testis once the urogenital ridge is formed. Following migration, somatic cells encompass the primordial germ cells that have migrated from the yolk sac. Ectopic migration of germ cells may give rise later to germ-cell tumours. The proximity of adrenal and gonad development is also attested to by the ectopic site of adrenal rests, commonly observed by surgeons during orchidopexies and hernia operations to be adjacent to the testes. In males with poorly controlled congenital adrenal hyperplasia, such adrenal rests can present as testicular tumours.

A unique feature of the early gonad is its bipotential nature of development. This indifferent stage changes at around six weeks' gestation, with the appearance in the male of Sertoli cells and seminiferous cords and the presence of a prominent coelomic blood vessel adjacent to the developing testis. Later, the interstitial cells differentiate into steroid-secreting Leydig cells. No such differentiation occurs in the developing ovary until weeks later. Unlike the testis, primordial germ cells are essential for fetal ovarian development, but the ovary *per se* is not essential for development of the female phenotype, and hence the concept that human fetal sex development is constitutively female.

The internal genitalia are also bipotential in the sense that the anlagen for development of the internal genital ducts are present initially in both sexes. Regression of the Müllerian ducts destined to form the uterus and Fallopian tubes occurs in the male though the action of anti-Müllerian hormone (AMH) produced by the Sertoli cells. Such action occurs only during a critical window between six and eight weeks' gestation, when AMH binds to the type II receptor in the Müllerian mesenchyme. Mutations in the AMH or AMH-receptor genes lead to remnants of Müllerian structures in otherwise normally developed males (Blackless *et al.* 2000). Androgens produced by the fetal testis in large concentrations and acting locally in a paracrine fashion stabilize the Wolffian ducts in the male to form the vas deferens, epididymis and seminal vesicles. The Wolffian ducts regress in the female in the absence of androgens.

The external genitalia also develop from a common anlage, with androgens playing a trophic role in differentiation of the genital tubercle into the penis, the urethral folds into the penile urethra, and the labioscrotal folds into the scrotum. The study of the human intersex syndrome 5-alpha-reductase deficiency has clarified the key role of dihydrotestosterone (a metabolite of testosterone) in masculinization of the external genitalia. The final step in male development requires the descent of the testis from its high intra-abdominal origin via a two-stage process of transabdominal and inguinal migration into the scrotum. Androgens are also key to testis descent (hypogonadotrophic hypogonadism – Kallmann syndrome – produces cryptorchidism), together with the role of the insulin-like peptide 3 and its receptor LGR8/GREAT. Gene disruption of these proteins in the mouse leads to cryptorchidism. Mutations in the human genes have been found in about 20 per cent of a series of patients with undescended

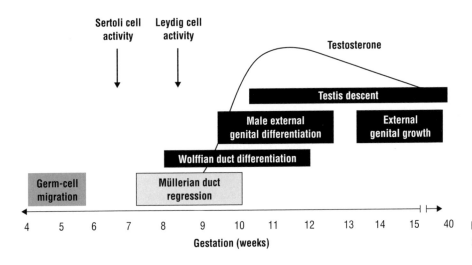

Figure 61.1 *Diagram depicting events in fetal male development.*

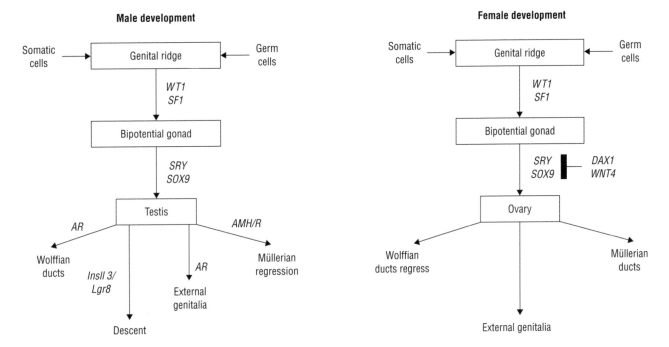

Figure 61.2 *Diagram depicting events in fetal female development.*

testes but who were otherwise normally developed and fertile. The events in fetal male development are summarized in Figure 61.1.

GENETIC AND ENDOCRINE CONTROL OF FETAL SEX DEVELOPMENT

An enormous number of genes have been identified as having a role in sex determination and sex differentiation, based on *Drosophila*, murine and human studies. Figure 61.2 shows those genes relevant to human fetal sex development together with the phenotypic counterpart. The *SRY* gene remains

leader of the pack for testis-determining genes. Inactivating mutations in *SRY* are found in 15–20 per cent of patients with complete XY gonadal dysgenesis leading to complete sex reversal. To date, no satisfactory explanation has been found for sex reversal in the majority of complete XY gonadal dysgenesis patients or indeed for the ten per cent of XX males who are *SRY*-negative. Most true hermaphrodites who have an XX karyotype (the most common karyotype in this form of intersex) are also *SRY*-negative. These observations indicate that a number of testis-determining genes remain to be identified and presumably are located on autosomes. The *SOX9* gene, for example, belongs to the same family of genes as *SRY*. *SOX9* not only is important in testis development but also has a key role in cartilage formation.

SOX9 mutations in humans result in the syndrome of campomelic dysplasia, a generally lethal skeletal malformation syndrome associated with sex reversal. Figure 61.2 also shows a schematic for female development. The genetic control in this sex classically has been regarded as 'neutral' in mammals, with female development occurring constitutively in the absence of testis determining genes. However, it is possible that genes such as *DAX1* and *WNT4* may act in the female as anti-testis genes; indeed, studies of Rokitansky syndrome suggest that *WNT4* may have a more direct role in ovarian development (Hughes 2004).

The endocrine control of sex differentiation is essentially relevant only in the male. Female fetal development occurs normally in the absence of estrogens, and hence the external genitalia in Turner syndrome at birth are normal. Male sex differentiation is dependent on an optimal production of androgens occurring from about 10–16 weeks' gestation. The fetal serum level of testosterone at this time reaches around 10 nmol/L, a value within the lower end of the normal adult range (Figure 61.1). Early androgen production by fetal Leydig cells may be autonomous before becoming dependent on placental human chorionic gonadotrophin (HCG). Placental insufficiency leading to suboptimal androgen production during this critical phase in sex differentiation may be a cause of idiopathic hypospadias and the association between intrauterine growth retardation and hypospadias. The pathway of androgen biosynthesis is illustrated in Figure 61.3. Both HCG and luteinizing hormone (LH) bind to the same membrane

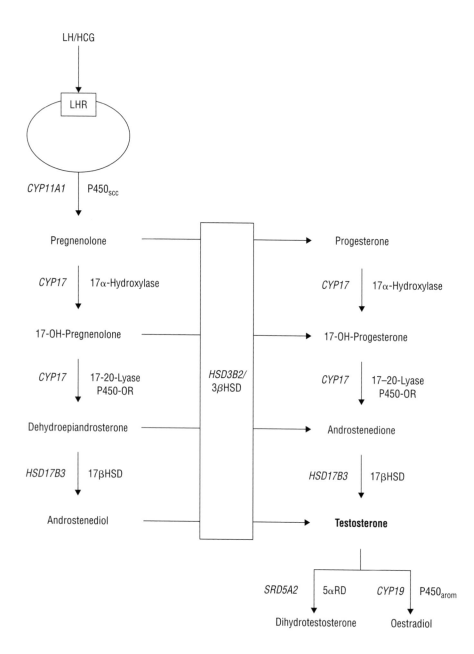

Figure 61.3 *Pathway of androgen biosynthesis.*

5αRD, 5-alpha-reductase; Arom, aromatase; 17βHSD, 17-beta-hydroxysteroid dehydrogenase; LHR, luteinizing hormone receptor; P450-OR, P450 oxidoreductase; SCC, side-chain cleavage.

receptor to initiate steroidogenesis, with androgen production becoming fetal pituitary-dependent during the second half of gestation. A male newborn with micropenis who develops hypoglycaemia is a constellation of signs strongly suggestive of congenital pituitary deficiency. Figure 61.3 shows that *CYP17* and cytochrome P450 oxidoreductase are key regulators of androgen. There is evidence from studies in the Tammar wallaby that the P450 oxidoreductase enzyme is used preferentially to synthesize dihydrotestosterone using substrates other than testosterone. Similar pathways may operate in the human fetus only to switch to the classical pathway of androgen biosynthesis postnatally (see later).

High-affinity binding to the intracellular androgen receptor (AR) mediates the action of androgens in target tissues. The AR is part of a large family of nuclear receptors that act as transcription factors when activated by ligands such as all steroids, thyroid hormones, retinoids and the thiotriglitazones. Figure 61.4 illustrates the basic mode of action of androgens in target cells and gives some examples of the biological actions that are mediated by androgens. Sex differentiation is one such effect, and the AR is expressed early in fetal tissues such as the Wolffian ducts and genital tubercle. Biological events such as prostate growth and spermatogenesis in later postnatal life are AR-dependent. While the AR is a transcription factor, little is known about the identity of androgen-responsive genes other than some that have been identified in the prostate, such as prostate-specific antigen. It is likely that some examples of XY intersex associated with androgen resistance but a normal AR ultimately may be found to be due to a mutation in an androgen target gene expressed in the male reproductive tract.

CAUSES OF AMBIGUOUS GENITALIA

The list of possible causes of abnormal genital development at birth is enormous. Table 61.1 provides a simple classification using a pragmatic approach to causation. By far the most common cause of newborn intersex is CAH due to 21-hydroxylase deficiency, leading to masculinization of an affected female fetus.

The masculinized female

CAH heads the list of causes of a masculinized female. CAH is not a true disorder of sex differentiation, as the gonads and internal genital ducts develop normally but the genital tubercle, urethral folds and labioscrotal swellings are stimulated by the excess production of androgens of adrenal origin. The most common defect is 21-hydroxylase deficiency, which leads to an accumulation of 17-OH-progesterone acting as a substrate for increased androstenedione production (Figure 61.5). This weak androgen is converted in the liver to the potent androgen, testosterone, whose concentrations in fetal serum in the CAH newborn may exceed the adult male range. The degree of masculinization can be severe enough in an affected female to result in an apparently normal 'male' at birth, but the absence of palpable gonads in the 'scrotal sac' should alert the clinician to investigate. Indeed, it is neglectful if a newborn male with non-palpable gonads is not investigated (see later). The majority of infants with 21-hydroxylase deficiency are also salt-losers, and it is essential to monitor serum and urinary electrolytes during the first weeks of life. About five per cent

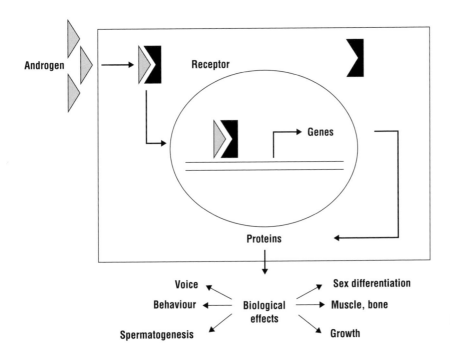

Figure 61.4 *Biological effects of mutations in the* AR *(androgen receptor) gene.*

of cases of CAH are due to 11β-hydroxylase deficiency. This defect also leads to an accumulation of excess androgens but not salt loss, because of the production of the potent salt-retaining hormone deoxycorticosterone (Figure 61.5).

Table 61.1 *Causes of ambiguous genitalia: functional classification*

Type/cause	Illustrative example
Masculinized female	
Fetal androgens, maternal androgens	CAH, placental aromatase deficiency, ovarian and adrenal tumours
Undermasculinized male	
Abnormal testis determination	Partial (XY) and mixed (XO/XY) gonadal dysgenesis
Androgen biosynthetic defects	LH receptor-inactivating mutations
Resistance to androgens	17β-OH-Dehydrogenase deficiency 5α-Reductase deficiency Androgen insensitivity syndrome variants
True hermaphroditism	
Presence of testicular and ovarian tissue	Karyotypes XX, XY, XX/XY
Syndromal	Denys–Drash, Frasier, Smith–Lemli–Opitz

CAH, congenital adrenal hyperplasia; LH, luteinizing hormone.

CAH is an autosomal recessive disorder. The molecular genetics of the different forms have been well-characterized. They include mutations of the *CYP21* gene located on the short arm of chromosome 6. The concordance between genotype and phenotype is close, so it is possible to predict a propensity to salt-wasting based on the genotype. It is now possible to prevent virilization of the external genitalia in an affected female by prenatal administration of dexamethasone to the mother. Clearly this can be offered only during a second or later pregnancy in an affected family and involves starting treatment as soon as the pregnancy is confirmed. An early start is necessary because excess adrenal steroid production is evident from about eight weeks' gestation. Dexamethasone is the glucocorticoid of choice. This does have a tendency to produce excess weight gain during pregnancy. A chorionic villus sampling is undertaken at around 10–12 weeks in order to check the karyotype and the *CYP21* genotype. It is essential that the index case and the family have been genotyped previously. If the karyotype based on chorionic villus sampling is 46,XY, then treatment is stopped, even if the male fetus is affected by CAH, based on *CYP21* genotype, because the external genitalia will be normal. Treatment is continued only in 46,XX affected fetuses. Affected females treated from early pregnancy are born with virtually normal external genitalia and do not require surgery. Outcome studies to date indicate that growth and development are normal, despite the early exposure to high doses of glucocorticoids.

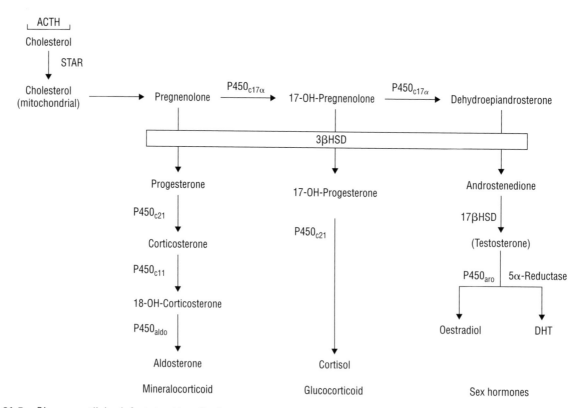

Figure 61.5 *Diagram outlining infant steroid synthesis.*
ACTH, adrenocorticotrophic hormone; DHT, dihydroxytestosterone; HSD, hydroxysteroid dehydrogenase; StAR, steroid adrenal receptor.

Apart from CAH, virilization in a female offspring may also be caused by the following:

- androgen-secreting tumours in the mother, including luteoma, arrhenoblastoma, hilar cell tumour and Krukenberg tumour of the ovary;
- maternal adrenal tumour (rare);
- rare mutations in the *CYP19* gene;
- mutations in the cytochrome P450 oxidoreductase enzyme.

Often in these situations, the fetus is protected from excess androgens by a remarkably efficient placental aromatase enzyme, which converts androgens to oestrogens. Even mothers with CAH can run quite high levels of testosterone without virilising a female fetus.

The undermasculinized male

The XY intersex infant is the result of a far greater number of diagnostic possibilities than is the case for the masculinized female. Nevertheless, it is useful to consider the possibilities in terms of a defect in testis formation (some form of gonadal dysgenesis), a defect in androgen production and a defect in androgen action.

In the case of gonadal dysgenesis, a number of causes have already been mentioned in describing the genetic control of gonad determination. Partial gonadal dysgenesis is inferred by the appearance of ambiguous genitalia in an XY infant with evidence of Müllerian remnants and inadequate androgen production. This implies Sertoli cell dysfunction, giving rise to inadequate AMH synthesis and, hence, the Müllerian remnants. A concomitant elevated follicle-stimulating hormone (FSH) is supportive of gonadal dysgenesis. Histology may show gonadal changes consistent with dysgenesis, such as underdeveloped seminiferous tubules with wide intertubular spaces, scanty germ cells, infantile Sertoli cells and a dense stroma containing psammoma bodies. However, this form of intersex is not categorized adequately and often is an assumption made after other causes have been excluded.

A better-characterized entity is mixed gonadal dysgenesis, which is associated with 45XO/46XY chromosomal mosaicism. Typically, there is a testis on one side and a streak gonad on the contralateral side. The resulting phenotype can be widely variable and is not a function of the percentage of cells bearing the XO line, at least in peripheral blood and fibroblasts. What probably is important is the proportion of 45,XO cell lines in the developing gonad. It is likely that the degree of masculinization is dependent on the amount of testosterone produced by the Leydig cells *in utero*. The paediatric endocrinologist and paediatric surgeon see a skewed population of XO/XY infants manifest as intersex, as more than 90 per cent of fetuses detected prenatally have normal male genitalia.

True hermaphroditism can be regarded as a defect in gonad formation, with histological confirmation of both testicular and ovarian tissue in the same individual being the key to the diagnosis. The prevalence of this form of intersex accounts for a large proportion of intersex cases in South Africa in view of the high incidence in the Bantu population. The most frequent karyotype in 46XX, with XX/XY mosaicism in a third of cases and a 46XY karyotype in less than ten per cent of cases. The most commonly found gonad is an ovotestis. The XX male generally is associated with normal male genitalia at birth, as is the case with Klinefelter syndrome (47XXY karyotype). However, hypospadias rarely can occur in both conditions. Infertility is invariable in adult life.

All of the enzyme steps shown in Figure 61.3 are essential for androgen biosynthesis, and a deficiency would result in varying degrees on undermasculinization. Some defects, such as steroid adrenal receptor (StAR) protein deficiency and 3β-hydroxysteroid dehydrogenase deficiency, are shared with the adrenal glands and, thus, lead to concomitant adrenal insufficiency. Two enzymes are unique to androgen production, and their deficiency gives rise to characteristic syndromes of XY intersex. The penultimate step in testosterone synthesis is mediated by 17β-hydroxysteroid dehydrogenase by reversibly converting androstenedione to testosterone. A type III isoenzyme catalyses this reaction, and mutations in the 17β-hydroxysteroid dehydrogenase (*17βHSD3*) gene give rise to severe undermasculinization at birth. Indeed, the condition can be missed, as the genitalia appear to be normal female. However, at puberty, there is a remarkable degree of virilization in the child raised as a girl, with deepening of the voice, increased body hair and musculature, and marked clitoromegaly. It has been difficult to explain the paradox of this 'double' sex reversal, other than to invoke the production of testosterone in peripheral tissues via other 17β-hydroxysteroid dehydrogenase isoenzymes acting at the time of puberty. A similar phenomenon also occurs with deficiency of the enzyme 5α-reductase, which converts testosterone to dihydrotestosterone. Mutations in the *SRD5A2* gene have been reported within discrete ethnic populations, such as in the Dominican Republic. Raised as females, these individuals virilize sufficiently at puberty to be changed to a male sex of rearing.

The prototype of a defect in androgen action is complete androgen insensitivity syndrome (CAIS), previously termed 'testicular feminization syndrome' (Hughes *et al.* 2002). CAIS is not strictly an intersex disorder, as the external genitalia are normal female and the infant is assigned a female sex at birth. Clinical presentation in infancy may occur through the appearance of inguinal swellings due to herniation of the testes. Bilateral inguinal herniae are much less common in female infants than in male infants, and it is debatable whether investigations such as karyotyping should be undertaken. There may be a family history of an older 'sister' who also had an inguinal hernia repair performed in infancy, since CAIS is an X-linked recessive disorder. The usual presentation of CAIS occurs later when an adolescent girl is investigated for primary amenorrhoea. Breast development is normal, as the elevated androgens are efficiently converted to oestrogens, which also give rise to the normal adult female body habitus. Pubic and axillary hair is either absent or scanty, and there are no menses, because of the lack of ovaries and a uterus. The partial form of the syndrome (partial androgen insensitivity syndrome, PAIS) is manifest as varying degrees of masculinisation such as isolated clitoromegaly, or severe hypospadias with micropenis, or normal male development other than some gynaecomastia in adolescence. There is an enormous spectrum of phenotypes consistent with PAIS being the most common cause of male undermasculinization. The pathophysiology of CAIS and PAIS is explained by a dysfunctional AR due to a spectrum of mutations in the *AR* gene (Figure 61.4). The majority of patients with CAIS have an identifiable mutation in this gene, but this is not the case in PAIS. This is despite a strict definition of PAIS based on normal testes producing age-appropriate amounts of androgens and other causes of XY intersex having been excluded. The pathway of androgen action is more complex than just binding of androgen to its receptor, and mutations in myriad hitherto unidentified genes may also underlie what is constituted as the PAIS phenotype.

Syndromes and the environment

A number of eponymous syndromes comprise genital anomalies such as hypospadias and micropenis as a component part. Examples include Smith–Lemli–Opitz syndrome, which is due to a defect in cholesterol metabolism. Variants in *WT1* mutations give rise to either Denys–Drash syndrome (genital anomalies, Wilms tumour, diffuse mesangial sclerotic nephropathy) or Frasier syndrome (gonadal dysgenesis resulting in almost complete XY sex reversal, a predisposition to gonadoblastoma and a nephropathy characterized by focal segmental glomerulosclerosis). The ATRX syndrome is a multisystem disorder characterized by XY gonadal dysgenesis, beta-thalassaemia, mental retardation and multiple congenital anomalies. The affected gene on the X chromosome is involved in chromatin remodelling.

Hypospadias is not an intersex disorder *per se*, but it is very common and, when severe, may form one end of the spectrum of an XY intersex disorder such as PAIS. Epidemiological studies have been conducted to determine whether there are associations between environmental factors and the occurrence of hypospadias. Certainly the intrauterine environment may play a part in the causation of isolated hypospadias, through the association with low birth weight for gestational age. It is likely that whatever mechanism operated to induce fetal growth retardation is also manifest in preventing optimal growth of the urethral folds and closure of the urethral plate. There is some evidence for an increase in the prevalence of male reproductive tract disorders being attributed to a testicular regression syndrome that has its origin in fetal life (Asklund *et al.* 2004). This is most persuasive for testicular cancer and perhaps for the observed decrease in sperm counts. Hypospadias trends are less certain because of inadequate epidemiological data, but there is a suggestion that the incidence of this birth defect may be increasing. This would

suggest an environmental effect, perhaps working in concert with a genetic predisposition to hypospadias. Polymorphisms such as that found in the *AR* gene for the number of glutamine residues are associated with hypospadias. Animal studies show that exposure to a range of chemicals classed as endocrine disruptors can disrupt development of the male reproductive tract and lead to anomalies such as hypospadias. These chemicals include pesticides, phthalates and ingested phyto-oestrogens in food. No clear-cut association with such environmental factors has yet been established in humans.

CLINICAL ASSESSMENT AND INVESTIGATIONS

Newborn infants with the following problems need to be investigated with reference to a possible disorder of sex development:

- ambiguous genitalia;
- severe hypospadias with or without undescended testes, micropenis, bifid scrotum/shawl scrotum;
- male with non-palpable testes;
- female with inguinal herniae;
- isolated clitoromegaly (mother as well);
- isolated labial fusion (more than adhesions);
- syndromal genital anomalies.

It has been estimated that genital anomalies occur in about one in 4500 births, whereas deviation from the genital anatomy of the 'ideal' male or female based on one literature search was estimated to be as high as two per cent of live births (Blackless *et al.* 2000). The so-called 'idealized' male newborn had a penile length between 2.5 and 4.5 cm, a normal position of the urethral meatus, testes fully descended in the scrotum and a 46XY karyotype. For the 'idealized' female newborn, the clitoris ranged in size from 0.2 to 0.85 cm, the reproductive tract was normal and the karyotype was 46XX. Such 'deviations' as sex chromosome aneuploidies, simple hypospadias and undescended testes included in this definition would not come even within a broad definition of intersex. The following details need to considered when assessing a newborn infant with genital anomalies:

- any relevant family history, particularly relating to features of CAH;
- size of the phallus and evidence of chordae;
- site of urethral opening (has a urine stream been observed?);
- number of external orifices on the perineum;
- development of labioscrotal folds, bifid scrotum, fused labia, skin rugosity and pigmentation;
- whether gonads are palpable, and their position.

It is useful to have some idea of the degree deviation from the normal genital anatomy. The Prader scoring system is applied to CAH, with a score of five indicating the most severe form of virilization of the female external genitalia, in which the urethra traverses to the tip of the enlarged clitoris and the labioscrotal folds are fused completely, like a scrotum. The degree of undermasculinization can be semi-quantified using a validated scoring system based on the presence or absence of a micropenis, the position of the urethral opening, whether the scrotum is bifid, and the position of the gonads. An attempt should be made to measure stretched penile length in order to identify true micropenis. This is defined as a value more than 2.5 standard deviations (SDs) below the mean for age. A measurement of 2.5 cm or less is often used to define micropenis in the newborn, but it may be necessary to consider ethnic variations in penile size. The physical examination of the infant should include any signs suggestive of a particular syndrome or associated adrenal insufficiency.

A list of the most relevant investigations is given in Table 61.2. The most common cause of ambiguous genitalia is CAH. A 46XX karyotype with a markedly elevated serum 17-OH-progesterone concentration and a uterus/cervix seen on ultrasound clinches this diagnosis. It then remains to establish whether the infant is also a salt-loser. Should CAH be excluded with a 46XX karyotype, then rarer disorders such as aromatase and oxidoreductase deficiencies may need to be considered. This will require specialized biochemical analyses and specific gene-mutation screens available in specialized units. The XY intersex infant usually requires more detailed investigation, and even then a definitive cause may not be established. Central to the investigation is the HCG stimulation test to assess the production of androgens by the testis. Measurement of androstenedione, testosterone and dihydrotestosterone provides information about any biosynthetic defect. Normal values for age are in keeping with some form of androgen resistance consistent with PAIS. The HCG test should be performed within the first few months of life when the pituitary-gonadal axis is active. The test is also valuable to indicate the presence or absence of testicular tissue, although measurement of serum AMH is also useful for this purpose. Imaging studies are useful in order to delineate the anatomy of the external genitalia and to locate the position of non-palpable gonads. It may be necessary to undertake magnetic resonance imaging (MRI) to find the gonads and, in due course, perform laparoscopy. This is also an opportunity to biopsy gonadal material for detailed histological examination and immunohistochemistry. When reconstructive surgery is performed for hypospadias repair, it is useful to obtain a pinhead-sized genital skin biopsy to establish a cell line for androgen binding studies as well as a source of deoxyribonucleic acid (DNA) and ribonucleic acid (RNA) for molecular analyses.

PRINCIPLES OF MANAGEMENT

The management of a newborn infant with ambiguous genitalia needs interdisciplinary skills exercised in specialized centres to which the family should be referred. Establishing a precise diagnosis may take time and, indeed, may never be achieved other than allocating the cause to a generic category of intersex. Such constraints should not impede reaching an early decision on sex assignment. The alteration of the phenotype to become congruent with that decision is not so urgent and can be delayed until the family has had access to all the professional skilled counselling needed for these conditions.

Management of the masculinized female as exemplified by CAH is straightforward in terms of sex assignment, even when the Prader score is five. Difficulties arise when the diagnosis is missed at birth in an apparent male newborn and comes to light only in later infancy or early childhood. Current practice tends towards maintaining the male sex assignment in such cases in view of the profound combined effects of prenatal androgens and early gender attribution on later psychosexual development. The medical aspects of early CAH management are constantly being revised and are not the subject of this chapter. The surgical aspects are discussed at the end of the chapter. Non-CAH causes of female masculinization are rare, but it is important to investigate them, as a disorder affecting the mother may be identified. It is possible that the problem may recur in subsequent pregnancies, and this should raise the distinct possibility of the cause being associated with a disorder of aromatase function.

The undermasculinized male is a more complex management problem that requires an orderly approach to the diagnostic possibilities by instituting appropriate investigations. This requires the use of specialized biochemical and molecular tests undertaken in recognized laboratories. Trials of androgen treatment during the first few months can provide useful information about androgen responsiveness and perhaps may be used to help sex assignment. Typical treatment regimens include a monthly injection of Sustanon® 25 mg

Table 61.2 *Investigating an infant with ambiguous genitalia*

Genetics	FISH (X-centromeric and *SRY* probes)
	Karyotype (high resolution, abundant mitoses
	Save DNA
Endocrine	17-OH-Progesterone, 11-deoxycortisol (plus routine biochemistry, *save serum!*)
	Renin, ACTH
	24-Hour urinary steroids (also check proteinuria)
	Testosterone, androstenedione, dihydrotestosterone
	LH, FSH, AMH, inhibin B
	HCG stimulation test (define dose, timing)
Imaging	Pelvic, adrenal, renal ultrasound
	MRI
	Cystourethroscopy, sinogram
Surgical	Laparoscopy
	Gonadal biopsies
	Genital skin biopsy (AR studies, extract DNA and RNA

ACTH, adrenocorticotrophic hormone; AMH, anti-Müllerian hormone; AR, androgen receptor; DNA, deoxyribonucleic acid; FISH, fluorescence *in situ* hybridization; FSH, follicle-stimulating hormone; HCG, human chorionic gonadotrophin; LH, luteinizing hormone; MRI, magnetic resonance imaging; RNA, ribonucleic acid.

(a mixture of testosterone esters). Even so, there has been a change towards raising XY infants as male despite the appearance of a severe micropenis at birth (see below). The family must be engaged fully in open discussions, including the prospect that a firm diagnosis may never be established, a significant drawback for any later genetic counselling. They must have the benefit of ongoing regular counselling, which includes the child at an appropriate stage in development.

SURGERY FOR AMBIGUOUS GENITALIA AND INTERSEX

Since the first edition of this textbook was published in 1998, there has been, and continues to be, considerable debate concerning the surgical management of this patient population. The nature of this debate includes the moral and ethical aspects of gender reassignment, the timing of surgery and the surgical techniques for all types of intersex condition. One polarized view has suggested that all decisions and surgery should be deferred until the affected person can make an informed choice for themselves (Diamond 1999). Traditionalists argue that the physical and psychological aspects of this non-intervention are unknown, and although they accept the need to modify current management regimens, they continue to advocate corrective surgery during childhood. With this intense interest, it became obvious that the quality of long-term follow-up was inadequate, and now increasing numbers of long-term series are appearing in the literature. It would seem that the results in terms of cosmetic, anatomical, functional and psychological outcomes are disappointing, and the optimism expressed in the first edition of this book was misplaced (Creighton and Minto 2001; Minto et al. 2003). The rationale behind early surgery was to normalize the genitalia, but recent reports suggest that the surgeon's ideas of normality are not matched by public perception when assessed by structured questionnaire and interview. This has led all but the most entrenched surgeons to reassess their approach to the surgical reconstruction of all patients with ambiguous genitalia and intersex. In this chapter, this modified approach will be reflected. However, because there is no sound evidence on which to base all decisions, it will undoubtedly still continue to reflect individual opinion and bias. As this field continues to change rapidly, it is important for the reader to realize that what is written in this section may rapidly become out of date.

There are two patient populations: those assigned a female gender and those assigned a male gender. The principles of surgery differ between these groups.

Surgery in the female

These patients include overvirilized females (CAH) and undervirilized males (mainly CAIH and PAIH). The components of surgery include the following:

GONADECTOMY

Gonadectomy is considered when the gonads are inappropriate for the sex of rearing or pose a risk of malignant degeneration. There is never an indication to consider gonadectomy in CAH.

The main group of patients is those with androgen insensitivity. In CAIS, there is a complete absence of androgen receptors, and the patient will not be affected by the normal levels of testosterone produced by the intra-abdominal testes. There is, therefore, no urgency to remove these testes, and there may be endocrine advantages to retaining them. Testosterone will be metabolized to oestrogen and thus will lead to breast development and will protect the bones from the early onset of osteoporosis, an increasing problem for patients with CAIS. The testes are not dysplastic and therefore carry a similar risk of malignant degeneration as any intra-abdominal testes (approximately one in 40), with the onset of malignancy in late teenage years or early adult life. Therefore, the decision for gonadectomy can be deferred safely until adolescence, when the patient can make an informed decision for herself. In patients with PAIS, some androgen receptors are present and the patient may respond to testosterone production in the first few months of life. It is generally accepted that cerebral imprinting can occur at this stage, so early gonadectomy is advisable.

There is also a case for the early removal of dysplastic gonads in conditions such as 46XY complete gonadal dysgenesis (Swyer syndrome), because of the very high risk of malignancy, with cases of gonadoblastoma being reported in infancy. The timing of gonadectomy in patients with mixed gonadal dysgenesis reared as females should be in infancy; in patients reared as males, the timing is a difficult decision (see below). Nowadays, a laparoscopic approach is favoured for removal of intra-abdominal gonads.

CLITORAL REDUCTION

In recent years, it has become apparent that the functional results of 'nerve-sparing' clitoral reduction are not as good as was hoped. Creighton and Minto (2001) have shown that the majority of women following clitoral surgery suffered from sexual dysfunction, and a significant proportion had anorgasmia. In addition, detailed surveys of sexually experienced women have shown that clitoral sizes greater than those that would be accepted by surgeons were thought to be the norm. Therefore, a more conservative approach to clitoral reduction is now advocated. During genitoplasty, it is possible to conceal the enlarged clitoris and avoid the need for formal clitoral reduction, except in the most severe cases. It is accepted that uncomfortable erections may occur with sexual arousal in later life, but the patient can then make an informed decision about clitoral reduction herself. In more severe cases, when formal surgery is required, partial (rather than complete) resection of the corpora cavernosa with preservation of the neurovascular bundles is recommended. If the glans needs to be reduced in size, then a wedge should be excised from the ventral aspect in the midline in order to preserve as many nerves as possible.

VAGINOPLASTY

The approach to vaginoplasty in the urogenital sinus has changed over recent years. If the confluence of the urethra and vagina is within 2.5 cm of the perineum, then the preferred approach is total urogenital mobilization (TUM). In TUM, the whole urogenital sinus is mobilized as far up as the bladder neck; this can then be pulled down to the perineum and the urogenital sinus can be excised, leaving separate urethral and vaginal openings. Although the long-term results of this approach are not available, it is hoped they will give superior results compared with previous approaches, where revision rates of 80 per cent were seen. In patients in whom the urogenital sinus confluence is over 2.5 cm from the perineum, a combination of TUM and the Passerini–Glazel procedure is the best approach, but there remains considerable debate regarding the timing of this surgery, with the extremes ranging from infancy to adolescence. However, it must be remembered that a persistent urogenital sinus may cause complications such as urinary infection and post-void urinary incontinence, necessitating early surgery.

In cases of gender reassignment, colovaginoplasty performed at an early age previously was recommended, but the results of long-term follow-up have been disappointing. One report described a high incidence of defunctional colitis, necessitating excision of the vagina in a significant number of cases. Therefore, vaginal surgery should be deferred until adolescence, when the patient can make an informed decision on what approach would be best for them. The choices include dilation, the Vechietti procedure, skin-flap or free skin graft vaginoplasty, and enterovaginoplasty using either small bowel or sigmoid colon.

FEMINIZING GENITOPLASTY

This involves reduction and separation of the labioscrotal folds and using some of the excessive clitoral skin to form the labia minora. In significantly virilized females, the author recommends that all patients should be afforded the opportunity of normalizing their external genitalia with a genitoplasty, concealing a moderately enlarged clitoris (clitoral reduction is recommended in only the most severe cases) and, in cases of a low-confluence urogenital sinus, TUM. Other forms of vaginoplasty should be deferred until adolescence if possible.

Surgery in the male

Many undervirilized males with mixed gonadal dysgenesis and true hermaphroditism will be reared as males. The principles of surgical reconstruction are as follows:

- Removal of all inappropriate gonadal tissue: in cases of true hermaphroditism, preservation of testicular tissue should be attempted when ovarian tissue is excised.
- Removal of inappropriate ductal structures: the utriculus needs to be resected only as far as can be conveniently

reached, since problems with the retained vaginal stump rarely arise.
- Correction of hypospadias: preoperative testosterone treatment is often required.
- Debate continues to surround the management of the dysgenetic testis in patients with mixed gonadal dysgenesis. There is a 30 per cent risk of gonadoblastoma, but the greatest risk is after puberty. Many of these testes produce adequate levels of testosterone that would allow spontaneous puberty, and it would seem to be inappropriate to remove these. Patients can be kept under clinical surveillance and following puberty can be involved in the decision as to whether to undergo gonadectomy. For patients with intra-abdominal testes that cannot be brought to the scrotum, early removal is best, as they have a higher risk of malignant change and endocrine function is usually impaired.

Long-term results

The long-term anatomical and functional results for patients with these conditions remain unclear. However, it is mandatory that careful long-term follow-up is put in place. Recent work has helped to identify the need for early and ongoing professional psychological input. In fact, patients have identified psychological support as one of their greatest and most unmet needs.

CLINICAL SCENARIO

Examination of a newborn term infant of birth weight 3240 g showed abnormalities confined to the external genitalia. A bifid scrotum showed the 'shawl' appearance of penoscrotal transposition. The right sac contained a palpable gonad resembling a testis; no gonad was palpable anywhere on the left side. The phallus was short with a severe chordae; an estimated stretched penile length was 1.9 cm. There was a single perineal opening.

Comment: The external genitalia are clearly ambiguous. It is likely that the palpable gonad in the right scrotal sac is a testis or possibly an ovotestis. All that can be assumed on the basis of the clinical examination is that CAH is not part of the differential diagnosis. Numerous possibilities include XY intersex (partial gonadal dysgenesis, androgen biosynthetic defect, PAIS), mixed gonadal dysgenesis and true hermaphroditism. Further progress can be achieved only by instigating appropriate investigations.

The following investigations were carried out:

- peripheral karyotype
- abdominal and pelvic ultrasound
- baseline serum LH and FSH

- three-day HCG stimulation test: 1500 units daily, with blood samples collected pre-HCG and 24 hours after the last HCG injection.

The ultrasound result was available immediately: two normal-sized kidneys for age were seen on abdominal ultrasound. There was a suggestion of Müllerian structures identified on pelvic ultrasound, but no gonad was visualized. The presence of a gonad resembling a testis was confirmed in the right scrotal sac, but no gonad was seen on the left side or in the left inguinal canal.

The karyotype was 45XO/46XY, with 60 per cent of cells carrying 45X (out of 100 mitoses examined).

At ten days of age, basal serum LH was 3.4 U/L and FSH was 10.2 U/L. At the same age, basal serum testosterone increased from 4.9 nmol/L to 15.4 nmol/L. Measurement of androstenedione and dihydrotestosterone was withheld.

Comment: The chromosome result enabled a straightforward diagnosis of mixed gonadal dysgenesis to be made to account for the genital anomalies. The cause in most cases is probably loss of the Y chromosome by non-disjunction after normal disomic fertilization. Baseline FSH was elevated slightly, in keeping with evidence of gonadal dysgenesis. There was a satisfactory testosterone response to HCG stimulation, suggesting the presence of active Leydig cell function and in keeping with the likelihood of the right gonad being a testis. The ultrasound findings were of limited value, despite suggesting that there was probably a streak gonad in the abdomen adjacent to what may be the remnants of a uterus and fallopian tube. There appeared to be no associated renal anomalies.

Sex assignment was male. At subsequent laparoscopy, a midline uterine remnant was identified and on the left side a nubbin of fibrous tissue attached to a fallopian tube. This was removed and histology showed ovarian-type stromal fibrous tissue with no follicles and consistent with a streak gonad. On the right side, a vas deferens and associated blood vessels were identified entering the right inguinal canal. A first-stage hypospadias repair was scheduled when the infant was about 15 months of age.

Comment: The findings at laparotomy and the subsequent histology are in keeping with the typical features of mixed gonadal dysgenesis. In this case, there appears to be a normal testis in the right hemi-scrotum, although a biopsy of this gonad will be required at some stage. The contralateral gonad was a streak gonad and needed to be removed because of the high risk of later malignancy. Adjacent Müllerian structures attest to the lack of AMH acting locally in early gestation. Hypospadias repair will be a staged process and may need preoperative testosterone treatment to enlarge the size of the phallus. The right gonad is in the scrotum and, hence, can be readily palpated during long-term follow-up. This monitoring can be complemented with serial ultrasound examinations and serum tumour markers. A testis biopsy would be recommended at puberty. It is expected that physical signs of puberty should occur spontaneously based on the results of the HCG stimulation test in infancy, but this test probably would be repeated just before puberty. The prospect for fertility cannot be predicted, as even XO/XY infants born as normal males may develop late-onset testis dysgenesis, leading to infertility.

REFERENCES

Asklund C, Jorgensen N, Kold Jensen T, Skakkebaek NE. Biology and epidemiology of testicular dysgenesis syndrome. *British Journal of Urology International* 2004; **93** (suppl 3): 6–11.

Blackless M, Charavastra A, Derryck A, *et al.* How sexually dimorphic are we? Review and synthesis. *American Journal of Human Biology* 2000; **12**: 151–66.

Creighton SM, Minto CL. Managing intersex. *British Medical Journal* 2001; **323**: 1264–5.

Diamond M. Pediatric management of ambiguous and traumatized genitalia. *Journal of Urology* 1999; **162**: 1021–8.

Grumbach MM, Hughes IA, Conte FA. Disorders of sex differentiation. In: Larsen PR, Kronenberg HM, Melmed S, Polensky KS (eds). *Williams Textbook of Endocrinology*, 10th edn. Philadelphia, PA: Saunders, 2003.

Hughes IA. Female development: all by default? *New England Journal of Medicine* 2004; **351**: 748–50.

Hughes IA, Lim HN, Ahmed SF. Clinical aspects of androgen insensitivity. *Clinical Pediatric Endocrinology* 2002; **11** (suppl 18): 9–15.

Minto CL, Liao LM, Woodhouse CRJ, Ransley PG, Creighton SM. The effect of clitoral surgery on sexual outcome in individuals who have intersex conditions with ambiguous genitalia: a cross-sectional study. *Lancet* 2003; **361**: 1252–7.

Ogilvy-Stuart AL, Brain CE. Early assessment of ambiguous genitalia. *Archives of Disease in Childhood* 2004; **89**: 401–7.

62

Paediatric and adolescent gynaecology

SARAH CREIGHTON

Learning objectives

- To understand common gynaecological problems in prepubertal girls.
- To understand common gynaecological problems in adolescents.
- To understand the presentation and treatment of ovarian cysts.
- To know the management of vaginal and uterine congenital anomalies.

INTRODUCTION

Serious gynaecological pathology in children and adolescents is rare. However, gynaecological symptoms are relatively common, and it is important that all clinicians dealing with children can make a correct assessment and plan appropriate management. Paediatric gynaecological problems are sometimes looked after poorly. Paediatricians and paediatric surgeons are often unfamiliar with the female genital tract, but additionally gynaecologists are not trained in looking after young children and their families.

This chapter will discuss management of some basic common gynaecological conditions that may present to a paediatric surgeon as well as the preliminary assessment of more complex problems.

COMMON GYNAECOLOGICAL PROBLEMS IN PREPUBERTAL GIRLS

Labial fusion

Labial fusion, also known as labial adhesions and labial agglutination, is common, with an estimated frequency in the population of 1.4 per cent (Christensen and Oster 1971). It usually presents from the age of one year. It is uncommon before this age, and it is never present at birth. The appearance is typical, with fusion of the labial skin extending from the posterior vaginal introitus towards the urethra. There is a clearly visible thin membranous line in the midline where the tissues join (Figure 62.1). In severe fusion, the urethral opening is visible as a pinhole opening. The aetiology is unknown but is thought to be due to mild vulvitis associated with a lack of oestrogen stimulation. Labial fusion is not caused by sexual abuse.

The majority of cases are asymptomatic. If present, symptoms are usually urinary. A small amount of urine may pool behind the adhesions, leading to post-micturition dribbling. This may cause urinary frequency and vulval soreness. There is also usually a high degree of parental anxiety, with concern about possible absence of the vagina.

The appearance is very typical, and the diagnosis is made on examination of the child. No other investigations are needed. However, if the parents are very anxious, then a pelvic scan to confirm the presence of a uterus may be helpful. Spontaneous resolution is common. If the child is asymptomatic, then treatment is not necessary. Reassurance that the condition will go away is all that is needed. If the child is symptomatic,

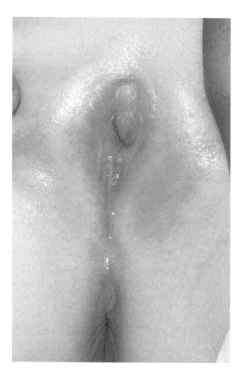

Figure 62.1 *Labial adhesions. There is midline fusion and the urethral opening is not visible.*

then treatment is usually with oestrogen cream. A small amount of oestrogen cream is applied to the labia in the midline daily for a period not longer than six weeks. The labia will start to 'buttonhole' and then separate. A normal vaginal opening will be seen, and this often provides great reassurance to the parents. Recurrence of the fusion after discontinuing the cream is common. Oestrogen cream cannot be used on a long-term basis, as a small amount is absorbed systemically, even with vaginal administration. Side effects can include breast swelling and tenderness and vaginal spotting. Surgical separation is needed rarely, unless urinary symptoms are severe and persistent. If this is performed, then oestrogen cream should be used postoperatively to prevent recurrence. Despite this, recurrence is common, even after surgery.

Labial adhesions have no implications for future gynaecological health and resolve completely as the child approaches puberty.

Vulvovaginitis

Persistent vaginal discharge or vulval irritation is the most common gynaecological presentation for a prepubertal child. The peak age for presentation is between three and seven years. The majority of patients will have a non-specific minor ailment, although a small percentage will have infection associated with systemic illness or child abuse.

Older children may complain of soreness and itch and may have associated dysuria. Younger children may appear fidgety or uncomfortable. The parents may have noticed discharge on the child's underclothes. The discharge may be greenish-yellow and offensive. The symptoms have usually been present for several weeks or months and can relapse and recur. Vaginal bleeding is not a sign of simple vulvovaginitis.

On examination, the vulva has a typical appearance, with a reddened 'flush' around the vulva and anus. The skin may be excoriated, and discharge may be seen collecting at the posterior fourchette. A low vaginal swab can be taken. Examination under anaesthetic is not indicated routinely unless a foreign body is suspected.

The most common cause of this group of symptoms is termed 'non-specific vulvovaginitis'. This is thought to be due to poor perineal hygiene combined with a lack of oestrogen stimulation, together with the anatomical features of the prepubertal vulva. The symptoms can be exacerbated by chemicals such as bubble-bath and detergents. Vaginal swabs may be normal. If positive, then the most common organisms identified are coliforms and other anaerobes, staphylococci and streptococci. The mainstay of treatment is conservative, with an emphasis on vulval hygiene. Broad-spectrum antibiotics can be helpful, but recurrence is common.

There are some other rarer causes that must be considered. The presence of a persistent watery discharge must raise suspicions of an ectopic ureter.

The presence of a foreign body in the vagina can cause vaginal discharge, although less commonly than thought previously. Vaginal bleeding or persistent foul-smelling discharge refractory to treatment, or any suspicion by the parents that the child may have inserted something into the vagina, means that an examination under anaesthetic is necessary.

Other specific systemic infections can cause vulvovaginitis, including systemic illnesses such as chickenpox and *Shigella* infection, as well as respiratory infections such as group A beta-haemolytic *Streptococcus* and *Streptococcus pneumoniae*. Threadworms are also a cause of vaginal and anal itching.

Persistent symptoms must also raise the possibility of sexual abuse. Detection of organisms usually transmitted by sexual intercourse, such as *Gonorrhoea*, *Chlamydia* and herpes, needs careful evaluation and appropriate referral.

COMMON GYNAECOLOGICAL PROBLEMS IN ADOLESCENTS

Pelvic pain

Adolescent girls with pelvic pain may present either to a surgeon or to a gynaecologist. It is important that the clinician assessing the girl takes a sexual history, and this is often best done in the absence of the parents. It is impossible to judge from her appearance whether a child is sexually active, and she may not admit to sexual activity in front of her parents. One in four girls in the UK is sexually active before the age of 16 years (Wellings 2001).

Gynaecological causes of pelvic pain in teenagers who are not sexually active include ovarian-cyst accidents such as torsion and haemorrhage. Ovulation pain can be severe

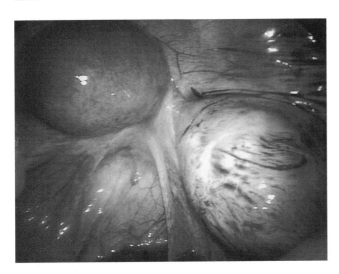

Figure 62.2 *Double uterus, with an obstructed non-communicating uterine horn on the right side. See also Colour Plate 17.*

and occurs mid-cycle. A rare cause is a non-communicating obstructed uterine horn (Figure 62.2), which presents with a history of increasingly painful periods and a pelvic mass. A pelvic ultrasound will be helpful. Vaginal examination is not necessary in girls who are not sexually active. If surgery is indicated, then this is usually performed laparoscopically.

Consensual sex and child abuse carry risks of infection and pregnancy. Pelvic inflammatory disease and complications of pregnancy, such as miscarriage and ectopic pregnancy, should not be forgotten. Ectopic pregnancy is still a significant cause of maternal death in very young women.

Ovarian cysts

In the past, neonatal ovarian cysts were considered rare. However, the advent of prenatal ultrasound has led to much more frequent detection. Neonatal cysts are of germinal or Graffian origin. Differential diagnosis includes urachal cysts, hydrocolpos and distal megaureter. The majority of these cysts resolve spontaneously during the neonatal period, as they are hormonally driven. As a general rule, asymptomatic cysts under 5 cm in diameter can be managed conservatively, with ultrasound follow-up. Larger cysts and those causing symptoms due to haemorrhage or infarction need to be removed. Ovarian tissue should be conserved if at all possible, unless torsion has already occurred. There is considerable debate as to whether it is important to prophylactically fix the contralateral ovary after one has torted and been lost. This is becoming less invasive surgically with the increasing expertise of therapeutic laparoscopy. The effect of sutures through normal ovarian structures is not clear. Routine practice currently does not involve fixation of the contralateral ovary.

Functional ovarian cysts can occur at any time of life. Follicular cysts are usually unilocular and lined with granulosa cells. Treatment is as described above, with expectant management being the most appropriate for smaller asymptomatic cysts. Corpus luteum cysts occur after puberty. They can

resolve spontaneously, but they are prone to rupture and bleeding and may present acutely. McCune-Albright syndrome is a condition in which precocious puberty is associated with polyostotic fibrous dysplasia of bone, café-au-lait spots and ovarian cysts, which may vary in size (Mauras and Blizzard 1986).

Ovarian tumours

The most common benign tumour in girls is teratoma. Ovarian teratomas are small and can be bilateral in up to 15 per cent of patients. The risk of malignancy is small but is present, and so the cyst should be removed. Ovarian tissue should be preserved if at all possible. Serous and mucinous cystadenomas are not common in children but may be found in older adolescents. They can be large and symptomatic and should be removed. Gonadoblastomas are rare and usually arise from dysgenetic gonads, often in a girl with an XY karyotype or Y chromosome fragment. They are usually benign, but they can contain germ cells, which can become malignant. Thecomas are rare; if they occur before puberty, they can cause precocious puberty due to oestrogen secretion.

Malignant ovarian tumours in childhood are usually of germ-cell origin. Correct treatment in a specialist centre is essential to achieve cure and also, if possible, to maintain fertility. Dysgerminoma is the most common; treatment is initially operative. The tumour, however, is very chemo- and radio-sensitive and the prognosis is good. Endodermal sinus tumours are less common; these are extremely aggressive, and treatment is surgical followed by aggressive chemotherapy.

VAGINAL AND UTERINE CONGENITAL ANOMALIES

Imperforate hymen

This can be recognized at birth if it causes obstruction of mucus and discharge, leading to a mucocolpos. Occasionally, this can be so large as to precipitate urinary obstruction. Treatment is by incision and drainage. Care must be taken to fully excise the membrane to prevent recurrence. If an imperforate hymen is suspected in an infant who is otherwise asymptomatic, with no collection of mucus, then surgery should be deferred. The child should be reviewed before menarche, and surgery can then be performed if necessary.

An imperforate hymen may also present in adolescence by causing a haematometria, with obstruction of the vagina and uterus. Symptoms are of cyclical pain but no bleeding. A pelvic and abdominal mass may be palpable, and inspection of the vagina reveals a bulging bluish appearance. Treatment is by incision of the membrane and drainage, usually with the release of a large amount of chocolate-coloured fluid. Again, it is important to ensure that enough of the membrane is excised to prevent recurrence.

Transverse vaginal septum

This can be an isolated finding or in association with other anomalies, as in McKusick–Kaufman syndrome, where it appears to be inherited recessively (McKusick *et al.* 1968). Presentation is with primary amenorrhoea and cyclical abdominal pain. It must be differentiated from an imperforate hymen, which has similar symptoms. Imperforate hymen is, however, easily diagnosed by a bluish bulge at the vagina, and simple surgical drainage is curative. With a transverse vaginal septum, the septum can be thick and treatment difficult. The approach to surgery depends on the position and thickness of the septum, which can be determined by ultrasound and magnetic resonance imaging (MRI) if necessary. If the septum is in the lower third of the vagina, then blind dissection may be adequate to reach the haematometria and drain it. The septum is then excised and the upper and lower parts of the vagina re-anastomosed. If the septum is high, then a combined abdominal and vaginal approach is necessary. Occasionally, the septum is so large that either intestinal transposition or skin grafting is necessary to bridge the gap between the upper and lower vagina. Fertility is possible in these patients, as long as the cervix is normal, and has been reported in the order of 40–50 per cent (Rock *et al.* 1982). Endometriosis may, however, be a significant problem and should be reduced by prompt diagnosis and treatment.

Duplication anomalies

Duplication anomalies arise from failure at some point of the fusion of the paired Müllerian ducts. The true incidence of such anomalies is unknown. Many are entirely asymptomatic and found by chance. The incidence is higher in women with infertility and recurrent miscarriage. Uterine anomalies can be isolated but are also associated with an increased incidence of renal anomalies. Uterine anomalies in particular duplication are almost universal in girls with cloacal anomalies. Diethylstilbestrol exposure also leads to an increased risk of Müllerian anomalies.

VAGINAL DUPLICATION

Management of these duplication anomalies depends on the type of anomaly and the symptoms. A longitudinal vaginal septum may not be diagnosed in childhood and may present only in later life, when it causes painful intercourse. This condition is usually diagnosed on vaginal examination, as it may be missed on ultrasound. Resection of the septum is straightforward and curative. Vaginal duplication is, however, often associated with a double uterus and cervix.

UTERINE DUPLICATIONS

A double uterus is not usually an indication for surgery. Successful pregnancy can occur in these women (Grimbizis *et al.* 2001). However, in some cases, there may exist a bicornuate or septate uterus, which may possess a non-communicating uterine horn. In this case, when menstruation starts, the non-communicating horn will fill with blood and result in a haematometria. This causes severe dysmenorrhoea and is associated with an increased incidence of endometriosis. Surgical options include either metroplasty (to join the two uteri) or resection of the obstructed horn. The decision as to the most appropriate procedure will depend on the size and position of the obstructed horn and the size of the remaining uterus and its potential for fertility. These procedures can now be performed laparoscopically. If the septum is thin and easily visualized hysteroscopically, then hysteroscopic resection may be possible.

Vaginal agenesis

Absence or shortening of the vagina can be an isolated abnormality or part of an intersex condition such as androgen insensitivity. Intersex conditions are discussed in Chapter 61 and are not addressed further here.

Vaginal agenesis is usually associated with an absent or poorly developed uterus. If a uterus is present but the vagina is absent or imperforate, then urgent problems with non-drainage of menstrual loss can arise. Presentation can be during childhood, particularly if part of a complex condition. However, presentation with primary amenorrhea in adolescence is also a common feature.

Mayer–Rokitansky–Kuster–Hauser syndrome

This is a rare condition with an estimated incidence of between one in 20 000 and one in 50 000. The most common presentation is with primary amenorrhoea. The external genitalia and pubertal development are normal. The vagina and uterus are absent, and the diagnosis is made on ultrasound scan. Laparoscopy is rarely necessary. Occasionally, the uterus may exist as very rudimentary horns lying either side of the pelvic wall (Figure 62.3). Further investigations will reveal a normal female karyotype and normal ovaries in terms of site and function. The aetiology of this condition is as yet known, although familial cases have been described. Up to 40 per cent of these women will also have urinary tract malformations, which may be minor or significant. In addition, skeletal anomalies are present in up to 12 per cent.

The psychological impact of this condition is enormous. The patient will not be able to bear children, and this may be deeply disturbing news to the patient and her parents. Initial management should be geared towards exploring and trying to come to terms with the diagnosis. The vagina is often short, and further intervention usually is necessary before a normal sex life is possible. The use of vaginal dilators is the first line of management before surgical vaginal replacement is considered. The repeated insertion of graduated dilators over a period of two to three months allows development of a vagina. The technique is to apply gentle pressure and use the dilators regularly

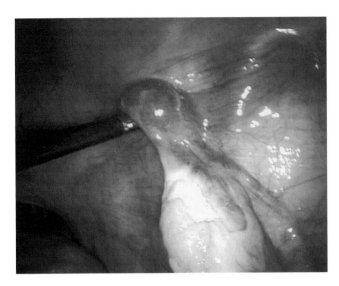

Figure 62.3 *Rudimentary uterine horn on the pelvic side wall. The vagina is absent. See also Colour Plate 18.*

for 30 minutes three times a day. Once the vagina is capacious enough to allow intercourse, the dilators can be discontinued, as intercourse itself will stretch the vagina. The main key to success is the motivation of the patient, and success rates of 78 per cent having 'normal sexual function' have been reported (Grimbizis *et al.* 2001). Failure with dilators leads to surgical options, which include creation of a neo-vagina and lining with either skin grafts or intestine.

CONCLUSION

Gynaecological conditions in children are not uncommon and can cause significant distress and worry to the child and her parents. Careful evaluation is essential, and in many cases simple reassurance and basic clinical remedies will be sufficient. In rarer cases, where surgical intervention is required, it is essential that the potential for sexual activity and fertility are not neglected whilst managing the presenting problem.

CLINICAL SCENARIOS

Case 1

A two-year-old girl was referred by her general practitioner with a diagnosis of absent vagina. The child is asymptomatic. The parents were highly anxious and had already looked up 'absent vagina' on the Internet. They were convinced that their daughter has an intersex condition and are prepared for major reconstructive surgery. On examination, the vaginal appearance was typical of labial adhesions, with a thin membrane fused in the midline. A pelvic scan confirmed the presence of a uterus. The use of oestrogen cream was discussed with the

family, who were keen to try it. After six weeks of use, the adhesions had disappeared and a normal vaginal introitus was visible. The family were reassured by this. They were advised to discontinue the oestrogen cream and were warned that recurrence is common until puberty.

Case 2

A 12-year-old girl presented with increasing severe pelvic and abdominal pain. Her periods had not started. A mass arising from the pelvis was palpable. Inspection of the vulva revealed a bulging bluish membrane. A pelvic ultrasound revealed haematocolpos. She was taken to theatre that day for incision and drainage of the vaginal membrane, after which she had normal menses.

Case 3

A 13-year-old girl presented with a two-day history of right iliac fossa pain. She also had a six-hour history of pain in the right hypochondrium and vomiting. She had been off her food and had not opened her bowels. She was pyrexial, and her white cell count was raised. On examination of the abdomen, she was tender in both iliac fossae, the right more so than the left. She was also tender over the liver. A more detailed history found that she had been sexually active for six months. Two weeks previously, she had had unprotected sexual intercourse with an older partner. A pregnancy test was negative. Following this, she had a vaginal examination by a gynaecologist. There was a purulent vaginal discharge, and endocervical swabs were taken. A diagnosis of pelvic inflammatory disease was made and she was started on antibiotics. The endocervical swabs subsequently confirmed *Chlamydia trachomatis*. She was followed up by the gynaecologist and was referred to the child protection team.

REFERENCES

Christensen EH, Oster J. Adhesions of labia minora (synechia vulvae) in childhood. *Acta Paediatrica Scandinavica* 1971; **60**: 709.

Grimbizis G, Camus M, Tarlatzis BC, Bontis JN, Devroey P. Clinical implications of uterine malformations and hysteroscopic treatment results. *Human Reproduction Update* 2001; **7**: 161–74.

Mauras N, Blizzard RM. The McCune–Albright syndrome *Acta Endocrinologica Scandinavica* 1986; **279**: 207–17.

McKusick VA, Weilbacher RG, Gregg CW. Recessive inheritance of a congenital malformation syndrome. *Journal of the American Medical Association* 1968; **204**: 113.

Rock J, Zakur H, Dlugi AM. Pregnancy success following surgical correction of an imperforate hymen and complete transverse vaginal septum. *Gynecology* 1982; **59**: 448.

Wellings K. Sexual behaviour in Britain: early heterosexual experience. *Lancet* 2001; **358**: 1843–50.

Urinary tract trauma

ALAN DICKSON

Learning objectives

- To understand how the urinary tract can be injured.
- To understand the principles of management of urinary tract injuries.
- To understand the application of imaging in urinary tract injuries.
- To understand the role of surgery in urinary tract trauma.
- To be able to describe the surgical technique for operation on an injured kidney.

INTRODUCTION AND RELEVANT BASIC SCIENCE

Urinary tract trauma is quite common in children, blunt trauma being the usual mode of injury. The severity of injury is usually mild, but injuries can be serious. When there is suspicion of significant injury tract injury, the child should be transferred to a centre where there is a specialist regional paediatric urology service.

Renal trauma heals well by secondary intention. Treatment therefore has become more conservative over the past decade, although some injuries still require specialized surgical intervention, either to facilitate healing or to remove the kidney. Injuries elsewhere in the urinary tract usually demand surgical treatment because of unremitting urinary leakage. After repair of the trauma, healing is by primary intention.

Renal trauma may be complicated by long-term renal scarring, which is liable to cause hypertension mediated through the renin–angiotensin system.

Infection is a risk in any trauma site where there is haematoma and fluid collection. Antibiotic treatment is mandatory in significant urinary tract trauma.

RENAL TRAUMA

The kidney is vulnerable to external blunt trauma in the child, being situated more superficially in the loin and not having the benefit of the generous muscle protection of adults. Penetrating renal injuries are seen rarely in the UK. Renal trauma may present as part of multiple trauma, most commonly following a road-traffic accident, due to either direct blunt trauma or a sudden acceleration/deceleration force. In the latter situation, the parenchyma may rupture or the renal vascular pedicle may tear, also damaging the renal pelvis.

A child with multiple injuries should have the urinary tract investigated as a matter of routine, with urinary assessment and abdominal computed tomography (CT) scanning. Isolated renal injury may occur following road accidents, but it is also quite likely to result from playing, cycling and sporting activities, the child typically presenting with either minor symptoms such as loin pain and/or haematuria but sometimes with systemic haemodynamic upset.

Minor blunt trauma may lead to significant kidney injury if the kidney has a pre-existing abnormality, such as hydronephrosis secondary to obstruction or reflux, cystic kidneys or Wilms tumour. A history of pre-existing urinary symptoms should, therefore, alert a clinician to the likelihood of underlying primary pathology. Standard conservative management principles in this situation are likely not to apply.

Presentation

The classic clinical features of renal trauma in children are identical to those in adults, including haematuria, loin pain, loin tenderness, a loin mass and local bruising over the kidney.

Children with suspected renal trauma should be admitted for observation and assessment. All should have urinalysis and blood analysis. Initial imaging should be with ultrasound scanning. Ultrasound evidence of kidney injury requires a CT scan to define the injury more clearly. Children presenting with multiple trauma should always have a CT scan of the abdomen, including the urinary tract. CT utilizing intravenous contrast is the investigation of choice, providing the best imaging of injured kidneys. It has replaced intravenous urography and arteriography.

Computed tomography grading

- *Renal contusion*: this accounts for over 90 per cent of all kidney injuries caused by blunt trauma. A contusion is an injury to the renal parenchyma, which becomes bruised and bleeds into the subcapsular area. These injuries present with varying degrees of flank pain and haematuria.
- *Renal laceration, with disruption of the renal capsule*: presentation is similar to that of renal contusions.
- *Renal laceration, with injury to the renal capsule extending into the renal collecting system*: these are more serious injuries, which can lead to the development of perirenal urinoma and/or haematoma, as well as severe blood loss, and may be associated with haemodynamic upset.
- *Renal transection*: in this situation, the kidney fractures. There is usually only a single fracture, but extensive multiple fragmentation may occur. These injuries are uncommon; a major UK centre might see one case per year. They are usually associated with haemodynamic upset and local signs of trauma.
- *Renal pedicle injury*: vascular injuries to the kidney are rare in children. They occur after either severe blunt trauma or rapid acceleration/deceleration injuries and may include intimal disruption or vessel transection. The presentation has the clinical features of renal injury listed above. The CT scan shows the kidney to be avascularized. The outcome for such kidneys is bleak.

Management

Renal injury must be managed in relationship to the general condition of the child. However, the following general principles apply:

- Children should be admitted, because stable children with grade 3 or above injuries can rapidly suffer significant bleeding and develop systemic shock. More commonly, children with renal injuries bleed more slowly, although possibly still leading to shock.
- Primary management of renal trauma is conservative, including circulatory support with intravenous fluids and possibly blood transfusion in grade 3 injuries or worse. Monitoring of vital signs and haemoglobin level is imperative, especially in injuries grade 3 and above. Follow-up scans will define whether there is ongoing haemorrhage or expansion of an urinoma.
- Indications for surgical management are not absolute, must be considered carefully in each patient, and usually occur after a period of conservative management.

Surgical management

- *Blood loss*: the indicator for acute intervention is systemic haemodynamic instability, which may occur in grade III and IV injuries. Open surgery generally is required. Sometimes, it may be possible to embolize a localized bleeding area.
- *Urinoma formation*: urine leakage into the perirenal area can take some time to produce symptoms. Small urinomas usually settle. If there is evidence of expansion, then placement of either percutaneous drains or double-J stents between the kidney and the bladder will aid resolution. If these fail and there is major disruption of the collecting system, then open exploration is required. If the kidney has good function, then attempts should be made to repair it, but the severity of the disruption may necessitate nephrectomy.
- *Evidence of pre-existing renal pathology*: in pre-existing pathology, it is unlikely that the kidney will settle with conservative management. Pre-existing abnormalities are usually clear on the CT scan. Early exploration should be performed to repair the kidney and the original abnormality. This may involve correction of an abnormality such as pelviureteric junction (PUJ) obstruction or placement of a stent from the bladder to the kidney to relieve a problem further down the urinary tract. The outcome for injured kidneys with pre-existing disease is good. Usually, the severity of the injury and the resulting disruption are minor. Reconstruction of a kidney with pre-existing disease is usually straightforward. Surgical repair of injured normal healthy kidneys is difficult.
- *Functional loss*: complete loss of function in all or part of a kidney usually occurs if the kidney has been severely

lacerated or ruptured, or if there is vascular injury. If only one fragment is avascularized, then this can be removed and the remainder of the kidney can be repaired. In most situations, however, total nephrectomy is required urgently to arrest haemorrhage or to encourage recovery. Nephrectomy may be required later because of non-function and a risk of hypertension.

Surgery of the injured kidney is challenging. It may be part of a general laparotomy for other intra-abdominal injuries. The kidney should be approached through the transperitoneal abdominal route. The usual operative finding is a massive retroperitoneal haematoma extending the length of the abdomen on the affected side. Surprisingly, it is usually possible to define the proximal aspects of the renal pedicle, obtaining vascular control of the major vessels with vascular slings or clamps before exposing the kidney. The posterior peritoneum can then be opened, the large blood clot mass evacuated, and the kidney exposed. It is important to try to interpret the operative findings in the light of the preoperative imaging in order to achieve optimum management. The injury often defines what surgical procedure is indicated and what reconstruction is possible. In a non-functioning kidney, nephrectomy is indicated. If part of the kidney is non-functioning, then partial nephrectomy with reconstruction of the residual part should be attempted. If the whole kidney is functional, then the injury should be repaired, if possible, although reconstructive procedures are not always feasible because of renal damage and resulting haemorrhage. In these circumstances, the kidney may be packed in order to achieve control of bleeding; a second procedure carried out 24–48 hours later after the haemorrhage has arrested generally will allow reconstruction if required, or even show that the injury is more limited than first thought.

Prognosis

The more severe the injury, the more likely there is to be resultant renal scarring and the more likely there is to be later development of hypertension. This is tested with a dimercaptosuccinic acid (DMSA) scan at least six months after the injury.

The prognosis for grade I or II injuries is excellent. The kidneys heal normally, and follow-up DMSA scans show no scarring. DMSA should not be performed in grade I injuries.

URETERIC TRAUMA

Ureteric trauma may occur following severe abdominal injury, usually related to a road-traffic accident. The most common cause of ureteric injury, however, is iatrogenic. Iatrogenic injuries occur in various surgical situations, including appendicectomy, bowel surgery, bladder surgery, hernia surgery, ureteric instrumentation and ureteric surgery itself.

Either disruption or complete division of the ureter occurs, with subsequent development of a urinoma. Generally, the history or circumstances raises the suspicion of the diagnosis, although the diagnosis may be suggested by visualization of the urinoma on ultrasound and then confirmed by retrograde ureterography, which demonstrates ureteric leakage or obstruction.

Ureteric trauma usually necessitates open surgical repair. In general, proximal ureteric injuries are managed by pyeloplasty type procedures and low ureteric injuries are managed by re-implantation procedures. Mid-ureteric injuries require careful end-to-end anastomosis over a JJ stent. Repair is fashioned using fine absorbable monofilament extramucosal sutures. Such anastomoses are liable to stenosis and require long-term follow-up after repair.

BLADDER TRAUMA

Bladder injuries in children may occur in blunt and penetrating trauma or may be a result of iatrogenic injury. Previously augmented bladders may also rupture spontaneously or following minor trauma.

Blunt trauma

The child complains of significant lower abdominal pain and is liable to have haematuria. Usually, the child has a history of pelvic injury. There may be evidence of a seatbelt injury or an associated pelvic fracture. Occasionally, the problem may be revealed only on CT scan or during laparotomy procedures for abdominal trauma. Diagnosis of bladder rupture can be suggested by ultrasound and confirmed by cystography. Cystography also reveals whether the injury is intraperitoneal or extraperitoneal, which will determine subsequent management.

In intraperitoneal urinary extravasation, laparotomy is required and the bladder is repaired with postoperative suprapubic catheter drainage. Surgical exploration can be avoided if the bladder rupture is lower on the viscus, with extraperitoneal urinary leakage. Such injuries generally settle following a period of seven to ten days of catheterization.

Bladder injuries require long-term follow-up to be sure that normal bladder function is restored.

Penetrating trauma

Penetrating trauma to the bladder is uncommon, but it does occur occasionally during assaults and accidental injury. All such injuries require surgical exploration and repair. It is essential to define the extent of the trauma at operation.

Iatrogenic injury

Iatrogenic injuries may occur during either during abdominal surgery or as a result of overfilling of the bladder. The injury may occur during cystography in neonates or when thin-walled diverticula are present in the bladder.

Most iatrogenic bladder injuries are obvious at the time of occurrence. If the abdomen is open when the injury occurs, then it is appropriate to repair it. The principles of management are otherwise the same as in relation to bladder injuries following blunt trauma. In general, iatrogenic injuries result in intraperitoneal leakage and require open repair.

Injury to the bladder or ureter has been reported during inguinal canal surgery. If the injury is noted at the time, then it should be repaired immediately. If, however, a child develops excessive abdominal pain or fluid leakage through the wound following an inguinal procedure, then bladder or ureteric injury should be considered. These injuries require open surgical management.

Rupture of enterocystoplasty

The complication of spontaneous bladder rupture following enterocystoplasty is a significant problem. A patient with an enterocystoplasty and presenting with abdominal pain should be considered as having bladder rupture until proven otherwise. Some of these perforations are perhaps spontaneous, but a careful history generally reveals an episode of blunt trauma or failure to empty.

Patients are often neuropathic and may present very ill hours or even days after the perforation occurs, with abdominal distension and/or abdominal pain. Investigation shows metabolic disturbance, including uraemia and acidosis. These patients require resuscitation and antibiotics before surgical management. The majority need surgery. The bladder rupture can be repaired and peritoneal toilet achieved. Sometimes, the leakage may be extraperitoneal, and management by bladder drainage is possible.

URETHRAL INJURY

Urethral injuries in children can occur in blunt perineal trauma, such as in straddle injuries; in association with pelvic fractures; as iatrogenic injuries from inappropriate instrumentation or catheterization; as a result of chronic damage due to prolonged urethral catheterization; and due to development of false passages in male patients performing intermittent catheterization.

Straddle injuries

Straddle injuries in females lead to vulval trauma, with bruising and tearing of the genitalia, extending around the urethral orifice. Usually there is no requirement for urethral repair, but a urethral or suprapubic catheter may be required to allow urinary drainage until local swelling resolves and spontaneous micturition becomes possible. Although vulval and clitoral injuries can appear severe, direct suturing usually repairs them easily.

Straddle injuries in males are more serious. The presentation usually includes urethral bleeding, with either haematuria or urinary retention. Acute management in this situation should be aimed at achieving bladder drainage. Attempts at catheterization by inexperienced doctors should be discouraged, so as to prevent further damage. Occasionally, acute direct cystourethroscopy by an experienced urologist can achieve urethral catheterization and continuity. The safest management is placement of a suprapubic catheter, allowing the urethral injury time to settle. Normal voiding may sometimes be re-established after a few days.

If micturition is not re-established, then generally the injury has been severe: the urethra has been disrupted significantly and then has healed by fibrosis and scarring. In this case, delayed corrective surgery should be performed usually after a delay of several months. Occasionally, if the stricture is short, it may be possible to open it up by endoscopic urethrotomy, but open urethroplasty is usually required. Urethroplasty in this situation is a demanding procedure and liable to recurrent problems, even in the most experienced hands. It is imperative to have preoperative imaging of the stricture. This will probably require both cystography through the suprapubic catheter and ascending urethrography. At operation, the stricture is approached through the perineum and posterior scrotum. It may be possible to resect the stricture and achieve end-to-end anastomosis, but if the stricture is long, then application of a pedicled or free graft is required. Nowadays, the material of choice is usually buccal mucosa.

Injuries to the posterior and membranous urethra

In males, injuries to the posterior and membranous urethra are usually associated with pelvic fracture. The principles of management are very similar to those of straddle injuries, as described above. Urethroplasty is required after a period of suprapubic drainage.

In females, injuries to the proximal urethra may extend into the bladder neck and can be complicated later by incontinence. Urethral catheterization may be achievable, but a suprapubic catheter is often required. In the longer term, continence or stricture problems may demand investigation and surgery.

Iatrogenic urethral damage

This usually occurs due to careless instrumentation, but it is unusual to cause serious injury. Normally, only superficial injuries mucosal tears and small false passages occur, and these settle spontaneously without therapy. Urethral and bladder neck rupture have, however, been reported with inappropriate dilation of the urethra following urogenital sinus reconstruction. Such damage is severe, leading to incontinence and necessitating eventual bladder neck reconstruction.

Prolonged urethral catheterization

Prolonged urethral catheterization can lead to urethral strictures in males. Although these strictures occur in any area in the urethra, they are more likely to occur in the bulbar and membranous urethra. Treatment options include urethral dilation and, if resistant, optical urethrotomy, incising the stricture with radial cuts. If the stricture is long or does not respond to these minor procedures, then urethroplasty is indicated.

Urethral injuries secondary to self-catheterization

Urethral injuries secondary to intermittent self-catheterization are common. Usually, the patient is male; he will first experience bleeding from the urethra, and thereafter difficulty with subsequent catheterization. Invariably, a false passage has been created. These problems are difficult to manage. In the acute situation, if urinary retention develops, then insertion of a suprapubic catheter is required; sometimes the problem will settle. Unfortunately, it is more common for urethral catheterization to be abandoned following such injuries, and a Mitrofanoff continent catheterizing stoma must then be fashioned. All children and their carers who practise intermittent catheterization should be trained carefully in order to avoid these complications.

GENITAL INJURY

Genital injuries occur commonly in children. They are usually minor. Injuries occur in a wide range of circumstances, including direct trauma, animal bites, bicycle crossbar injuries and falls. Injuries may occur to the penis during careless closure of a zip. Injuries to the male external genitalia have even occurred during maternal episiotomy at childbirth.

It is extremely unusual for these injuries to be severe or for deep tissues to be injured. Because of the area involved in the injury, it is usually advisable to admit these children and give intravenous antibiotics. Injury of any severity requires examination under general anaesthesia in order to allow proper cleansing and debridement of the wound and inspection of the underlying tissues. Good reconstruction of the genitalia can be achieved, even when the initial appearance may suggest major disruption.

The most severe injuries that occur to the genitalia follow ritual circumcision. Ritual circumcision is normally achieved very competently without complication. Complications do occur, however, including major haemorrhage, glanular trauma and loss of part or all of the shaft skin. After resuscitation, these acute injuries generally require formal arrest of haemorrhage and surgical reconstruction. Even in the most severe external appearances, however, it is usually possible to achieve good skin cover. Amputation of part of the glans penis may be repaired by conversion to a hypospadias abnormality,

with a view to subsequent reconstruction. Alternatively, the raw area of the glans can be grafted with buccal mucosa, although this leaves an unusually shaped glans.

Significant penile trauma may result from a tourniquet injury, secondary to wrapping of thread or string around the base of the penis. This can result in penile damage. Management involves immediate release of the offending tourniquet material followed by observation to determine whether there is permanent injury. Reconstruction may be required in due course.

Childhood genital injuries immediately raise the question of sexual abuse. The history of the injury and the general physical examination are extremely important. Every genital injury should be investigated carefully and appropriately to ascertain the circumstances of the injury. Although in most situations it is clear that abuse is not an issue, in others the help of a paediatrician or child protection team to analyse the background circumstances of the child is essential.

CLINICAL SCENARIOS

Case 1

A seven-year-old girl presents acutely after being hit on the left side by a car. She is in severe pain, and there is bruising in the left flank. On arrival, her blood pressure is 130/70 mmHg and her pulse rate is 125/min. There is no evidence of other injury. An intravenous infusion is established. After giving a bolus of crystalloid and pain relief, maintenance fluids are maintained. After one hour, her blood pressure is 115/65 mmHg and her pulse rate is 100/min. Ultrasound scan shows her spleen to be normal, but there is a collection of fluid around the left kidney. She is admitted and monitored. For a short period, the blood pressure falls to 80/50 mmHg, and a further bolus of crystalloid is administered. CT scan shows a laceration across the mid-zone of the left kidney and haematoma/urinoma formation around the kidney. She is soon feeling better and is able to eat. Two days later, follow-up ultrasound shows that the collection has enlarged by 50 per cent, but the girl is well. The following day, she is in pain and has developed a flank mass, but she remains haemodynamically stable. Ultrasound shows a very large collection. She is taken to theatre, where a JJ stent is placed, and she is subsequently maintained on bedrest. Thereafter, serial ultrasound shows gradual shrinkage of the collection. She is discharged after ten days. Follow-up DMSA scan at four months demonstrates the left kidney to be scarred across the mid-zone and contributing 36 per cent of her total renal function.

Case 2

An 11-year-old boy presents at the accident and emergency department after being stabbed in the abdomen. He is bleeding from the suprapubic stab wound and has haematuria.

He seems well, except for abdominal tenderness. An intravenous infusion is commenced and analgesia is administered. Abdominal X-ray is normal. The boy is taken to theatre and the bladder is explored. There is perforation of the anterior and posterior walls of the bladder. The peritoneum is then opened to reveal perforation of the sigmoid colon and faecal leakage into the pelvis. All injuries are repaired, a suprapubic catheter is left to drain the bladder, and the boy goes home well six days later.

Case 3

A three-year-old boy presents with a swollen bleeding penis. His father informs the doctor that the family dog attacked the child. The doctor notices multiple bruising on the child's body and neck and calls the child protection team.

FURTHER READING

Brown SL, Elder JS, Spirnak JP. Are paediatric patients more susceptible to major renal injury from blunt trauma? *Journal of Urology* 1998; **160**: 138–40.

Connor JP, Hensle TW. Trauma to the urinary tract. In: O'Donnell B, Koff SA (eds). *Pediatric Urology*, 3rd edn. Oxford: Butterworth-Heinemann, 1997; pp. 696–724.

Heyns CF. Renal trauma: indications for imaging and surgical exploration. *British Journal of Urology, International* 2004; **93**: 1165–70.

Kardar AH, Sundin T, Ahmed S. Delayed management of posterior urethral disruption in children. *British Journal of Urology* 1995; **75**: 543–7.

McAninch JW, Safir MH. Genitourinary trauma. In: Weiss RM, George NJR, O'Reilly PH (eds). *Comprehensive Urology*. London: Mosby, 2001; pp. 637–50.

Adolescent and adult care of patients with congenital urological abnormalities

SUZIE VENN, RACHEL LEAVER AND CHRISTOPHER WOODHOUSE

Learning objectives

- To understand the conditions requiring long-term follow-up.
- To understand the problems of adolescents and adults with these conditions.
- To understand the long-term complications of urinary reconstruction.
- To understand the effects of these conditions on fertility and the risk of inheritance.

INTRODUCTION

With advances in neonatal and paediatric care, children born with complex urological abnormalities are surviving through adolescence and into adult life. Adolescence is now appreciated as a separate stage in development, requiring a different approach to care, as abnormal body image and the practical demands of a congenital condition worsen the normal trials of the teenage years.

The aims in childhood and adolescence are to produce an adult who can function successfully in society – working, forming relationships and procreating. The success of paediatric urologists in reconstructing their patients has resulted in young people who, rightly, expect to achieve these goals. Specialist input in adult life is required to continue the medical management and to assist in the achievement of social goals.

ADOLESCENCE

Adolescence is always a difficult time, as the child passes through puberty and matures into an independent adult.

The child during adolescence aims to develop in a number of areas into an adult. These include:

- achieving more mature relationships;
- starting sexual relations;
- achieving a social role;
- accepting one's body/physique;
- achieving emotional independence;
- achieving assurance of economic independence;
- preparing for an occupation.

These milestones are a cause of anxiety for all teenagers, but especially for those with congenital abnormalities. Achieving independence is particularly difficult for children with disabilities.

Preparation for independence must begin in childhood. Even severely affected children should be encouraged to undertake some of their own care and share in normal household chores. It is too late to begin in adolescence. However, as the child moves through adolescence, the parents should encourage a progression in freedom, responsibility and duties.

Physical independence may not be possible when full-time parental care is required. Even so, aiming to do some things independently of the parents may help to raise the adolescent's self-esteem and, conversely, allow more freedom for ageing parents.

Emotional independence is also difficult for many reasons: physical differences and lack of time spent with their own peers may mean these people have poor social skills. In addition, parents may find it harder than normal to 'let go', as they have often made huge personal sacrifices to care for the child. Loss of schooling due to time spent in hospital may have resulted in poor examination results, so that opportunities for a career are limited.

There is often a conflict over the extent to which adolescents with disabilities are allowed to undertake dangerous or stressful occupations or hobbies. The ambitions of patients usually far outstrip those that the parents would contemplate (although the same may be said for normal teenagers). A distinction should be drawn between undertakings that would be demonstrably harmful to the medical condition and those that are just stressful to parents and adolescents in general. Once the former have been ruled out (and there are surprisingly few of them), then the latter should be encouraged. It is particularly important that disabled people should be helped to achieve those things that they are able to do.

Acceptance of body image is a key stage of adolescence and is worsened by surgical scars, abnormal genitalia and alternative voiding systems. A further feature of adolescence is the need for the person to fit in with his or her peers; therefore, compliance with treatment and attendance at clinics may be poor.

It is now acknowledged that adolescence is a stage of development separate from both childhood and adulthood. Most paediatric specialties will now have a transition phase before passing on patients to colleagues in adult clinics. In some conditions, such as diabetes and asthma, the medical problems in adult life are the same as those encountered by patients whose illness began after maturity. Having passed through the traumas of adolescence, care in a conventional adult specialist is appropriate. For children with congenital abnormalities, and especially those of the genitourinary system, there is no parallel in adult life: adults do not acquire exstrophy or posterior urethral valves.

It is also acknowledged that separate child, adolescent and adult areas are needed for inpatient care and a more appropriate approach is needed for adolescent management. These young people do not want to be seen in clinics with children or nursed on wards with adults. Adolescent areas have a more relaxed approach to care by the nursing staff and also a multidisciplinary team with, for example, a psychologist to assist both the patient and the parents. In the clinic, there is a gradual transfer of responsibility from parent to adolescent, with time and opportunity to discuss issues of accommodation, occupation and sex. When compliance is poor, the aim is to keep the patient 'medically safe' until he or she is ready to take full responsibility for their own care.

ADULT LIFE

With the hopefully successful transition from child to adult through adolescence, young adults with congenital abnormalities, and in particular those with complex reconstructions, will need care for the rest of their life. Adult life brings new emotional and psychological challenges, including fertility, pregnancy and concerns about inheritance of their condition. As few of the major genitourinary anomalies can be 'cured' in the accepted sense of the word, there is the additional anxiety of ongoing medical care and future complications. Specialist input is needed, both medically and with nursing support. These patients' conditions are rare, so experience with their management can be gained only in specialist clinics.

This also applies to backup services such as radiology, where liaison with an experienced uroradiology team is essential. The input of a nephrologist is also important. Many adolescents have renal damage that, over a lifetime, may lead to hypertension or renal failure. Prophylactic treatment to protect the kidneys usually will have to be started earlier and be more aggressive than would be used in older adults. Hyperperfusion of surviving nephrons is a potent cause of late renal morbidity.

Often, the only clinician seeing these patients in secondary care is a urologist, so a knowledge of the bowels, bones and brains – or, at least, access to an interested specialist – is needed. The instant advice that is often needed may best be given by a dedicated nurse specialist, especially for problems related to the reconstructed urinary tract. Finally, these patients need time in the clinic and continuity of care, which is not provided easily in a busy general urology clinic.

MEDICAL MANAGEMENT

Although there are a variety of congenital urological conditions that require long-term follow-up, there are a number of similarities in their medical care. Renal impairment is not uncommon, requiring close surveillance. The reconstructive procedures performed are not disease-specific, and so the follow-up and complications apply to all patients.

Upper urinary tract

It is unfortunately common for there to be a degree of renal impairment in patients with congenital urological conditions. The kidneys may have failed to develop, or the damage may have occurred *in utero* and after birth due to a neuropathic bladder or as a consequence of surgery. The principles of management in adolescence and adult life are to avoid further damage from obstruction and to slow the progress of chronic renal failure.

At handover in adolescence, usually the patient is stable, but imaging is needed for comparison if their ongoing care is at another institution. The mainstay of management is ultrasound. In the presence of dilation, a renogram is required to exclude obstruction. Once there is established follow-up, in the hands of an experienced uroradiologist, routine imaging can be by ultrasound. A baseline glomerular filtration rate (GFR) is very useful at handover, so that any change in dilation can be assessed against change in GFR. A further GFR is required after puberty and then at five-year intervals in patients with bladder reconstruction or high-risk conditions such as posterior urethral valves.

All patients with mild renal impairment need at least annual measurement of blood pressure and urine analysis to exclude proteinuria with ACE inhibitors. Early treatment of hypertension and proteinuria slows the development of renal failure, which is the most critical medical factor in the management of these patients. They can be managed predominantly in one or other clinic to avoid duplication of appointments, provided that both clinicians are aware of the investigations required by the other.

The 'bladder'

A considerable number of patients who require follow-up have had their bladders reconstructed. This varies from an augmentation of the bladder to complete replacement with a segment of intestine. The follow-up is dictated largely by the complications that occur. These are similar, although of varying frequency, depending on the amount and type of bowel used and other factors such as the method of emptying the neo-bladder. The long-term complications of using bowel in the urinary tract can be divided into those caused by removal of a portion of intestine from the intestinal tract and those due to the presence of bowel in the urinary tract.

Complications caused by removal of a portion of intestine from the intestinal tract include the following:

- *Bowel disturbance:* it is now accepted that between 25 and 50 per cent of adult patients suffer a troublesome change in their bowel habit after enterocystoplasty. The aetiology is not clear, but malabsorption, altered bacterial flora and underlying neuropathic bowel dysfunction have been proposed.
- *Vitamin B12 deficiency:* this is known to occur in some patients after surgery. Patients generally present with insidious symptoms but may develop irreversible neuropathy if not recognized. Serum vitamin B12 must be measured annually, and supplements must be given when the level approaches the lower limit of normality. Some centres give all patients a regular supplement on the grounds that it is cheaper than doing the test and eliminates the risk of missing a serious deficiency.

Complications of bowel in the urinary tract include:

- *Metabolic acidosis* when measured by arterial blood gases is very common but rarely causes symptoms. The concerns of resultant growth failure in children have not

been shown to occur, but long-term risk of loss of bone density remains a concern.
- *Clean intermittent self-catheterization (CISC):* although this should be considered a consequence rather than a complication of surgery, the incidence does increases with time.
- *Urinary tract infection (UTI):* asymptomatic bacteriuria is very common, with symptomatic infection in 20 per cent of patients. Infection raises the levels of nitrosamines in the urine, which may be a factor in the pathogenesis of malignancy.
- *Stones:* these are very common, increasing with emptying the pouch via a continent catheterizable stoma to nearly 100 per cent.
- *Mucus:* this does not decrease with time and may cause stones, difficulty with catheterization and increased numbers of symptomatic UTIs.
- *Carcinoma:* this remains an undefined but possible risk.
- *Perforation:* this is a potentially life-threatening problem, particularly in adolescents who may forget to empty their neo-bladder.

The 'urethra'

The reconstructed bladder often needs to be emptied by catheter, either using the native urethra or via a continent catheterizable stoma (CCS) such as a Mitrofanoff. Complications occur with both methods, and easy access to specialized help for these patients is essential. Complications include the following:

- *Stomal stenosis:* initially, simple dilation is effective in up to 21 per cent of patients. If this fails, then revision of skin stoma using VQ-, VQQ- or VQZ-plasties may be required.
- *Urinary leakage:* in general, this requires revision of the catheterizable channel to extend its length and/or the bladder/neo-bladder tunnel.
- *Stomal prolapse:* this requires excision of the prolapsed segment and revision of skin anastomosis.
- *Bladder-level stenosis:* this requires excision of the stenotic segment, with revision of the tunnel into the bladder/neo-bladder and lengthening of the channel if necessary.
- *Angulation of catheterization channel or diverticulum, causing catheterization difficulties:* this is seen most commonly in Monti channels. A change of catheterization technique may be all that is required to overcome this problem; if this fails, then formal channel revision with reduction in extravesical length is required.

Difficulties with urethral CISC may require a change in catheterization technique, urethrotomy and a period of catheterization or formation of a CCS if the native urethra becomes impassable.

Pregnancy

Urine stored in an intestinal reservoir is altered in some way so that the conventional 'blue-line' pregnancy tests are often falsely positive (even in men). False-negatives have not been seen. Women wishing to confirm a pregnancy must, therefore, have the serum human chorionic gonadotrophin (HCG) level measured.

Increasing numbers of girls with complex reconstructions now are becoming pregnant. With more experience, a few observations can be made. A number will develop obstruction of the upper tract during the second trimester, and so close imaging is required during this period. Difficulties with catheterization may occur during pregnancy. Early treatment of UTI is advisable in order to avoid miscarriage. Patients with repeated UTIs should be kept on prophylactic antibiotics that are 'safe' in pregnancy. Vaginal delivery is probably advisable, unless there is an obstetric indication, but a planned caesarean section is a better option than an emergency caesarean section. It is sensible to have the presence of a urologist who understands the anatomy of the reconstructed bladder; delivery in a specialized unit therefore may be advisable. Babies of exstrophy mothers are often breech presentation and so commonly require caesarean section.

SPECIFIC CONGENITAL UROLOGICAL CONDITIONS

Due to limited space, only a few specific comments will be made on each of the more common conditions.

Reflux nephropathy

Although the current aggressive management of reflux in childhood may reduce this problem, at present approximately 17 per cent of patients are entering dialysis programmes due to reflux nephropathy. Children who enter adolescence with significant renal damage need to be followed up either in a specialized clinic or by a nephrologist. In the past, it was advised that girls with persistent reflux should be re-implanted to avoid problems during pregnancy, but conflicting results have left this issue unresolved. Pregnancy does carry a higher risk of miscarriage than in the normal population and has been shown to accelerate renal damage. The risk of inheritance of this condition is one in three, so the fetus should be screened to exclude reflux. The risk of hypertension is high in patients with reflux nephropathy, reaching about 25 per cent by age 25 years and rising with increasing age.

Neuropathy

Patients with spina bifida are probably the most challenging in this group. These patients change from being children who are light in weight, mobile on callipers and with educational support to wheelchair-bound adults who are difficult to nurse due to their size and increasing kyphosis, living at home with ageing parents, socially isolated and unable to find work. They are the most severely affected of neuropathy patients; other neuropathy patients lead independent and fulfilled lives. Social attitudes need to alter to help such individuals find suitable housing and work. The improvement in their morale once they are working is of immeasurable value.

Medically, it is necessary to consider these factors when planning any reconstruction. There is little point aiming for urethral voiding if it is not possible to transfer to the toilet without assistance. Stomas must be sited high on the abdomen, as kyphosis will increase with time. All the generic medical care already discussed is needed for these patients. Bowel function continues to be a problem in adolescence and adult life. Formation of a stoma to perform antegrade continence enemas (ACE), with either bowel or a percutaneous tube, may be appropriate. It appears rare in adult life to have problems with hydrocephalus, but assistance with access to computed tomography (CT) scanning and neurosurgeons may be needed. Sexual function varies from normal to absent. The opportunity and time to discuss these patients' sexual concerns must be made available in the clinic. The risk of inheritance is increased, so sexually active girls should be advised of the importance of preconception folic acid and booking into the antenatal clinic early when pregnant, if they would consider termination of an affected fetus.

Exstrophy

This group of patients on the whole do extremely well and are often high achievers in society. No doubt this is because the condition affects only the genitourinary tract. Medical management depends on reconstruction and care of renal function. An additional factor is that these patients carry an increased risk of malignancy in the bladder remnant, which if possible should be screened.

The major problem with exstrophy girls and boys is the appearance of the genitalia. Boys have short broad penises, often with a dorsal curve. Surgical correction of the curvature is possible, ideally using a graft to reduce further shortening. There is, unfortunately, no successful method of lengthening the penis, and therefore it is necessary for these people to accept and work around the limits of their length. Once they have accepted their lot, they generally form long-lasting successful relationships. Fertility may be impaired due to blocked ejaculatory ducts following bladder neck surgery.

In girls, the genitalia lie on the lower abdominal wall, rather than in the perineum. There is an abnormal distribution of pubic hair and non-fusion of the clitoris and labia. Surgery can correct this appearance. The girls are fertile and generally have no problems conceiving. They are prone to uterine prolapse (procedentia), which occurs in up to half of the patients after pregnancy. Surgery for repair is complex, the most successful being a Gore-Tex™ wrap around the cervix to secure it to the sacrum. Inheritance is reported to occur in one in 70 pregnancies. Antenatal diagnosis is difficult, as the only feature on ultrasound is a bladder that does not fill at 18–20 weeks.

Posterior urethral valves

These boys need close and regular follow-up, as their bladders cannot be trusted. Follow-up is as described previously, but a flow rate may also be of help to exclude obstruction. Fertility is often impaired due to slow ejaculation and abnormal sperm count.

FURTHER READING

Greenwell TJ, Venn SN, Mundy AR. Augmentation cystoplasty. *British Journal of Urology International* 2001; **88**: 511–25.

Nguyen HT, Peters CA. The long-term complications of posterior urethral valves. *British Journal of Urology International* 1999; **83**: 23–8.

Woodhouse CRJ. Adolescent urology. *British Journal of Urology International* 1999 (suppl 3): iv.

Woodhouse CRJ. The fate of the abnormal bladder in adolescence. *Journal of Urology* 2001a; **166**: 2396–400.

Woodhouse CRJ. Prospects for fertility in patients born with genitourinary anomalies. *Journal of Urology* 2001b; **165**: 2354–60.

Index